NEUROSCIENCE SECRETS

NEUROSCIENCE SECRETS

MARGARET T. T. WONG-RILEY, PhD

Professor
Department of Cell Biology, Neurobiology, and Anatomy
Medical College of Wisconsin
Milwaukee, Wisconsin

HANLEY & BELFUS, INC. / Philadelphia

Publisher: HANLEY & BELFUS, INC.
                  Medical Publishers
                  210 South 13th Street
                  Philadelphia, PA 19107
                  (215) 546-7293; 800-962-1892
                  FAX (215) 790-9330
                  Web site: http://www.hanleyandbelfus.com

Note to the reader: Although the information in this book has been carefully reviewed for correctness of dosage and indications, neither the authors nor the editor nor the publisher can accept any legal responsibility for any errors or omissions that may be made. Neither the publisher nor the editor makes any warranty, expressed or implied, with respect to the material contained herein. Before prescribing any drug, the reader must review the manufacturer's current product information (package inserts) for accepted indications, absolute dosage recommendations, and other information pertinent to the safe and effective use of the product described.

Library of Congress Cataloging-in-Publication Data

Neuroscience secrets / edited by Margaret T. Wong-Riley.
        p.   cm. — (The Secrets Series®)
    Includes bibliographical references and index.
    ISBN 1-56053-316-1 (alk. paper)
    1. Neurosciences Miscellanea.   I. Wong-Riley, Margaret T. T.
II. Series.
    [DNLM: 1. Nervous System Physiology Examination Questions. WL
18.2 N946 1999]
RC343.5.N48   2000
612.8'076—dc21
DNLM/DLC
for Library of Congress   99-34312
                                            CIP

NEUROSCIENCE SECRETS   ISBN 1-56053-316-1

Last digit is the print number: 9   8   7   6   5   4   3   2   1

CONTENTS

CONTRIBUTORS

Neal H. Barmack
Senior Scientist, Neurological Sciences Institute, Oregon Health Sciences University, Portland, Oregon

Janice M. Burke, PhD
Marjorie and Joseph Heil Professor, Departments of Ophthalmology and of Cell Biology, Neurobiology, and Anatomy, Medical College of Wisconsin, Milwaukee, Wisconsin

William E. Cullinan, PhD
Assistant Professor of Anatomy and Neurobiology, Department of Biomedical Sciences, Marquette University; Adjunct Assistant Professor, Department of Neurosurgery, Medical College of Wisconsin, Milwaukee, Wisconsin

Kathleen M. Donahue, PhD
Assistant Professor, Deparment of Radiology, Medical College of Wisconsin, Milwaukee, Wisconsin

Frank M. Faraci, PhD
Associate Professor, Departments of Internal Medicine and Pharmacology, University of Iowa, Iowa City, Iowa

Troy Hackett, PhD
Research Associate, Department of Psychology, Vanderbilt University, Nashville, Tennessee

Harold H. Harsch, MD
Associate Professor, Department of Psychiatry, Medical College of Wisconsin, Milwaukee; Associate Medical Director, Froedtert Memorial Lutheran Hospital, Milwaukee, Wisconsin

Robert F. Hevner, MD, PhD
Assistant Adjunct Professor, Department of Psychiatry, University of California, San Francisco, California

Neeraj Jain, PhD
Research Assistant Professor, Department of Psychology, Vanderbilt University, Nashville, Tennessee

Jon H. Kaas, PhD
Professor, Department of Psychology, Vanderbilt University, Nashville, Tennessee

Linda J. Larson-Prior, PhD
Associate Professor, Division of Basic Sciences, Touro University College of Osteopathic Medicine, Vallejo, California

Pat R. Levitt, PhD
Thomas Detre Professor of Neuroscience and Chair, Department of Neurobiology, University of Pittsburgh School of Medicine, Pittsburgh, Pennsylvania

Julian H. Lombard, PhD
Professor, Department of Physiology, Medical College of Wisconsin, Milwaukee, Wisconsin

BethAnn McLaughlin, PhD
Research Associate, Department of Neurobiology, University of Pittsburgh School of Medicine, Pittsburgh, Pennsylvania

Carolanne E. Milligan, PhD
Assistant Professor, Department of Neurobiology and Anatomy, Wake Forest University School of Medicine, Winston-Salem, North Carolina

Michelle Mynlieff, PhD
Assistant Professor of Biology, Department of Biology, Marquette University, Milwaukee, Wisconsin

Jay Neitz, PhD
Associate Professor, Department of Cell Biology, Neurobiology, and Anatomy, Medical College of Wisconsin, Milwaukee, Wisconsin

Hershel Raff, PhD
Professor of Medicine, Deparment of Medicine, Medical College of Wisconsin; Director, Endocrine Research Laboratory, St. Luke's Medical Center, Milwaukee, Wisconsin

Diane Daly Ralston, PhD
Associate Professor, Department of Anatomy and Neurological Surgery, University of California, San Francisco, California

Henry J. Ralston, III, MD
Professor, Department of Anatomy and Neurological Surgery, University of California, San Francisco, California

Linda Rinaman, PhD
Assistant Professor of Neuroscience, Department of Neuroscience, University of Pittsburgh, Pittsburgh, Pennsylvania

Chris G. Sobey, PhD
Senior Research Officer, Department of Pharmacology, University of Melbourne, Parkville, Victoria, Australia

Elliot A. Stein, PhD
Professor, Department of Psychiatry, Pharmacology, and Cell Biology; Professor, Biophysics Research Institute, Medical College of Wisconsin, Milwaukee, Wisconsin

Iwona Stepniewska, PhD
Assistant Professor, Department of Psychology, Vanderbilt University, Nashville, Tennessee

Sara J. Swanson, PhD, ABPP-Cn
Assistant Professor, Department of Neurology, Medical College of Wisconsin, Milwaukee, Wisconsin

John L. Ulmer, PhD
Associate Professor, Department of Radiology, Medical College of Wisconsin, Milwaukee, Wisconsin

Patrick R. Walsh, MD, PhD
Professor, Department of Neurosurgery, Medical College of Wisconsin, Milwaukee, Wisconsin

Margaret T.T. Wong-Riley, PhD
Professor, Department of Cell Biology, Neurobiology, and Anatomy, Medical College of Wisconsin, Milwaukee, Wisconsin

PREFACE

This is the first book in The Secrets Series® on neuroscience. Over the past 30 years, it has become apparent that neuroscience is not a single discipline, but rather an amalgamation of multiple fields: neuroanatomy, neurophysiology, neurochemistry, neuroembryology, neuroendocrinology, and neurobehavioral science, to name just a few. Topics can range from invertebrates to vertebrates and from molecules to systems. No single book can cover all of these topics, and so the focus is restricted to those that may be of greatest interest and relevance to our special audience: medical students, graduate students, residents, postdoctoral fellows, and anyone interested in the neurosciences.

With so many "neuro" books on the market, why do we need another basic science book? That is a legitimate question. We have tried to create a different perspective, a new way of looking at a familiar object, and an integration of traditional and new ideas. We hope to ask probing questions, and to stir the minds of our readers to think and to ponder. We may not have all the correct answers, and some of our answers may need to be revised in the future. Nevertheless, we hope that most of the questions raised will be "timeless."

In organizing this book, I drew upon my 5 years of experience as the Co-Director of the Integrated Medical Neuroscience Course at the Medical College of Wisconsin. The goal of the course was to integrate structure, function, and clinical relevance into each lecture, and to cover topics ranging from cellular and molecular neurobiology to systems neuroscience. *Neuroscience Secrets* is organized in a similar fashion: from individual neurons and synaptic transmission, through the various sensory and motor systems, to neural plasticity and the neurobiology of behavioral disorders. It is by no means all encompassing, but it covers most of the essential topics in neuroscience. This book is meant as a supplement to, not as a substitute for, standard textbooks in the neurosciences.

In recruiting authors for the chapters, my main goal was to find individuals who have a passion for teaching and are good communicators. Of course, these neuroscientists are also specialists in their fields. In these days of tight grant funding and research competitiveness, it is a rare individual who sets aside precious time from his or her busy schedule to devote to this educational endeavor. And so, I salute all of my colleagues who contributed to the writing of this book. I hope that it has been a fun journey for all of them, and I hope that our readers find the book interesting, informative, and educational.

Margaret Tze Tung Wong-Riley, Ph.D.
EDITOR

Dedication

To

Our Past and Present Teachers

and

Our Present and Future Students

As long as the brain is a mystery, the universe, the reflection of the structure of the brain, will also be a mystery.

~ Santiago Ramón y Cajal

A

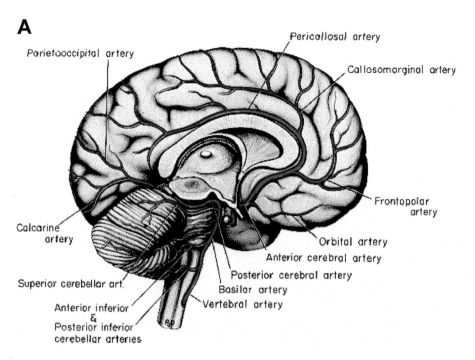

Parietooccipital artery

Pericallosal artery

Callosomarginal artery

Frontopolar artery

Calcarine artery

Orbital artery

Anterior cerebral artery

Posterior cerebral artery

Superior cerebellar art.

Basilar artery

Anterior inferior & Posterior inferior cerebellar arteries

Vertebral artery

B

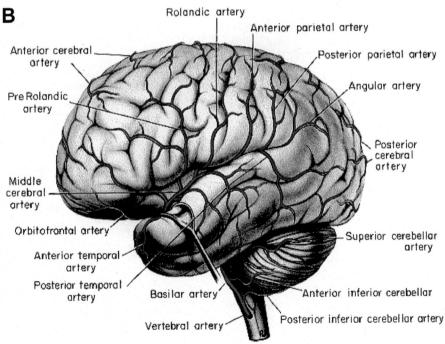

Rolandic artery

Anterior parietal artery

Anterior cerebral artery

Posterior parietal artery

Pre Rolandic artery

Angular artery

Posterior cerebral artery

Middle cerebral artery

Orbitofrontal artery

Superior cerebellar artery

Anterior temporal artery

Posterior temporal artery

Basilar artery

Anterior inferior cerebellar

Posterior inferior cerebellar artery

Vertebral artery

Chapter 18, Figure 2.   See page 261.

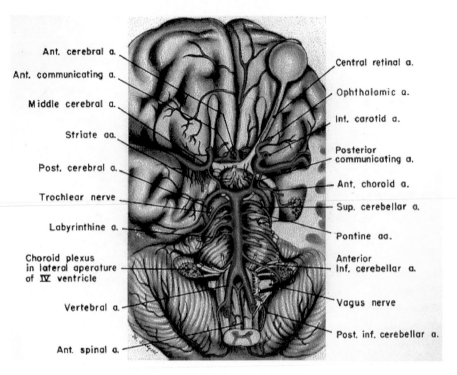

Ant. cerebral a.

Ant. communicating a.

Middle cerebral a.

Striate aa.

Post. cerebral a.

Trochlear nerve

Labyrinthine a.

Choroid plexus
in lateral aperature
of IV ventricle

Vertebral a.

Ant. spinal a.

Central retinal a.

Ophthalamic a.

Int. carotid a.

Posterior
communicating a.

Ant. choroid a.

Sup. cerebellar a.

Pontine aa.

Anterior
Inf. cerebellar a.

Vagus nerve

Post. inf. cerebellar a.

Chapter 18, Figure 3. See page 262.

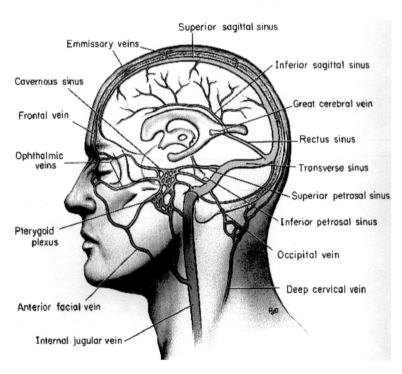

Superior sagittal sinus

Emissary veins

Cavernous sinus

Frontal vein

Ophthalmic
veins

Pterygoid
plexus

Anterior facial vein

Internal jugular vein

Inferior sagittal sinus

Great cerebral vein

Rectus sinus

Transverse sinus

Superior petrosal sinus

Inferior petrosal sinus

Occipital vein

Deep cervical vein

Chapter 18, Figure 4. See page 263.

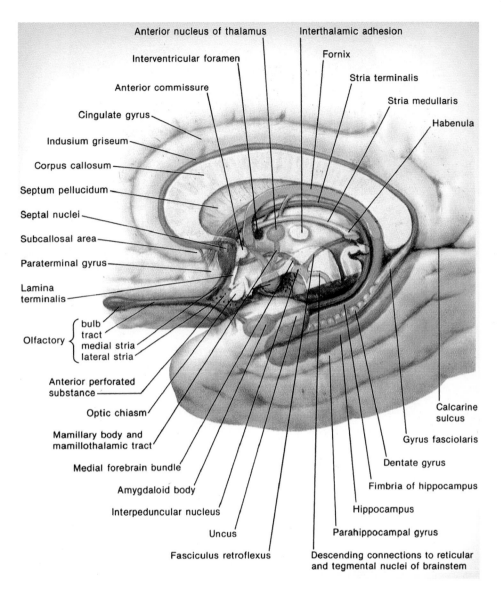

Anterior nucleus of thalamus

Interthalamic adhesion

Interventricular foramen

Fornix

Anterior commissure

Stria terminalis

Stria medullaris

Cingulate gyrus

Habenula

Indusium griseum

Corpus callosum

Septum pellucidum

Septal nuclei

Subcallosal area

Paraterminal gyrus

Lamina
terminalis

Olfactory { bulb
tract
medial stria
lateral stria

Anterior perforated
substance

Calcarine
sulcus

Optic chiasm

Gyrus fasciolaris

Mamillary body and
mamillothalamic tract

Dentate gyrus

Medial forebrain bundle

Fimbria of hippocampus

Amygdaloid body

Hippocampus

Interpeduncular nucleus

Parahippocampal gyrus

Uncus

Fasciculus retroflexus

Descending connections to reticular
and tegmental nuclei of brainstem

Chapter 19, Figure 1. See page 279.

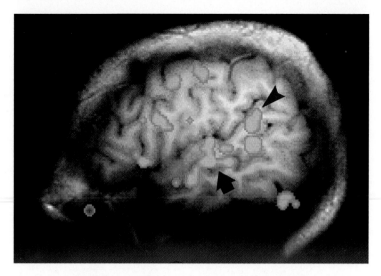

Chapter 22, Figure 5. See page 328.

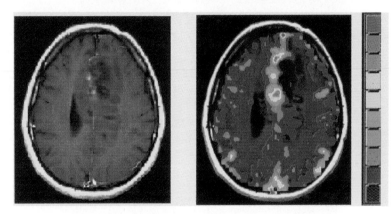

Chapter 22, Figure 18. See page 344.

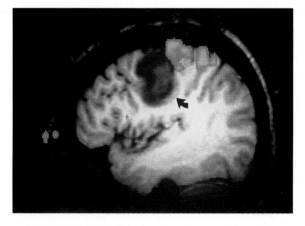

Chapter 22, Figure 19. See page 345.

1. NEURONS AND GLIA: STRUCTURE AND ELECTRICAL PROPERTIES

Margaret T. T. Wong-Riley, Ph.D., and Julian H. Lombard, Ph.D.

Our central nervous system is made up of at least 100 billion neurons, as many as there are stars in the sky. Neurons are unique in that they can receive, conduct, and transmit signals. We see, hear, touch, smell, and taste with our neurons; we sense our external and internal environments with neurons; and we react with action, emotions, and hormonal secretions that are controlled by neurons. Neurons enable our master computer, the brain, to process, compute, integrate, transmit, and store information. All of these remarkable abilities make us what we are.

NEUROCYTOLOGY

1. Who is the recognized father of neuroanatomy?

One cannot begin the study of neuroscience without recognizing an eminent forefather of this discipline, Santiago Ramon y Cajal (1852–1934). He was a Spanish physician and neurohistologist who made outstanding contributions to our understanding of the cellular organization of the nervous system. From his studies of neurons in many regions of the brain and in a number of animal species, Cajal was able to develop theories on nervous system function that remain largely valid. In 1906, Cajal and his Italian contemporary, Camillo Golgi, whose silver staining technique he avidly used, shared the Nobel Prize in Medicine and Physiology.

2. What is the Neuron Doctrine?

The Neuron Doctrine was proposed by Cajal at the turn of the 20th century. He believed that neurons were individual cells that communicated with each other by contact (the synapse). Golgi, on the other hand, proposed that neurons formed a continuous syncytium, the so-called Reticular Theory. Although they shared the Nobel Prize, Cajal's theory triumphed in the end.

3. What is meant by "dynamic polarization"?

Cajal proposed that the functional building blocks of the brain, the neurons, were structurally and functionally polarized such that the input enters one end, the dendrites, and the output exits from the other end, the axon. This dynamic polarization exists regardless of sizes and shapes of neurons. Contacts are made between individual neurons through synapses.

4. How is a neuron distinguished from other cell types?

Neurons are specialized in three major ways:

1. They possess an electrically excitable membrane.

2. They are able to communicate with each other and with effector organs through chemical, electrical, or gaseous synapses.

3. They contain a special type of intermediate filament known as neurofilament.

The first feature is not unique, as muscle cells also are electrically excitable and can propagate action potentials. Smooth muscles and cardiac muscles have gap junctions and are able to fire synchronously. However, neurons have a variety of morphologic and physiologic features that enable them to communicate effectively not only with neighboring cells, but also with distant neurons and effector organs. The cytoskeletal proteins—neurofilaments—are unique to neurons, and this can be verified by an antibody test against neurofilaments. It is the combination of all three properties that distinguishes a neuron from the other cell types.

5. How many different types of neurons are there?

Neurons can be classified in many ways:
- Size (small, medium, and large, with somal sizes of 5–150 μm in diameter)
- Shape (unipolar, pseudounipolar, bipolar, multipolar (Fig. 1); chandelier; granule; horizontal; pyramidal; spindle; stellate)
- Axon length (projection/relay neurons or Golgi type I, interneurons or Golgi type II)
- Neurotransmitter/neuromodulator type (cholinergic, adrenergic, dopaminergic, serotonergic, GABAergic, glutamatergic, peptidergic)
- Function (excitatory, inhibitory, modulatory, sensory, motor, commissural)

The size and shape of the soma are related to the length and number of processes. Typically, the cell body contains less than 1/10 of the cell's total volume.

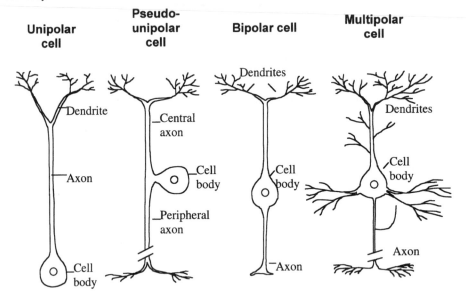

Figure 1.   The number of processes arising from the neuronal cell body determines whether the neuron is unipolar, pseudounipolar, bipolar, or multipolar.

6. What is the difference between the axon hillock and the initial segment?

The *axon hillock* is actually that part of the cell body (perikaryon, soma) that is devoid of Nissl substance (or rough endoplasmic reticulum). It identifies the site where the axon originates. The *initial segment* is the start of the axon where action potentials are initiated. It is devoid of myelin and is characterized by a dense undercoating beneath the axolemma and an array of microtubules streaming down the axon.

7. How are dendrites different from axons?

Characteristics of Dendrites and Axons

DENDRITE	AXON
Can be single or multiple extensions of the cell body	Single extension from the cell body or from a dendrite
Can contain all cytoplasmic organelles except for Golgi apparatus, especially in proximal dendrites	Can contain most cytoplasmic organelles except for Golgi apparatus, rough endoplasmic reticulum, and ribosomes

Table continued on facing page

Characteristics of Dendrites and Axons (Continued)

DENDRITE	AXON
Tapers in a proximodistal direction; can branch profusely and can have dendritic spines; spines contain spine apparatus and receive the bulk of the synapses	Trunk stays cylindrical, can branch profusely; terminals enlarge to form boutons that contain synaptic vesicles; varicosities can occur along the trunk for en passant synapses
Almost never myelinated	Can be myelinated or unmyelinated
Usually ramify close to the cell body	Can ramify close to or far away from the cell body
Responds with graded depolarization or hyper-polarization that decrements spatially and temporally; some can generate action potentials	Action potentials are generated at the initial segment of axons, propagated along the axonal trunk (up to 100 m/s), and transmitted at the axon terminals
Major receptive site of synapses (postsynaptic), but may also be presynaptic (e.g., dendro-dentritic synapse)	Major effector site of synapse (presynaptic), but may also be postsynaptic (e.g, axo-axonal synapse)
Structurally absent in unipolar cells	May be absent (e.g., amacrine cells)
Major energy-consuming portion of a neuron	Energy consumption is low in the axon trunk, but may be low, moderate, or high in axon terminals

m/s = meters per second

8. What subcellular features are prominent in neurons?

Neurons are highly active in both transcription and translation. The presence of euchromatin (active DNA) in the nucleus and stacks of rough endoplasmic reticulum (Nissl substance) in the cytoplasm (Fig. 2) exemplify this. There are more genes expressed in the brain than in any other organ in the body. As much as one-third of the entire genome may be devoted to brain-specific genes.

To maintain shape and assist in intracellular transport, neurons also have a rich supply of cytoskeletal proteins, including microtubules, microfilaments, and the specialized intermediate filaments known as neurofilaments.

The other organelles found in neurons, such as the Golgi apparatus, mitochondria, smooth endoplasmic reticulum, ribosomes, and lysosomes, are common to various cell types. Mitochondria are the energy powerhouse of the cell and are particularly active in neurons, especially in dendrites. Lysosomes are involved in neuronal membrane turnover (synthesis and degradation). Lipofuscin are pigmented inclusions thought to be large, end-stage lysosomes that contain indigestible material. They are more prominent in the aging brain.

9. What is so special about the neuronal plasma membrane?

The plasma membrane maintains the electrical voltage gradient (membrane potential or E_m) between the inside and the outside of a cell. It contains ion pumps and ion channels that form the basis of electrical excitability (see the chapter Synaptic Transmission). The protein composition of the plasma membrane varies among different compartments of a neuron (cell body, dendrites, and axon). At active sites of synapses, especially the postsynaptic sites, there is a greater density of specialized ion channels and receptor proteins.

The integral membrane proteins have hydrophobic, membrane-spanning segments and hydrophilic segments that face the extracellular and/or the intracellular space (amphipathic). The pore of an ion channel is formed in the center (by a special arrangement of the amino acids and/or their charge groups) and allows charged ions to pass through the membrane.

10. What features are common to ion channels and ion pumps?

Both ion channels and ion pumps allow the passage of charged ions through the lipid bilayer of the membrane. They both contain subunit domains and transmembrane segments. The central pore is formed by special segments of each channel protein (see the Neurophysiology section on page 8 and the chapter Synaptic Transmission).

Characteristics of Ion Channels and Pumps

TYPE	SUBUNIT TYPE	DOMAINS	TRANSMEMBRANE SEGMENTS
Voltage-gated Na$^+$ channel	2 (α,β)	4/α (I–IV); β1 β2	6 segments/α domain (S1–S6); 1/β
Nicotinic ACh receptor (ion channel)	4 ($\alpha,\beta,\gamma,\delta$)	5 ($\alpha,\alpha,\beta,\gamma,\delta$)	4 segments/domain (M1–M4)
Gap junction (ion channel)	2 (connexons)	6 (connexins)	4 segments/connexin
Na$^+$/K$^+$ATPase (ion channel and ion pump)	2 (α,β)	2 (α,β)	10 segments/α (H1–H10); 1/β

ACh = acetylcholine, ATP = adenosine triphosphate

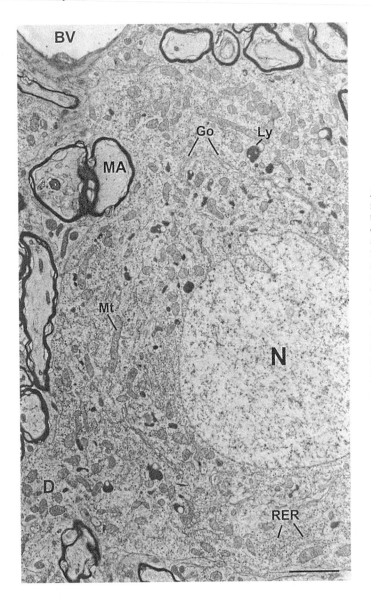

Figure 2. An electron micrograph of a neuron in the CNS. Note that the nucleus (N) has euchromatin, and the cytoplasm contains the usual organelles, such as Golgi apparatus (Go), mitochondria (Mt), rough endoplasmic reticulum (RER), lysosomes (Ly), and cytoskeletal proteins. A dendrite (D) is seen arising from the cell body at the lower left corner. In the neuropil (area outside of neuronal cell body) are blood vessels (BV), myelinated axons (MA), and synaptic complexes.

11. How does the cell maintain a normal ionic gradient across its membrane?

An enzyme known as Na$^+$/K$^+$ATPase performs the important function of maintaining the resting membrane potential in all cells, with the inside more negative than the outside. It is an integral protein of the plasma membrane and serves both as an ion channel and an ion pump. It utilizes energy from the hydrolysis of ATP to pump three Na$^+$ ions out of the cell for every two K$^+$ ions into the cell. The Danish physiologist Jens C. Skou won the Nobel Prize in 1997 for its discovery.

Na$^+$/K$^+$ATPase is particularly concentrated in those regions of the neuron where frequent membrane depolarization demands greater pumping activity for membrane repolarization, such as the postsynaptic dendrites (see the Neurophysiology section on page 11 and the chapter Synaptic Transmission).

12. What proteins typically are associated with the cytoplasmic side of the plasma membrane?

The spectrin and ankyrin families of proteins often are associated with the cytoplasmic side of the membrane. These and other proteins link the cytoskeleton to the plasma membrane.

13. How do neurons maintain their shape?

Neurons maintain their shape by specialized groups of proteins that form their skeleton, known as cytoskeleton. These proteins often exhibit patterns peculiar to neurons, so as to accommodate the variety of shapes assumed by neurons and their processes.

14. What components make up the cytoskeleton of a neuron?

The cytoskeletal components of a neuron include actin microfilaments (~ 5–8 nm in diameter), neurofilaments (~ 10 nm), and microtubules (~ 24 nm) (Fig. 3). Only neurofilaments are unique to neurons; the other two components are common to various cell types.

MICROFILAMENT

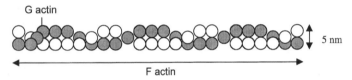

NEUROFILAMENT

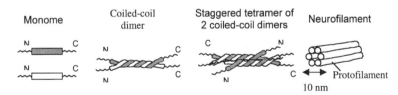

MICROTUBULES

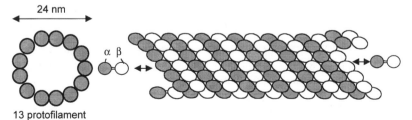

Figure 3. Three major types of cytoskeletal proteins are found in neurons.

15. What are microfilaments? What do they do?

Microfilaments are polar polymers made up of globular actin monomers (Fig. 3). Imagine two strands of pearls twisted together in a helical fashion to form a braid. Each pearl is a globular actin monomer (**G actin**), and each braid is a flexible actin microfilament (**F actin**). The polymerization of G-actin to F-actin depends on the binding of G actin to ATP.

Actin probably is the most abundant protein in all cell types and is found in the cytoplasm throughout the neuron. The actin gene family encodes α (skeletal muscle), β, and γ actins. Neuronal actin is a mixture of β and γ, which differ from α-actin by only a few amino acid residues.

Microfilaments are important in changing and/or maintaining cell shape. The polarized structure of F actin (with a slow-growing minus end and a fast-growing plus end) also provides for a treadmilling mechanism of locomotion used by migrating cells.

16. Why are drugs that prevent *or* stabilize microfilament polymerization toxic to cells?

A cell's viability depends on a dynamic equilibrium between G and F actin. Drugs that prevent polymerization of actin (e.g., cytochalasin B) by binding to the plus end of a microfilament alter the shape of cells and inhibit their movements. On the other hand, drugs that stabilize microfilaments and prevent their depolymerization (e.g., phalloidins from poisonous mushrooms) by binding tightly all along their sides also block cell movements that require the turnover of microfilaments. In both cases, the cell's viability is seriously threatened.

An old remedy for mushroom poisoning is to eat a large quantity of raw meat rich in actin, which will compete for the binding of phalloidin.

17. What is so special about neurofilaments?

Neurofilaments are **neuron-specific** intermediate filaments found throughout the neuron, especially in axons. They are of special interest because neurofibrillary tangles (modified neurofilaments) are the hallmarks of neurodegenerative disorders, especially of Alzheimer's disease.

Neurofilaments are made up of fibrous monomers that are twisted to form coiled-coil dimers and then tetramers (Fig. 3). Because the tetramers are formed by antiparallel dimers, neurofilaments are not polarized (i.e., the two ends are the same, unlike actin and tubulin). Tetramers are then packed together in a helical array to form the protofilament, and multiple protofilaments form the 10-nm neurofilament. Three types of polypeptide subunits make up the neurofilaments: 70 kDa, 140 kDa, and 210 kDa (known as NF-L, NF-M, and NF-H for low, middle, and high molecular weight neurofilaments).

18. What happens when the regulation of neurofilaments is disrupted?

The number, length, position, and assembly of neurofilaments are regulated by neurons. When this regulation is disrupted, abnormal filamentous tangles may form. Such is the case with neurofibrillary tangles, which are bundles of abnormal filaments made up of paired helical filaments (two filaments in a helix) containing a type of microtubule-associated protein known as tau. Neurofibrillary tangles are found not only in Alzheimer's disease, but also in Down's syndrome, postencephalitic Parkinsonism, dementia pugilistica, and a variety of degenerative, metabolic, and viral disorders. A small number of them also are found in the normal, aging brain.

19. What do we know about microtubules in neurons?

Neuronal microtubules (neurotubules) are hollow tubes (24 nm in diameter) whose walls are made up of 13 protofilaments (Fig. 3). Each protofilament is a linear series of tubulins, and each tubulin is a heterodimer of globular α-tubulin and β-tubulin. Imagine that the α-tubulin and β-tubulin each forms a spiral staircase around the hollow cylinder, and these spirals alternate with one another. In this manner, a spiral of α-tubulin tends to face the rapidly growing, plus end of the microtubule, while the β-tubulin spiral faces the slow-growing, minus end. In axons, microtubules are all oriented with their plus ends away from the cell bodies; in dendrites, their polarity is mixed.

Microtubules are found throughout each neuron. They form bundles with cross-bridges at the initial segments of axons and are important in axonal and dendritic transport. Secretory vesicles, for example, move toward the plus end of microtubules and are carried to the nerve terminals where they function.

20. How do microtubules change their lengths?

Microtubules elongate by **polymerization** and shorten by **depolymerization.** Each heterodimer of α-tubulin and β-tubulin has a nonhydrolyzed GTP bound to it. When it binds a second exchangeable (hydrolyzable) GTP, which neutralizes the positive charge, polymerization is favored. When GTP is hydrolyzed to GDP, it changes the subunit conformation and weakens the bond, thereby promoting depolymerization. Polymerization and depolymerization are regulated by different neuronal signals.

21. How do certain anticancer drugs interact with microtubules?

Drugs that depolymerize microtubules (e.g., colchicine) or stabilize microtubules (e.g., taxol) kill cells by disrupting normal microtubular functions. They often are used as chemotherapeutic drugs against cancer because they prevent mitosis, which is dependent on microtubules. One of the common side effects of these drugs, however, is sensory nerve paresthesia (abnormal sensation).

22. What are MAPs?

MAPs are **microtubule-associated proteins** that anchor microtubules to one another and to other parts of the neuron. There are two major classes of MAP: high molecular weight proteins (200–300 kDa), which include subtypes of MAP-1 to MAP-5, and low molecular weight tau proteins (55–62 kDa). High molecular weight MAPs help in cross-linking microtubules with one another and with other cytoskeletal elements and organelles. Both high and low molecular weight MAPs stabilize microtubules by preventing the dissociation of tubulin from their ends. Dephosphorylated tau proteins are found only in axons, while the phosphorylated tau are found in both axons and dendrites. Conversely, MAP-2 is found in cell bodies and dendrites, but not in axons.

23. How do MAPs help with the transport of material along neuronal processes?

Two types of high molecular weight MAPs serve as motors or ATPases, and they utilize the energy of ATP hydrolysis to propel material along the microtubules: **kinesins** are motors that are plus-end directed (i.e., move material from the cell body toward the axon terminals; anterograde transport), while **dyneins** are minus-end directed (i.e., move material from the axon terminals toward the cell body; retrograde transport) (Fig. 4). Cytoplasmic dynein also is known as MAP-1C.

Both kinesin and dynein are composed of two heavy chains and several light chains. The heavy chain has a globular ATPase head that binds to the microtubules and a rodlike tail that binds to specific cargoes to be transported. These two motors essentially "walk" their cargoes toward their destinations.

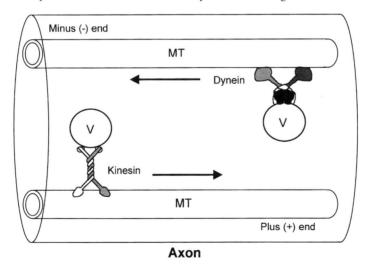

Axon

Figure 4.   Axoplasmic transport within an axon. Kinesin is plus-end–directed and transports organelles, such as synaptic vesicles (V), along the microtubules (MT) from the cell body toward the axon terminal. Dynein is minus-end–directed and is responsible for retrograde transport.

24. What are the various ways by which subcellular components are transported within the axon?

The cell body is the major site of macromolecular and organellar synthesis. Axons lack the synthetic machinery (no ribosomes or rough endoplasmic reticulum) and depend on the soma for their supply of newly synthesized components. At the same time, degraded proteins and membranes must be returned to the cell bodies for recycling or degradation.

There are two major rates of transport along the axon: slow and fast. Slow transport (0.2–2.5 mm/day) moves only in the anterograde direction, while fast transport moves in both the anterograde (~ 400 mm/day) and retrograde (~300 mm/day) directions. Only the fast process is ATP-dependent; it utilizes ATPases (kinesin and dynein side arms) to hydrolyze ATP and propel the transported material along the microtubules.

Slow axoplasmic transport or flow moves soluble proteins and components of microtubules and neurofilaments. Fast axoplasmic transport moves a complex mixture of proteins, including actin and neuronal myosin, metabolic enzymes, calcium-binding proteins such as calmodulin, and organelles such as mitochondria and vesicles of smooth endoplasmic reticulum. Synaptic vesicle precursors move primarily in the anterograde direction. Recycled membranes and lysosomes containing materials for degradation move primarily in the retrograde direction.

25. Why is retrograde axonal transport relevant to both clinicians and researchers?

Retrograde axonal transport enables the delivery of material from the extracellular space surrounding the axon terminals to the cell bodies. Such material includes useful substances such as nerve growth factors as well as viruses (e.g., herpes, rabies, and polio) and toxins (e.g., tetanus and cholera). Damage to neuronal cell bodies can lead to severe clinical manifestations.

Researchers can capitalize on retrograde axonal transport by microinjecting labeled tracer substances in the vicinity of axonal terminals and following the label to the cells of origin. Major neuronal pathways can be traced in this fashion. Neuronal pathways also can be traced by following the injected tracer transported in an anterograde direction from the cell bodies to the axon terminals.

26. Do dendrites also perform transporting functions?

Yes. The components and rates of transport are similar to those of axonal transport. For example, all newly synthesized membranous organelles are delivered to the dendrites from the cell bodies by anterograde dendritic transport.

NEUROPHYSIOLOGY

27. What is the membrane potential?

The difference in electrical potential (voltage) across the plasma membrane of excitable cells.

28. Why is it important?

The membrane potential is essential for all local and propagated electrical signals generated by the cell because transmission of signals between excitable cells depends on changes in membrane potential.

29. What causes the membrane potential?

The membrane potential is caused by the diffusion of ions across the membrane, down their respective electrochemical gradients. This diffusion results in a separation of charge (potential difference) across the membrane. The membrane potential is a function of the concentration of specific ions inside and outside of the cell, and the permeability of the cell membrane to these ions.

30. Which ions contribute to the membrane potential?

Resting membrane potential is determined primarily by K^+ ions, but also by Na^+ ions to a much lesser extent (and by any other ion that is not passively distributed across the cell membrane). During the action potential, sodium ions become the major contributor to the membrane potential in most neurons. As the permeability to sodium increases and Na^+ ions cross the membrane, they approach their equilibrium potential, which is highly positive (around + 60 millivolts

[mV]). In some excitable cells (notably smooth muscle and some neurons), Ca^{2+} ions are responsible for the action potential in a manner similar to that described for Na^+ ions.

31. Why are Ca^{2+} ions important for nerve function?
- They carry ionic current in some neurons.
- Extracellular Ca^{2+} ions can decrease the excitability of a nerve cell membrane by binding to membrane proteins, thereby increasing the threshold potential.
- They are essential for the release of neurotransmitters at synapses, as well as neurosecretory products such as hormones and releasing factors.
- Intracellular Ca^{2+} also can increase K^+ conductance in many cell types.

32. What are the clinical consequences for neurons of electrolyte imbalances?
The elevated K^+ (hyperkalemia) that can occur with end-stage renal disease causes a reduced excitability of neurons (as well as cardiac and skeletal muscle cells) by depolarizing the cell membrane and eventually inactivating some of the Na^+ channels. Severe and rapid increases in K^+ can cause hyperexcitability by depolarizing membrane potential toward threshold. This condition can cause cardiac arrest and death via direct effects on the cardiac muscle cells that produce lethal arrhythmias. The hypokalemia that can occur in patients on diuretic drugs causes the resting membrane potential to become more negative (hyperpolarization) and can reduce the excitability of neurons, as well as muscle cells.

Increases in plasma Ca^{2+} levels (hypercalcemia) can cause decreased neuromuscular excitability by interfering with the ability of the neuron to reach threshold for activation of the fast Na^+ channel. Reductions in plasma Ca^{2+} levels (hypocalcemia) that can occur in response to vitamin D_3 deficiency, hypoparathyroidism, or severe alkalosis can cause intermittent contraction of skeletal muscle (hypocalcemic tetany) as a result of an increased excitability of motor nerves and skeletal muscle cells.

Reduced plasma Na^+ (hyponatremia), occurring as result of conditions such as inappropriate antidiuretic hormone secretion in small cell carcinoma of the lung, leads to neurologic changes such as weakness and confusion.

Increased levels of hydrogen ions block Na^+ channel function by combining with negatively charged amino acids in the channel. This is the basis for depressed neuronal activity and reduced CNS function during conditions of severe acidosis such as diabetic coma, metabolic inhibition, and impaired renal function.

33. What does it mean when we say that an ion is passively distributed across the cell membrane?
An ion is passively distributed when it is not actively transported. The equilibrium potential of a passively distributed ion is the same as the membrane potential. If the membrane potential changes due to changes in the electrochemical gradient or the permeability of the membrane to ions that are not passively distributed, the intracellular concentrations of passively distributed ions change so that the equilibrium potential of each ion is equal to the new membrane potential. Cl^- ions are passively distributed in many cells, such as skeletal muscle.

34. What factors regulate the contribution of each permeable ion to the diffusion potential?
- The concentration difference of each permeable ion across the membrane
- The electrical potential difference across the membrane
- The relative permeability of the membrane for that ion

For example, during resting conditions, the diffusion of K^+ ions down their electrochemical gradient causes the inside of the membrane to become negatively charged relative to the outside, opposing the further diffusion of K^+ ions. During the action potential in a mammalian motoneuron, Na^+ permeability increases dramatically, and the membrane potential is determined primarily by the diffusion of Na^+ ions down their electrochemical gradient.

35. What is the equilibrium potential for an ion?
The equilibrium potential for a specific ion is the potential difference when the diffusion of the ion down its concentration gradient is exactly balanced by the electrical potential difference across

the membrane. Under these conditions, the ion is at its equilibrium potential, and the net electro-chemical gradient (sum of the potential energy of electrical and chemical forces) is zero. An ion can reach its equilibrium potential if the membrane is permeable to only that ion.

36. What is the Nernst equation?

The Nernst equation is the equation that describes the equilibrium potential for a given ion. It is named after the 19th century chemist, Walter Nernst, who derived it in 1888. For a monovalent cation, e.g., K^+, the Nernst potential (equilibrium potential) is described as follows:

$$E_K = -\frac{RT}{ZF} \ln \frac{[K^+]_i}{[K^+]_o} \qquad \text{or} \qquad -60 \log \frac{[K^+]_i}{[K^+]_o} \quad \text{at } 37° \text{ C}$$

where E_K is the membrane potential value at which K^+ is in equilibrium, R is the gas constant, T is the absolute temperature (in degrees-Kelvin), Z is the valence of the ion, and F is the Faraday constant.

37. Can the membrane potential be described by the Nernst equation?

No, because the membrane is not permeable to only one ion. Therefore, under normal condi-tions, no individual ion can be at its equilibrium potential, and the membrane potential is affected by any ion that is not passively distributed. As a result, the membrane potential primarily is a steady-state diffusion potential in which the concentrations of the contributing ions are maintained by mem-brane transport systems. Although a small component of the membrane potential is due to the action of the electrogenic Na^+/K^+ pump, the **diffusion potential** component is responsible for the majority of the membrane potential.

38. Is there a valuable equation to describe the diffusion potential component of the mem-brane potential?

Yes, there are two. The classic diffusion potential equation for electrically excitable membranes is the **constant field equation**, also known as the **Goldman, Hodgkin, Katz (GHK) equation**:

$$E_m = -\frac{RT}{ZF} \ln \frac{P_K [K^+]_i + P_{Na} [Na^+]_i + P_{Cl} [Cl^-]_o}{P_K [K^+]_o P_{Na} [Na^+]_o + P_{Cl} [Cl^-]_i}$$

The GHK equation describes the membrane potential as a function of the distribution of all monova-lent cations and anions that are not passively distributed across the plasma membrane. In some cen-tral nervous system neurons, Cl^- is actively transported and contributes to the membrane potential as shown in the equation. If Cl^- ions ares not actively transported (as in skeletal muscle), P_{Cl} and the chloride concentration terms would not appear in the GHK equation.

The other valuable equation is the **chord conductance equation.** The chord conductance equa-tion describes the membrane potential as a function of the conductances and the equilibrium poten-tials for the various ions contributing to the membrane potential in a specific tissue:

$$E_m = \frac{gK}{\Sigma g} (E_K) + \frac{gNa}{\Sigma g} (E_{Na}) + \frac{gx}{\Sigma g} (E_x)$$

where gK and gNa are the K^+ and Na^+ conductances, respectively; E_K and E_{Na} are the K^+ and Na^+ equilibrium potentials, respectively; gx is the conductance for any other ion that is not passively dis-tributed across the membrane; E_x is the equilibrium potential for that ion; and Σg is the sum of the membrane conductance for all ions that are not passively distributed across the membrane. An ad-vantage of the chord conductance equation is that it can express the contribution of divalent ions, specifically Ca^{2+}, to the membrane potential. This is important in tissues such as smooth muscle and some neurons, where Ca^{2+} is an important current-carrying ion.

39. What is the Na^+/K^+ ATPase, and why is it important?

The Na^+/K^+ ATPase, sometimes known as the "sodium pump" or the "Na^+/K^+ pump,"is a mem-brane-bound protein that hydrolyzes ATP while transporting Na^+ ions out of the cell and K^+ ions into the cell against their electrochemical gradients. In addition to generating the electrogenic component of the membrane potential (see Question 41), the Na^+/K^+ pump is crucial for maintaining the ionic gradients across the plasma membrane that are responsible for the diffusion potential component of the membrane potential. Without the Na$^+$/K$^+$ ATPase to transport these ions across the cell membrane, their concentrations would equalize, and the membrane potential would be lost. This state would cause the loss of cell function. (See also Question 11.)

40. What are the major regulators of Na$^+$/K$^+$ ATPase activity?

The major regulators of Na$^+$/K$^+$ pump activity are the internal Na$^+$ concentration and the external K$^+$ concentration. Active extrusion of Na$^+$ from the cell is coupled with active uptake of K$^+$ into the cell. Both Na$^+$ and K$^+$ are obligatory for pump function, since pump activity ceases when external K$^+$ is removed experimentally or when internal Na$^+$ is zero. In addition, the Na$^+$/K$^+$ pump requires ATP to function. Therefore, Na$^+$/K$^+$ transport ceases when ATP stores are exhausted due to conditions such as anoxia or ischemia.

41. Is the membrane potential only a diffusion potential?

No. Part of the membrane potential results from the activity of Na$^+$/K$^+$ ATPase, which is electrogenic. This means that the activity of the Na$^+$/K$^+$ ATPase leads to a separation of charge that contributes to the potential difference across the membrane. Charge separation occurs because the Na$^+$/K$^+$ ATPase transports more Na$^+$ ions out of the cell than K$^+$ ions in. The ratio of Na$^+$ ions transported out to K$^+$ ions transported in is 3Na$^+$:2K$^+$. The contribution of the Na$^+$/K$^+$ ATPase to the membrane potential (electrogenic portion of membrane potential) varies from a few mV to as much as 20 mV in some cells. The higher the leak rate for Na$^+$ into the cell and for K$^+$ out of the cell, the larger the electrogenic component of the membrane potential. In neurons, the increased [Na]$_i$ and increased [K$^+$]$_o$ in the vicinity of the cell membrane, which results from repetitive action potentials, activates the Na$^+$/K$^+$ ATPase and hyperpolarizes the membrane (makes the membrane potential more negative) until internal Na$^+$ concentration has returned to normal values.

42. What are the molecular components of the Na$^+$/K$^+$ pump?

The Na$^+$/K$^+$ pump (Fig. 5) consists of two subunits or polypeptide chains (α and β). The catalytic α-subunit has ten membrane-spanning sequences, and the regulatory β-subunit has one membrane-spanning sequence plus an extracellular segment. The α-subunit has intracellular binding sites for Na$^+$ and ATP and extracellular binding sites for K$^+$ and ouabain. The β-subunit is closely associated with the α-subunit and is required for normal α-subunit function, possibly by insuring that the α-subunit is positioned properly in the cell membrane.

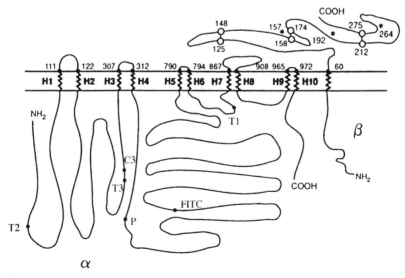

Figure 5. Molecular structure of the Na$^+$/K$^+$ pump in the cell membrane. (From Sperelakis N (ed): Cell Physiology Source Book, 2nd ed. San Diego, Academic Press, 1998; with permission.)

43. What is ouabain?

Ouabain is a specific, competitive inhibitor of the Na^+/K^+ pump that binds to an external site on the Na^+/K^+ pump and stearically hinders K^+ binding.

44. What is an action potential?

An action potential is a rapid, transient, and reversible depolarization of an electrically excitable cell (Fig. 6).

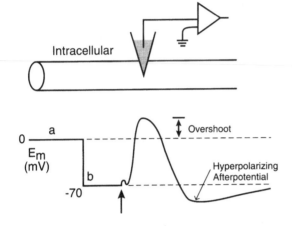

Figure 6. Neuronal action potential recorded with an intracellular microelectrode. Note the positive overshoot and the hyperpolarizing afterpotential. The rate of rise is the change of voltage per second from the start of the action potential to the peak of the overshoot. The small potential change prior to the action potential is the stimulus artifact. (From Sperelakis N, Banks RO (eds): Essentials of Physiology, 2nd ed. Boston, Little, Brown, 1996; with permission.)

45. What are the characteristic parameters of an action potential?

• Overshoot
• Duration
• Rate of rise

These parameters are characteristic for each type of excitable cell and are determined by changes in ion conductance that give rise to the action potential.

46. What is the overshoot in the action potential?

The overshoot (Fig. 6) is an increase in membrane potential to positive values during an action potential. The overshoot demonstrates that membrane permeability to a positive ion increases, allowing it to move down its electrochemical gradient from the outside to the inside of the cell. Historically, this led to the discovery of the importance of the Na^+ ion in contributing to the action potential.

47. What is the hyperpolarizing afterpotential (positive afterpotential)?

The hyperpolarizing afterpotential (Fig. 6) occurs at the end of the action potential and is the undershoot of the membrane potential to values that are more negative than the original resting membrane potential. It is due to a slow return of K^+ conductance to its resting value during the action potential. As a result, K^+ conductance is still somewhat elevated at the end of the action potential, and the membrane potential becomes hyperpolarized as it approaches the K^+ equilibrium potential.

The hyperpolarizing afterpotential sometimes is called the positive afterpotential. This designation can be confusing, since the neuronal cell membrane is hyperpolarized during the "positive" afterpotential. The term arose because the voltages measured by *extracellular* recordings during this part of the action potential are more positive than the resting value.

48. How are action potentials initiated?

Action potentials are initiated by depolarization of the cell membrane. In most cases, excitatory neurotransmitters released at the synapse cause changes in ionic conductance, leading to membrane depolarization. If this depolarization is of sufficient magnitude, an action potential is initiated at the **initial segment** of the axon, which is the region of a neuron that has the lowest threshold potential. In some neurons and other excitable cells (particularly smooth muscle), spontaneous pacemaker activity occurs, in which automatic changes in ionic conductance lead to alternating phases of depolarization and repolarization, producing spontaneous electrical activity.

49. What causes an action potential?

An action potential is caused by sequential changes in the permeability of the cell membrane to different ions, resulting in initial depolarization followed by a subsequent repolarization (Fig. 7). The *depolarization* is caused by increased membrane permeability to ions whose equilibrium potential is less negative than the resting membrane potential. In most cases, action potentials are due to a sudden explosive increase in the permeability of the membrane to Na^+, which has an equilibrium potential of approximately +60 mV under normal conditions. The initial activation of Na^+ conductance is caused by depolarization to a **threshold potential**, which is the membrane potential at which the activation of Na^+ channels becomes self-sustaining. This initial activation is followed by a slower, automatic return of Na^+ conductance to its resting level, which prevents the membrane potential from completely reaching the Na^+ equilibrium potential during the overshoot of the action potential. This is termed *inactivation of sodium conductance*.

The *repolarization* phase of the action potential is due to an increase in K^+ conductance, which causes the membrane potential to return toward the K^+ equilibrium potential. This increase is activated by the depolarization that occurs during the action potential. The repolarization of the membrane by the increase in K^+ conductance is aided by the inactivation of the Na^+ conductance.

In some neurons, calcium-dependent potentials occur due to increases in membrane permeability to Ca^{2+}. The influx of Ca^{2+} ions causes the membrane potential to approach the Ca^{2+} equilibrium potential, leading to depolarization.

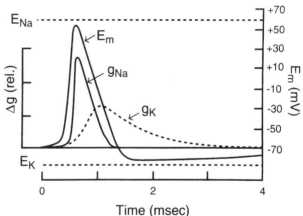

Figure 7. Time course of voltage change (E_m), relative sodium conductance (g_{Na}) and relative potassium conductance (gk) during an action potential. E_{Na} represents the sodium equilibrium potential. (From Sperelakis N, Banks RO (eds): Essentials of Physiology, 2nd ed. Boston, Little, Brown, 1996; with permission.)

50. What is the refractory period?

The refractory period (Fig. 8) is the time following an action potential during which a second action potential either cannot be elicited regardless of stimulus strength (**absolute refractory period**), or a higher than normal stimulus strength is required to elicit a second action potential (**relative refractory period**). The duration of the refractory period differs among excitable cells, and determines the maximum frequency of action potentials that can be generated in the cell.

51. How are action potentials propagated?

Action potentials are propagated over nerve cell bodies and down the axon by the spread of current through the cytoplasm, through the extracellular fluid, and across the cell membrane (Fig. 9). When the membrane is depolarized to the threshold value, action currents flow longitudinally in the extracellular fluid and in the intracellular cytoplasm that make up the circuit. These currents flow from the normally polarized region ahead of the action potential into the active region of the action potential, and from the repolarized region behind the action potential back into the active region.

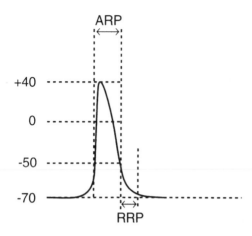

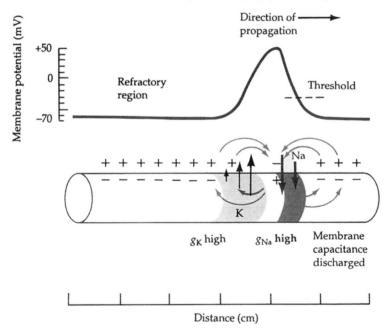

Figure 8. Duration of absolute refractory period (ARP) and relative refractory period (RRP) during an action potential in a neuron. (From Sperelakis N, Banks RO (eds): Essentials of Physiology, 2nd ed. Boston, Little, Brown, 1996; with permission.)

They draw the capacitative charge off of the membrane (see Question 52), causing the membrane potential in the region ahead of the active site to reach threshold for the self-sustaining increase in Na^+ conductance. As a result, the action potential is propagated down the fiber. The increase in K^+ conductance behind the action potential balances the depolarizing influence of current flowing behind the active site, insuring that the action potential is propagated in only one direction.

Figure 9. Current flow in a nerve fiber during the propagation of an action potential. (From Nicholls JG, Martin AR, Wallace BG (eds): From Neuron to Brain: A Cellular and Molecular Approach to the Function of the Nervous System, 3rd ed. Sunderland, Massachusetts, Sinauer Associates, Inc., 1992; with permission.)

52. What is membrane capacitance? Why is it important?

Membrane capacitance refers to the ability of the cell membrane to store an electrical charge. It is important because the capacitative charge on the cell membrane has to be "drawn off" in order to depolarize the membrane to the threshold potential. When an area of membrane is depolarized, for example during the propagation of an action potential, current flows into the depolarized area, reducing the capacitative charge and producing depolarization in the surrounding areas. The presence of a membrane capacitance also means that the changes in membrane potential that result from current flow across the membrane during a subthreshold stimulus are not instantaneous, but instead change in an exponential manner (Fig. 10). This effect of membrane capacitance is important in determining the **time constant** of the membrane (see Question 58).

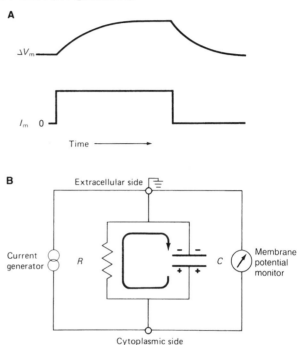

Figure 10. Capacitance function of a nerve cell membrane. **A**, The relationship of the change in membrane potential (ΔV_m) and current across the membrane (I_m). **B**, The equivalent circuit diagram for the nerve cell membrane. Because the membrane capacitance (C) is parallel with the membrane resistance (R), the membrane potential does not change instantaneously with membrane current. (From Kandel ER, Schwartz JH, Jessell TM (eds): Principles of Neural Science, 3rd ed. New York, Elsevier Science, Inc., 1991; with permission.)

53. Why does the cell membrane act like a capacitor?
The bimolecular lipid layer serves as an insulator between the cytoplasm and the extracellular fluid, which can conduct ionic currents. Because of its insulating properties, the membrane can store charge when there is a voltage difference across it (Fig. 10). The capacitance of the membrane of electrically excitable cells is approximately $1 \mu F/cm^2$.

54. What is a subthreshold depolarization?
A small depolarization that does *not* reach the threshold value (at which the activation of Na^+ conductance becomes self-sustaining, producing an action potential).

55. What is an electronic potential?
A local, nonpropagated change in membrane potential that occurs in response to a subthreshold stimulus. Electronic potentials decay exponentially as a function of time and distance from the point of application as a result of the passive electrical properties (**cable properties**) of the membrane (see Question 56).

56. What determines the passive electrical properties of the neuronal membrane?
The passive electrical properties of the neuronal membrane are determined by the membrane resistance, membrane capacitance, extracellular resistance, and intracellular (axoplasmic) resistance. With small (subthreshold) changes in voltage across the membrane, the change in the membrane

potential with distance and the amount of time required for the membrane potential to change are functions of the cable properties of the membrane. The exponential change of membrane potential with *distance* is determined by the division of current as it flows across the cell membrane, through the axoplasm, and along the extracellular fluid bathing the outside of the membrane (Fig. 11). The *time* required for passive changes in membrane potential to be completed is determined by the capacitance of the cell membrane and by the membrane resistance.

A

Current generator

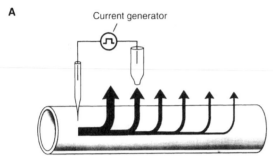

B

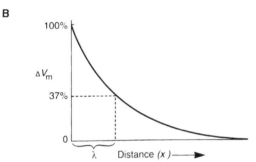

Figure 11. **A**, Current flow across a nerve fiber during a subthreshold depolarization. **B**, Change in membrane voltage (ΔV_m) with distance from point of stimulation. λ is the length constant. (From Kandel ER, Schwartz JH, Jessell TM (eds): Principles of Neural Science, 3rd ed. New York, Elsevier Science, Inc., 1991; with permission.)

57. What is the length constant?

The length constant (λ) describes the distance along the axon membrane (cm) at which a subthreshold change in membrane potential has been passively attenuated to 37% of its initial value (Fig. 11). The length constant is a function of membrane resistance (R_m), extracellular resistance (R_O), and intracellular resistance (R_i), according to the following equation:

$$\lambda = \sqrt{\frac{R_m}{R_O + R_i}}$$

58. What is the time constant?

The time constant (τ) describes the time required for a subthreshold change in membrane potential to decay to 37% of its initial value when the stimulus is terminated, or to reach a point that is 63% of its peak value (within 37% of the final value) when a subthreshold stimulus is applied to the membrane.

The membrane potential fails to change instantaneously with time when a stimulus is applied or withdrawn because the cell membrane acts as both a resistor and a capacitor (Fig. 10). If the cell membrane were purely a resistor, the change in voltage with an applied stimulus would be instantaneous as the current flowed across the membrane. However, since the membrane functions as a capacitor by storing charge, the current that flows when the stimulus is initially applied goes into one "plate" of the membrane capacitor. This occurs rapidly at first, and then the current flowing into the membrane capacitor falls exponentially as voltage increases across the capacitor. Eventually, all of the current is flowing through the membrane resistance, and the change in membrane potential reaches its full value. When the stimulus is terminated, there is an exponential fall of current and voltage across the membrane capacitor and the membrane resistance, as the capacitor discharges through the resistor. The time constant is expressed in seconds, and can be described by the following equation:

$$\tau = R_m C_m$$

where τ is the time constant (seconds), R_m is the membrane resistance, and C_m is the membrane capacitance.

59. What is the physiologic significance of the length constant and time constant?

The exponential decay of nonpropagated subthreshold changes in membrane potential with time (described by the time constant) and with distance (described by the length constant) are important in the summation of local changes in membrane potential to: (1) reach threshold for action potential generation, as in the case of subthreshold depolarizations of the membrane, or (2) hyperpolarize the membrane and render it less excitable, as in the case of the local membrane hyperpolarization that occurs during inhibitory postsynaptic potentials. The larger the value of the time constant, the easier it is for repeated subthreshold depolarizations to add together to trigger an action potential (**temporal summation**). The greater the length constant, the easier it is for the excitatory postsynaptic potentials occurring simultaneously at different points in the postsynaptic membrane to add together to initiate an action potential (**spatial summation**). In addition, the greater the length constant, the faster the conduction velocity of the nerve fiber. This is because a larger area is depolarized by local circuit currents in fibers with a greater length constant. As a result, the threshold for initiating action potentials is reached at points that are farther down the membrane, leading to a higher conduction velocity.

60. What factors affect the velocity of impulse propagation?
- The time it takes to depolarize the membrane ahead of the action potential to the threshold value (inversely proportional)
- The magnitude of the length constant of the membrane (directly proportional)

61. How does fiber diameter affect conduction velocity?

The larger the fiber, the faster the conduction velocity. This primarily is due to the presence of a lower internal (axoplasmic) resistance in the large fibers. In contrast, small fibers have slower conduction velocities.

62. What is a compound action potential?

A compound action potential is a wave of depolarization and repolarization recorded from extracellular electrodes. This combination wave is possible because currents resulting from electrical changes in neurons and other cells can be conducted through the extracellular fluid. The shape of the compound action potential is a function of the sizes of the fibers within the nerve trunk. Compound action potentials obtained during electroneurograms can be used to detect pathologic changes, e.g., demyelinating diseases, in peripheral nerves.

63. What is the strength-duration curve?

It is a plot of the parameters (strength and duration) of an applied current pulse that are necessary to bring the membrane to threshold (Fig. 12). The longer the current pulse, the smaller the current intensity required to excite the membrane to threshold. The strength-duration curve is a hyperbolic relationship. The **rheobase** is the asymptote parallel to the x-axis and represents the lowest intensity of current capable of producing an action potential, even when the current is applied for an infinite amount of time. The **minimal stimulation time** is the asymptote parallel to the y-axis and represents the shortest duration of stimulus that can produce excitation, even when large current pulses are applied. The **chronaxie** is the time that a stimulus of double the rheobase strength must be applied to reach threshold. The shorter the chronaxie, the more excitable the fiber. The chronaxie is important because some nerve disorders in humans can be detected by changes in this parameter.

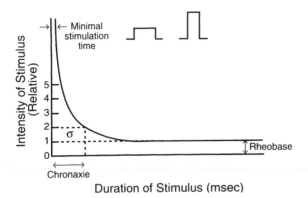

Figure 12.   Strength-duration curve for nerve stimulation. (From Sperelakis N, Banks RO (eds): Essentials of Physiology, 2nd ed. Boston, Little, Brown, 1996; with permission.)

64. What is accommodation?

The loss of sensitivity of a neuron or other excitable cell to an applied stimulus. Accommodation occurs because a slow depolarization of the membrane toward the threshold value activates some Na⁺ channels, but not enough to trigger the self-sustaining increase in Na⁺ conductance that produces an action potential. These activated channels then inactivate spontaneously and cannot be reactivated until they return to the resting state, which requires the membrane to repolarize to a more negative value of membrane potential. As a result, these channels are lost from the pool of available Na⁺ channels. In addition, some voltage-gated K⁺ channels are opened during the depolarization. This increases K⁺ conductance and reduces the excitability of the cell, since these open K⁺ channels exert a hyperpolarizing influence that opposes the depolarization of the membrane to the threshold value.

65. What is depolarization blockade?

In most electrically excitable cells, the maintenance of a membrane depolarization well above the threshold value (i.e., towards zero mV) maintains an "inactivated" state for Na⁺ conductance. This is known as depolarization blockade, and it is due to the fact that the fast Na⁺ channels can be activated only from their resting state, which is restored after the membrane potential has returned to more negative values. If the membrane remains depolarized, the Na⁺ channels remain in their inactivated state and do not allow Na⁺ permeability to increase. As a result, the ability of the neuron to generate action potentials is lost. Local anesthetics produce a depolarization blockade by combining with the amino acids that form the intracellular mouth of the Na⁺ channel; this prevents further channel activity, resulting in loss of neuron function.

66. What is an ion channel?

An ion channel is a protein in the cell membrane that provides a pathway (the "pore" component of the channel) for charged particles (ions) to cross the lipid layer of the cell membrane. Other parts of the channel protein confer ion selectivity to the channel and determine the channel's gating properties.

67. Which ion channels are important for the function of neurons?

In most neurons, fast Na⁺ channels and various types of K⁺ channels are responsible for the function of the neuron. In some neurons, Ca²⁺ channels and Cl⁻ channels also play a role.

68. What is the basic molecular structure of the sodium channel?

The Na⁺ channel is an alpha helical polypeptide (260–270 kDa) consisting of approximately 2000 amino acids (Fig. 13). It has four homologous domains (I–IV), each consisting of six membrane-spanning segments that are composed of hydrophobic alpha helical proteins. The domains are arranged in a circular fashion in the membrane. The walls of the ion channel (or pore) are formed by a combination of specially angled chain segments between the fifth and sixth membrane-spanning segments, which allow ions to pass through the membrane and appear to contribute to ion selectivity. Positively charged voltage sensors are located in the S4 transmembrane segments.

In the mammalian brain, the alpha subunit is associated with a β_1 subunit (36 kDa) and a β_2 subunit (33 kDa). In skeletal muscle, the alpha subunit is associated only with a β_1 subunit. The beta subunits are integral membrane proteins that interact with the phospholipid bilayer. The β_1 subunit has a noncovalent attachment to the alpha subunit, while the β_2 subunit is covalently attached to the alpha subunit by a disulfide bond. Both the β_1 and β_2 subunits are heavily glycosylated. Glycosylation appears to be required for normal biosynthesis and assembly of the Na^+ channel in neurons.

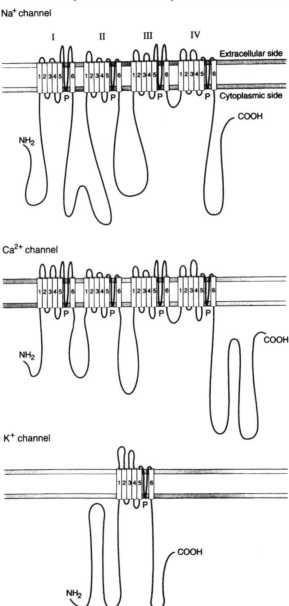

Figure 13. The molecular structures of the alpha subunit of the fast Na^+ channel *(upper panel)*, slow voltage-gated Ca^{2+} channel *(middle panel)* and voltage-activated K^+ channel *(lower panel)*. (From Kandel ER, Schwartz JH, Jessell TM (eds): Principles of Neural Science, 3rd ed. New York, Elsevier Science, Inc., 1991; with permission.)

69. Are there calcium channels in nerve cell membranes? What do they do?

Yes. In some nerve cells, depolarization of the membrane activates slow (L-type) calcium channels, leading to an influx of Ca^{2+} ions that cause the membrane to depolarize the cell toward the Ca^{2+} equilibrium potential. In some cases, Ca^{2+} influx causes regenerative action potentials with slow rise times.

70. Describe the calcium channel's structure.

The structure of the L-type Ca^{2+} channel (Fig. 13) is very similar to that of the Na^+ channel. It also is an alpha helical protein (approximately 2000 amino acids) containing four homologous membrane subunits consisting of six membrane-spanning sequences of amino acids, with connecting loops of amino acids on the extracellular and intracellular sides of the cell membrane. The membrane-spanning segments of the Ca^{2+} and Na^+ channels are quite alike. The main differences between the two channel types are in the extracellular and intracellular amino acid sequences and in the intracellular loop between the fifth and sixth transmembrane sequence. These differences are responsible for the ion selectivity of the different types of channels.

71. What is the structure of the voltage-gated potassium channel?

The voltage-gated K^+ channel is a delayed rectifier K^+ channel (Fig. 14). It consists of four separate and heterologous alpha helical polypeptide chains, which comprise about 600 amino acids. Each chain has six membrane-spanning sequences. The four domains are aggregated in the membrane in an arrangement that is similar to the large, connected domains of the subunits that form Na^+ and Ca^{2+} channels. The pore portion of the K^+ channel is made up of four homologous repeat chains of amino acids between the fifth and sixth sequences in each of the independent domains. In addition to the alpha subunits, K^+ channels have various beta subunits, which may maintain structural stability of the channel pore and regulate the gating properties of the channel. The delayed rectifier K^+ channel is responsible for the repolarization of the cell membrane following an action potential.

Neurons also contain a variety of other K^+ channels, such as Ca^{2+}-activated K^+ channels, inward rectifier K^+ channels, and ATP-sensitive K^+ channels. These have different conductances, different voltage dependencies, different mechanisms of regulation, and, in some cases, a different structure from the delayed rectifier K^+ channel.

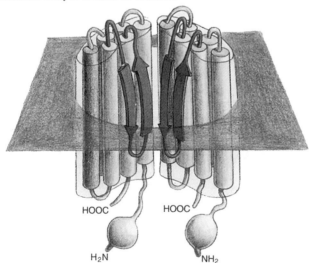

Figure 14. Voltage-gated K^+ channel in the nerve cell membrane. The pore portion of the channel is composed of four homologous repeat chains of amino acids *(arrows)* between the fifth and sixth membrane-spanning sequences. The amino terminus (NH_2) is important in voltage inactivation of the channel via a "ball and chain" mechanism that blocks the pore. (From Alberts B, Bray D, Lewis J, et al: Molecular Biology of the Cell, 3rd ed. New York, Garland Publishing, Inc., 1994; with permission.)

72. What is voltage-dependent activation of an ion channel?

The activation or opening of an ion channel due to a change in membrane potential. During voltage-dependent activation, depolarization of the cell membrane can cause the displacement of positively charged amino acids within the transmembrane pore, leading to activation or opening of the channel.

73. What is channel inactivation?

Closing of the channel so that it can no longer pass ionic current. This appears to involve the movement of amino acids into positions that prevent the movement of ions through the channel.

74. How are the gating properties of fast Na^+ channels, Ca^{2+} channels, and K^+ channels different?

Fast Na^+ channels and slow Ca^{2+} channels have a double gating mechanism, with both an activation gate and an inactivation gate. If either gate is closed, the channel cannot conduct ionic current. The activation gate is closed at the resting potential and the inactivation gate is open. When the membrane is depolarized, opening of the activation gate leads to a regenerative increase in Na^+ conductance during the rising phase of the action potential. The inactivation gate, which is open at resting membrane potential, closes slowly upon depolarization, and is responsible for spontaneous inactivation of Na^+ conductance. The membrane has to be repolarized to reopen the inactivation gate. Ca^{2+} channels also are activated and subsequently inactivated by membrane depolarization.

In contrast, the K^+ channel that is responsible for repolarization and recovery following the action potential has only an activation gate. The gate is activated by membrane depolarization, and the kinetics of gate opening are much slower than those of the Na^+ channel's gate. Consequently, the K^+ efflux that is responsible for the repolarization of the membrane during the action potential begins after the Na^+ conductance is inactivated. The K^+ channel is inactivated by the return of the membrane potential to normal values.

GLIA

75. Since the central nervous system basically lacks connective tissue, how are neurons supported and held together?

Neurons are held together by supporting cells called glia (Greek; means "glue"). They outnumber neurons by about 10:1. However, they occupy only about 50% of the central nervous system's (CNS) volume. Glial cells have processes, but they do not form synapses, and they are not known to conduct action potentials. They provide support, insulation, and nourishment to neurons.

76. Which is more likely to give rise to tumors in the CNS: neurons or glia?

Since neurons are postmitotic cells, while glial cells retain their ability to divide, CNS tumors are caused more often by glia than by neurons. The mitotic property of glia, however, permits the repair of CNS lesions by the formation of a glial scar (gliosis).

77. What are the major types of glia?

There are five major types of glia: astrocytes, oligodendrocytes (CNS), Schwann cells (peripheral nervous system [PNS]), microglia, and ependymal cells (Fig. 15).

78. What are the distinguishing features of astrocytes?

Astrocytes (star-shaped) are the largest and most numerous type of glial cells. There are two major forms: **fibrous astrocytes** have long, thin processes and are found in the white matter; **protoplasmic astrocytes** have shorter, thicker processes and are found in the gray matter. Both types have vascular "end-feet" or "foot processes" that contact and surround blood vessels. These processes also line the ventricles as well as contact neurons.

Astrocytes (and Schwann cells) possess special cytoskeletal intermediate filaments called glial fibrillary acidic proteins or GFAP. These are 50 kDa, vimentin-like proteins identifiable with antibodies against GFAP.

79. What are the main functions of astrocytes?

• *Support and repair:* Astrocytes are the "connective tissue of the CNS." They fill most of the spaces not occupied by neurons and blood vessels and provide both mechanical and presumably metabolic support for neurons. When neurons die or are damaged, astrocytes proliferate and form a glial scar to fill in the empty space.

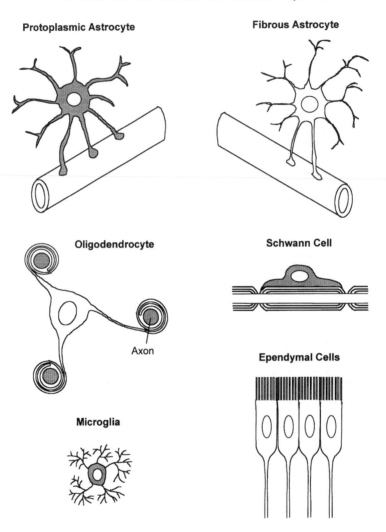

Figure 15.   Major types of glial cells found in the nervous system: protoplasmic astrocytes, fibrous astrocytes, oligodendrocytes, Schwann cells, microglia, and ependymal cells.

- *K^+ buffering:* K^+ ions that are released by spiking neurons are taken up by astrocytes. This helps to control the ionic composition of the extracellular fluid surrounding the neurons and assists neurons in maintaining their membrane potential. Glial cells have only K^+ channels, so they respond to changes in extracellular K^+ with changes in V_m, but they are *not* excitable.
- *Neurotransmitter removal:* Astrocytic processes surround synapses and actively take up some neurotransmitters with high affinity, removing them from the synaptic cleft. These processes assist in the rapid termination of the synaptic signal.
- *Nutrition of neurons:* This role is suggested by the presence of astrocytic "end-feet" on blood vessels and the proximity of astrocytes to neurons. However, there are no solid data on the nutritional role of astrocytes for neurons.
- *Reception of neurotransmitters:* Recently, astrocytic membranes were found to possess neurotransmitter receptors that can trigger electrical and biochemical events inside the glial cells.

80. How do the electrical properties of glial cells compare with those of neurons?
- Glial cells behave passively in response to electrical current.
- Glial cells do not conduct impulses.
- The membrane potential of glial cells is more negative than that of neurons.
- Glial cells are linked by low-resistance connections that permit direct passage of ions and small molecules between the cells.
- Changes in glial cell membrane potentials in different extracellular K^+ concentrations can be predicted exactly by the Nernst equation for K^+. Changes in Na^+ and Cl^- concentration do not produce significant changes in the membrane potential of astrocytes, indicating that the contribution of ions other than K^+ to the membrane potential of these cells is negligible.

81. Do neurons and astrocytes interact?

It is likely that astrocytes interact with neurons. Trains of action potentials in a nerve lead to a depolarization of the surrounding astrocytes. The magnitude of this depolarization depends on the number of nerve fibers activated, and a large depolarization of astrocytes can last for some time after the train of impulses in the nerve has ceased.

The depolarization of the astrocytes in response to action potentials in the surrounding neurons is due to the accumulation of K^+ ions in the interstitial space during the repolarization phase of the neuronal action potential. Astrocytic membrane potentials recover to normal values as the K^+ concentration in the interstitial space decreases, due to uptake and diffusion of K^+ ions by the astrocytes and neurons.

82. How do astrocytes interact with each other?

Because of the low-resistance pathways connecting astrocytes, the depolarization of astrocytes in a specific area draws current from those in unaffected areas. As a result, K+ ions enter the astrocytes in the depolarized regions and leak into the interstitial space in regions where $[K^+]_o$ is normal.

83. How do astrocytes regulate extracellular K^+ concentration? Why is this important?

Astrocytes separate groups of neurons. The arrangement of the astrocytes allows the local K^+ concentration to rise, rather than diffuse into surrounding areas following impulses in the neurons. Thus, K^+ buildup is localized, and cross talk between neurons is prevented. This regulation function is important because the astrocytes can act as conduits for the rapid uptake of K^+ from the interstitial space and help maintain a constant extracellular environment.

84. Are neurons and astrocytes connected?

No. Neurons and astrocytes are separated by an extracellular space of about 20 nm in width. This space prevents currents generated by action potentials in individual neurons from spreading into neighboring cells. Electrophysiologic experiments also fail to demonstrate any connection between neurons and astrocytes.

85. Do neurons influence astrocytes?

Yes. The release of K^+ into the extracellular space by neurons during the repolarization phase of the action potential leads to K^+ accumulation, which depolarizes the membrane of the astrocytes. Membrane potential changes in astrocytes contribute to the changes in potential that can be measured during extracellular recordings, such as an electroencephalogram.

In astrocytes, K^+ conductance is not uniformly distributed along the surface of the cell. The end feet of the astrocytes that contact blood vessels and the pial membrane have a much higher K^+ permeability than the rest of the membrane, allowing the excess K^+ that was taken up elsewhere on the cell surface to be extruded from the end feet. This extrusion may be important in allowing the astrocytes to regulate arterial diameter, by causing a vasodilatation that increases oxygen delivery and blood flow during periods of increased neuronal activity.

86. What are the major functions of oligodendrocytes?

Oligodendrocytes are smaller than astrocytes and have fewer processes (Fig. 15). Their chief function is to myelinate axons in the CNS (see Question 87). One oligodendrocyte may myelinate many axons by extending individual processes to wrap around individual axons or segments of axons.

87. How are Schwann cells different from oligodendrocytes?

Schwann cells, which are derived from the neural crest, are the PNS counterpart of oligodendrocytes because they myelinate peripheral axons (Fig. 15). A single Schwann cell myelinates only a single axon or a segment (internodal segment) of a single axon, whereas one oligodendrocyte may myelinate many axons (up to 50 or more axons or internodal segments of axons). A single axon in the PNS can be myelinated by as many as 500 Schwann cells. Schwann cells surround all peripheral axons, whether myelinated or not, while oligodendrocytic processes do not surround unmyelinated axons in the CNS. Processes of a single Schwann cell may surround many unmyelinated axons. Finally, Schwann cells are covered by a **basal lamina**, whereas oligodendrocytes are not.

88. What is myelin? How does it form?

Myelin is simply the plasma membrane of oligodendrocytes or Schwann cells wrapped tightly around individual axons, much like the end of a tube of toothpaste wrapped concentrically around a pencil. The cytoplasmic content of myelin-forming cells (by analogy, the toothpaste) is squeezed out in the process. The resultant myelin sheath has a structure of alternating **major dense lines** (formed by apposing cytoplasmic faces) and **minor dense lines** or **intraperiod lines** (apposing extracellular faces of plasma membrane of myelin-forming cells) (Fig. 16A). The **inner mesaxon** is where the intraperiod line first forms next to the axon trunk. In the PNS, there also is an **outer mesaxon**, where the intraperiod line is clearly demarcated by the expanding Schwann cell cytoplasm. There is no outer mesaxon in central myelin.

Similar to the plasma membrane, myelin is made up of 70% lipid and 30% protein. It is rich in cholesterol and phospholipid as well as in a specialized group of proteins known as **myelin basic proteins**.

89. What are clefts of Schmidt-Lanterman?

The clefts (or incisures) of Schmidt-Lanterman are "splits" between major dense lines of myelin that are filled with Schwann cell cytoplasm (Fig. 16B). They usually occur obliquely across the width of the myelin sheath in the PNS only. Their function is not known, but they may provide a pathway for metabolites to diffuse to the depths of the myelin sheath.

Henry Schmidt was an American pathologist who described the clefts in 1874, 3 years before a similar description by A.J. Lanterman, a German anatomist.

90. What is the function of myelin?

The main function of myelin is to insulate axons so as to decrease ionic flux across the axolemma and increase the membrane resistance (producing a greater length constant). The larger the axon, the thicker the myelin. Ensheathed portions of axons are no longer excitable, but they have excellent cable properties (i.e., a low capacitance and a high resistance to current leakage).

A myelin sheath on an axon increases its conduction velocity. However, conduction of action potentials along a myelinated axon depends on the presence of nodes of Ranvier.

91. What are nodes of Ranvier?

These are periodic unmyelinated portions of a myelinated axon trunk where there is a greater current density. They typically occur every 0.5–2 mm (internodal distance) along the axon trunk; the larger the axon, the longer the internode. In the PNS, Schwann cell processes shield the nodes, but in the CNS the nodes are exposed to the extracellular fluid without a shield (Fig. 16C).

The absence of myelin and the presence of a high concentration of voltage-gated Na^+ channels (~ several thousand channels/μm^2) at the node enable current to flow easily across it. This flow allows the membrane potential to reach threshold at these points, causing the action potentials to jump from node to node (saltatory conduction) in a myelinated axon and greatly increasing their conduction velocity (up to 120 m/sec). Unmyelinated fibers conduct at < 2 m/sec.

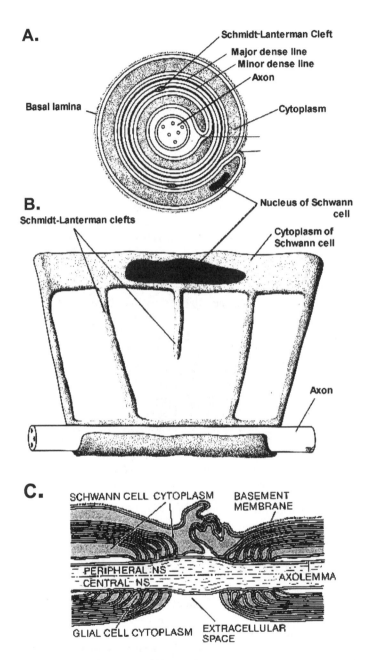

A.

Schmidt-Lanterman Cleft
Major dense line
Minor dense line
Axon

Basal lamina

Cytoplasm

B.
Schmidt-Lanterman clefts

Nucleus of Schwann cell

Cytoplasm of Schwann cell

Axon

C.
SCHWANN CELL CYTOPLASM   BASEMENT MEMBRANE

PERIPHERAL NS
CENTRAL NS   AXOLEMMA

GLIAL CELL CYTOPLASM   EXTRACELLULAR SPACE

Figure 16. **A**, Myelin around a peripheral axon showing the major dense line, the minor dense line, the inner mesaxon, and the outer mesaxon. **B**, Formation of the Schmidt-Landerman incisure (or cleft) by the cytoplasm of a Schwann cell. **C**, A node of Ranvier covered by Schwann cell cytoplasm in the peripheral nervous system (upper part) and one that is bare in the central nervous system (lower part). (Images A and B are modified from Snell RS: Clinical Neuroanatomy for Medical Students, 3rd ed. Boston, Little, Brown and Company, 1992; with permission. Image C is modified from Kuffler SW, Nichols JG: From Neuron to Brain. Sunderland, MA, Sinauer Associates, Inc., 1976; with permission.)

92. Are all axons myelinated?

No. Only axons with diameters greater than 1 μm usually are myelinated.

93. When does myelination normally begin and end?

The process of myelination normally starts during late fetal development and continues through the first postnatal year.

94. How do demyelinating diseases affect conduction velocity?

Demyelinating diseases lead to a slowing of action potential propagation along the fiber, and the loss of normal circuit functions in the neurons.

95. What is multiple sclerosis?

Multiple sclerosis is a demyelinating disease of the CNS with inflammatory features. Both sensory and motor axons are affected, and gliosis (sclerosis) after demyelination occurs at multiple sites in the brain, spinal cord, and optic nerve. Patients often complain of weakness, incoordination, paresthesias (abnormal sensations), speech impairment, and visual disturbance. There is a marked slowing as well as abnormal conduction of action potentials, which may lead to paralysis. The course of the disease is characterized by repeated periods of remission and relapses over many years. Etiology is unknown, but is postulated to be an autoimmune response against the CNS myelin.

96. What is Guillain-Barré syndrome?

This is a demyelinating disease of the PNS, also known as acute febrile polyneuritis. It is an autoimmune response against one's own PNS myelin, and it may follow mild infections and inoculations. Patients suffer from disturbances in sensory perception and motor coordination, which are caused by a slowing or failure of conduction of action potentials in peripheral nerves that innervate skin and muscles.

George Guillain and Jean Alexandre Barré were French neurologists who lived in the late 19th and early 20th centuries.

97. Do axons and Schwann cells influence each other?

Yes. Following axotomy, Wallerian degeneration of distal axons induces a down-regulation of myelin gene expression. Functional regeneration of peripheral nerves causes a reinduction of myelin gene expression. Remember that myelin forms from the plasma membrane of Schwann cells.

Schwann cells, in turn, influence the local properties and viability of axons because when there is profound myelin degeneration, previously myelinated axons deteriorate.

98. Is there a special name for the junction between CNS glia and Schwann cells?

Yes. The PNS interfaces with the CNS at the glial-Schwann junction, also known as the **Obersteiner-Redlich area**. This junction is formed on both the dorsal and ventral spinal nerve roots. On the dorsal root, it is proximal to the sensory ganglion (i.e., the sensory ganglion is part of the PNS).

Heinrich Obersteiner and Emil Redlich were Austrian neurologists who lived during the late 1800s and early 1900s.

99. What are microglia? What is their main function?

Their name indicates that they are very small cells (Fig. 15). Under normal conditions, microglia have tiny, oval cell bodies with many short processes and are relatively few in number. However, when neurons undergo degeneration, microglia increase in size (hypertrophy) and number (hyperplasia). Their main function is to phagocytize degenerated debris in the CNS.

100. What are ependymal cells? Why are they important?

Ependymal cells are cuboidal or columnar epithelial cells that line the inside of the neural tube (ventricles of the brain and central canal of the spinal cord) (Fig. 15). They also line the surface of the choroid plexus, which is the source of cerebrospinal fluid (CSF). Some ependymal cells are ciliated and may aid in CSF circulation. Their microvilli may engage in secretory or absorptive functions.

Ependymal cells have desmosomes (zonula adherens) and some gap junctions, but no tight junctions (zona occludens). Thus, substances in the CNS can penetrate the brain. *Modified* ependymal cells that form the choroid plexus epithelium *do* have circumferential tight junctions (see Question 101).

Ependymal cells also are involved in directing cell migration during embryonic development of the brain.

101. What makes up the choroid plexus?

The choroid plexus is composed of capillary endothelial cells of the pia mater covered by a layer of modified ependymal cells, known as the choroid plexus epithelium. Together, the cells protrude into the cavities of the lateral, third, and fourth ventricles and produce CSF. The epithelial cells have numerous microvilli that greatly expand their surface area. The choroid plexus has both secretory and filtration functions. The epithelial and endothelial cells have different sets of transporters. For example, the transport of vitamin C is much more active in the epithelial cells than in the endothelial cells.

102. What is the composition of cerebrospinal fluid?

CSF is clear, watery, and of low density. It contains very little protein, with an ionic composition similar to that of blood plasma. Glucose and amino acids that are needed by the brain move down their concentration gradients by facilitated diffusion, whereas other molecules probably are actively secreted. The entire volume of CSF (~ 150 ml) is replaced three to four times a day.

103. Why do we need cerebrospinal fluid?

CSF serves several important functions. It:
- Maintains a fluid environment that is comparable in composition to that of the extracellular space
- Cushions and protects the brain from mechanical impact with the skull
- Effectively reduces the weight of the brain in situ to less than 50 g due to its buoyancy property
- Serves as a lymphatic system for the brain
- Allows for the movement of peptide hormones secreted by the hypothalamus to remote sites for action
- Affects cerebral blood flow and pulmonary ventilation via pH levels..

104. How does the cerebrospinal fluid flow through the brain?

CSF flows from the two lateral ventricles to the third ventricle through the two interventricular foramina of Monro (Fig. 17). It then passes through the cerebral aqueduct of Sylvius to the fourth ventricle. From there it flows through the two lateral foramina of Luschka and the medial foramen of Magendie into the subarachnoid space. This space bathes the cortex as well as the brain stem and the spinal cord. A limited amount of CSF also flows through the central canal of the spinal cord.

105. What are arachnoid villi?

These are protrusions of arachnoid membrane into the superior sagittal sinus (Fig. 17). Arachnoid villi act as one-way valves for the flow of CSF from the subarachnoid space to the venous sinus. This one-way flow is an important means by which harmful metabolites from the brain are removed.

106. What is the Virchow-Robin space?

It is a perivascular subarachnoid space formed by the invasion of blood vessels into the parenchyma of the cerebral cortex (Fig. 18). This space is filled with CSF and is lined by the pia mater. It facilitates diffusion of small solutes between the extracellular fluid of neural tissue and CSF of the subarachnoid space as well as of the ventricular system.

Rudolf Ludwig Karl Virchow was a German pathologist and Charles Phillipe Robin was a French anatomist. Both lived in the 19th century.

107. What is the blood-cerebrospinal fluid barrier?

The epithelial cells of the choroid plexus have circumferential tight junctions that form the blood-CSF barrier. Active transport of solutes is mediated by carriers.

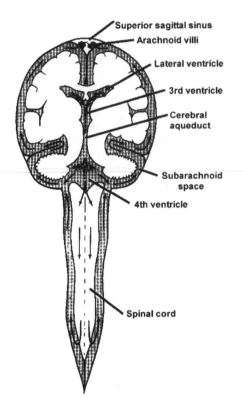

Figure 17. Circulation of the cerebrospinal fluid through the ventricular system and the subarachnoid space. (Modified from deGroot J, Chusid JG: Correlative Neuroanatomy, 20th ed. East Norwalk, CT, Appleton & Lange, 1988.)

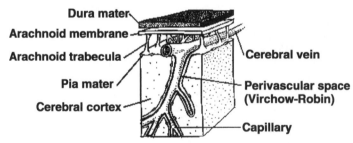

Figure 18. Dura mater, arachnoid mater, and pia mater. The perivascular space is known as the Virchow-Robin space. (Modified from Kandel ER, Schwartz JH, Jessell TM: Principles of Neural Science, 3rd ed. New York, Elsevier, 1991.)

108. What is the blood-brain barrier?

Unlike capillaries elsewhere in the body that have fenestrated endothelium, those of the CNS have **tight junctions** between endothelial cells that are resistant to the passage of ions and small molecules (Fig. 19). Moreover, there is no evidence of fluid-phase or receptor-mediated endocytosis by brain endothelial cells. Astrocytic glial cells that form endfeet around the capillaries also contribute to such a barrier.

The blood-brain barrier protects the brain from many toxins as well as potential antigens. There is relatively little immune response in the CNS, and the brain is regarded as "immunologically privileged."

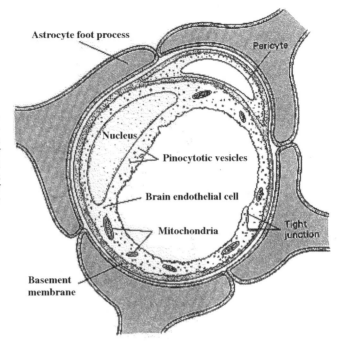

Figure 19. The blood-brain barrier is formed primarily by tight junctions between endothelial cells of CNS blood vessels. (Modified from Kandel ER, Schwartz JH, Jessell TM: Principles of Neural Science, 3rd ed. New York, Elsevier, 1991.)

109. Are there areas of the brain that do not have a blood-brain barrier?

Indeed there are leaky areas. These include the **posterior pituitary** and **circumventricular organs** (CVO), such as the area postrema, median eminence, choroid plexus, and subfornical organ. The leakiness is caused either by fenestrated capillaries or by numerous cytoplasmic vesicles that transport their contents across the endothelial cells.

The absence of a blood-brain barrier is necessary in the posterior pituitary because neurosecretory products have to reach the blood stream. The chemoreceptive subfornical organ requires transcellular transport for water balance and other functions.

Special ependymal cells known as **tanycytes** line the CVOs. Interestingly, the tanycytes have tight junctions that prevent free exchange between the CVOs and the CSF.

110. What are the cell types in the peripheral ganglia?

Craniospinal ganglia (dorsal root ganglia, cranial nerve sensory ganglia)
- *Pseudounipolar neurons* with no dendrites
- *Satellite cells* that are homologous to Schwann cells and are of neural crest origin. They surround neurons and have no processes.
- *Fibrocytes* (capsule cells) that synthesize connective tissue in the ganglia

Autonomic ganglia (e.g., intramural, paravertebral)
- *Postganglionic neurons* (multipolar)
- *Satellite cells* that synapse on ganglionic neurons
- *Capsular fibrocytes*

NON-NEURAL AND NONGLIAL COMPONENTS

111. What are the three membranes of the meninges?

The meninges protect the CNS from direct contact with the bony skull and vertebral column. They are three membranes: the dura mater, arachnoid, and pia mater (Fig. 18).

The **dura mater** (Latin; hard mother) is a tough, fibrous membrane that forms the outermost cover of the brain and the spinal cord. It has an outer *periosteal* layer that attaches to the bone and an inner *meningeal* layer that encloses the venous sinuses and partitions the brain (falx cerebri, tentorium cerebri, falx cerebelli, and diaphragma sellae).

The **arachnoid** (Greek; spider) is a thin, avascular, spider web–like membrane that forms a trabecular meshwork underneath the dura. The CSF flows in the subarachnoid space. Arachnoid granulations are groups of arachnoid villi (see Question 105) that lead from the subarachnoid space into the venous sinuses. They increase in size and number and tend to calcify with advancing age.

The **pia mater** (Latin; tender mother) is a thin membrane made up of reticular, elastic, and collagenous fibers. It follows the contours of the brain to the depths of fissures and sulci, and it carries the blood vessels with it. It forms the tela choroidea of the third and fourth ventricles, and it combines with the ependyma to form the choroid plexus of the ventricular system.

112. What makes up a peripheral nerve?

A peripheral nerve is made up of nerve fibers, connective tissue, and blood vessels (*vasa nervorum*). A given nerve may contain both myelinated and unmyelinated axons, and both sensory and motor nerve fibers. A *nerve fiber* is an axon plus its Schwann cell sheath (either myelinated or unmyelinated).

113. What makes up the connective tissue in a peripheral nerve?

There are three parts to the connective tissue of a peripheral nerve (Fig. 20):
- **Endoneurium** is a delicate, loose connective tissue that surrounds axons and their associated Schwann cells. It is made up of collagen and reticular fibers and the vasa nervorum forms a loose capillary plexus within it.
- **Perineurium** is a moderately dense, fibrous connective tissue that divides groups of nerve fibers into fascicles.
- **Epineurium** is a dense, fibrous connective tissue sleeve that surrounds the entire nerve. This tissue is thick enough to be sutured in nerve repair operations.

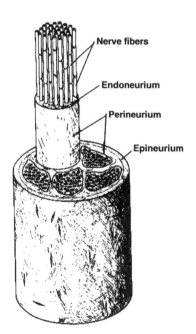

Nerve fibers

Endoneurium

Perineurium

Epineurium

Figure 20.   The peripheral nerve is surrounded by connective tissues consisting of the innermost endoneurium, the perineurium, and the outermost epineurium. (From Snell RS: Clinical Neuroanatomy for Medical Students, 3rd ed. Boston, Little, Brown and Company, 1992; with permission.)

BIBLIOGRAPHY

1. Alberts B, Bray D, Lewis J, et al: Molecular Biology of the Cell, 3rd ed. New York, Garland Publishing, Inc., 1994.
2. Bear MF, Connors BW, Paradiso MA: Neuroscience: Exploring the Brain. Baltimore, Williams and Wilkins, 1996.
3. Berne RM, Levy MN: Physiology, 4th ed. St. Louis, Mosby, 1998.
4. Guyton AC, Hall JE: Textbook of Medical Physiology, 9th ed. Philadelphia, W.B. Saunders Company, 1996.
5. Kandel ER, Schwartz JH, Jessell TM (eds): Principles of Neural Science, 3rd ed. New York, Elsevier Science, Inc., 1991.
6. Kandel ER, Schwartz JH, Jessell TM (eds): Essentials of Neural Science and Behavior. Norwalk, Appleton and Lange, 1995.
7. Lodish H, Baltimore D, Berk A, et al: Molecular Cell Biology, 3rd ed. New York, Scientific American Books, 1995.
8. Nicholls JG, Martin AR, Wallace BG (eds): From Neuron to Brain: A Cellular and Molecular Approach to the Function of the Nervous System, 3rd ed. Sunderland, MA, Sinauer Associates, Inc., 1992.
9. Raff H (ed): Physiology Secrets. Philadelphia, Hanley & Belfus, Inc., 1998.
10. Ross MH, Romrell L, Kaye GI: Histology: A Text and Atlas, 3rd ed. Baltimore, Williams and Wilkins, 1995.
11. Siegel GJ, Agranoff BW, Albers RW, Fisher SK, Uhler MD (eds): Basic Neurochemistry: Molecular, Cellular, and Medical Aspects, 6th ed. Philadelphia, Lippincott-Raven, 1999.
12. Sperelakis N (ed): Cell Physiology Source Book, 2nd ed. San Diego, Academic Press, 1998.
13. Sperelakis N, Banks RO (eds): Essentials of Physiology, 2nd ed. Boston, Little, Brown and Company, 1996.

2. SYNAPTIC TRANSMISSION

Michelle Mynlieff, Ph.D.

1. What are the two types of synapses?

Synapses are either electrical or chemical in nature. In an **electrical** synapse, the pre- and post-synaptic cells are connected by ion channels, allowing direct flow of current from one cell to the next. In a **chemical** synapse, excitation of the presynaptic cell leads to release of a neurotransmitter that diffuses to the postsynaptic cell. The postsynaptic cell has receptors for the transmitter. Activation of these receptors causes some type of postsynaptic change.

2. What are the characteristics of each type of synapse?

Electrical synapses provide a means of instantaneous transmission, since the cells in question are electrically coupled. This coupling allows rapid and synchronous firing of interconnected cells in regions where a rapid response is mandatory for survival. This type of synapse usually occurs between a *large* presynaptic fiber and a *small* postsynaptic cell, because the presynaptic cell must produce a substantial enough change in the postsynaptic cell to fire an action potential. Electrical coupling is not ideal for all synapses due to these structural limitations. Chemical synapses are much more structurally flexible. They generally are slower than electrical synapses, but are useful when long-term changes in cellular function are desired. Electrical synapses have a high threshold for firing because the effective resistance for each cell is decreased due to the electrical coupling. According to Ohm's law ($V = IR$), it takes a larger amount of current to reach threshold; thus, electrically coupled cells are well suited for all-or-nothing responses, such as the release of a protective cloud of ink from *Aplysia*. Also, the large channels in an electrical synapse allow moderately sized organic compounds such as second messengers to cross from one cell to the next.

3. Describe the structure of an electrical synapse.

Electrical synapses consist of a zone of very close apposition (3.5 nm) between two neurons, called a **gap-junction**. The normal distance between cells is approximately 20 nm. The gap is bridged by specialized channels called gap-junction channels, which allow flow of both cations and anions between the two cells. These channels consist of a pair of cylinders called **connexons**. There is a connexon in the "presynaptic" membrane and another in the "postsynaptic" membrane. The terms presynaptic and postsynaptic are relative in an electrical synapse, since transmission is bidirectional. Each connexon is called a hemichannel. The channel formed by two connexons is approximately 1.5–2 nm in diameter.

4. What is currently known about the molecular structure of the channels in an electrical synapse?

Each connexon consists of six 7.5-nm-long **connexins** arranged in a circle to form the pore in the membrane (Fig. 1). Each connexin has four hydrophobic, membrane-spanning regions, two extracellular loops, and two cytoplasmic loops. The four membrane-spanning regions are highly conserved in different tissues. The two extracellular loops also are highly conserved and are thought to be the recognition sites for opposing connexons. The two cytoplasmic loops show a great deal of sequence variability when genes from different tissues are compared. This variability allows differential regulation of the channels in different tissues.

5. Is it possible to regulate the conductance of the channels in an electrical synapse?

The gap-junction channels typically have a very large conductance of approximately 100 picosiemens (pS) but are known to be regulated by voltage, pH, and internal calcium concentration.

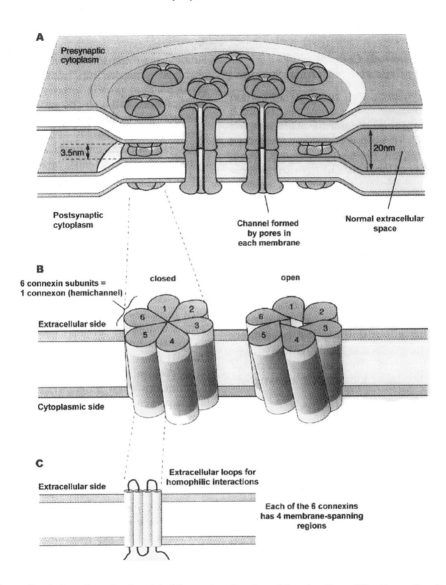

Figure 1. A three-dimensional model of the gap-junction channel, based on X-ray diffraction studies. **A**, A gap-junction channel is actually a pair of hemichannels, one in each cell, that match up in the gap of the extracellular space by means of homophilic interactions. **B**, Each hemichannel, or connexon, has a characteristic hexagonal outline due to the arrangement of its six protein subunits, called connexins. **C**, A single connexin is thought to have four membrane-spanning regions. (Adapted from Kandel ER, Schwartz JH, Jessell TM: Essentials of Neural Science and Behavior. Norwalk, CT, Appleton & Lange, 1995.)

6. Suggest a mechanism by which the channels in an electrical synapse physically open and close.

One theory is that the hemichannels rotate slightly in relation to one another, opening and closing in a manner similar to a camera shutter. The pore is exposed by a concerted tilting of the connexins at 0.9-nm rotation of the cytoplasmic base.

7. Are electrical synapses found in all types of organisms?

Most of the studies on gap junctions have been performed in invertebrates, but there are many electrical synapses present in vertebrates as well. Although many gap junctions in vertebrates only exist early in development, others continue to play an important role later in vertebrate life. For example, it recently has been shown that a particular form of familial deafness in humans is caused by a mutation in one of the connexin genes.[9]

8. Describe the structural features of a chemical synapse.

At the site of communication—the synapse—there are morphological specializations that can be visualized with electron microscopy. The typical intercellular space between neurons of approximately 20 nm widens slightly to 20–40 nm at a chemical synapse. The space between the two neurons is called the synaptic cleft. The presynaptic terminal has a fuzzy, dark thickening of the membrane termed the active zone, which is thought to be the area where the vesicles dock for release. The terminal is filled with neurotransmitter-containing synaptic vesicles (Fig. 2).

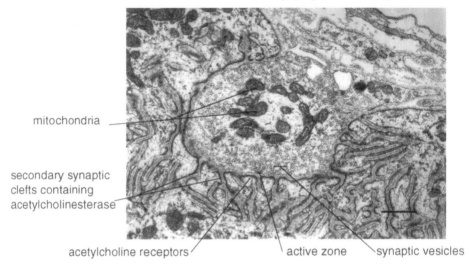

Figure 2.   Electron micrograph of the neuromuscular junction. The motor nerve terminal lies in the primary synaptic cleft and contacts the postsynaptic membrane of the soleus muscle fiber. Bar = 0.6 μm. (Image courtesy of Danny A. Riley.)

9. What is the sequence of events preceding release of neurotransmitters?

An action potential invades the presynaptic terminal, causing a depolarization of the membrane. The depolarization leads to the opening of voltage-dependent calcium channels in the presynaptic membrane. An influx of calcium causes vesicles to dock and release their contents into the synaptic cleft. Neurotransmitters diffuse across the cleft to bind postsynaptic receptors, thereby activating the receptors and leading to a postsynaptic response. The response varies in character depending on the neurotransmitter released, the postsynaptic receptor subtype, and the nature of the postsynaptic cell. The action of the neurotransmitter is terminated either by enzymatic degradation, as in the case of acetylcholine (ACh), or by a specific transporter-mediated uptake into glia and neurons.

10. What is the quantal theory of synaptic transmission? What evidence is there for this theory?

Quantal theory states that neurotransmitters are released in discrete packets. Evidence for this has come from a number of well-known studies. Fatt and Katz demonstrated tiny spontaneous postsynaptic potentials of 0.5–1 millivolts (mV) in the frog neuromuscular junction. Since the evoked postsynaptic response in the neuromuscular junction was termed an end-plate potential, these spontaneous potentials were designated as miniature end-plate potentials (MEPPs). Their data showed that MEPPs had the same time course and drug sensitivities as end-plate potentials; both were blocked by cholinergic antagonists, and both time courses could be lengthened by the application of acetylcholinesterase (AChe) inhibitors. Del Castillo set out to determine if a single molecule of ACh could account for a MEPP. He was able to produce a response much smaller than 0.5 mV, providing evidence against this theory. Furthermore, Katz and Miledi showed that the ion flux through a single cholinergic channel was 0.3 microvolts (μV), which is only 1/2000 of the amplitude of a MEPP. Since two ACh molecules are necessary to activate the cholinergic channels, and some neurotransmitter probably is lost in the cleft due to diffusion, it is assumed that a minimum of 5000 molecules of ACh are necessary to produce a single MEPP. This amount has been confirmed by direct chemical measurement of ACh released.

Experiments on end-plate potentials in low-calcium solution have substantiated the quantal theory. Since a typical end-plate potential is about 70 mV, the response to an individual quantum (~0.5 mV) is too small to substantially change the end-plate potential. However, the contribution of a single quantum is visible in a low-calcium solution, where end-plate potentials are decreased to 0.5–2.5 mV in amplitude. Moreover, it has been shown that the amplitude varies from one stimulation to the next. Stimulation of the nerve in low-calcium and/or high-magnesium solution often fails to produce an end-plate potential at all. MEPPs also can be measured under these conditions, and it has been discovered that the end-plate potential is a multiple of the MEPP amplitude (Fig. 3).The size of individual MEPPs is not affected by the low-calcium solution.

Although all of the initial work on the quantal theory of transmission was performed in the neuromuscular junction, the quantal nature of transmission also has been demonstrated in the majority of central synapses tested. In central synapses the miniature responses are called miniature excitatory postsynaptic potentials (mEPSPs) or miniature inhibitory postsynaptic potentials (mIPSPs). In the voltage clamp mode of recording, these are called currents instead of potentials (mEPSCs or mIPSCs).

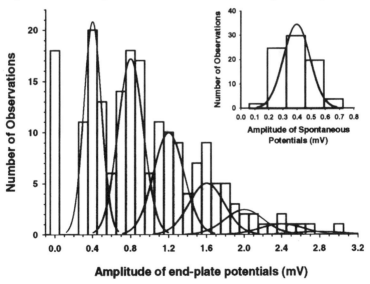

Figure 3.   Histograms of end-plate potential and spontaneous potential amplitude distributions in a fiber in which mammalian neuromuscular transmission was blocked by increased magnesium concentration in the extracellular solution. Peaks in end-plate potential distribution occur at 1, 2, 3, and 4 times the mean amplitude of the spontaneous potentials (0.4 mV). A Gaussian curve was fit to the spontaneous potentials. Multiple Gaussian curves were generated to fit the histogram of the evoked potentials about a mean amplitude xv with a variance of σ^2, where v and σ^2 are the mean and variance of the spontaneous potential amplitude distribution. (Adapted from Boyd A, Martin AR: The end-plate potential in mammalian muscle. J Physiol 132:74–91, 1956.)

11. What is the evidence that a single vesicle is equivalent to a single quantum?

Evidence that a single quantum represents a single vesicle comes from freeze fracture studies of the neuromuscular junction. Frozen tissue is fractured under a high vacuum and coated with platinum and carbon. This procedure offers a view of the intermembrane structures, since the path of membrane cleavage usually is between the two hydrophobic layers of the membrane. One to two rows of large intramembranous particles, thought to be calcium channels, were discovered along the dense bar of the active zone. The density of the particles was $1500/\mu m^2$, which is the approximate number necessary for release. It has been assumed that the calcium channels regulating release must be very close to the release site, because the interior of the cell has great calcium-buffering capacities. Quick-freezing of the tissue in the act of release, by treating it with 4-amino pyridine (a potassium channel-blocker known to broaden the action potential), revealed deformations in the membrane along the row of calcium channel particles. These deformations are thought to represent the fusion of vesicles. They do not persist after neurotransmitter release has ceased, and statistical analysis of this process has shown that the vesicles fuse independently. Further evidence for the fusion of vesicles has been provided by electrophysiological analysis of membrane capacitance. Since the capacitance is directly proportional to the membrane surface area, capacitance should increase as vesicles release their contents. Patch clamp techniques have allowed careful measurement of the membrane capacitance, demonstrating an increase with release and a decrease as the membrane is recycled into new vesicles.

12. How has calcium dependence of release been shown?

External calcium is known to be necessary for neurotransmitter release. The amplitude of the postsynaptic potential exhibits a deep dependence on the extracellular calcium concentration on the order of a third to fourth power function.[2,4] The calcium channels regulating release probably are located close to the docking sites for the synaptic vesicles, to counter the calcium-buffering capacity inside the cell. Quantification of calcium concentrations within the presynaptic terminal with fura-2 fluorescence suggests that the internal concentration need only be raised 10- to 20-fold from an approximate resting level of 5 nM. It is likely that the spatial compartmentalization of the presynaptic terminal exceeds the limitations of current calcium imaging techniques. Theoretical calculations of the buffering capacity of the presynaptic terminal suggest that the calcium concentration near the calcium channels must be about 100 μM. Recordings in hair cells using calcium-dependent potassium channels as an assay for calcium concentration also suggest a concentration of 100 μM upon depolarization.

13. How does the calcium increase in the presynaptic terminal?

It is the concentration of calcium in the presynaptic terminal rather than the source of the calcium that is important in triggering neurotransmitter release. Calcium enters the presynaptic terminal through voltage-dependent calcium channels that are activated by depolarization. The channels can be broadly defined as low-voltage-activated and high-voltage-activated calcium channels. It is assumed that the high-voltage-activated channels are the ones mediating release. These channels can be further subdivided into four groups: L, N, P/Q, and R channels. Which of these channels mediates release of neurotransmitters is not entirely agreed upon. Various tissues use different channels to mediate release. In secretory cells, L channels play a large role; in neurons, the N and P/Q classes play the most significant roles. In addition to channel identity varying within different tissues, there are species differences. In the frog neuromuscular junction, for example, the N channels play the predominant role, whereas in mammalian neuromuscular junctions, the P/Q channels seem to be the predominant channels controlling release.

14. Name the major proteins associated with the synaptic vesicle.

PROTEIN	DESCRIPTION
Cysteine string protein	Peripheral membrane protein that is palmitoylated on more than 10 cysteines and contains a DNA-J homology domain. Function unknown.
Cytochrome b561	Electron transport protein required for intravesicular mono-oxygenases in subsets of secretory vesicles. Required for dopamine-β-hydroxylase and peptide amidase activity.

Table continued on facing page.

PROTEIN	DESCRIPTION
Neurotransmitter transporters	Transporters specific for the neurotransmitter contained in a particular cell accumulate neurotransmitter in vesicles.
Rab proteins	Rab 3A, rab3C, rab5, and rab7. Regulation of docking and fusion.
Rabphilin-3A	Binds to rab3A and rab3C as a function of GTP.
Secretory carrier membrane proteins	Ubiquitous integral membrane proteins of secretory and transport vesicles. Function unknown.
SV2s	Highly glycosylated proteins containing 12 transmembrane regions and homology to bacterial and eukaryotic transporters. Function unknown.
Synapsins Ia, Ib, IIa, and IIb	Fibrous phosphoproteins that link vesicles to the cytoskeleton and each other.
Synaptobrevins (VAMPs; vesicle-associated membrane proteins)	Small proteins that are cleaved by tetanus toxin and by botulinum toxins B, D, F, and G.
Synaptogryn	Polytopic protein. Function unknown.
Synaptophysins	Polytopic proteins that bind to synaptobrevins. Function unknown.
Synaptotagmins	Bind calcium and phospholipids and interact with neurexins, AP2, and syntaxins. May function as the calcium sensor in fast calcium-dependent release.
Transport proteins (channels) for chloride and zinc	Mediate chloride flux for glutamate uptake and zinc uptake.
Vacuolar proton pump	Proton complex of more than 12 subunits. Establishes electrochemical gradient for neurotransmitter uptake.

GTP = guanosine triphosphate, SV2 = synaptic vesicle protein 2, AP2 = adaptor protein 2.
Adapted from Siegel GJ, Agranoff BW, Albers RW, et al: Basic Neurochemistry, 6th ed. New York, Raven Press, 1999.

15. What are the major proteins mediating the docking of the synaptic vesicles associated with the plasma membrane?

PROTEIN	DESCRIPTION
Munc 13	Mammalian homologs of the *Caenorhabditis elegans unc-13* gene that is essential for exocytosis. Function unknown.
Neurexins	Include one of the receptors for α-latrotoxin and may function in cell-cell recognition between neurons.
SNAP-25	Synaptosome-associated protein of 35K that binds to syntaxin and is cleaved by botulinum toxin A and E.
Syntaxins	Cleaved by botulinum toxin C1 and binds synaptotagmins, SNAP-25, synaptobrevins, complexins, munc 13a, SNAPs, calcium channels, and munc 18 proteins.
Voltage-gated calcium channels	Mediate calcium influx for neurotransmitter release at the active zone.
RIM	Binds to rab3 in a GTP-dependent manner and may mediate rab3 action in regulating fusion.

RIM = Rab-interacting molecule, GTP = guanosine triphosphate.
Adapted from Siegel GJ, Agranoff BW, Albers RW, et al: Basic Neurochemistry, 6th ed. New York, Raven Press, 1999.

16. Name the soluble proteins involved in synaptic vesicle docking.

Munc 18 proteins are mammalian homologs of the *C. elegans unc*-18 gene and sec1, sly1, and slp1 products of yeast, and they bind tightly to syntaxins. N-ethylmaleimide-sensitive factor (NSF) and α/β/γSNAPs (soluble NSF attachment proteins) bind synaptobrevin and syntaxin to form the docking complex.

17. What is the current theory on how vesicle docking occurs?

Prior to release, the synaptic vesicles are kept near the active zone by synapsin and rab3A. Synapsin binds to the cytoskeleton, inhibiting the release of the vesicles. Rab3A is thought to be necessary for localization to the active zone, since mutations of the rab3A gene cause the vesicles to be randomly distributed throughout the terminal. Upon calcium influx, synapsin is phosphorylated by calcium-calmodulin–dependent (CAM) kinase, leading to the release of the vesicle from the cytoskeleton. In low-calcium synaptotagmin, synaptobrevin and syntaxin form a complex. Synaptotagmin has two calcium binding sites and acts as the sensor for calcium influx. When calcium enters the cell, synaptotagmin binds to it and displaces it from the synaptobrevin/syntaxin complex. Once synaptotagmin is removed, α-SNAP can bind to the complex with NSF and cause fusion of the vesicle with the presynaptic membrane (Fig. 4).

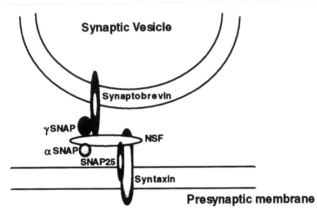

Figure 4. Upon binding to calcium, synaptotagmin in the vesicular membrane becomes unbound from the synaptobrevin/syntaxin complex, allowing the soluble factors in the cytosol to bind to the complex.

18. What do the terms SNAPs and SNARE refer to?

SNAPs (synaptosome-associated proteins) are soluble NSF-attachment proteins that in conjunction with other soluble proteins, such as NSF and munc 18, are involved in assembling the fusion, or SNARE (soluble NSF-associated protein receptor), complex. The concept of a SNARE complex generally is linked to the hypothesis of vesicle docking outlined in question 17. The SNARE hypothesis requires four components:

1. A vesicle membrane protein (v-SNARE; synaptobrevin and synaptotagmin)
2. A target membrane protein (t-SNARE; syntaxin and SNAP-25)
3. A cytosolic protein required for membrane fusion (NSF)
4. Adapters for NSF (SNAPs).

19. How are vesicles recycled?

There are two different theories on how vesicles are recycled. The first resembles the mechanism in secretory cells, where clathrin-coated pits mediate recycling of the vesicles. Clathrin is a fibrous protein that in its purified state consists of a three-limbed triskelion. Each limb comprises a heavy (180,000 Dalton) and light (35,000–40,000 Dalton) chain. The clathrin polymerizes into a lattice along the cytosolic face of the membrane, causing endocytosis. The coated region expands inward, forming a clathrin-coated pit that pinches off to form a new vesicle. A chaperone protein rapidly removes the clathrin coat, and the vesicle fuses with endosomes to recycle into synaptic vesicles.

The second hypothesis is termed the "kiss-and-run" hypothesis. In this model, intact vesicles are rapidly retrieved from the presynaptic membrane after releasing their contents via a fusion pore. After immediate refilling with neurotransmitter, they re-enter the releasable pool of vesicles. This second mechanism is thought to occur on a faster time scale than the first mechanism. In reality, both mechanisms may be at work in the presynaptic terminal, with the two processes feeding different populations of vesicles.

20. What are temporal and spatial summation of synaptic responses?

A single synaptic potential may not be sufficient to cause a postsynaptic cell to reach threshold. If the presynaptic cell is fired rapidly enough (i.e., before the postsynaptic response is over), the postsynaptic responses can summate to reach a higher postsynaptic potential. This is called temporal summation. In addition, it is possible to have different synaptic inputs on various parts of the cell. If these inputs are activated at the same time, their responses can summate to produce spatial summation. In the case of the vertebrate neuromuscular junction, only a single motoneuron synapses on each muscle fiber, but in the central nervous system, neurons receive both excitatory and inhibitory inputs from many different cells. It is the sum of all of these synapses that ultimately determines the behavior of the postsynaptic cell.

21. Are there any structural differences between excitatory and inhibitory synapses?

Two morphological types of synapses were described by E. George Gray: Gray's Type I and Gray's Type II (also referred to as "asymmetric" and "symmetric," respectively). **Type I synapses** most often are excitatory. The synaptic cleft typically is wide (~ 30 nM), with a 1–2 μm^2 synaptic area. The presynaptic terminals contain round vesicles and prominent dense projections. There is an extensive dense region on the postsynaptic side of the synapse. The **Type II synapses** most often are inhibitory. They typically have a more narrow synaptic cleft (~ 20 nm) and a smaller synaptic area (< 1 μm^2). The vesicles in the presynaptic terminal are oval (or "pleomorphic"), and the presynaptic membrane specializations are less obvious. The postsynaptic density typically is less in the Type II synapses than in the Type I (Fig. 5). These morphological features give an indication of the identity of the synapse, but should not be taken as proof. Immunocytochemical analysis aimed at determining the neurotransmitter type in the presynaptic terminal provides more substantial evidence for classifying a synapse as inhibitory or excitatory.

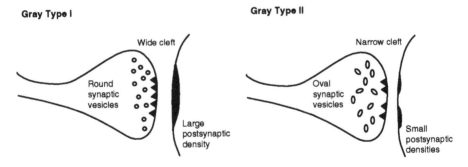

Figure 5.   Two morphological types of synapses help with inhibitory or excitatory classification.

22. Besides shape, are there any other identifying features of synaptic vessels that might giver a clue to their identity?

Vesicles containing neuropeptides and monoamines, such as catecholamines and indoleamines, tend to show as dense-core vesicles in electron micrographs.

23. Do vesicles contain a single neurotransmitter type?

Classic neurotransmitters such as amino acids or biogenic amines frequently are co-localized with neuroactive peptides or purinergic compounds such as adenosine triphosphate (ATP).

24. Discuss the differences between the innervation of a muscle fiber and a central nervous system neuron in vertebrates.

In vertebrates, muscle fibers are innervated by a single motoneuron (this is not true in invertebrates), but central neurons usually receive both excitatory and inhibitory input from a number of cells. The synapses on a central neuron can occur on the dendrites (axodendritic), axon (axoaxonic), or cell body (axosomatic). Because of the life-sustaining function of the neuromuscular junction in controlling respiration, this synapse has a large safety factor: a single stimulation of a motoneuron typically releases 150 quanta, whereas a central neuron releases 1–10 quanta upon a single stimulation. The synapse at the neuromuscular junction is huge (2000–6000 μm^2), and the central synapses are tiny (2 μm^2). In contrast to central synapses, the postsynaptic membrane at the neuromuscular junction contains junctional folds.

25. What was the first direct demonstration of a neurotransmitter effect?

In 1892, J. N. Langley demonstrated that transmission through the mammalian ciliary ganglion was blocked selectively by nicotine, suggesting a chemical form of communication between neurons. Scientists in the early half of this century continued to build upon this idea of chemical transmission. Otto Loewi found in 1921 that stimulation of the vagus decreased the heart rate of a frog. Furthermore, the fluid from the inhibited heart decreased the heart rate of an unstimulated heart. This action was mimicked by the application of exogenous ACh. In the 1930s, Feldberg established ACh as the neurotransmitter in autonomic ganglia, while Dale and his colleagues demonstrated that motoneurons released ACh in skeletal muscles to exert their action.

26. What are the criteria for a neurotransmitter?

In order to show that a substance acts as a neurotransmitter in a particular synapse, the following criteria must be met:

• It must be synthesized within the presynaptic neuron. Antibodies against enzymes for the production of a certain neurotransmitter often are used as immunohistochemical markers for particular neuron types.

• Sufficient amounts of the substance must be released from the presynaptic terminal to produce a postsynaptic response.

• Exogenous application of the compound must mimic the effect of synaptic release.

• There must be a mechanism for action termination and removal of the compound. In the case of ACh in the neuromuscular junction, the action is terminated through enzymatic degradation by AChE. The resulting acetate and choline are then transported back into the neuron to act as substrates for future ACh synthesis. The actions of the majority of neurotransmitters are terminated by high affinity uptake systems, which are specialized for each neurotransmitter. These transporters are a common site of drug action (e.g., antidepressants, cocaine). Following uptake, the neurotransmitter is degraded within the neuron.

27. What are the two types of neurotransmitter receptors? How do they function to produce a postsynaptic response?

Receptors are either ionotropic or metabotropic in nature. **Ionotropic receptors** have an ion channel incorporated directly into their structure. Binding of the ligand opens the associated ion channel. **Metabotropic receptors** are more complicated and offer more flexibility in terms of changing cell function. Metabotropic receptors activate an enzyme, either directly—as in the case of certain peptide receptors that have intrinsic enzymatic activity (i.e., epidermal growth factor, fibroblast growth factor, nerve growth factor, and insulin)—or through the activation of a second messenger cascade. Typically, the receptor is linked to a G-protein that can stimulate activity of intracellular enzymes, releasing a second messenger. The second messenger may go on to activate yet another enzyme or may directly affect channel function or even gene transcription rates. Thus, metabotropic receptors can profoundly affect cellular function, and though they often take longer to produce an effect, the results last longer than for ionotropic receptors.

28. Describe the main excitatory neurotransmitter and its receptors in the central nervous system.

The main excitatory neurotransmitter in the central nervous system is glutamate. This excitatory amino acid can activate both N-methyl-D-aspartate (NMDA) and non-NMDA ionotropic glutamate receptors. The non-NMDA receptors can be broken down further into multiple classes. These receptors are permeable to cations, with certain molecular species having a preference for sodium and others a preference for calcium. They mediate fast excitatory transmission.

The NMDA receptors show a voltage dependence: binding of glutamate alone is not sufficient to cause an opening of this cation channel due to a blockage by magnesium. If the membrane is depolarized for a sufficient period of time, the magnesium leaves the channel pore, allowing calcium and sodium to flow into the cell. The NMDA receptor also has a binding site for glycine and requires a minimum glycine concentration for activation. Influx of calcium through this channel seems to be the most important mediator of its effects. The NMDA channel has been implicated in many studies on synaptic plasticity. Since behavioral studies show that continual repetition facilitates learning, it is reasonable to think that the continual stimulation necessary to remove magnesium from the pore of the channel correlates with learning.

In addition to the ionotropic receptors for glutamate, there are a number of metabotropic receptors, which are linked to various G-protein systems.

29. Describe the main inhibitory neurotransmitters and their receptors.

Glycine and GABA (γ-aminobutyric acid) are the two main inhibitory neurotransmitters. Both glycine and GABA have ionotropic receptors that are permeable to chloride. In addition to its ionotropic receptor, $GABA_A$, GABA also has two metabotropic receptors called $GABA_B$ and $GABA_C$.

30. What are the molecular features of ionotropic receptors?

Ionotropic receptors share similarities with voltage-gated ion channels and gap junction ion channels. All three types of channels have multiple membrane-spanning regions. The ionotropic channels are multimeric structures, and each subunit contains four membrane-spanning regions, M1–M4. M2 lines the channel pore (Fig. 6).

The nicotinic ACh receptor, the $GABA_A$ receptor, and the glycine receptor belong to the same family. The nicotinic ACh receptor consists of five subunits: α, α, β, δ, and either an ε (adult form) or γ (embryonic form). The α subunits bind ACh. The $GABA_A$ receptor consists of a multimeric structure composed of α, β, and γ subunits, which can bind GABA with varying affinities; the α and β subunits bind barbiturates, and only the α subunit binds benzodiazepines. To date, only two subunits of the glycine receptor have been identified. The α and β subunits also form a pentameric structure, although the precise stoichiometry is still questioned.

The glutamate ionotropic receptors have a similar general structure as the other ionotropic receptors, but belong to a different family. Like the GABA receptors, NMDA receptors bind a number of different ligands in addition to the main ligand for the receptor. There are binding sites on the channel for glycine, magnesium, zinc, and phencyclidine (PCP).

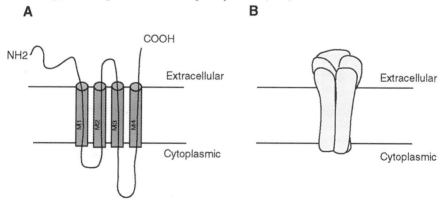

Figure 6. **A,** Each subunit of an ionotropic receptor has four hydrophobic membrane-spanning regions (M1–M4), with the carboxyl and amino terminals located on the extracellular side of the membrane. **B,** Ionotropic receptors typically are pentameric in structure. The stoichiometry of the various subunits depends on the receptor subtype.

31. What are the molecular features of G-protein–coupled receptors?

G-protein–coupled receptors are globular glycoproteins whose structures are based on a bundle of seven membrane-spanning, hydrophobic helices connected by hydrophilic loops. The glycosylated amino terminal is on the extracellular side of the membrane, and the carboxyl terminal is on the cytoplasmic side. The most highly conserved regions in this family of receptors are the hydrophobic membrane-spanning domains. The amino and carboxyl terminals as well as the cytoplasmic loop between membrane-spanning sequences 5 and 6 are the most varied.

32. Is it possible to have a depolarizing inhibitory potential?

Typically one thinks of depolarizing potentials as excitatory and hyperpolarizing potentials as inhibitory. While this generally is true, the most important aspect of the synaptic effect is whether it makes it easier or harder for the postsynaptic cell to fire an action potential. Since depolarizations take a cell closer to threshold, and hyperpolarizations take a cell further from threshold, the typical understanding seems logical. However, there are scenarios where depolarizations can be inhibitory. For example, in a cell whose membrane potential is slight hyperpolarized in comparison to the equilibrium potential for chloride, opening chloride channels would cause a slight depolarization—yet the response would still be inhibitory. The slight depolarization would not be sufficient to bring the cell anywhere near threshold for firing an action potential. The decrease in resistance actually would make it harder for another synaptic input to bring the cell to threshold ($V = IR$). In some synapses there might even be a general decrease in resistance without any significant change in membrane potential, making it harder to fire an action potential in that cell. This effect is called **shunting**.

Another example of a depolarizing inhibitory response can be found in axoaxonal connections in the spinal cord. An interneuron synapses on the presynaptic terminal of a Group Ia afferent neuron, where it produces a depolarizing response. The depolarization decreases the amplitude of any action potentials invading the terminal partly because they will arise from a less negative potential, and partly because of the increase in potassium conductance and slight inactivation of sodium channels caused by the depolarization. Since the amount of neurotransmitter released from the terminal is directly proportional to the action potential amplitude, the depolarization will be inhibitory.[5]

33. What are the neurotransmitter and receptor in the vertebrate neuromuscular junction?

The vertebrate neuromuscular junction neurotransmitter is ACh, which acts upon nicotinic ACh receptors. These are ionotropic receptors that are nonspecific for cations.

34. What are the broad categories of modulatory transmitters?

Transmitters that bind to metabotropic receptors are often thought of as modulatory because they don't produce a fast ionic current. The ultimate result of activation of these receptors, however, is often the turning off or on of ionic currents. In addition to their effects on ionotropic receptors, ACh, GABA, and glutamate all bind to metabotropic receptors to produce slower, longer-lasting postsynaptic effects. Another broad class of small-molecule transmitters is the biogenic amines, which include the catecholamines, dopamine, norepinephrine and epinephrine, indoleamine, serotonin, and histamine. Purines such as ATP, ADP, uridine triphosphate, and adenosine are active at purinergic receptors. There are also a large and growing group of neuroactive peptides that have been categorized.

35. How do the receptors of modulatory transmitters cause postsynaptic changes?

The modulatory transmitters act through a second-messenger cascade. The transmitter is the first messenger, which binds to a receptor activating a transducer. The transducer affects the activity of a primary effector, leading to the production of a second messenger. The second messenger can then affect a second effector. The scheme can stop at any point depending on the receptor and cell type.

36. How does the synthesis of biogenic amines differ from the synthesis of neuroactive peptides?

The catecholamines (epinephrine, norepinephrine, and dopamine) are all part of the same enzymatic pathway that begins with L-tyrosine and stops at a specific point to produce the neurotransmitter of choice. Each neuron contains only the enzymes necessary to reach that point in the synthetic cascade. The indoleamines (serotonin and melatonin) follow a similar cascade that begins with tryptophan. Histamine and GABA are produced from histidine and glutamate, respectively. In contrast, neuroactive peptides begin as prohormones. Prohormones are long peptides that often contain multiple copies of a single peptide or even multiple neuroactive peptides in a single sequence. They are enzymatically degraded to the appropriate peptides in a cell-specific fashion.

37. What is a G-protein?

G-proteins are the main type of transducer used in second-messenger cascades. A G-protein consists of an α, β, and γ subunit and is so-named because it binds guanine nucleotides. Before binding of a ligand to its receptor, the α subunit of the G-protein binds to GDP. Binding of the ligand promotes the exchange of GDP for GTP. When the α subunit is bound to GTP it can more readily dissociate from the β and γ subunits. Once the subunits dissociate, they can affect the primary effector. The α subunit has a slowly activating, intrinsic GTPase activity that allows it to convert the bound GTP to GDP and reassociate with the other subunits to turn off the cascade (Fig. 7). Many different versions of the G-protein subunits have been cloned to date.

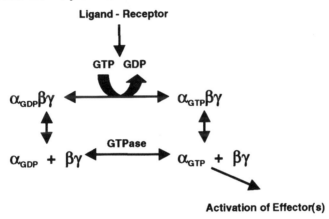

Figure 7.   Scheme for G-protein activation and inactivation.

38. Describe four biochemical tools that are used to study G-protein–mediated responses.

Two nonhydrolysable guanine nucleotides typically are used to probe the involvement of G-proteins in a particular response. Due to their nonhydrolysable nature, these compounds bind irreversibly to the G-protein, inhibiting the exchange of GTP and GDP. GTPγ-S is an analogue of GTP that maintains the protein in the activated state. GDPβ-S is an analogue of GDP that maintains the protein in the inactivated state. Two neurotoxins also are commonly used in elucidating the role of G-proteins. The toxins are specific for certain categories of G-proteins, and they modify the G-proteins by adding an ADP-ribose moiety from intracellular NAD^+ to the α subunit. Pertussis toxin, the toxin responsible for whooping cough, ADP-ribosylates the G-proteins of the Gi and Go families, thereby permanently inactivating the G-protein. Cholera toxin, the toxin responsible for cholera, ADP-ribosylates G-proteins of the Gs family, and the G-protein is permanently activated.

39. Describe the adenylate cyclase second-messenger system.

A ligand such as norepinephrine binds its receptor, causing activation of the Gs form of G-protein. Gs stimulates adenylate cyclase, increasing the production of cyclic adenosine monophosphate (cAMP) in the cell. The cAMP can go on to produce a number of intracellular effects: some channels are directly gated by cAMP; there is a cAMP-dependent protein kinase; and there are cAMP response elements on DNA that can affect transcription rates.

40. Are there other mechanisms by which cAMP levels can be modulated?

cAMP levels are regulated by the balance between adenylate cyclase, which synthesizes cAMP, and phosphodiesterase, which metabolizes it. Activation of a receptor can lead to changes in phosphodiesterase activity, often through changes in calcium levels.

41. Is cAMP the only cyclic nucleotide important in transduction of synaptic signals?

No, cyclic guanosine monophosphate (cGMP) also plays an important role.

42. What are the consequences of phospholipase C activation?

Phospholipase C catalyzes the breakdown of phosphoinositol-4,5-biphosphonate into inositol 1,4,5-triphosphate (IP_3) and diacylglycerol (DAG). IP_3 is soluble and binds to a receptor in the endoplasmic reticulum to open calcium channels. This binding leads to an increase in internal calcium concentration from intracellular stores. The calcium can regulate enzyme functions directly or can interact with calmodulin or other calcium-binding proteins to indirectly activate or inactivate a host of enzymes within the cell. One enzyme whose activity is modulated by calcium concentrations is protein kinase C (PKC). DAG remains in the membrane and directly affects the activity of PKC by lowering its requirement for calcium. DAG also can be further broken down by phospholipase A_2 into arachidonic acid. Arachidonic acid can have activity of its own or can be metabolized to eicosanoids that include various prostaglandins and leukotrienes. Eicosanoids are important in the inflammatory response as well as in the regulation of ion channel functions, receptors, neurotransmitter release, synaptic plasticity, and neuronal gene expression. They have dual roles as messengers modulating cell functions and participants in the nerve tissue's response to injury.

43. Do all first messengers act through receptors?

No. In addition to classic neurotransmitters and neuroactive peptides, gases represent a relatively new class of first messengers. Nitric oxide (NO) and carbon monoxide can diffuse from one cell to the next, allowing for communication in both directions, without the use of receptors. NO was first described as endothelial-derived relaxing factor. It is known to be synthesized in neurons in response to calcium influx through NMDA receptors and has been implicated as a significant player in long-term potentiation. One mechanism by which NO produces an effect is stimulation of guanylyl cyclase activity.

44. What is the clinical presentation of a patient with myasthenia gravis?

There are three main clinical manifestations of myasthenia gravis (MG). The first involves the **motor systems**, with weakness in extraocular muscles, facial muscles, and muscles of mastication, bulbar-innervated muscles, and respiratory muscles. Clinically, the muscle weakness presents as ptosis (drooping eyelids), facial weakness, dysarthria (stammering), dysphagia (incomplete language function, inability to articulate), difficulty chewing, respiratory failure, and weakness of extremity muscles. The weakness worsens with continued muscle activity (fatigability). The second involves the **thymus gland**, with thymic hyperplasia (70% of young people with MG), thymoma (epithelial tumor), or thymic carcinoma. The third involves the **peripheral immune system**, with circulating antibodies and other autoimmune disorders.

45. What is the mechanism underlying the symptoms of myasthenia gravis?

MG is an autoimmune disease in which the immune system makes antibodies against the nicotinic form of the ACh receptor. Since the nicotinic receptors in the brain are protected by the blood-brain barrier, the main symptoms are due to loss of nicotinic receptors in the neuromuscular junction. The antibodies bind to the receptors and ultimately lead to their destruction.

46. How is myasthenia gravis treated?

Dialysis can alleviate the symptoms of MG by removing the antibodies to the nicotinic receptors, but frequent dialysis is required; thus, this method is impractical. The most common form of treatment is the administration of AChE inhibitors. This treatment allows the neurotransmitter to be present in the synaptic cleft for longer periods of time, thereby activating as many functional receptors as are present. The safety factor built into the neuromuscular junction ensures success for this method: even with a 30% loss of receptors, a muscle can still reach threshold if the neurotransmitter is present long enough to activate the remaining receptors. The dose of these compounds must be carefully monitored to avoid side effects due to overactivation of the parasympathetic nervous system.

47. What is botulism?

Botulism is food poisoning caused by the ingestion of botulinum toxins, which are produced by the anaerobic bacteria *Clostridium botulinum. C. botulinum* spores commonly are found in soil and, therefore, on vegetables and edible fungi—but the spores do not harm a normal, healthy individual because toxins are produced only when the bacteria are exposed to anaerobic conditions. Moreover, most of the spores are destroyed by stomach acid, and any remaining living spores are unable to cross the gastrointestinal tract. However, *C. botulinum* can present a serious problem in canned goods that have not received proper heat sterilization: the anaerobic environment of the can is ideal for the production of the botulinum toxin. Another common source of *C. botulinum* spores is raw honey. Raw honey should never be fed to infants under 1 year of age because their gastrointestinal tract is more permeable to large molecules (to allow for antibody absorption from breast milk).

48. How do botulinum toxins and tetanus toxins interfere with synaptic transmission?

Botulinum toxins and tetanus toxin are zinc-dependent metalloproteases that cleave synaptobrevins (vesicle-associated membrane proteins; VAMPs) located in the vesicle membranes. The synaptobrevins are intimately involved in the docking of the vesicles for neurotransmitter release.

49. Can botulism be treated?

There is an antidote available for botulinum toxin, but it is only effective if taken before the symptoms of botulism appear.

BIBLIOGRAPHY

 1. Augustine GJ, Adler EM, Charlton MP: The calcium signal for transmitter secretion from presynaptic nerve terminals. Ann NY Acad Sci 635:365–379, 1991.
 2. Augustine GJ, Charlton MP, Smith SJ: Calcium entry and transmitter release at voltage-clamped nerve terminals of squid. J Physiol 369:163–181, 1985.
 3. Boyd A, Martin AR: The end-plate potential in mammalian muscle. J Physiol 132:74–91, 1956.
 4. Dodge Jr FA, Rahamimoff R: Cooperative action of calcium ions in transmitter release at the neuromuscular junction. J Physiol 193:419–432, 1967.
 5. Eccles JC, Eccles RM, Magni F: Central inhibitionary action attributable to presynaptic depolarization produced by muscle afferent volleys. J Physiol 159:147–166, 1961.
 6. Goda Y: SNAREs and regulated vesicle exocytosis. PNAS 94:769–772, 1997.
 7. Kandel ER, Schwartz JH, Jessell TM: Essentials of Neural Science and Behavior. Norwalk, CT, Appleton & Lange, 1995.
 8. Kandel ER, Schwartz JH, Jessell TM: Principles of Neural Science, 3rd ed. Norwalk, CT, Appleton & Lange, 1991.
 9. Kelsell DP, Dunlop J, Stevens HP, et al: Connexin 26 mutations in hereditary nonsyndromic sensorineural deafness. Nature 387:80–83, 1997.
10. Lodish H, Baltimore D, Berk A, et al: Molecular Cell Biology. New York, W.H. Freeman and Company, 1995.
11. Palfrey HC, Artalejo CR: Vesicle recycling visited: Rapid endocytosis may be the first step. Neuroscience 83:969–989, 1998.
12. Siegel GJ, Agranoff BW, Albers RW, et al: Basic Neurochemistry, 6th ed. New York, Raven Press, 1999.

3. DEVELOPMENT OF THE VERTEBRATE NERVOUS SYSTEM

Pat Levitt, Ph.D.

1. How does the nervous system arise?

The nervous system forms from one of the primary germ layers, the **ectoderm**. All vertebrate embryos derive from a blastocyst that eventually produces three distinct layers of cells, the ectoderm, mesoderm, and endoderm. These germ layers form during the period of gastrulation, when cells move in complex ways to form different layers of cells. The mesoderm gives rise to skeletal tissues, such as muscle, cartilage and bone, vasculature, and internal organs such as the kidneys. The endoderm gives rise to internal organs of the digestive system and germ cells. The embryonic ectoderm forms the outer-most layer of cells, and will form the integument as well as the nervous system.

2. What terminology is routinely used by developmental biologists to describe events that relate to the formation of specific tissues, such as the nervous system?

Biologists speak and write of *determination, commitment, specification, fate, lineage and clonal-relatedness, differentiation,* and *de-differentiation* in describing the state of an individual cell or groups of cells during certain periods of development. Oftentimes, these terms are applied to cells that give rise to differentiated tissue, the stem and progenitor cells of the embryo. There are subtle differences between these two types of cell.

Stem cells are self-renewing precursors of any tissue in the organism. They have the ability, under different conditions, to generate any cell type.

Progenitor cells (or progenitors, precursors) form from stem cells. They usually do not exhibit specific phenotypic traits of a tissue. Progenitors give rise to the population of mature cell types in any particular tissue. In the nervous system, progenitor cells give rise directly to neurons and macroglia (astrocytes and oligodendrocytes). Progenitors continue to divide until giving rise to differentiating cells. Thus, progenitors have the ability to maintain an undifferentiated state during cell division, increasing the population of precursors that are necessary to produce a certain number of differentiated cells. Progenitors are restricted in their ability to produce specific cell types and eventually are exhausted during development.

3. What is commitment?

Commitment refers to the particular fate of a cell that is defined during development. Commitment suggests that the cell has already expressed a certain gene program and/or has been acted upon by extrinsic signals that place the cell on a path of differentiation to which it remains committed. In the past, commitment was subdivided further into irreversible and reversible states, but these subdivisions have been discarded because commitment implies irreversibility of state.

4. Define cell fate.

Fate refers to the potential end-stage of differentiation that the cell will attain if normal development proceeds. Fate is determined by position of the cell in the embryo (its exposure to unique environmental factors) and the lineage of the cell.

5. What is specification?

Specification of a cell is flexible, and reflects the potential for a cell to still be acted upon by its environment to change its fate.

6. What is determination?

Determination refers to cells that have decided irreversibly to express a particular set of well-defined traits or phenotypes (fate). Determination occurs through a combination of the readout of specific programs of gene expression and responses to environmental cues.

7. Define differentiation.

Differentiation refers to the molecular and structural state of a cell that is beginning to express certain key features. These features allow identification of the cell as a specific type.

8. Define lineage.

Lineage of a cell refers to the strictly inheritable traits that allow a cell to express a specific phenotype.

9. What is clonal-relatedness?

Clonal-relatedness refers to the lineage relationship of a cell to a predecessor of previous generations. It may be evaluated by labeling a progenitor with a marker that is faithfully inherited through cell generations, such as a dye or nonvirulent virus strain.

10. What is induction?

Induction of a state of differentiation or specification refers to the actions of extrinsic cues that change the expression of genes that control further development of the target cell. These extrinsic cues effect change via direct contact (through the membrane) or diffusible substances (nuclear receptors).

11. When does the ectoderm become committed to forming nervous system structures?

The cells that comprise the ectoderm migrate actively through well-delineated regions of the blastocyst during gastrulation. Biochemical activities in these regions are involved in neural induction, the process by which the ectodermal cells are induced to form the neural plate. Hilde Mangold and Hans Spemann discovered this process in the 1930s. Experimental evidence in mammals, frogs, and chicks indicates that commitment by the ectodermal cells to form structures of the nervous system occurs during the cells' migration, prior to settling as a primary germ layer.

12. How is neuroectoderm formed?

Blastocyst cells migrate through a region of the embryo, where cells produce molecules able to induce changes in gene expression. These changes ultimately promote differentiation of the nervous system. In chicks and mammals, Hensen's node is the region of the embryo that contains the inductive activity. In amphibians, the homologous region is the dorsal lip of the blastopore. The final outcome of the migration and induction is the formation of a sheet of cells that serves as the forerunner of the neuroectoderm, with an underlying accumulation of cells into a solid tube of mesodermal cells that forms the notochord. The notochord expresses molecules that diffuse to the overlying neuroectoderm to control the differentiation of cell populations within the central nervous system (CNS).

13. What molecules control the formation of neuroectoderm?

Polypeptide members of the transforming growth factor-beta (TGF-β) family of diffusible molecules are produced by cells in the region of Hensen's node and dorsal lip of the blastopore. In vivo and explant experiments demonstrate that different family members can induce cells from any region of the blastocyst to differentiate into neuroectoderm. The nervous system forms through a series of complex inductive events, relying on the interactions of somatic mesoderm, prechordal and chordomesoderm (notochord), and non-neural (lateral) ectoderm with the overlying ectoderm that is located along and apposed to the midline of the embryo.

14. What events occur to produce the first recognizable structures of the nervous system?

Neurulation results in the formation of a broad, thin collection of cells, the neural plate, which is comprised of a columnar neuroepithelium. This neuroepithelium can be distinguished from the lateral ectoderm, which eventually will form the epidermis. Through differential cell proliferation and constriction of the apical borders of neuroectodermal cells, the plate begins to fold at two lateral hinge regions and one medial hinge region of the neural plate. The thickened lateral lips move dorsally to fuse into a tube. Cells that reside in the lips end up most dorsally and pinch off to form the neural crest. The neural plate fuses dorsally to form the neural tube first at the level of the midbrain, then rostrally and caudally. Two principal axes, anteroposterior and rostrocaudal, define the organization of the nervous system.

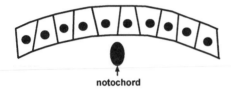

notochord

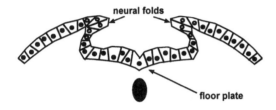

neural folds

floor plate

The process of neurulation. Ectoderm is induced by underlying mesoderm to undergo a molecular and morphological transformation, forming the neuroectoderm. In the second stage, neural folds form by an invagination of the neuroectoderm. When the neuroectoderm rounds up to form the neural tube, the cells of the neural fold *(open circles)* eventually pinch off to form the neural crest *(gray circles)*. The ventral midline of the neuroectoderm becomes the floor plate.

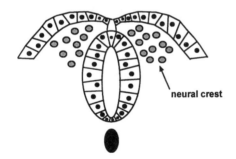

neural crest

15. How are cells within the neural tube organized?

Cells of the neural tube organize into a pseudostratified epithelium around the lumen. The basal lamina forms along the external side of the tube, where the meninges covering of the brain develops from neural crest cells. The neural tube itself does not contain a basal lamina, but does produce extracellular matrix proteins that are secreted into the rather large extracellular spaces. Initially, the neuroepithelial cells, known as progenitor or precursor cells, have their cell bodies situated within the inner three-quarters of the tube, in the ventricular zone (also termed the germinal matrix). The basal processes of the cells extend to the basal lamina, forming a cell-free marginal zone. In almost all CNS regions, cells move from their locations of origin in the neural tube to find their final position in the brain or spinal cord (exceptions include granule neurons of the olfactory bulb and hippocampus).

16. What are the structural units that subdivide the early neural tube?

Vesicle formation in the neural tube defines the major subdivisions of the neuraxis. Morphogenetic changes, in the form of bulges or swellings termed neuromeres, are evident from the dorsal and ventral surfaces. The bulges are established through differential proliferation of neuroepithelial cells. **Rhombomeres**, the bulges that form the hindbrain, have been established as true, repeated, segmented units. **Prosomeres** in the forebrain, though not truly segmented units, do represent distinct regions of the neural tube from which major brain subdivisions will form. Establishment of the rhombomere structural units is thought to restrict cell movement between domains and provide a lineage-based mechanism for specialization of different regions of the CNS. This has not been shown for prosomere regions of the forebrain.

The regionalization process is completed by 7 weeks in humans, 8.5 days in mice, and approximately 10 days in rats. The columnar epithelium becomes pseudostratified as cell proliferation occurs rapidly.

17. What are the primary morphogenetic events that occur to produce different major regions of the CNS?

Initially, there are three vesicles (forebrain, midbrain, and hindbrain) that form the middle and rostral end of the neural tube. The spinal cord forms the caudal half of the neural tube. A series of bulges in the brainstem appear, forming the segmented rhombomeres that extend from the border of the caudal end of the mesencephalon through the spinal cord. The anterior end of the single forebrain vesicle extends forward bilaterally, forming the prosencephalic vesicles. This region contains the developing tel- and diencephalon, and the lumen serves as the precursor of the lateral ventricles and the single third ventricle. The mesencephalon remains as a single vesicle, with the lumen serving as the conduit between the third ventricle and the fourth ventricle of the hindbrain. This conduit is termed the **cerebral aqueduct**. The hindbrain forms the two additional vesicles, the metencephalic and myelencephalic vesicles. These are the forerunners of the pons and cerebellum, and medulla, respectively.

The flexures of the brainstem form during this three-vesicle stage. The cephalic flexure forms at the border between the mesencephalon and hindbrain, bending to move the forebrain vesicle ventrally. The cervical flexure forms at the junction between the hindbrain and spinal cord, bending the caudal neural tube ventrally.

At the five-vesicle stage, the pontine flexure forms at the pontine-medullary junction, bending ventrally. The pontine and cervical flexures eventually straighten out, but the rostral cephalic flexure maintains its orientation, thus permanently changing the longitudinal axis of the brainstem with respect to the forebrain axis.

Lengthening of the spinal cord and of the vertebral column do not occur at the same rate during fetal development. At midgestation, the spinal and vertebral levels are comparable. At birth, the spinal cord (S4) ends at the third lumbar vertebrate. In the adult, the spinal cord only reaches the L1 vertebral segment. (L3-4 subarachnoid space serves as the target for cerebrospinal fluid collection).

During histogenesis, a modest sulcus, termed the **sulcus limitans**, extends longitudinally in the mediolateral plane of the spinal cord, marking the boundary between the sensory (dorsal) and motor (ventral) regions. It turns to extend longitudinally in the dorsoventral plane from the floor of the 4th ventricle to separate the medial regions (motor) from the lateral regions (sensory) of the brainstem. In the diencephalon, the dorsal, medial, and ventral sulci of His separate the dorsal, ventral thalamus and hypothalamus, respectively. The sulci are most evident as indentations along the third ventricle.

18. What molecular mechanisms contribute to axial patterning?

During formation of the embryo, genes that are responsible for pattern formation are expressed in all germ layers. These genes encode proteins that are known to regulate the transcription of other genes that are downstream and control cellular differentiation. In the hindbrain and spinal cord, homeobox *(Hox)* genes are expressed in distinct patterns and are thought to control anteroposterior patterning. As in drosophila, where the *Hox* genes were first identified, the overlapping patterns of expression in different segments in the vertebrate hindbrain, spinal cord, and peripheral nervous system neurons (ganglia) form a *Hox* code for regional specification. The spatial order of gene expression in the tissue is reflected in an orderly distribution of the genes on specific chromosomes. The disruption of the pattern of *Hox* gene expression can result in the transformation of the tissue into another segment, or the loss of an entire rhombomere segment that is supposed to give rise to certain neuronal populations.

19. What molecular mechanisms are responsible for regionalizing the brain and spinal cord into dorsal and ventral structures?

Diffusible signals from the notochord (such as the protein sonic hedgehog) induce midline neuroectoderm to form specialized cells, the floor plate. The floor plate serves as the source of sonic hedgehog that begins the process of ventralizing the neural tube rostrally, up to the level of the diencephalon. In **ventralization**, cell groups in the CNS form that typify the ventral half of the CNS, such as motor neurons in the brainstem and spinal cord, substantia nigra in midbrain, hypothalamus in the diencephalon, and basal ganglia in the forebrain. Prechordal mesoderm also secretes sonic hedgehog to ventralize the telencephalon.

Non-neural ectoderm secretes fibroblast growth factor 8 and different bone morphogenic proteins that act in a complex fashion with other factors to dorsalize the neural tube. In **dorsalization**, cell populations in the CNS form that typically are found in the dorsal half of the CNS, such as sensory neurons in the spinal cord and brainstem, tectum in the midbrain, dorsal thalamus in the diencephalon, and cerebral cortex in the telencephalon.

These inductive events regulate the overall fate of neuroepithelial populations by controlling complex patterns of transcription factors expression, which in turn regulate differential gene expression of newly generated neurons along the entire neuraxis.

20. What cells contribute to the formation of the peripheral nervous system?

The cells of the neural crest form all components of the peripheral nervous system (PNS), including sensory, sympathetic, and parasympathetic ganglia; Schwann cells; head mesenchyme; and pia-arachnoid. The migratory routes of neural crest cells, from the dorsal neural tube, define the environment through which the cells move. The environment, in turn, regulates cellular phenotype through inductive interactions with different non-neural tissues.

Transplantation experiments of Le Douarin demonstrated that the host environment dramatically regulates cellular differentiation. Thus, head neural crest, which normally contributes to the ciliary ganglion, can differentiate into neurons of the sympathetic chain when transplanted into the trunk region of a host.

21. What structures are formed by the neural crest that arises from the head?

The PNS in the head region is formed from neural crest cells and cells arising from ectodermal placodes, thickenings of the ectoderm that also form peripheral sensory structures. Neural crest cells in the head region migrate along three ventrolateral pathways from the dorsal neural tube, passing underneath the ectoderm to reach the branchial arches. These cells contribute to cranial nerve (trigeminal, facial, acoustovestibular) and parasympathetic ganglia. Head neural crest also forms the major portion of skeletal and connective tissues.

22. What structures are formed by the neural crests that arise from the trunk?

Neural crest cells that migrate ventrally through the trunk somites form dorsal root and sympathetic ganglia and adrenal chromaffin cells. Schwann cells of the entire PNS also are produced from trunk neural crest. Neural crest that migrates dorsally in the trunk just under the overlying ectoderm forms melanocytes of the skin. The enteric nervous system is formed from neural crest cells that migrate into the gut from the vagal (anterior) and sacral (posterior) regions of the embryo.

23. What five stereotyped cellular events are principally responsible for the development of the nervous system?

Precursors of the nervous system undergo a stereotyped pattern of development that includes cell *proliferation, migration* from their point of origin to their final position, and cellular *differentiation*, in which specific gene products are expressed that contribute to unique phenotypes.

Differentiation for neurons involves the formation and growth of axons and dendrites. For glia, differentiation involves formation of proteins and proteolipids that are critical for their function.

The fourth key event involves *synaptogenesis*, the formation of synapses between specific target populations. A fraction of all populations of cells that contribute to the nervous system undergo *naturally occurring cell death*, a process that is important in establishing appropriate quantitative relationships among neuronal populations.

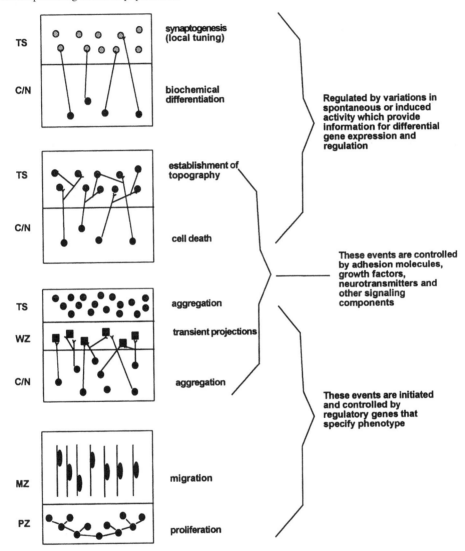

Key events in development of the CNS, from proliferation through synaptogenesis. PZ = proliferative zone, MZ = migratory zone, C/N = cortex or nucleus, WZ = waiting zone for early synapses, TS = target structure. (Modified from Meineke D: Neural development. In Koslow SH, et al (eds): The Neuroscience of Mental Health II: Status and Potential for Mental Health and Mental Illness. Washington, DC, NIH, 1995.)

24. What is meant by neuronal polarity? How is polarity established?

Neurons produce two distinct processes, dendrites and axons, that serve as the message receiving and sending components of the neuron, respectively. Dendrites are essentially extensions of the neuronal soma. Thus, a neuron is described as polarized because of the asymmetry in information processing and, at the subcellular level, in the distribution of proteins and organelles that form dendrites and axons.

Polarity is evident when the neuron first arises, with dendrite- and axon-specific proteins expressed during the time when neurons begin to migrate from their places of origin to their final positions in the CNS or PNS. It is thought that unique peptide sequences are responsible for trafficking organelles and proteins to the dendritic or axonal compartment. Dendrites grow slowly over many weeks and months, whereas axons grow several orders of magnitude more rapidly, reaching target areas in some instances prior to the neurons reaching their their final resting positions.

25. How are neurons produced?

The progenitor cells of neurons are situated in the ventricular and subventricular zones. They exhibit an initial cell cycle time of approximately 8–12 hours. In all vertebrates, the first neurons leave the cell cycle in the mesencephalic/pontine region of the brainstem. Once a neuron leaves the cell cycle, it no longer has the ability to divide. Thus, this exit is considered the neuron's "time of origin." Incorporating a tag (^{3}H-thymidine or bromodeoxyuridine) into the DNA of cells in S-phase allows investigators to determine when a cell leaves the cell cycle. Cells that continue to divide will dilute the tag.

The nuclei of progenitor cells translocate within the ventricular zone through different stages of the cell cycle. The cells that reside next to the surface are in M-phase. If they re-enter the cycle (G_1), the nucleus moves away from the surface. The nucleus reaches the outer margins of the ventricular zone in S-phase and then moves towards the lumen again as the cell proceeds through G_2 and M. The specific reasons for this movement are not known.

There are gradients of neurogenesis in all brain areas, such that neurons that reside in one region will be born before or after those in another region. For example, in the spinal cord, there is a ventral-to-dorsal gradient of neurogenesis, with the ventralmost motor neurons being born before the sensory neurons of the dorsal horn. In the thalamus, there is a lateral-to-medial gradient of histogenesis. Thus, the first neurons migrate to the edge of the dorsal diencephalon, and the next neurons migrate to a position medially. In general, large projection neurons are generated before smaller interneurons.

26. When and where are astrocytes generated in the CNS?

Progenitor cells of macroglia of the CNS reside in the ventricular and subventricular zones. In general, glia are produced after neurons, but neurogenesis and gliogenesis overlap temporally and spatially. In fact, specialized glial cells, the **radial glia**, which are responsible for the structural integrity of the CNS, are produced at the same time that the first neurons are generated. Radial glia reside in all areas of the CNS. Their cell bodies remain in the ventricular zone, and they extend long processes to the pial surface, where they form endfeet. Radial glia provide guides for neurons that undergo radial migration from the ventricular and subventricular zones to their final positions. After migration is completed, radial glia either die or undergo morphological transformations to form astrocytes.

Most astrocytes arise from progenitor cells in the ventricular and subventricular zones. They are produced towards the end of neurogenesis, appearing when levels of the epidermal growth factor receptor increase dramatically in progenitors. Astrocytes migrate into grey and white matter, forming intimate relationships with the pia-arachnoid, blood vessels, and synapses. Astrocytic precursors also migrate into these regions, and can divide in situ under a variety of conditions to form more astrocytes, even in the adult brain. Cell lineage studies indicate that depending upon the region of the developing CNS, a small percentage of neuronal progenitors also can produce astroglia.

27. When and where are oligodendrocytes generated in the CNS?

Oligodendrocytes arise late prenatally and throughout postnatal development, originally from progenitors in the subventricular zone. Oligodendrocytes and their precursors migrate mostly into white matter to differentiate into myelin-forming cells. Cell lineage studies using retroviral markers indicate that astroglia and oligodendroglia can share common progenitors.

28. When and where are brain microglia generated?

Microglia and brain macrophages arise from peripheral cells that enter the CNS vasculature to seed the embryonic nervous system. They appear to be present from the onset of angiogenesis. The cells originate from connective tissue blood cells during development. Microglia undergo extensive proliferation pre- and postnatally in regions of the brain that undergo naturally occurring cell death and remodeling. Thus, during development, microglia generally are found in proliferative zones and axon tracts.

29. How do neurons migrate in the CNS?

The cell soma of the postmitotic neurons moves away from the ventricular zone initially by translocating the nucleus away from the luminal (ventricular) surface, toward the pia. In nonlaminated structures, such as the diencephalon, brainstem, and spinal cord, the new zone that contains the cell bodies of postmitotic neurons is termed the **mantle zone**. This zone continues to grow during histogenesis, housing the motor, sensory, and association nuclei of different brain regions.

At middle and late stages of development, when the mantle zone grows to more than a few cells thick, the early postmitotic neurons that are generated from the ventricular zone migrate along specialized radial glia. The **radial glia** set up tracks of fibers that extend from their cell bodies in the ventricular zone to their endfeet along the pial surface. The fibers contain a high concentration of intermediate filaments, comprised of glial fibrillary acidic protein. The radial glia tracks in large brains, such as gyrencephalic animals, form as early as the first neurons.

Neurons also may migrate in a direction tangential to the radial axis. For example, interneurons that arise from the ganglionic eminence in the basal telencephalon migrate tangentially for long distances to enter and populate the entire neocortex. Neurons can migrate in this tangential direction along developing axons. In the brainstem, neurons from the dorsal rhombic lip migrate along the edge of the brainstem within axon tracts to populate the inferior olive and pontine nuclei.

30. What unique patterns of cell migration contribute to the special histological organization of the neocortex?

Histogenesis in the cerebral cortex has been studied most extensively. The mature neocortex is a six-layered structure, and its formation follows a well-defined pattern. The first neurons that are generated move out toward the pial surface, forming a single layer of cells, called the **preplate**, that is situated between the ventricular and marginal zones. The marginal zone becomes cortex layer I. The next neurons that are produced (for the cerebral cortex proper) migrate along radial glia and split the preplate into a superficial layer of scattered neurons (Cajal-Retzius cells), which reside along the deep aspect of the marginal zone, and scattered neurons in a **subplate**, which is situated between the newly formed cortical plate (the cerebral cortex proper) and the ventricular zone.

The subplate is a transient structure that appears to participate in the guidance of axons to the appropriate regions of the cerebral cortex. In gyrencephalic animals, some of the subplate neurons survive and reside in the white matter as interstitial neurons. Their function is unknown.

The axons that originate from cortical neurons as they migrate, along with cortical afferents, grow into an **intermediate zone** that resides below the subplate and above the ventricular zone. The intermediate zone is the forerunner of the cortical white matter. As neurogenesis proceeds, neurons that will reside in the deepest layers of the cortex (V, VI) take up residence in the cortical plate.

The neurons born next, which will reside in more superficial layers (II–IV), must migrate past the earlier generated neurons to their final positions. This reflects the "inside-out" gradient of neurogenesis and migration that characterizes the development of the cerebral cortex. Interestingly, mutation of the *reelin* gene (encodes an extracellular matrix protein) in mice results in an abnormal outside-in pattern of migration. The neurons destined for layers VI, V, and IV are produced from progenitor cells in the ventricular zone.

At about this time, a new, superficial zone of progenitor cells termed the subventricular zone (SVZ), forms. The nuclei of these progenitor cells maintain a position away from the ventricular surface through all phases of the cell cycle. Thus, pulse-labeling of dividing cells with ^{3}H-thymidine at this stage of development results in the labeling of two zones of cells. The SVZ produces the later-generated neurons destined for the superficial layers of the cerebral cortex and most of the macroglial cells (astrocytes and oligodendrocytes). The SVZ remains in a restricted region along the rostroventral end of the lateral ventricle as a region of progenitor cells that can produce new neurons and glia in adults. It is unique to the telencephalon (cerebral wall and ganglionic eminence of the basal forebrain). At the end of neurogenesis, the SVZ produces only macroglia and ultimately becomes exhausted in most regions of the telencephalon. A small number of multipotential progenitors remain and produce most glia and some neurons, and pluripotential stem cells produce any cell type.

31. What unique patterns of cell migration contribute to the special histological organization of the cerebellar cortex?

The cerebellar cortex is a laminated structure with an inner granule cell layer, middle Purkinje cell layer, and superficial molecular layer. The latter contains the well-known esplanade dendrites of Purkinje cells and the millions of granule cell axons that synapse on the Purkinje cells.

During development, the roof of the 4th ventricle contains in the ventricular zone progenitors that give rise to the deep cerebellar nuclei and the Purkinje cells. The Purkinje cells migrate along radial glia to reside superficially next to the pial surface. Specialized radial glia (Bergmann glia) translocate their somata to the Purkinje cell layer and maintain extended fibers to the pial surface. Simultaneously, the lateral edges of the 4th ventricle, at the level of the pons, thicken and produce the progenitor cells that migrate rostromedially just underneath the pial surface to reside superficial to the Purkinje cells. This structure, termed the external granule cell layer, forms the progenitor cell population that gives rise to the granule neurons. The granule neurons leave the cell cycle and migrate down the Bergmann glial processes, past Purkinje cells, to form the internal granule cell layer.

This development pattern, known as an "outside-in" pattern of histogenesis, is distinct from the cerebral cortex. A large number of spontaneous mutations that alter the development of the cerebellar cortex (*staggerer, leaner, weaver, tottering, reeler*) have been identified in the mouse.

32. How do axons find their appropriate target?

A combination of local guidance cues (*contact attraction* and *repulsion*) and long-range guidance cues (*chemoattraction* and *chemorepulsion*) act in concert to mediate directed growth. In general, axons grow in specific patterns along stereotyped pathways to innervate specific target areas. Axons use their tips, or **growth cones**, to sense cues along their route to grow to the proper target structures. It is clear that growth cone behavior can be influenced by intermediate cues from guidepost structures that provide directional information for growing in certain patterns at key decision-making junctures. Thus, axon guidance is a directed and not a random process.

In most brain areas, axon growth into appropriate target structures occurs well before extensive dendritic development. In mammals, only 1–10% of adult synapse numbers are present at birth in the CNS, although the establishment of axon pathways and innervation of targets is completed well before birth in most species.

33. How do growth cones function as the guiding ends of axons?

Growth cones are broad extensions of axons that contain broad lamellipodia and fine filopodia extensions. Growth cones and axons differ in composition. Neurofilaments are present in axons, but do not extend into growth cones. Microtubules extend into the body of the growth cone and into one or two lamellapodia, but not into filopodia. Actin microfilaments are a prominent feature of axons and growth cones, extending into all lamellapodia and filopodia.

Growth cones are structurally diverse, which may be a reflection of their highly active and changing growth patterns as they read cues in their microenvironment. It is hypothesized that growth cones advance through the interaction of membrane receptors with growth-permissive molecules in the microenvironment and a dynamic control of actin polymerization and depolymerization at the leading edge of the growth cone. Nonpolymerized actin that is not tethered to membrane receptors intracellulary does not impact on the direction of growth cone movement and is recycled retrogradely by interacting with myosin-based motors.

34. What are the major molecular activities that contribute to axonal pathfinding?

Two molecular activities, **chemoattraction** and **chemorepulsion**, are thought to provide the major cues responsible for guiding the growth of axons along specific pathways to appropriate target regions. Additionally, cues that facilitate or promote axon outgrowth participate in the process of axon pathfinding, but may not provide directional cues to the growth cones. In many instances, a single molecule may influence axon growth by serving both as a chemoattractant and chemorepulsive molecule. This dual activity highlights the fact that each guidance molecule can interact with different membrane receptors that mediate the activation of different intracellular signaling pathways, ultimately resulting in a specific pattern of axonal growth.

The pattern of expression of molecules that are attractive and/or repulsive, and the patterns of expression of their receptors by specific cell populations in the nervous system, are thought to contribute to patterns of axon pathfinding.

35. What major classes of molecules mediate chemoattraction and chemorepulsion?

The expression of guidance activity may occur in the form of diffusible, extracellular matrix- or membrane-bound molecules. The netrin, semaphorin, and collapsin families provide the molecular basis of axon guidance achieved by secreted cues arising from a distance. **Netrins** are large polypeptide molecules closely related in structure to laminin-1, a nondiffusible extracellular matrix protein. It was first shown that netrins are produced by cells of the floor plate, which helps guide axons to the midline before they cross. **Semaphorins** comprise a large family of secreted and transmembrane proteins that bind to neuropilin receptors to generate attractive and/or repulsive activities. **Collapsin-I** was the first collapsing (repulsive) activity isolated, in chicken, and is identical to members of the Sema III subfamily.

Tyrosine kinase receptors (Eph) and their ligands (ephrins) form a major class of membrane-bound molecules that require cell contact for signaling. They typically are distributed in gradients. The role of the Eph system in rectinotectal axon guidance is well-elucidated, with Eph A3 serving principally as a repulsive cue when interacting with two different ligands expressed in the tectum, Ephrins A2 and A5.

Membrane-bound adhesion molecules comprise the cadherin (REF), integrin (REF), and Ig superfamilies. **Cadherins** interact homophilically in a Ca^{++}-dependent fashion with identical cadherins. **Integrins** serve as dimeric receptors (α and β polypeptides) for a variety of extracellular matrix proteins in the presence of Mg^{++} and Ca^{++}, including laminin, fibronectin, collagens, and proteoglycans. **Ig superfamilies** exhibit structurally-related immunoglobulin loops and may contain fibronectin or epidermal growth factor receptor domains. These molecules exist in transmembrane and glycosyl phosphatidylinositol (GPI)–anchored forms. Ig superfamily members can bind homophilically to the identical molecule or heterophilically to other Ig superfamily members and perhaps other membrane receptors.

None of these major families are solely attractive or repulsive; individual molecules may express both activities.

36. What contribution does cell death make to the development of the nervous system?

Progenitor cells and neurons undergo naturally occurring cell death as part of a normal process of reducing cell populations. The extensive nature of cell death in progenitor cells was recently revealed with sensitive tags of cell death, and documented specifically in a knockout mouse that eliminated the gene for a protein that is crucial for cell death. In the mouse, there was an enormous increase in the number of progenitors and neurons that normally would have died. Thus, progenitor cell death may control the degree to which neurogenesis produces populations of a certain size.

Neurons die during development in a process that is thought to reflect two aspects of cellular interaction. There appears to be competition between neurons in their targets for synaptic space and trophic support. There also appears to be a need for balance between input and output for neurons; creating a physiological or anatomical imbalance causes neurons to die. As much as half of the neurons in a specific CNS region may die to produce the final complement of mature neurons. All populations of neurons appear to undergo some degree of cell death (see Chapter 24).

37. How do synapses form in the PNS?

Synaptogenesis in the periphery occurs between neurons and between neurons and non-neural targets. Much of our understanding of synapse formation comes from studies of the neuromuscular junction, which arises upon contact of the axonal growth cone with the membranes of muscle fibers. Synaptogenesis involves the formation of specialized membrane folds, the so-called junctional folds, on the target cells; a concentration of neurotransmitter receptors (acetylcholine; Ach) at the folds; and a synaptic basal lamina that contains signals for synaptic differentiation and maintenance. During neuromuscular development, multiple axons may innervate one muscle fiber, but during a period of synapse elimination, a 1:1 relationship is established between axon and muscle fiber.

Neurons, Schwann cells, and muscle cells contribute to the basal lamina. In experiments in which the muscle cell is removed and the peripheral axon is forced to form a new synapse, the original junctional basal lamina contains sufficient molecular cues for the growth cone to find the original location of the synapse. A complex molecular cascade, which includes neuregulins, agrin, muscle-specific kinase, and rapsyn, is responsible for synapse differentiation, including the clustering of Ach receptors on muscle cells.

38. How and when do synapses form in the CNS?

There is an extensive and extended period of synaptogenesis that occurs in the brain and spinal cord. Different regions undergo peak levels of synapse formation at different times postnatally. In the brainstem, peak formation in rodents occurs within the first week after birth, whereas in the cerebral cortex, the peak occurs during the second and third weeks postnatal, prior to adolescence. All brain areas exhibit a late development period of synapse loss to modify quantitatively the relationships between neuronal populations.

The molecular cascade responsible for the formation of central synapses is unknown. However, specialized proteins with unique molecular domains, called PDZ domains, bind to and maintain synapse-specific proteins in clusters at synapses. The PDZ domain proteins form bridges by interacting with both the synaptic proteins and structural proteins such as tubulin. Clustered proteins include certain kinases, actin and actin-binding proteins, PDZ proteins such as PSD-95 gephyrin and GRIP, and neurotransmitter receptors, for example AMPA, NMDA, mGluR, and glycine, which contain amino acid domains that bind specifically to PDZ domains.

39. Why are synapses eliminated?

Both the numerical relationship between neuron and target and the refinement of maps require reorganization, withdrawal, and elimination of synapses toward the end of development. The molecular mechanism remains a mystery. In general, neurons synapse with more target cells in the immature than in the mature nervous system. Synapse elimination occurs over a protracted period of time. In the cerebral cortex of humans, for example, synapse elimination and reorganization may occur over 3–5 years, just prior to and during puberty.

In most instances, it appears that competition between presynaptic elements drives synapse withdrawal. It is thought that some forms of synapse elimination are activity-dependent processes, because experiments in which tetrodotoxin is used to silence neurons result in failed synapse elimination. Activity may stabilize the synapse, or may provide an advantage during the competition for molecules that cannot be shared but are essential for synapse maintenance.

Synapse elimination has been studied best at the neuromuscular junction, where the multiple innervation of muscle fibers is reorganized, and in the visual system, where retinotropic maps are refined by elimination of synapses from neurons that initially terminate in inappropriate zones of the tectum or lateral geniculate nucleus. The role of competition between synapses in remodeling developing neural connections is exemplified in studies of the formation of ocular dominance columns in the visual cortex of animals with binocular vision. Left and right eyes, whose projections form initially in overlapping zones, reorganize into separate domains through physiological competition.

40. What is developmental plasticity?

Manipulation of binocular experience during a certain period of development helped to define the concept of a "sensitive" and a "critical" period of developmental plasticity. **Sensitive period** refers to the time in development when an experimental manipulation is able to alter the normal course of development. For example, the closing of one eye at birth in a monkey or cat results in failed development of binocular vision, which is reflected in the spreading of synapses of the open eye into closed eye territories, and the loss of synapses from the closed eye in its normal territory. The closing of one eye late postnatally or in the adult does not elicit such changes, indicating that the sensitive period of developmental plasticity in the visual system has passed. Opening the closed eye during a certain period of development allows binocular vision to develop normally. The time after which eye reopening fails to elicit normal development defines the **critical period** for synaptic plasticity, when the specific system is amenable to reversal of the manipulation that would cause abnormal development.

Note that different systems in the CNS and PNS have temporally distinct sensitive and critical periods.

BIBLIOGRAPHY

1. Goodman CS: Mechanisms and molecules that control growth cone guidance. Annu Rev Neurosci 19:341–377, 1996.
2. Goodman CS, Shatz CJ: Developmental mechanisms that generate precise patterns of neural connectivity. Cell 72:77–98, 1993.
3. Jessel TM, Lumsden A: Inductive signals and the assignment of cell fate in the spinal cord and hindbrain: An axial coordinate system for neural patterning. In Cowan WM, Jessel TM, Zipursky SL (eds): Molecular and Cellular Approaches to Development. Oxford, Oxford University Press, 1997, pp 290–333.
4. Katz L, Shatz CJ: Synaptic activity and the construction of cortical circuits. Science 274:1133–1138, 1996.
5. LeDourain NM: The Neural Crest, 1st ed. Cambridge, Cambridge University Press, 1982.
6. Levitt P: Experimental approaches that reveal principles of cerebral cortical development. In Gazzaniga MS (ed): The Cognitive Neurosciences. New York, MIT Press, 1994, pp 147–163.
7. Lillien L: Neural progenitors and stem cells: Mechanisms of progenitor heterogeneity. Curr Opin Neurobiol 8:37–44, 1998.
8. Rubenstein JLR, Shimamura KS, Martinez S, Puelles L: Regionalization of the prosencephalic neural plate. Ann Rev Neurosci 21:445–477, 1998.
9. Sidman RL, Rakic P: Neuronal migration with special reference to the human brain: A review. Brain Res 62:1–35, 1973.
10. Tessler-Lavigne M, Goodman CS: The molecular biology of axon guidance. Science 274:1123–1133, 1996.
11. Zigmond MJ, Bloom FE, Landis SC, et al: Fundamental Neuroscience, 1st ed. San Diego, Academic Press, 1999.

4. THE SOMATOSENSORY SYSTEM

Jon H. Kaas, Ph.D.

1. What is the somatosensory system?

The somatosensory system is a division of the nervous system that allows us to make accurate inferences about the outside world by using information from receptors that respond to touch and vibrations, our own movements, temperature, and noxious (painful) stimuli. Our ability to recognize objects and surfaces by touch depends on this system. We not only recognize the shapes of objects, but also determine if they are soft or hard, moving or still, cool or hot, and whether they can cut or burn. Although shapes can be perceived passively when objects touch the skin, touch usually is an active process involving exploration of objects with our fingers or—as is observed in babies—with our lips and tongue. Adults typically use their fingers to learn about the world.

2. What are the parts of the somatosensory system?

Much of the somatosensory system consists of brain structures that are activated by either sensitive mechanoreceptors in the skin that signal surface contact or from deeper receptors in muscles and joints that signal limb movements and position (Fig. 1). Since object recognition can depend on information gathered over short periods of time and on the relative locations of skin receptors on the changing position of the fingers during active touch, information is needed about both the types and locations of skin contact and the positions of skin surfaces during contacts. Other parts of the somatosensory system are specialized to mediate aspects of pain and temperature sense. Information is transduced and transformed into a neural code by receptors in the skin and deeper tissues, conducted over afferents to the spinal cord and brain stem, and relayed first to the somatosensory thalamus and then to the somatosensory cortex. At each stage, there are several specialized subdivisions of the system in the brainstem nuclei and cortical areas. In cortex, the somatosensory system starts to interact with other systems so that the information can be used. Most notably, the somatosensory areas of cortex project to motor areas of cortex to help guide and control movements. Many of the subcortical outputs of somatosensory cortex also relate to motor performance.

3. Are all somatosensory systems alike?

All humans probably have very similar somatosensory systems, unless they experienced some early trauma or body malformation that interfered with the normal development of the system. Small modifications of the system are expected to occur, especially in cortex, as a result of sensory experience and training. For example, great musicians and athletes may have fine-tuned parts of the processing system to allow the precise discriminations that are important in their performances. Major differences in the system exist between different species of mammals. Fish, amphibians, and reptiles have systems that are less similar to ours than to other mammals. Finally, insects, worms, and starfish have quite different somatosensory systems.

4. How does the somatosensory system differ in the various species of mammals?

There are two major types of differences. First, species of mammals explore the environment in different ways, and the somatosensory system has been modified to help each species perform well by using proportionately more of the total system for the parts of the body used for obtaining tactile information. We use our fingers and mouth the most and the skin of the middle of our back very little. Thus, tactile receptors are concentrated in the fingers, lips, and tongue, and there are few on the back. Sheep have hard hoofs that are not very useful in exploring the environment, and sheep obtain most of their information with their face, lips, and tongue. Thus, these body parts have many receptors, and large parts of the somatosensory system are devoted to these receptors in sheep. Rats explore their environment with the long whiskers that are in rows on the muzzle of the upper face. These whiskers are moved back and forth to contact objects, and most of the somatosensory system is devoted to the

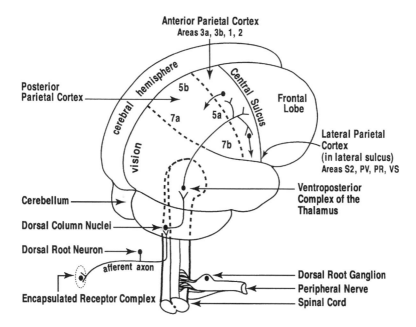

Figure 1. The basic components of the somatosensory system on a posterolateral view of a human brain. Somatosensory afferent neurons course from receptors in the skin or deeper tissues and enter the spinal cord or brain stem of the same side. Second-order neurons cross to the opposite side of the central nervous system and ascend to the thalamus, where third-order neurons project to somatosensory areas of anterior parietal cortex. Somatosensory information is distributed from anterior parietal cortex to lateral parietal cortex and posterior parietal cortex. Dashed lines = hidden parts of the brain stem and boundaries of posterior parietal cortex; numbers in parietal cortex = Brodmann's areas; S2 = second somatosensory area; PV = parietal ventral area.

whiskers on the face. Many animals use whiskers or lips to obtain information and a few, such as humans, monkeys, and raccoons, use their hands or paws the most. Other mammals have various specializations, such as the highly sensitive, grasping tail of the spider monkey or the trunk of an elephant. The highly sensitive bill of the duck-billed platypus may even have developed another sense—electrosensation—to detect the electrical activity generated by the muscles of its swimming prey in dark, murky water.

The other way that somatosensory systems differ is in complexity. Humans probably have the most complex systems, with vast regions of the cerebral cortex devoted to processing somatosensory information. Thus, we are able to use this information in many ways, and learn and acquire astonishing skills. Rats and mice have small brains, and they can't devote so much tissue to processing somatosensory information. They do have comparable somatosensory structures at the early stages of processing in the spinal cord and brain stem, but these parts, of course, are much smaller. At the level of cerebral cortex we not only have larger somatosensory areas, but more somatosensory areas.

5. What are the receptors for tactile information?

Receptors are specialized nerve cell ends in the skin and other tissues. The nerve cells have long axons to conduct information to the central nervous system. Specialized tissue may surround the receptor endings to help them respond to stimuli, or unspecialized endings, called free nerve endings, may be present. Free nerve endings generally are less sensitive, and they are relatively unimportant in coding tactile information. Free nerve endings respond to mechanical deformations when the skin is touched; chemical signals released by injury in the case of pain receptors; and temperature changes for temperature coding.

The sense of touch is more critically subserved by four different types of highly sensitive mechanoreceptors that have encapsulated endings in the skin. That is, the nerve cell endings that are receptive to tactile stimuli are aided in their sensitivity and selectivity for certain types of stimuli by being closely associated with specialized non-neural cells in the skin to form a receptor complex. These receptors have various names, but they also are classified by how they respond to a sudden indentation of the skin. They most often are studied in the glabrous or non-hairy skin of the palm surface of the hand or lips. However, these receptors and variations of these receptors also occur in hairy skin. Mechanoreceptors typically are associated with the roots of hairs, where they use the stresses associated by hair movements to generate signals. Of course, most of our hairy skin is not very hairy, and receptors surrounding hair roots are not as important to us as for mammals with fur and whiskers.

NERVE TERMINALS IN THE GLABROUS SKIN

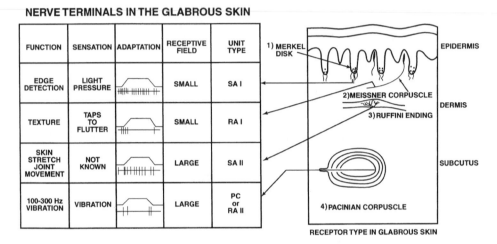

FUNCTION	SENSATION	ADAPTATION	RECEPTIVE FIELD	UNIT TYPE
EDGE DETECTION	LIGHT PRESSURE		SMALL	SA I
TEXTURE	TAPS TO FLUTTER		SMALL	RA I
SKIN STRETCH JOINT MOVEMENT	NOT KNOWN		LARGE	SA II
100-300 Hz VIBRATION	VIBRATION		LARGE	PC or RA II

RECEPTOR TYPE IN GLABROUS SKIN

Figure 2. Receptor types and characteristics of afferent fibers from the glabrous skin of the hand. Afferents are rapidly adapting (RA) types I and II and slowly adapting (SA) types I and II. The ramp in the adaptation column indicates the onset, maintenance, and offset of a skin indentation of one second. The vertical marks on the horizontal line indicate neuronal spikes in the afferent (hertz or vibration cycles per second).

6. What are the four main tactile receptors and afferents of the glabrous skin?

Four functionally distinct classes of low-threshold receptors that are sensitive to skin deformation have been described in the glabrous skin (Fig. 2). In the superficial skin, a class of *slowly adapting* afferents terminate in association with specialized receptor cells to form receptor sites called **Merkel disks**. These afferents are classified as slowly adapting (SA) because they continue to respond throughout the duration of skin indentation with a probe. They are called SA type I to distinguish them from a less common type II, which has larger receptive fields and responds especially well to skin stretch. SA-I receptors are especially concentrated in the finger tips and they are very important in identifying objects pressed against the skin. When single SA-I afferents are electrically stimulated in humans, they produce a sensation of light, uniform pressure at a particular skin location corresponding to the receptive field. Increases in the rate of electrical stimulation increase the magnitude of the sensation. Abilities such as Braille reading critically depend on this receptor.

The endings of a second class of slowly adapting afferents, SA-II, are encapsulated to form receptor complexes known as **Ruffini corpuscles**, which are deeper in the skin than Merkel disks. Ruffini corpuscles also are found in deeper tissues, such as ligaments and tendons. Movement of the skin, tendon, or ligament stretches the corpuscle, causing a response as long as the stretch is maintained. The functional role of SA-II receptors is not completely clear, but they appear to help signal limb and digit positions.

The most common receptor afferent of the glabrous hand is the *rapidly adapting* (RA) I type. RA-I endings terminate to form encapsulated **Meissner corpuscles** in the superficial skin. Meissner corpuscles are constructed so that skin deformations stretch the corpuscle and activate the afferent; they respond only to changes in skin indentations and not to steady indentation. Hence, their response is rapidly adapting to a maintained stimulus, and these receptor are not well suited to signaling a steady state. They provide information about shape and the intensity of contact during active touch, and information about the texture of rubbed surfaces. Electrical stimulation of an RA-I afferent is felt as a light tap for each electrical pulse that merges into a flutter at high frequencies.

The fourth class, the RA-II afferents, terminate in the highly laminar **Pacinian corpuscles** deep in the skin and other tissues. They are highly sensitive to skin indentations, but the layers of the corpuscle dampen the effects of maintained pressure so that Pacinian corpuscles only signal transitions. Because of their deeper locations and high sensitivity, they respond to stimuli at some distance from the receptor, and thus they have large, poorly defined receptive fields. Pacinian corpuscles respond to vibrations, such as those felt by your hand on a lightly tapped table. They appear to have little role in object identification, but seem to have a major role in signaling and roughly locating sudden skin deformations produced by ground and air vibrations and skin contacts.

7. What is a receptive field?

The receptive field for tactile afferents is the region of skin where light to moderately light contact produces a response in the afferent. The measured response in the afferent is the electrical current as the receptor and afferent depolarize and send a traveling wave or spike to the central nervous system. The timing and number of spikes and the pattern of spikes across afferents form the neural code—the source of information for analysis by the central nervous system. Because pressure on the skin can distort skin tissue for some distance, the precise receptive field can be difficult to determine. Thus, light contact, to reduce the spread of skin distortion, is used to most accurately determine the sizes of receptive fields.

8. Are other receptors important in object recognition?

Objects are identified best during active touch. Thus, the nervous system needs to keep track of the relative positions of all skin surfaces in contact with the explored object. Finger position may be signaled in part by SA-II afferents, which respond to stretches of the skin as the fingers bend and move. Ruffini corpuscles and Golgi tendon organs in joints also could be important, but they are not critical since position sense survives joint removal and replacement with artificial joints. Instead, the most important receptor for position sense (kinaesthesia) is likely to be the **muscle spindle receptor**, which signals information about the lengths of muscles and indirectly about the positions of limbs and fingers. They also have important reflexive roles in muscle contraction and movement control via spinal cord connections, and via a relay of muscle spindle information to the cerebellum.

9. What are the afferents for pain and temperature?

Afferents in peripheral nerves can be classified according to their conduction rates of spikes to the spinal cord. A fibers are fast, with A-delta fibers slower than A-alpha fibers, and C fibers are slow (B fibers are efferents to muscles). Pricking pain appears to be mediated by A-delta afferents and nociceptors and burning pain by C-polymodal nociceptors. Since thick A-delta afferents conduct much faster than C-fibers, you can feel two pains separated in time, a first and second pain with a burn. Afferents that respond to tactile stimuli with increases of discharge rate into the painful range are polymodal (touch and pain) and are sometimes referred to as wide dynamic range neurons. Low-threshold thermoreceptive afferents respond to either warming or cooling temperatures in the skin, while being unresponsive to tactile stimuli. Other thermoreceptive afferents are polymodal, and they signal heat in the painful range.

10. How do afferents get to the spinal cord and brain stem?

Afferents typically branch in the skin to form several adjacent endings or receptors. The afferents bundle as they travel toward the spinal cord, and they soon join efferent axons from the motor neurons of the spinal cord that are coursing outward to muscles. The mixture of sensory afferents and motor efferents form the converging branches of peripheral nerves that finally separate into the dorsal (posterior) sensory and ventral (anterior) motor roots of nerves that enter (dorsal) or leave (ventral) the spinal cord between the separate vertebrae. The afferents that enter at any single dorsal root innervate a narrow strip of skin, called a dermatome, from the midline of the back to the midline of the belly or down the arm or leg. Although the afferents in one dermatome overlap those in adjacent dermatomes somewhat, the concept is useful in that a loss of sensation in any dermatome suggests a spinal injury that compresses a specific dorsal root. The neurons that make up the afferents of peripheral nerves have a cell body or soma near the spinal cord in the dorsal root ganglion. The part of the neuron sending information toward the cell body is called a **dendrite** for neurons in the central nervous system, and the part conducting spikes (action potentials) away from the cell body is called an **axon**. For peripheral afferents, however, the "dendrite" looks like an axon and functions like an axon, so it is usually called an axon. Afferents from the face enter the lower brain stem via the trigeminal nerve. (See figure on following page.)

11. After the afferents enter the spinal cord and brain stem, where do they go?

Afferents enter the dorsal (posterior) spinal cord, where they branch to terminate on neurons in the dorsal (posterior) horn of the grey matter of the spinal cord or join fiber (axon) tracts (the dorsal or posterior columns) to terminate on neurons in the lower brain stem. Afferents that enter the brain stem terminate on neurons that are functionally comparable to those in the dorsal horn of the spinal cord or within trigeminal nuclei of the lower brain stem, which combine with those innervated by spinal cord afferents to form the dorsal column—trigeminal complex of nuclei. Afferents that mediate pain and temperature and aspects of crude touch do not send branches to the lower brain stem, but instead terminate only in the dorsal horn or the brain stem equivalent.

12. What do the terminations in the spinal cord do?

Afferents terminate on neurons in the dorsal horn to contribute to local spinal cord processing and reflexes mediated in the spinal cord. Some of these neurons send axons into the dorsal columns or course more laterally in the white matter to join peripheral afferents and terminate in the lower brain stem. Others cross to the white matter of the opposite side of the spinal cord to form the ventrolateral spinothalamic path and course toward the thalamus. The spinothalamic path includes information relayed from nociceptors, thermoreceptors, and polymodal afferents, but not the low-threshold SA and RA afferents or the muscle spindle afferents, which course in the dorsal columns. Thus, damage to the primary afferents in the dorsal columns or to the second order afferents in the crossed ventrolateral spinothalamic tract produces quite different deficits in sensation.

13. Describe the deficits produced by damage to the dorsal columns or spinothalamic tract.

Damage to the spinothalamic tract impairs temperature and pain sensibilities, but partial recoveries often occur due to incomplete lesions and the relay of information over chains of spinal cord neurons. Dorsal column damage impairs fine tactile discriminations and discriminations involving the temporal aspects of stimuli. For example, the direction of stimuli moving on the skin is not detected. The loss of sensory information also impairs the guidance of fine motor movements. Nevertheless, tactile stimuli still can be localized, using information in the spinothalamic tract and higher-order relays of spinal cord information, and many other simple discriminations remain possible.

14. What is the dorsal column–trigeminal nucleus complex?

The dorsal column–trigeminal nucleus complex consists of associated groups of neurons in the lower brain stem and upper spinal cord that receive inputs from ipsilateral (same side) low-threshold mechanoreceptors and project to the contralateral (opposite side) ventroposterior nuclear complex via a fiber tract known as the medial lemniscus (Fig. 3). Afferents from the head and body merge to form a systematic representation of the body across three main groups of cells or nuclei. Afferents originating from the leg and lower body terminate most medially in the **gracile "nucleus"** (actually, a subnucleus) of the complex, while those from the hand and arm terminate in the **cuneate nucleus**. Those from the face and head terminate most laterally in the principal **trigeminal nucleus**. These

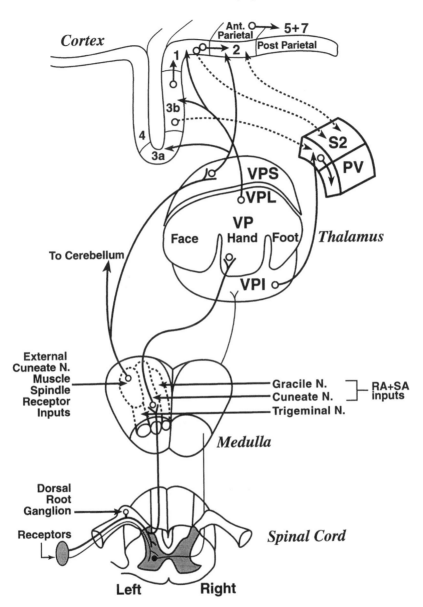

Figure 3. Somatosensory pathways from receptors to the cortex. Sections of spinal cord, lower brain stem, thalamus, and cortex are shown, but not to scale. N = nucleus; RA = rapidly adapting; SA = slowly adapting; PV = parietal ventral area; S2 = second somatosensory area; VP = ventroposterior nucleus; VPI = ventroposterior interior nucleus; VPS = ventroposterior superior.

nuclei are elongated in the rostrocaudal dimension of the brain stem. The RA-1 and SA classes of cutaneous afferents appear to terminate in the middle of these nuclei, RA-II (Pacinian) afferents may terminate caudally, and muscle spindle afferents terminate separately in the external cuneate nucleus (for the forelimb) and associated cell groups (for the rest of the body). Thus, much of the information in the separate classes of receptors is quite distinct.

Some processing goes on in the complex, as 20–25% of the neurons within the complex are local inhibitory neurons. In addition, there are descending inputs from cortex that modify the output. Nevertheless, the neurons that project from the complex to the thalamus closely reflect the response properties of the afferents that terminate in the complex.

15. Which structures are included in the somatosensory thalamus?

Various proposals have been made on how to divide the somatosensory thalamus, and different names have been applied to the same structures. It is now common to distinguish a large ventroposterior nucleus (VP) by neurons that are activated by the SA and RA low-threshold mechanoreceptors (see Fig. 3). VP systematically represents the body from tongue medially to foot laterally, with digits pointing down (ventral) and the trunk at the top (dorsal). In humans VP is sometimes called nucleus ventralis caudalis. The medial part of VP representing the face often is distinguished as a separate nucleus (actually, it is a subnucleus), called the medial ventroposterior nucleus (VPM), and the lateral part representing the rest of the body is called the lateral ventroposterior nucleus (VPL).

The ventral posterior superior (VPS) nucleus caps VP. VPS has been included in VP by many investigators, but VPS contains a separate representation of mainly muscle spindle receptors, and VPS is architectonically distinct from VP. A thin ventroposterior inferior nucleus (VPI) under and behind VP is more commonly recognized. VPI receives spinothalamic inputs, and subregions of this nucleus appear to be related to temperature and pain. Parts of the medial thalamus also are involved in nociceptive functions. Finally, the anterior pulvinar and parts of the lateral posterior thalamus are interconnected with regions of somatosensory cortex, and thus have somatosensory functions.

16. What does the somatosensory thalamus do?

A major function of the somatosensory thalamus is to receive ascending inputs from the medial lemniscus and the spinothalamic tract and distribute this information to an array of cortical areas. Other structures, such as the anterior pulvinar, receive information from cortex and distribute it back to cortex. However, neural processing in the thalamus also alters the content of the distributed information. All somatosensory nuclei receive major inputs from areas of somatosensory cortex, and these inputs modify the output. In addition, about 25% of the neurons in the somatosensory thalamus are local inhibitory neurons rather than relay neurons. Nevertheless, the response properties of neurons in VP and VPS closely reflect those of their inputs (SA and RA mechanoreceptors for VP; muscle spindle receptors for VPS). Separate clusters of neurons in VP have SA or RA response properties. Projections from VPI to cortex are widespread, and these inputs appear to modulate rather than activate neurons in cortex.

17. How are pain and temperature relayed to cortex?

Pain and temperature information via the spinothalamic tract terminates in parts of VPI, which projects to anterior and lateral portions of parietal cortex, including S2 (see Fig. 3). Other inputs are to the posterior part of the ventromedial nucleus of the thalamus, which relays to insular cortex of the lateral fissure. Inputs to the ventral caudal portion of the medial dorsal nucleus of the medial thalamus relay to limbic (emotional) cortex of the medial wall of the cerebral hemisphere (area 24C of Brodmann).

18. Which regions of cortex are involved in somatosensory processing?

Cortical areas early in the sequence of somatosensory processing are in anterior parietal cortex of primates, which contains the **four cytoarchitectonic fields** of Brodmann: areas 3a, 3b, 1, and 2. Collectively, these four fields are commonly referred to as primary somatosensory cortex, or S1, although only area 3b is homologous to S1 of rats and other mammals. Higher-order somatosensory processing takes place in Brodmann's areas 5 and 7 in posterior parietal cortex; the second somatosensory areas, S2; and associated fields of lateral parietal cortex in the lateral (Sylvian) fissure. Brodmann's theories of how cortex of various mammals is divided into functional areas were published at length in German in 1909. Brodmann gave areas both names and numbers, but only the numbers are now in common use.

19. What is the relationship between S1 and the four cytoarchitectonic fields?

Anterior parietal cortex or postcentral parietal cortex includes the areas on the posterior bank of the central sulcus and the gyrus just behind the central sulcus. Early attempts to determine the functional organization of this cortex in humans depended on the sensory and motor effects of electrically stimulating various sites in this cortex (Fig. 4). Electrical stimulation produced a feeling of numbness or tingling that was localized to various parts of the body, depending on the site of stimulation. Investigators concentrated on the locations of sensations as stimulation sites progressed from medial to lateral in cortex, and they paid little attention to aspects of organization in the anterior-posterior direction. Thus, the complete region was considered to be a single representation of the body.

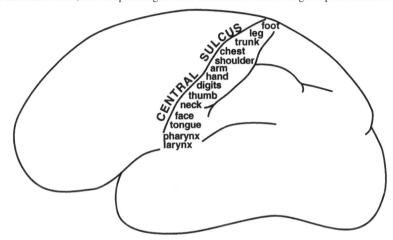

Figure 4. The order of representation of body receptors in postcentral or anterior parietal cortex of humans based on the sensory effects of electrical stimulation of cortex. (Modified from a 1931 illustration by O. Forester.)

Subsequent recordings with electrodes placed on the surface of the brain in monkeys as parts of the body were tapped with probes did not change this impression at first, and this whole region was called primary somatosensory cortex, S1. Later, microelectrode recordings from the middle layers of cortex produced detailed maps of anterior parietal cortex in monkeys, and it became clear that the S1 region actually contains four strip-like, parallel representations of the body, all proceeding from foot to tongue in mediolateral sequences (Fig. 5). Each of these representations corresponds to one of the classic cytoarchitectonic fields: areas 3a, 3b, 1, or 2. Some investigators now restrict the term S1 to the representation in area 3b, but the use of S1 to refer to all four fields is common.

20. Why are there four primary or primary-like representations?

Each of the four areas performs different functions. Areas 3b, 1, and 2 can be thought of as three serial levels of cortical processing. SA and RA inputs from VP of the thalamus are first processed in area 3b, where neurons have the smallest receptive fields and the simplest response properties, closely reflecting those of the SA and RA inputs from VP of the thalamus. Area 3b projects to area 1, where processing is continued and neurons have larger receptive fields and more complex response properties. Area 1 also receives modulating thalamic inputs from VP. Area 1 projects to area 2, where neurons also receive muscle spindle receptor thalamic inputs from VPS. Neurons in area 2 thus have information from skin receptors and from receptors that signal digit and limb positions. Area 2 neurons have large, complex receptive fields, and the neurons are most responsive in active touch. Thus, area 2 has a unique and important role in processing information for object identification.

Area 3a neurons also receive muscle spindle information from VPS of the thalamus, and somatosensory information from areas 3b, 1, and especially 2. Because area 3a projects strongly to motor cortex, and its neurons combine tactile and muscle receptor inputs, area 3a seems to have a special role in informing motor cortex and guiding motor behavior.

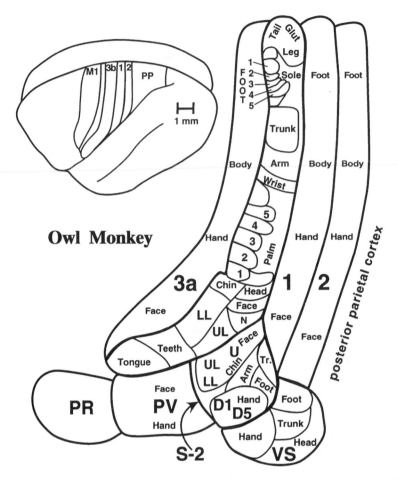

Figure 5. Subdivisions of somatosensory cortex in a New World monkey. The areas are similar to those in humans, but easier to illustrate in a monkey without a central sulcus. An outline of a dorsolateral view of the left cerebral hemisphere on the left shows the lateral and superior temporal fissures. The four somatosensory fields of anterior parietal cortex are enlarged with associated fields on the right. Note that area 3b systematically represents the body from tail to tongue in a mediolateral cortical sequence. Areas 3a, 1, and 2 represent the body in a similar sequence (not shown in detail). The parietal rostral (PR), parietal ventral (PV), ventral somatosensory (VS) areas, and S2 form additional representations, but the internal structures of only S2 and VS are shown. Areas PR, PV, S2, and VS have been unfolded from the cortex of the lateral nucleus so they can be seen. Digits of the hand and foot are numbered. LL = lower lip; UL = upper lip; N = nose; glut = gluteal skin. Note the large proportions of 3b devoted to hand and face.

21. Why does area 1 also receive inputs from the ventroposterior nucleus?

VP projects to layer 4 of area 3b and to layer 3 of area 1 (and to a lesser extent, area 2). The VP inputs to area 3b activate neurons, while the inputs to area 1 have the role of modulating neurons that are activated by inputs from area 3b. Thus, we see aspects of serial and parallel processing in area 1. The processing sequence from VP to area 3b and then area 1 is serial, while the projections from VP to both area 3b and area 1 are parallel. Combinations of serial and parallel inputs are common in cortical areas.

22. Does somatosensory cortex have a columnar organization?

The idea that somatosensory cortex has a columnar organization stems from the early research and conclusions of Vernon Mountcastle in the 1950s and 1960s. All cortex has a **laminar organization,** and the middle layer 4 receives activating inputs and has neurons with the simplest response properties. All cortex has a **vertical organization**, with rows of neurons from the surface to the white matter having features in common as a result of strong vertical interconnections. In anterior somatosensory cortex, all neurons in a vertical row respond to the same location on the body. This vertical organization has been repeatedly demonstrated, and it is not in question.

Unfortunately, the well-known vertical organization is often confused with the concept of columnar organization, a third type of organization that has been proposed for cortex. In columnar or modular organization, neurons in groups of adjacent vertical rows share features that differ from neighboring groups. Several different types of columnar organization have been most studied in visual cortex of monkeys. Probably all cortical areas have a columnar organization, but it has been difficult to determine the nature of this organization for somatosensory areas. However, there is evidence that SA and RA thalamic inputs terminate separately in patch-like modules or columns in area 3b. The early idea that a mosaic of columns of neurons, related to either cutaneous or deep (muscle spindle or joint) receptors, exists in primary somatosensory cortex has not been supported.

23. What impairments occur with lesions of anterior parietal cortex?

Lesions produce impairments in tactile discriminations, texture discriminations, and discriminations of shape and manipulative skills. Impairments especially include those of fine finger movements, and processing in areas 3a and 2 is especially important in guiding skilled movements. Remarkably, with small lesions, there may be no obvious lasting impairment due to the extensive plasticity of somatosensory cortex, so that neurons can be reassigned to new tasks. In addition, many simple somatosensory discriminations do not depend on somatosensory cortex.

24. How is lateral somatosensory cortex organized?

The organization of cortex in the lateral sulcus is not fully understood, but this cortex contains several higher-order fields that are thought to provide important processing steps in object identification. One of these areas, the second somatosensory area (S2) has been long known from animal studies, and much of the cortex of the lateral sulcus was thought to be S2. S2 is a small oval of cortex containing a systematic representation of the surface of the contralateral body as a result of converging inputs from areas 3a, 3b, 1, and 2. The receptive fields are large, and response properties are complex. Another representation, the parietal ventral area (PV) has been more recently established. PV has inputs from anterior parietal cortex and S2, and seems to be the next step above S2 in processing. The proposed parietal rostral and ventral somatosensory fields are less well understood, but they appear to be additional somatosensory areas of the lateral cortex. Some of these fields access entorhinal cortex and then the hippocampus, so that tactile memories can be formed.

25. What do areas of lateral somatosensory cortex do?

An old idea was that S2 and associated regions of cortex are involved in pain perception. Now the prevailing view is that these fields are critically involved in identifying objects and surfaces by touch, and in storing memories for such objects and surfaces. These areas, undoubtedly, are also important in guiding and informing motor cortex, since they project extensively to motor, premotor, and working-memory areas of the frontal lobe. S2 is no longer considered to have a significant role in pain perception. However, S2 does receive major inputs from VPI of the thalamus, which receives most of the spinothalamic projections. Insular cortex of the lateral sulcus also receives a relay of spinothalamic information, and this cortex may have a role in pain perception.

26. How is posterior parietal somatosensory cortex organized?

The organization of this cortex is even less well understood than that of lateral somatosensory cortex. Traditionally, this region has been divided into the cytoarchitectonic regions 5 and 7 of Brodmann, and each of these regions has been divided into parts a and b, but these distinctions have no precise functional meaning. More caudally in posterior parietal cortex, there has been some progress in defining areas of cortex devoted to processing visual and visuomotor information, such as the medial, lateral, and ventral intraparietal areas.

27. What does posterior parietal cortex do?

There are several levels of processing and probably a range of functions in posterior parietal cortex. Neurons closest to anterior parietal cortex in area 5 have properties that are similar to those in area 2, and they appear to represent a next step in serial processing. Posterior parietal cortex as a whole is thought to be very important in providing information for motor control, and connections with the supplementary motor area and other premotor fields are prominent. Visual information from the occipital lobe may combine in posterior parietal cortex with limb position information from anterior parietal cortex to guide the positions of hands for appropriately grasping objects. Posterior parietal cortex is thought to be more involved with locating objects than identifying them. Lesions of the posterior parietal cortex, especially the right side, cause contralateral neglect, so that touch on the parts of the body contralateral to the lesion is less apparent than touch on the ipsilateral body. Regions of posterior parietal cortex connect with limbic cortex on the medial wall of the cerebral hemisphere, and these connections may play a role in attention.

28. What are the response properties of neurons in posterior parietal cortex?

Neurons in different subdivisions have different properties. Many neurons combine visual and somatosensory inputs. Neural activity in the medial intraparietal area, for example, reflects limb movement and position, but the responses of neurons also are modulated by visual stimuli and direction of gaze. Area 5 neurons are less complex, and they reflect limb position and movement.

29. Are there somatosensory areas on the medial wall of the parietal lobe?

Penfield and Jasper in the 1950s postulated the existence of a supplementary sensory area on the medial wall, but there has been only limited evidence for such an area. Nevertheless, there is evidence that posterior cingulate cortex has an evaluative role and somatosensory functions.

30. Do the somatosensory areas of the two cerebral hemispheres communicate?

The somatosensory system is a highly lateralized system in that peripheral nerves subserve one side of the body or the other, with little or no overlap at the body midline. Peripheral nerve inputs terminate on the same side of the spinal cord or brain stem. Second-order neurons cross to the other side of the spinal cord or brain stem to terminate in the thalamus and form representations almost exclusively of the contralateral half of the body (some limited bilateral representation of skin of the mouth occurs). The anterior parietal areas are activated by thalamic projections related to the contralateral half of the body.

However, each cortical area has interconnections via the corpus callosum with its matched area in the other hemisphere and two or three adjacent representations. In anterior parietal cortex, these callosal connections do not seem to participate in the excitatory receptive fields of most neurons, so that receptive fields are confined to the contralateral body and are not bilateral. Some parts of the representations, especially the hand portion of area 3b, are almost devoid of callosal connections, while the higher-order field, area 2, has more callosal connections. Anterior parietal and posterior parietal fields have more evenly distributed and often dense callosal connections, and neurons in some of these areas have bilateral receptive fields that are activated from both sides of the body. Clearly, such neurons are important, as we often need to compare stimuli on both sides of the body, and the hands may explore objects together. In addition, perceptual skills learned with one hand transfer to the other, and this transfer depends on the corpus callosum.

BIBLIOGRAPHY

1. Kaas JH: The somatosensory system. In Paxinos G (ed): The Human Nervous System. New York, Academic Press, 1990, pp 813–844.
2. Kaas JH: The functional organization of somatosensory cortex in primates. Ann Anat 175:509–518, 1993.
3. Kaas JH, Pons TP: The somatosensory system of primates. In Steklis HP (ed): Comparative Primate Biology, Vol. 4: Neurosciences. New York, Alan R. Liss, Inc., 1988, pp 421–468.
4. Mountcastle VB: Perceptual neuroscience: The cerebral cortex. Cambridge, MA, Harvard University Press, 1998.

5. THE VISUAL SYSTEM

Janice M. Burke, Ph.D., Jay Neitz, Ph.D., and Margaret T. T. Wong-Riley, Ph.D.

The visual system has long been regarded as a model for understanding the structural and physiologic bases of sensory processing. It is exquisitely organized into a receptive surface (the retina), a relay station (the lateral geniculate nucleus), and a site for perception (visual cortex). Additional structures in the eye assist with light transmission, and other subcortical and cortical centers help process various visual functions. The relative positions of the two eyes provide for a sizeable binocular visual field, and the effect of monocular perturbation can be analyzed and compared with a convenient internal control, the unperturbed eye. For these reasons, the visual system is probably the most studied among the sensory systems.

NON-NEURONAL TISSUES OF THE EYE

1. How does light reach the retina?

Starting from the outside world, light passes through the following series of transparent tissues before reaching the retina: cornea, anterior chamber (which contains aqueous humor), lens, and vitreous. Each tissue is highly specialized to maintain transparency; loss of transparency results in pathologies that can reduce vision or cause blindness. Light also passes through all the inner layers of the retina before reaching the outer segments of the photoreceptor cells, where the light-sensitive visual pigments are found.

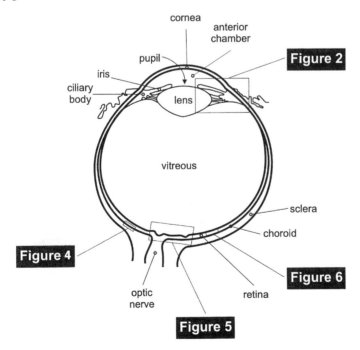

Figure 1. The human eye and its major structures.

2. Which tissues in the light path are responsible for light refraction?

The major refractive tissue of the eye is the **cornea**. Its refractive power is due to its curvature and to the difference in index of refraction between air (1.0) and the tissue (1.38). Second in refractive power is the **lens**, which can change shape to focus light on the retina.

3. How does the lens change its focus?

The lens is covered on its anterior surface (toward the front of the eye) by a single-layered epithelium, while the body of the lens is composed of elongated lens fiber cells. The entire lens is encased in a capsule of extracellular matrix. Radiating from the capsule at the perimeter of the biconvex lens are fibrils called the **zonules** (or zonules of Zinn—one of the great names in biology). The zonules connect to finger-like processes of the ciliary body, which suspend the lens behind the pupil. The muscles of the ciliary body hold the lens under constant tension, flattening it. When focusing on a near object (accommodation), the ciliary muscles relax, which releases tension on the lens and allows it to become more rounded due to its natural elasticity. With aging, lens elasticity decreases, reducing near vision (a condition called presbyopia).

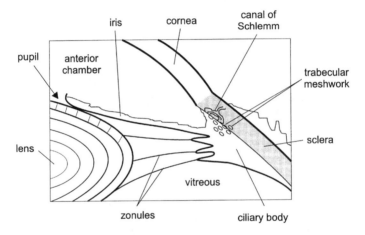

Figure 2. Part of the anterior segment of the eye, showing the supporting structures of the lens and the anterior chamber angle, which is the site of aqueous humor outflow. (Refer to Figure 1.)

4. What is the pupil and how does it work?

The pupil is a central hole in the iris. The iris contains two muscle groups: a sphincter around the pupil margin, which is under parasympathetic control, and dilator muscles radiating from the pupil rim, which are controlled by the sympathetic nervous system. With light stimulus, some retinal axons go to the visual reflex center in the pretectal nuclei, which stimulates sphincter muscles to control pupil diameter and thereby regulate light entry into the eye. In concert with its control of pupil size, the visual reflex center in the midbrain also controls extraocular muscles for eye movement and ciliary muscles for lens focus.

5. What determines differences in eye color?

The iris is the colored portion of the eye. Blue-eyed and brown-eyed people do not have different iris pigments; the pigment in all eyes is **melanin**. Eye color differs depending upon the *number* of melanocytes (pigment-containing cells) and the *ratio* of melanocytes to blood vessels in the iris stroma. Brown eyes have large numbers of melanocytes; hazel/green eyes have intermediate numbers; and blue eyes have fewer pigment-containing cells. There is a posterior epithelium on the iris that is similarly pigmented in all eyes.

6. How is corneal transparency maintained?

The cornea consists of three tissue layers: an outer stratified epithelium, an inner monolayer endothelium, and the central stroma. The **stroma** is a thick connective tissue layer with few cells (keratocytes) and a large amount of extracellular matrix consisting predominantly of type I collagen fibrils and highly sulfated proteoglycans. The collagen fibrils are organized into layers that form mutually perpendicular (orthogonal) strata from anterior to posterior in the corneal stroma. The spacing of these collagen layers is precise to allow the unimpeded passage of the wavelengths of light in the visible range. This spacing is maintained by regulation of tissue hydration; if the water content increases, the tissue swells, and the cornea becomes opaque.

7. What causes loss of corneal transparency?

There are two major causes of loss of corneal transparency: damage to the endothelium and damage to the stroma.

Damage to the endothelium is the most common cause because it leads to corneal swelling. Water normally leaks into the stroma from the aqueous humor and is continuously pumped out by the endothelium. The water pumping function of the endothelium is due to its plasma membrane Na+/K+ ATPase (sodium pump). The continuous pumping process maintains normal stromal hydration and transparency. Since endothelial cells do not normally divide, damage to the endothelium that reduces cell number also reduces the overall pumping capacity of the tissue, resulting in corneal decompensation. The endothelium can be damaged or lost by viral infection, aging, intraocular surgery, and even long-term contact lens wear.

Wounds resulting from damage to the stroma heal, but the remaining scar is opaque because of the disorganization of the collagen matrix. If the corneal scar is large or in the central light path to the retina, vision will be impaired.

8. Is there a treatment for irreversible loss of corneal transparency?

Yes, the cornea can be transplanted. In the procedure, full- or partial-thickness cornea from a donor is grafted to the center of the host cornea, which is partially or completely removed. The surface epithelium and stroma of the graft are repopulated by host cells. Rejection of a corneal transplant is infrequent because the cornea, like the other transparent tissues of the eye, lacks blood vessels, limiting access of immune cells to the graft. In full-thickness grafts, the endothelium also is transplanted, and surgical success is largely determined by the health of the endothelium, which must continue to pump water from the cornea to maintain transparency.

9. What is the effect on the cornea of refractive surgery to reduce the need for spectacles?

Refractive surgery is an elective procedure performed to change the shape of the cornea and reduce the need for eyeglasses, primarily for people with moderate myopia. LASIK (laser in situ keratomileusis) is the current preferred technique. In LASIK, a partial-thickness cut is made in the cornea, allowing a lamellar flap of tissue to be moved aside so that part of the central cornea can be ablated with an excimer laser. After the flap is replaced and the wound has healed, scarring usually is minimal, and corneal curvature typically is closer to normal. Thus, the need for corrective lenses is reduced. All refractive surgical techniques, especially LASIK, are relatively new, and long-term effects are unknown. One possible future concern is that the rates of corneal decompensation will be higher in people who have had refractive surgery, increasing the need for corneal transplantation as they age.

10. Does the lens use the same mechanism as the cornea to maintain transparency?

No, the tissue structure of the lens is quite different. At an early stage in its embryonic development, the lens is a fluid-filled epithelial sphere. Later, the posterior epithelium develops into lens fiber cells, which elongate in the anterior-posterior direction as they differentiate, filling the sphere. In lens fiber cells, organelles are lost, and the cytoplasm fills with proteins called **crystallins**. Lens transparency, therefore, is due to several structural features: the absence of extracellular matrix between lens fibers; the lack of intracellular organelles within lens fibers; and the presence of lens crystallins. The latter proteins form aggregates of small particle size that do not impede light passage.

11. What is a cataract?

A cataract is an opacity of the lens. Cataracts can be broadly divided into two types: central nuclear, which are most common in the aging eye, and non-nuclear (cortical or posterior subcapsular). Cataracts of mixed phenotype also are common. Indeed, cataracts are the most frequent cause of blindness world-wide. In industrialized nations, cataracts are considered an ocular disease of aging, but cataracts also are found in children, and the incidence of childhood cataracts is especially high in the developing world.

12. What causes a cataract?

There is no acceptable answer to this question yet, but preliminary answers to two questions re-garding cataract etiology might be attempted:

A. What are the risk factors for cataracts?

Cataracts have multiple risk factors, and sorting out the contribution of each to the complex pathology is a formidable task. The evidence is overwhelming for some cataract risks, such as time (aging), trauma, and intraocular inflammation. Undernutrition also is a cataract risk factor. Whether antioxidants are the missing nutrients remains to be established, although this is a tempting theory because there appears to be an oxidative component to cataract formation. Ultraviolet light (espe-cially UV-B radiation), systemic or topical steroids, diabetes, and smoking also are cataract risk fac-tors. A genetic component to cataracts is indicated from twin studies and sibling correlational analyses, and from the existence of congenital cataracts in both humans and animals. In animals, several mutations in crystallin genes have been implicated in cataractogenesis.

B. What happens at the cellular/molecular level to make the lens opaque?

Proteins expressed at high levels in the mammalian lens are the α-, β-, and γ-crystallins. The α-crystallins are both structural proteins and molecular chaperones that stabilize crystallins and other enzymes under conditions of stress (e.g., heat or UV radiation) and prevent the formation of protein aggregates. Interactions among normal crystallins maintain them in a closely packed, yet soluble, form, but during cataract formation the lens becomes opaque as a consequence of increased **protein insolubility**. Lens proteins may become insoluble due to limited proteolysis by the action of cal-pains, which are calcium-dependent enzymes that cleave peptide groups responsible for normal crystallin oligomerization. Protein insolubility also increases due to the oxidation of cysteine sulfhydryls, producing disulfide crosslinks.

Elevated levels of oxidants (e.g., hydrogen peroxide) and diminished levels of antioxidants (e.g., glutathione) in cataractous lenses implicate **oxidation** in cataract formation. Aside from rendering crystallins insoluble, oxidation also may impair the chaperone function of α-crystallins. The region of the αA-crystallin molecule that is responsible for its chaperone function contains cysteine residues that are oxidized during cataractogenesis, perhaps affecting protein chaperone activity and increasing the formation of protein aggregates.

The molecular changes that lead to cataracts are many and complex, but the result is that mech-anisms to maintain lens transparency are overwhelmed, and opacities develop.

13. Why is the vitreous transparent?

The vitreous owes its transparency to a virtual absence of cells and to a low content of protein, in-cluding matrix macromolecules (the vitreous is 99% water). The major macromolecules of the vitre-ous are hyaluronic acid and type II collagen. The macromolecules form a loose network in the center of the vitreous and a denser web in the vitreous cortex adjacent to the retina. Overall, the vitreous has the consistency of a soft gel. The few cells in the vitreous, which are in the cortex, appear to be macrophages that continuously transmigrate the vitreous. As shown in animal studies, macrophages enter the anterior vitreous from the blood vessels of the ciliary body, and leave the vitreous through retinal vessels. In intraocular inflammations, the number of vitreous cells may increase dramatically.

14. If the vitreous is mostly water, does that mean that it is functionally inert?

When it was discovered many years ago that the vitreous could be surgically removed and re-placed with buffers with few adverse clinical consequences, it was assumed that the vitreous did not perform essential functions. However, that view has changed. After removal of the vitreous, the macromolecular composition appears not to be restored, but the soluble components are restored. The soluble fraction of the vitreous may function as both a nutrient source and a waste product sink for the adjacent retina. Since the vitreous is a reservoir for products secreted or released by the surrounding retina, its composition provides information about the metabolic activity of normal or diseased tissue. For example, potentially angiogenic growth factors such as fibroblast growth factor and vascular endothelial cell growth factor have been found in the vitreous of eyes with neovascular disease (e.g., proliferative diabetic retinopathy). This finding is consistent with the view that these factors contribute to undesirable blood vessel growth in the eye.

15. What are the "vitreous floaters" that can be seen when looking at a homogeneous bright scene (e.g., a clear sky)?

With aging, the vitreous undergoes **syneresis**, in which the collagen-hyaluronic acid network collapses, separating the vitreous gel into coarse strands of matrix separated by liquid pools. As the eye moves, the strands can float into the visual axis. With aging, the vitreous also separates from the retina (posterior vitreous detachment). The separation occurs within the cortical vitreous matrix or between the cortex and the inner limiting lamina, which is the basement membrane of the retinal glial cells that forms the interface between the retina and vitreous. Posterior vitreous detachment can be incomplete, and retained sites of vitreous attachment can put traction on the retina, producing retinal holes. This traction may even completely detach the retina.

16. The transparent tissues of the eye use many different mechanisms to remain transparent. Are there any mechanisms in common?

Yes, the transparent tissues of the eye all contain unidentified factors that inhibit blood vessel growth, which contributes to tissue transparency by making normal tissues avascular. Researchers take advantage of the absence of vessels in the cornea to test putative angiogenic substances. In the assay, a pellet of the test substance is inserted into a pocket in the cornea. The cornea is then examined over time to determine whether blood vessels invade from the surrounding **limbus** (junction between the clear cornea and adjacent vascularized sclera).

17. Which tissues in the eye are vascularized, and what is the blood supply?

The major vascularized tissues of the eye form the uveal tract that lies between the dense connective tissue sclera and the transparent tissues on the light path to the retina. In the anterior segment of the eye, the uveal tissues are the iris and ciliary body. Posterior to the ciliary body is the vascular choroid, which surrounds the entire retina. The outer third of the retina lacks intraretinal vessels, so choroidal vessels provide oxygen and nutrients for this portion of the tissue, which includes the photoreceptors. The inner two-thirds of the retina contain intraretinal vessels, which enter the eye at the optic nerve. The retina, therefore, has two blood supplies. Vascular occlusions, depending upon their site, can differentially affect the inner and outer retina.

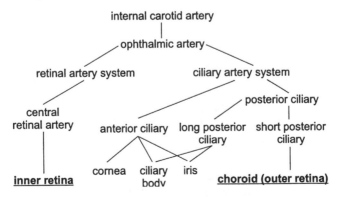

Figure 3. The ocular circulation, with dual blood supply to the retina.

18. If the outer retina does not have blood vessels of its own, how is nutrient and gas availability to the photoreceptors controlled?

The outer segments of the photoreceptors are closely associated with the apical microvilli of an adjacent epithelium, the **retinal pigment epithelium** (RPE). The RPE monolayer and its underlying matrix (Bruch's membrane) lie between the photoreceptor cells and the capillary bed of the choroid (choriocapillaris). Since the endothelium of choroidal capillaries is fenestrated, the movement of gases, nutrients, and waste products between photoreceptors and choroidal vessels is regulated not by the endothelium but by the RPE. Tight junctions between RPE cells have a barrier function, restricting paracellular movement of molecules, while the transport activities of the RPE cells regulate transcellular movement. These properties of the RPE give the tissue its function as the outer blood-retinal barrier. (The inner blood-retinal barrier is at the level of the nonfenestrated endothelium of intraretinal capillaries.)

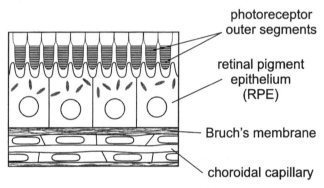

photoreceptor
outer segments

retinal pigment
epithelium
(RPE)

Bruch's membrane

choroidal capillary

Figure 4. The retinal pigment epithelium, with the overlying photoreceptors of the retina and the underlying extracellular matrix (Bruch's membrane) and capillaries of the choroid. (Refer to Figure 1.)

19. Does the retinal pigment epithelium perform other functions in support of photoreceptors?

Yes, the outer segments of photoreceptors and the apical surface of the RPE layer have a close physical association to facilitate several essential functions performed by the RPE in support of photoreceptor function and survival.

The transmembrane transport of metabolites by RPE cells requires a sodium gradient generated by the RPE Na^+/K^+ ATPase. This ion transporter is highly enriched in the RPE apical plasma membrane, where it also helps regulate sodium and potassium homeostasis in the environment of the photoreceptors, as required for membrane hyperpolarization with photic stimulation.

It can be argued that RPE pigment (melanin) exists to refine the function of photoreceptors as visual cells. Stray light that is not captured as it passes through the photoreceptor outer segments is absorbed by RPE melanin. This absorption reduces light scatter within the eye, increasing visual resolution.

One of the most important functions performed by RPE cells for photoreceptors is participation in the complex process of **photoreceptor renewal**. Photoreceptor disc membranes (comprised largely of visual pigments) are continuously replaced with the light-dark cycle. For example, with the onset of light, the tips of rod photoreceptor outer segments detach, and the packets of discs (containing the pigment **rhodopsin**) are then phagocytized by the RPE. Within RPE cells, the phagosomes fuse with lysosomes, producing phagolysosomes, and the contents are degraded. Some of the degradation products are shuttled to the apical surface of the RPE cells for transport back to the photoreceptors for biosynthesis of new disc membranes. Components of disc membranes also are transported from the blood by RPE cells. Of particular importance is the metabolism and transport by RPE cells of retinoids, vitamin A derivatives which become the chromophore that complexes with the visual pigment proteins (**opsins**). RPE participation in the process of photoreceptor renewal is essential not only for disc turnover, but also for photoreceptor survival. In the Royal College of Surgeons strain of rat, for example, photoreceptor degeneration occurs as a consequence of a genetic defect in the RPE cells that inhibits photoreceptor renewal by preventing internalization of shed photoreceptor tips.

20. What is a retinal detachment?

A retinal detachment is a separation of the sensory retina, at the level of the photoreceptor outer segments, from the RPE. Retinal detachments can have many causes, including trauma or traction on the retina from a partially detached vitreous. Although the outer segments of photoreceptors and the apical microvilli of RPE cells are in close apposition, there are no known attachment proteins forming junctions between the membranes. Rather, the small cleft between the plasma membranes (called the subretinal space) is filled with an interphotoreceptor matrix (IPM). Adhesion to the IPM is relatively weak, which makes the photoreceptor-RPE interface a site of potential separation. Because the RPE performs many support functions for photoreceptors that require close cell-cell apposition (see Question 19), photoreceptor cell function and survival decline with retinal detachment. Detachment results in a visual field loss (**scotoma**) that can reduce vision if the scotoma is large or involves the portion of the retina used for high acuity vision. Detached retinas can be surgically reattached; the goal is to restore normal photoreceptor-RPE interactions.

21. Do photoreceptors and retinal pigment epithelium recover after surgical reattachment of a detached retina?

Yes, and no. Visual recovery after retinal reattachment is variable and is affected by many factors, including the size, position, and duration of the detachment. However, even rapid repair of a "simple" detachment does not necessarily result in fully restored vision, suggesting that defects remain at the RPE-photoreceptor interface. When the retina detaches, some photoreceptors are damaged and some RPE cells detach from their substrate, exposing Bruch's membrane. Recovery of the RPE after retinal detachment therefore requires repair of a wound in the epithelium. Animal studies show that RPE cells, which do not normally proliferate, heal a wound by dividing and migrating to reform a contiguous monolayer. However, the RPE cells at the site of a repaired detachment may not reacquire the **polarized epithelial morphology** that is required for support of photoreceptor function or survival, perhaps contributing to permanent visual defects.

A normal RPE-photoreceptor interface at a retinal reattachment site also requires restoration of the intervening interphotoreceptor matrix (IPM). The IPM contains interphotoreceptor retinoid binding protein, which binds several retinoids and participates in shuttling retinoids within the subretinal space in the process of photoreceptor renewal. The IPM is known to contain several bioactive molecules such as basic fibroblast growth factor (bFGF), inhibin (a member of the transforming growth factor β superfamily), and pigment epithelium-derived factor (PEDF), a member of the serine protease inhibitor family. bFGF and PEDF have neurotrophic activity, raising the possibility that failure to restore the biological activity of the IPM is another contributor to diminished photoreceptor survival after retinal reattachment.

22. What are the major age-related ocular diseases?

The incidence of several ocular pathologies increases with age. The most common aging eye diseases with the greatest impact on vision are cataract, glaucoma, and age-related macular degeneration.

23. What tissue changes occur during age-related macular degeneration (AMD)?

The **macula,** which is centered approximately 3 mm temporal to the optic nerve, has a high density of the photoreceptors (cones) that are responsible for high acuity and color vision. Defects of the macula therefore have a prominent effect on vision. AMD is a progressive, degenerative disease involving a complex of macular tissues: photoreceptors, RPE, Bruch's membrane, and underlying choriocapillaris.

In the earliest clinically detectable disease, **drusen** (tissue debris) accumulates in focal patches in Bruch's membrane, possibly signaling functional changes in the RPE. Eyes with drusen may progress to develop the "dry" (non-neovascular) form of the disease, in which cell changes are detected in all tissues of the macular complex, although vision loss may not be severe. In about 10% of patients with AMD, the disease progresses further to the "wet" (neovascular) form, in which choroidal blood vessels grow through Bruch's membrane under the RPE, or also through the RPE layer into the subretinal space. The new vessels are fragile and often bleed. Neovascular growth may be accompanied by the development of fibrous tissue membranes that distort the retina, producing detachments. Significant photoreceptor degeneration accompanies neovascular AMD, accounting for 80% of the severe vision loss associated with the disease.

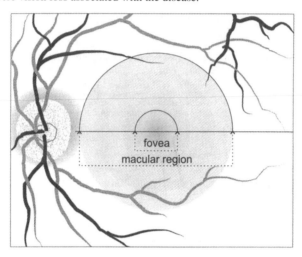

Figure 5.   The posterior fundus of the eye, showing the macular region and adjacent optic nerve. (Refer to Figure 1.)

24. What causes the macular region of the retina to degenerate with aging?

There is no satisfactory answer to this question. Like many diseases of aging, the causes are expected to be multiple and interrelated.

Some causes of AMD might be inferred from epidemiologic data. Several positive risk associations for AMD have been identified, including hyperopia, smoking, elevated serum cholesterol, arteriosclerosis and cerebrovascular diseases, greater caloric intake, and use of antihypertension medications. Positive association of AMD with light iris color and greater elastotic degeneration of the dermis (coupled with animal studies suggesting that UV and blue light exposure predisposes to retinal degeneration) implicates light exposure in the etiology of AMD. Several AMD risk associations taken together point to oxidative tissue damage as a cause of the disease. This view is supported by studies that appear to show reduced risk of AMD in individuals with a diet high in antioxidants, or with higher blood levels of antioxidants such as carotenoids.

Family history predicts as many as 20% of AMD cases, suggesting a genetic component to the disease. Identification of gene mutations that contribute to AMD involves first identifying the genetic basis for heritable diseases that exhibit a similar macular degeneration. These genes might prove to have other mutations, which predispose to late-onset macular degeneration. Recently, genes for three forms of inherited macular degeneration have been found: Sorsby fundus dystrophy (SFD), Stargardt disease, and Best macular dystrophy. Mutations in the SFD gene, which encodes tissue inhibitor of metalloproteinases-3, do not appear to contribute to AMD. Whether mutations in the Stargardt gene, which encodes an ATP-binding cassette transporter, contribute to AMD is still controversial. It also has not been determined whether bestrophin, the gene with the mutation that causes Best's disease, is a candidate gene for AMD. Knowledge of AMD genetics is still in its infancy, and it is likely that mutations in several genes contribute to increased risk.

25. Are there any treatments for age-related macular degeneration?

There are no therapies for non-neovascular AMD.

For the 10% of cases that progress to develop subretinal neovascular membranes, laser photocoagulation of the blood vessels has been shown to slow further visual loss when compared to untreated eyes. However, the chance of recurrence of neovascular membranes is 50% even with laser treatment.

In the absence of any acceptable treatment for AMD, there are several experimental therapeutic approaches that are in various stages of testing. A trial is underway to determine whether micronutrient supplementation (e.g., antioxidants, zinc) protects against the disease, which is believed to have a dietary component. Surgical removal of subretinal neovascular membranes has been attempted, but the benefit of this procedure has not been shown. Antiangiogenic agents may have a future place in treating or preventing neovascular AMD. Another possible treatment is RPE transplantation. The rationale for this protocol comes from evidence indicating that AMD is at least partially an aging disease of RPE cells, which over years may fail to provide adequate support for photoreceptors to maintain their function and survival. The goal therefore would be to replace aged, defective RPE cells with more functionally active, younger tissue. However, there are many challenges to developing the technique of transplantation therapy, not the least of which is producing a graft in which the RPE cells are structurally and functionally normal.

26. What is glaucoma?

Glaucoma is a heterogeneous group of diseases characterized by optic nerve damage leading to peripheral visual field losses that can progress to blindness. Glaucoma also usually features elevated intraocular pressure (IOP), which is the most common clinical sign and risk factor for glaucoma. Elevated IOP forces the optic nerve to cup backwards against a constriction point where the nerve passes through the sclera. Pressure on the optic nerve circulation and on axons, which blocks retrograde axonal transport, leads to axonal loss and ganglion cell death.

There are two main types of glaucoma: open angle and angle closure. **Primary open angle glaucoma** can have a juvenile or adult (after age 40) time of onset; chronic, adult-onset, open angle glaucoma is the most common form of the disease. It is expected to affect as many as 67 million people worldwide by the year 2000. In open angle glaucoma there is no obvious physical blockage to the angle of the iris where aqueous humor leaves the anterior chamber (see Question 27), but outflow appears to be impeded, leading to increased IOP. In **angle closure glaucoma**, the outflow pathway is physically blocked. For example, with intraocular hemorrhage, blood cells can block the angle. Another type of angle closure glaucoma is pupillary block glaucoma, in which an obstruction of the pupil leads to aqueous accumulation behind the iris, forcing it forward so that it occludes the trabecular meshwork and interrupts aqueous outflow.

Glaucomas may be treated surgically and/or with medications. The goal of treatment is to reduce IOP by reducing aqueous production or increasing aqueous outflow, with an aim of limiting pressure-induced optic nerve damage.

27. What is the tissue source and function of aqueous humor?

Aqueous humor is produced by the epithelium of the ciliary body, which filters blood plasma and secretes molecules to produce a fluid that is compositionally similar to cerebrospinal fluid. After production, aqueous humor moves anteriorly through the pupil into the anterior chamber, then out of the anterior chamber at the angle of the iris. At the angle, fluid enters the trabecular meshwork, the canal of Schlemm, and then the veins of the sclera (see Fig. 2). The balance of continuous production and outflow of aqueous humor determines intraocular pressure, which maintains the turgidity of the eye. In addition to maintaining intraocular pressure, aqueous humor may also have a nutritive function for the avascular tissues (cornea and lens) bordering the anterior chamber.

28. What causes primary open angle glaucoma (POAG)?

There is no complete answer to this question, but a high proportion of cases have a genetic basis. Genetic studies have thus far mapped one gene locus for juvenile-onset POAG and two loci for chronic adult-onset POAG. Mutations in these genes in affected families are beginning to be identified. Most extensively studied is the MYOC/TIGR gene (myocilin/trabecular meshwork–inducible glucocorticoid response). In situ RNA hybridization shows high expression levels of the MYOC gene in trabecular meshwork cells and in the anterior portion of the sclera. The gene encodes a 57 kD protein, myocilin, of yet unidentified function. The expectation is that myocilin mutations will be shown to affect aqueous outflow, elevating intraocular pressure and contributing to the pathogenesis of glaucoma. It also is expected that mutations in many genes will be found to confer an increased risk of glaucoma.

As for other ocular diseases that increase in frequency with aging, genetic risk factors for glaucoma act in concert with unidentified physiologic factors to cause disease. One physiologic factor that has been implicated in POAG is an age-related increase in oxidative injury to cells in the aqueous outflow pathway. Oxidative damage to enzymes and structural proteins, perhaps mediated by hydrogen peroxide, may increase aqueous outflow resistance by modifying the extracellular matrix macromolecules secreted by trabecular meshwork cells.

29. How are lasers used in the eye?

Lasers are applied in many specialties of medicine, but they are particularly heavily used in ophthalmology. Some lasers are used as cutting tools, and several other types are used to treat retinal pathologies. For the latter types, laser energy passes through the clear tissues of the eye, allowing noninvasive treatment of intraocular structures.

An example of a laser used in the eye as a cutting tool is the excimer laser, which can ablate tissue in corneal refractive surgery. Another example is the neodymium:YAG laser, which is used to remove posterior lens capsule opacifications that can develop following cataract extraction.

An example of a retinal application laser is the argon laser, which can be used for panretinal photocoagulation to treat diabetic retinopathy. By unknown mechanisms, this treatment leads to regression of the newly formed vessels that characterize the proliferative disease. Lasers also are used to ablate the new vessels that develop in the macula in the wet form of age-related macular degeneration (AMD). Argon or (if close to the fovea) krypton lasers are used for this purpose. Laser treatment of eyes with AMD does not restore the vision that was lost due to previous photoreceptor degeneration, but it slows the further progression of the disease. Lasers also may be used as an adjunct to retinal reattachment surgery, to produce a local scar that acts as a "spot weld" to help keep the retina from redetaching.

30. What is the tissue response in the retina when it is lasered?

The laser energies in the retina usually are absorbed by naturally occurring pigments, such as hemoglobin in blood or melanin in the RPE. The tissue effects of laser are due largely to the heat that is generated as the energy is absorbed; the heat spreads to surrounding cells, producing focal injury. Cell death then induces an inflammatory response, which is followed by local proliferation and, ultimately, a return to growth quiescence. If the laser injury is confined to the retina and RPE, the result may be a gliotic scar within the retina. If the tissues of the choroid also are involved, the choroid and retina may be interconnected by a scar that forms a chorioretinal adhesion. Lasers of different types and different energies are used to control the extent of tissue injury to obtain a particular therapeutic outcome while limiting ancillary damage to retinal neurons. The molecular events accompanying the complex process of retinal wound repair after laser treatment are poorly understood; thus, the mechanism whereby a desirable outcome results often is unknown.

31. Are eye diseases of aging inevitable?

Perhaps, but only if you are very long lived. Most diseases with a late-in-life onset (such as aging forms of cataract, glaucoma, and macular degeneration) appear to have both a genetic component and a toll-of-years component. People who lack significant genetic risk factors may be spared ocular diseases of aging for decades. Indeed, aging eye diseases are not ubiquitous, even in people in their 90s. However, the passage of time, during which cellular aging occurs, takes a toll on everyone. Each species has a maximum life span, which is the documented age of the longest-lived member of that species. For humans, the maximum life span is about 125 years. It is likely that anyone who lives to this advanced age will have some loss of vision, resulting from functional declines in ocular tissues.

THE RETINA

32. Is it true that humans have two kinds of photoreceptors, one kind for black-and-white vision and one for color vision?

No. This is a common misconception. Human vision is based on two kinds of light-sensitive receptor cells: rods and cones. The **rod photoreceptors** are specialized for vision under very dim light, and they do not take part in vision under normal daylight. Thus, for most activities, vision is based on cone photoreceptors. When only the rods are operating, such as at night when the only illumination is the moon and stars, we do not see color because rods do not provide any color vision. During the day, when only the cones are operating, we see in color. However, these facts should not be misunderstood to imply that the rod photoreceptors provide black-and-white vision during the day. The cone photoreceptors allow perception of both black-and-white and color during the day.

In people with normal color vision, there are **three classes of cone photoreceptors**. Very roughly, one class of cones is most sensitive to blue light, one to green, and one to red light. Our color vision is a result of these three classes. If we had only one class of cones, we would see only in black and white. There are several distinct differences between the blue cones and the red and green cones. First, defects in the genes that encode the photopigments in the red and green cones occur with high frequency and are the cause of the common forms of color blindness (see Question 34). A second difference is that the vast majority of the cones in the normal eye are red and green, while blue cones are relatively few in number (about 7% of the total number of cones). Thus, our vision is much more critically dependent on the red and green cones, and the small number of blue cones are present principally to provide an extra dimension of color vision.

33. How does light that falls on the retina get transduced into an electrical signal?

Photopigment molecules are members of an extremely large family of receptor molecules called G-protein–coupled receptors. It is believed that all members of this family originally evolved from a single common ancestor. However, the different members have diverged to serve an enormous variety of signaling functions in the human body. Most members of this receptor family are activated by interaction with a ligand molecule. For example, the dopamine receptor molecule is activated by the neurotransmitter dopamine. The photopigment molecules are unique G-protein–coupled receptors in that they are activated by light.

G-protein–coupled receptors act through a series of biochemical steps to accomplish their ultimate actions. The first step is always to activate a messenger molecule called a G-protein. G-proteins are so named because they bind to guanine-based nucleotides. The activated photopigment molecule can activate several hundred G-protein molecules, known as transducin in the retina, within a period of 100 milliseconds after being activated by light. The activated transducin in turn activates an enzyme, cyclic G phosphodiesterase (cG PDE). The activated cG PDE breaks down an intracellular signaling molecule, cyclic guanosine monophosphate (cGMP).

The important role cGMP has in the photoreceptor cell is that it acts on cGMP-gated sodium channels in the plasma membrane of the photoreceptor. When cGMP is bound to the channel, it is open to the passage of sodium ions into the cell. When the photoreceptor is in the dark, cGMP levels are high and there are ample numbers to bind to the sodium channels and hold them open. The movement of the positive sodium ions into the cell depolarizes it. Thus, the photoreceptors are relatively depolarized in the dark. Light acts through the phototransduction cascade to break down cGMP. When light falls on the cell, the cGMP levels drop, fewer molecules are available to bind to the channels, the channels close, and the photoreceptor hyperpolarizes.

34. What causes color blindness?

Congenital red-green color vision defects are extremely common. In the U.S. they occur in 8–10% of men and nearly 1% of women. There are two major categories, with important differences between them, and a wide range of severity for red-green color vision defects. Almost all red-green color vision defects are caused by the absence of one class of light-sensitive receptor in the eye. People who are missing the receptors most sensitive in the *middle* part of the spectrum are termed

deutan; those missing the receptors most sensitive toward the *red end* are termed **protan**. Normally, the absence of one class of photoreceptor from the eye affects only color vision. These are stationary genetic disorders; they do not get better or worse.

Most people with color vision defects, even though they are missing one class of photoreceptor, have some degree of residual variability in one of their two remaining classes. Small differences in sensitivity to different colors among the remaining photoreceptors form the basis for a reduced form of color vision called **color anomaly**. The degree of color vision impairment for color vision anomalies varies from mild to severe. About two-thirds of all people diagnosed with red-green colorblindness have some form of color anomaly.

The most severe form of red-green color vision deficiency is called **dichromacy**. About one-third of red-green colorblind people have this most severe form. The word dichromat literally means "two colors." To give an illustration, a color television mixes three primary colors (red, green, and blue) to produce the full gamut of colors we see in the real world. Dichromats only need two primary colors for a TV to acceptably simulate all the colors of the real world. If the green color "gun" was burned out on a TV, so that only mixtures of red and blue remained, a person with normal trichromacy would find the resulting images bizarre and intolerable. However, the dichromat could adjust such a two-color TV so that it looked acceptably like the real world to his or her eye, and could do the same if only the green and blue colors were available. Similarly, colorblind people may choose clothes or makeup in color combinations that appear bizarre to most of us but look perfectly fine to them.

Even though the color vision of people with the most severe forms of red-green colorblindness is dramatically different than normal, they still are not completely colorblind. Complete colorblindness would allow acceptance of a color TV with all but one of the colors burned out as adequately representing the real world. This kind of complete colorblindness is extremely rare.

35. Are there any treatments for colorblindness?

At the present time, colorblindness cannot be treated or cured. Medications and special diets are ineffective. Additionally, beware of claims that specially tinted sunglasses or contact lenses can be used to give people with color vision defects improved color vision: this is untrue. These claims are based on improved scores on some standard color vision tests. Some people who dispense these lenses are wrongly convinced that they are helping people see better. Even when scores dramatically improve, what is really happening is that the lenses make some of the colors in a color vision test appear darker or lighter than other colors, allowing a colorblind person to differentiate. Colored lenses effectively help people "cheat" on some colorblind tests. However, there are many tests for which the glasses are not helpful, and the lenses do not significantly improve color vision in the real world.

36. What causes retinitis pigmentosa?

Retinitis pigmentosa (RP) is an inherited, progressive, degenerative disorder of the retina. It is estimated to affect as many as 1 in 4000 people in the U.S. The earliest visual symptoms are losses of peripheral vision. As the disease progresses, the visual loss becomes more central. The final stage is a complete loss of vision.

The progression of the disease is associated with differential distribution of rods and cones in the retina. The cones are concentrated in the central retina in a region called the **fovea**. There are no rod photoreceptors in the center of the fovea. Cone density falls off very quickly outside the central fovea, such that within just a few millimeters from the center, the rods outnumber the cones. In general, rods outnumber cones by about 20:1 in the peripheral retina.

Autosomal RP has been found, so far, to be associated with defects in three different proteins that are specifically expressed in the rod photoreceptors. There are still many cases of RP in which the genetic locus of the disease has not been identified, but this is an active area of research. The best-characterized genetic mutations that cause RP are defects in the genes that encode the rod photopigment, rhodopsin. Since absorption of light by the photopigment molecules is the first step in vision, it is not surprising that mutations in rhodopsin genes cause visual impairment. However, it is not clear why the mutations cause death of the photoreceptors and retinal degeneration. Nor is it clear why the degeneration eventually progresses to destroy the cones in the fovea.

37. What causes night blindness?

Night blindness is caused by a *stationary* defect in the rod photoreceptors, in contrast to retinitis pigmentosa (see Question 36), which is a progressive, degenerative disorder. Deleterious mutations in the genes that encode proteins involved in visual transduction cause congenital stationary night blindness (CSNB). The mutant proteins cause the rod photoreceptor cells to be either active or inactive (see Question 33). Proteins found to be defective in CSNB include rhodopsin (photopigment), transducin, and phosphodiesterases (G-proteins). Why some mutations in visual transduction proteins cause the photoreceptors to degenerate while others cause a loss of visual function without degeneration is not well understood. This is an area of active scientific investigation.

38. Certain drugs, for example Viagra, are said to cause alterations in color vision. How do they act?

Viagra (sildenafil citrate) is an oral therapy for erectile dysfunction. The erection of the penis involves release of nitric oxide (NO) in the erectile tissue (corpus cavernosum). The NO activates the enzyme cyclic guanosine monophosphate (cGMP; see Question 33), which acts indirectly to allow the flow of blood into the tissue. Viagra enhances the effect of NO by inhibiting the enzyme phosphodiesterase type 5 (PDE5), which breaks down cGMP.

A side effect of Viagra is that it causes mild, transient impairment of color vision. This side effect is a sufficient concern to have caused the airlines to recently place restrictions on the use of Viagra by airline pilots. There are many color cues, especially at night and under adverse flying conditions, that must be correctly interpreted by the pilot. While Viagra has a high specificity for PDE5, it also has an inhibitory effect on PDE6, which is involved in phototransduction in the retina. Moreover, both PDE and cGMP are important molecules for intracellular signaling in many neurons, including higher-order neurons in the visual pathway.

Drug-induced color vision manifestations may be caused by an alteration in phototransduction or effect on signaling at a higher level in the visual system, either in second-order neurons in the retina, which are responsible for early visual processing, or in the more central visual system.

39. During embryogenesis the retina originates from an expansion of the neural tube. Neural epithelium eventually becomes the retina. Usually we think of the brain and central nervous system as being what originates from the neural tube. Does this imply that the retina is a true part of the brain?

Yes, it can be considered to be so, based on a number of the retina's characteristics. There is a blood-retinal barrier, like the blood-brain barrier, that restricts movement of certain molecules from the blood vessels into the retina. Like the brain's glia, retinal glial cells (called Muller glia) fill the space between adjacent neurons. In addition, the retinal neurons form layers in a manner similar to neurons in the cerebral cortex.

There are five major neuronal cell types in the retina (Fig. 6). Information is transmitted synaptically from photoreceptors to bipolar cells and from bipolar cells to ganglion cells (whose axons form the optic nerve). In addition to these pathway cells, which carry visual information from the receptor to the brain, there also are two types of interneurons: the horizontal cells and amacrine cells. These interneurons allow for the lateral sharing of information within the retina.

The layering of the retina is more distinct than many brain centers. There are three nuclear layers, and they contain the cell bodies of the neurons. The outer nuclear layer contains cell bodies of the photoreceptors. The ganglion cell layer contains the perikarya of the ganglion cells. Between these two layers is the inner nuclear layer, which contains cell bodies of the bipolar, horizontal, and amacrine cells. Synapses in the retina are made in two plexiform layers, the outer plexiform layer, where photoreceptors synapse with bipolar and horizontal cells, and the inner plexiform layer, where the bipolar cells synapse with amacrine and ganglion cells.

The retina is the "brain" area where the first stage of visual processing takes place. At this early stage, the patterns of connections among the cell types form circuits that give individual ganglion cells specialized properties for responding to stimulus attributes such as form, color, and motion.

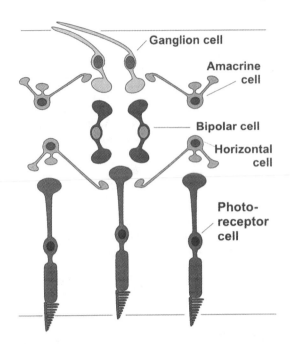

Figure 6. Major neural cell types in the retina. The great variety in dendritic arborization and connectivity within each of the major classes of neurons is not illustrated here. Different patterns of interconnectivity give rise to different types of ganglion cells that are selectively responsive to specific attributes of the visual stimulus. (Refer to Figure 1.)

Labels (top to bottom): Ganglion cell; Amacrine cell; Bipolar cell; Horizontal cell; Photo-receptor cell

40. Do all the nerve fibers in the optic nerve carry the same kind of information, just from different parts of the eye?

No. The fibers in the optic nerve are the axons from the ganglion cells in the retina. Distinctly different kinds of ganglion cells extract very different kinds of information from the retinal image. It is said that parallel pathways carry visual information. Two kinds of visual information are extracted by two major classes of retinal ganglion cells, M cells and P cells. About 90% of the retinal ganglion cells are P cells, and 10% are M cells. These are named because they have different patterns of connections in the magnocellular and parvocellular layers of the lateral geniculate nucleus of the thalamus. The P cells have tiny dendritic fields and carry information necessary for high acuity vision. The M cells have large dendritic fields and are specialized to carry information required for the perception of motion.

41. The electroencephalogram (EEG) and electrocardiogram (EKG) are examples of field or gross potentials. These potentials are recorded from the body's surface, but they represent the summed electrical activity from a population of cells within the body (heart cells, EKG; brain cells, EEG). These measurements are important clinically in the evaluation of heart and brain function. Is there anything similar that can be used to evaluate eye function?

Yes. One potential that can be measured from the eye is the electroretinogram (ERG). The ERG is a valuable tool for evaluating retinal and visual function for clinical diagnosis. One electrode—a fine conducting thread or a smooth foil or wire incorporated into a contact lens—is positioned on the surface of the cornea. A second (reference) electrode is placed elsewhere on the head. Potentials generated by cells in the retina are recorded each time the eye is stimulated by a flash of light (Fig. 7a). For the ERG, voltage changes are plotted as a function of time after the onset of the flash. The ERG is a complex waveform composed of several components (Fig. 7b). There is an initial a-wave that represents, in part, potentials generated by the photoreceptors. It is followed by a b-wave that reflects neural activity generated proximal to the photoreceptors. Two other components, the c- and d-wave, are seen under some recording conditions. The c-wave reflects voltage changes at the level of the retinal pigment epithelium, and the d-wave is an off-potential generated at the cessation of the stimulus. The ERG can be used to determine if the source of a vision disorder is at the level of the retina or in some higher center and, in a limited way, it can be used to determine which cell types in the retina are involved in the disorder.

a.

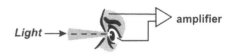

Light →   amplifier

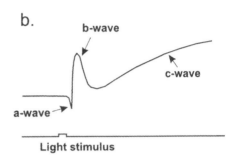

Figure 7. The electroretinogram (ERG). **A**, Conditions for recording. **B**, An example of an ERG waveform like that elicited by a brief flash. The d-wave is not evident in this trace.

b.

b-wave

c-wave

a-wave

Light stimulus

42. What causes amblyopia, and how is it treated?

Most people have known someone who has been diagnosed with amblyopia (sometimes called lazy eye). It is the most common cause of visual loss in young children in the U.S. Amblyopia is a nervous system disorder, but the problem is not with the retina. Amblyopia is formally defined as a unilateral decrease in visual acuity without detectable organic disease of the neural components of the eye (the retina and optic nerve). The most common cause is a cross-eye or wall-eye. However, it is not the nonparallel eye that is ultimately the problem. The root of the disorder is an acuity loss in the deviated eye that does not recover when the cross- or wall-eye is corrected. When a young child has a cross-eye, images from the two eyes are not properly in register. This abnormal visual experience leads to a loss of the normal connections in the central visual system from that eye. Any problem that interferes with the normal registered images from the two eyes can cause amblyopia. Thus, a cataract in one eye or even extreme far- or near-sightedness in one eye can cause it.

The treatment is to first correct image registration. Then a regimen of eye patching is used. Basically, the unaffected eye is patched so that the child is forced to use his amblyopic eye. The eye patching must be monitored carefully to avoid keeping the patch on the "good" eye too long, causing it to become amblyopic while the amblyopic eye takes over. The changes that cause amblyopia are a form of neural plasticity and occur mainly in childhood. The susceptibility is highest at 2–4 years of age, and the plasticity (and susceptibility to amblyopia) is largely over by about ages 7–9.

CENTRAL VISUAL PATHWAYS

The central pathways for conscious visual perception include the dorsal lateral geniculate nucleus, the primary and secondary visual cortices, and a number of higher-order visual areas in the occipital, parietal, and temporal lobes.

Subcortical centers that are involved in visual reflex behavior include the pretectum and the superior colliculus. Both are located in the midbrain.

43. What happens to fibers that leave the retina?

Fibers from the retinal ganglion cells form the optic nerve that leaves the retina. The nasal fibers decussate at the optic chiasm, and the temporal fibers remain on the same side. Both fibers then form the optic tract, which terminates mainly in the lateral geniculate nucleus of the thalamus. About 10% of the fibers project to the pretectum and the superior colliculus of the midbrain. A limited number of fibers project to a few small nuclei in the brain stem as well as to the hypothalamus.

44. What is a receptive field?

The receptive field is the area of the retina in which an image can modify the discharge (excitatory and/or inhibitory) of a visual neuron at different levels of the optic pathway. Receptive fields vary in size and shape. Neurons that process information from the central visual region have receptive fields that are much smaller than those representing more peripheral regions. Receptive fields of retinal ganglion cells, lateral geniculate neurons, and neurons at the first stage of cortical processing are circular, with a concentric and antagonistic center-surround organization. Receptive fields of cortical neurons beyond the first stage are rectangular, with straight-line borders between antagonistic zones.

45. Which aspect of the visual stimulus is most important to the visual system?

Our visual system does not faithfully transmit the absolute light intensity falling on the eye; rather, it is concerned with local differences in intensity. That is, **contrast**—luminance or chromatic—is the key. Each cell signals whether the center of its receptive field is illuminated differently from its surround, but gives little or no signal when both regions are illuminated equally. Thus, receptive fields can be subdivided into ON-center/OFF-surround, OFF-center/ON-surround, Red-ON-center/Green-OFF-surround, and so forth. This principle holds for retinal ganglion cells, lateral geniculate neurons, and visual cortical neurons.

46. What is the role of the pretectum?

The pretectum is involved in the control of pupillary size in response to light or to conscious visual accommodation. The pathways are as follows:

bright light to one eye → optic nerve, optic tract → pretectal nuclei → bilateral Edinger-Westphal (parasympathetic nuclei) → oculomotor preganglionic nerve → bilateral ciliary ganglia → postganglionic nerve → constrictor pupillae muscle of the iris → constriction of both pupils

The response in the stimulated eye is called **direct light reflex**, while the response in the unstimulated eye is known as **consensual light reflex**.

47. What is involved in visual accommodation?

Accommodation is a voluntary act initiated in the cortex (extrastriate and formal eye field [area 8]) and relayed via the superior colliculus and the pretectum. It involves three processes:

• Convergence of eyes by the contraction of both medial recti muscles
• Change of lens shape in both eyes to more convex, due to the contraction of ciliary muscles, which relaxes the suspensory ligament of the lens
• Constriction of both pupils when the pretectal/tectal area, under the direction of the cortex, mediates the reflex.

48. What is Argyll-Robertson pupil?

In this condition the pupils are constricted (miotic), and they respond to accommodation but not to bright light, indicating that the two processes are dissociable. The exact location of the lesion is not known, but it is thought to be in the pretectum of the midbrain. The condition commonly is associated with central nervous system syphilis (tabes dorsalis) and was first described in 1869 by Douglas Argyll Robertson.

49. What is the function of the superior colliculus?

The superior colliculus (SC) is involved in coordinating eye and head movements to track, capture, and maintain a visual image onto the central retina, especially the fovea. Visual information is coordinated with somatosensory and auditory information within the SC to allow proper tracking of environmental stimuli. SC cells are not responsive to diffuse illumination, but are excited by any local change or motion confined to the cell's receptive field. Cells in the deeper layers actually fire in bursts before saccadic eye movements.

50. What is meant by retinotopy?

Retinotopy is an orderly representation of the retina by higher visual centers, such that the retinal surface is "reproduced" onto the surface of these centers. The reproduction often is skewed in favor of a much larger (magnified) representation of the central retina; hence, the central visual field.

LATERAL GENICULATE NUCLEUS

51. How do fibers from the two eyes come together to provide for a single vision?

Nature has devised an ingenious way to bring information seen by each eye together to form a single vision. Fibers from the right half of each eye, which sees the left half of the visual field (because of the inversion of the image by the lens), project to the right dorsal lateral geniculate nucleus (LGN), and fibers from the left half of each eye project to the left LGN. These fibers are aligned in a precise, retinotopic fashion, such that not only do adjacent retinal fibers from the same eye project to adjacent sites in the LGN, but fibers from both eyes that represent the same point in the binocular visual field are aligned vertically in adjacent laminae of the LGN. Thus, a column of cells through the six layers of the LGN (much like a toothpick through a club sandwich) "sees" a single point in the visual field. Adjacent columns "see" adjacent points in the visual field and project to adjacent sites in the primary visual cortex. This topographical overlap is a structural first step toward binocular single vision.

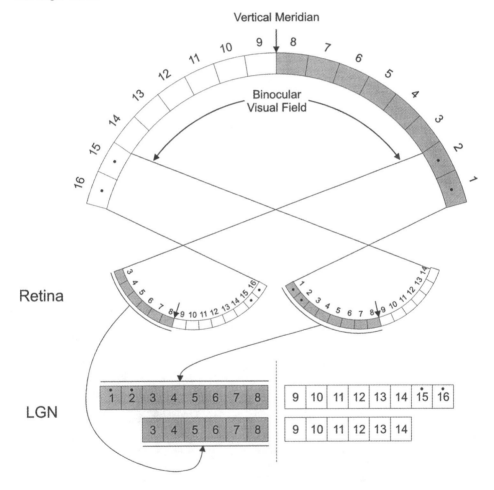

Figure 8. Visuotopic representation in the retina and the lateral geniculate nucleus (LGN). The right half of the visual field *(shaded)* is represented by the left halves of the two retinas *(shaded)*, which project to the left LGN *(shaded)*. Adjacent points in the visual field register to adjacent portions of the LGN (only two of the six major LGN layers are illustrated).

52. What are the consequences of abnormal optic nerve crossing?

Normally, only fibers from the nasal half of each retina cross over to the contralateral LGN to align with ipsilaterally projecting fibers from the temporal half of each retina. If some of the latter fibers decussate to the opposite LGN, they will align with fibers representing different, rather than the same, points in the visual field. The result is double vision or **diplopia**. This abnormal crossing of retinogeniculate fibers occurs in human (and animal) ocular **albinism** that results from a defect in the tyrosinase gene. Tyrosinase is the enzyme that catalyzes the oxidation of tyrosine to form melanin. The lack of pigment in the retinal pigment epithelium results in a misrouting of fibers from about the first 20° of the temporal retina, and this defect is not associated with generalized pigment deficiency. Infants with ocular albinism do not benefit from surgery, because the neural substrate for cortical binocularity is absent.

Guillery RW: Visual pathways in albinos. Sci Am, May 1974, pp 44–54.

Creel D, O'Donnell FE, Witkop CJ: Visual system anomalies in human ocular albinos. Science 201: 931–933, 1978.

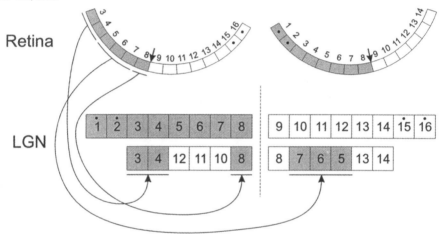

Figure 9.   Disrupted visuotopic representation due to misrouting of the retinogeniculate fibers, a common defect in retinal albinism. Adjacent points in the visual field are no longer represented in adjacent portions of the LGN. This condition frequently leads to diplopia and strabismus.

53. Why are there six major layers in the dorsal lateral geniculate nucleus?

This is an interesting question to which there is no known answer. However, a plausible explanation is as follows: We need at least two layers to segregate the larger relay cells (magnocellular) from the smaller ones (parvocellular) that process different aspects of visual stimuli. Each of the two layers has to separate fibers coming from the two eyes, necessitating four layers. A third division into predominantly ON-center and OFF-center channels (increased response to an increment or a decrement of light, respectively, in the center of the cell's receptive field) for the parvocellular layers requires a minimum of six layers.

Organization of the Major LGN Laminae*

LAMINA	TYPE	PROJECTION	SPECIALIZATION
1	Magnocellular	Contralateral	Mixed ON-center and OFF-center
2	Magnocellular	Ipsilateral	Mixed ON-center and OFF-center
3	Parvocellular	Ipsilateral	Predominantly OFF-center
4	Parvocellular	Contralateral	Predominantly OFF-center
5	Parvocellular	Ipsilateral	Predominantly ON-center
6	Parvocellular	Contralateral	Predominantly ON-center

* Based on studies of macaque LGN; human LGN is similar, except that ON-OFF segregation is assumed but not proven.

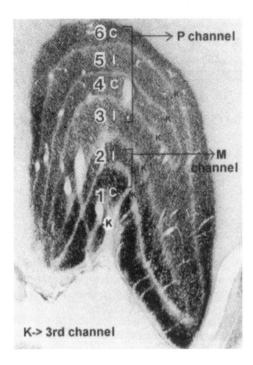

Figure 10. The dorsal LGN of a macaque monkey has laminar organization similar to that of humans. This section has been reacted for a mitochondrial enzyme, cytochrome oxidase, to show differences in metabolic activity. The major layers are numbered 1 to 6 ventro-dorsally. Laminae 1, 4, and 6 receive contralateral (C) retinogeniculate projections, while laminae 2, 3, and 5 receive ipsilateral (I) ones. Layers 1 and 2 form the magnocellular (M) channel, and layers 3 to 6 form the parvocellular (P) channel. Small cells ventral to each of the major laminae form the koniocellular (K) or third channel.

54. What are the koniocellular layers?

In addition to the six major laminae, there also are scattered small cells that form the interlaminar nuclear groups (also called intercalated or koniocellular layers) ventral to each principal layer. These cells are immunoreactive for the α subunit of type II calmodulin-dependent protein kinase (αCaM II kinase) and the 28 kDa vitamin D–dependent calcium-binding protein, calbindin. They project to cytochrome oxidase-rich puffs in the primary visual cortex (see Question 62). They form the so-called "third channel" of geniculocortical projections (in addition to the magnocellular and parvocellular channels).

Hendry SHC, Yoshioka T: A neurochemically distinct third channel in the macaque dorsal lateral geniculate nucleus. Science 264:575–577, 1994.

55. What are the physiologic characteristics of lateral geniculate neurons?

As with retinal ganglion cells, LGN neurons have receptive fields that are of concentric, antagonistic, center-surround organization, but they respond less to diffuse light and more transiently to changes in illumination than ganglion cells. The physiologic properties of LGN relay neurons are dictated not only by their size, shape, and neurochemicals, but also by the input they receive from the retina, visual cortex, and brainstem and locally from interneurons. In general, magnocellular neurons are concerned with high-sensitivity vision of form and contour, but are somewhat colorblind and lack the resolution for fine detail. Parvocellular neurons are slower and less sensitive to light, but they can resolve color and fine details. Most of the time, both systems contribute to vision. Only at the extremes of high flicker or resolution does one system become dominant.

Signals from the retina are modified in the LGN such that the LGN can no longer be considered as a simple relay station.

Receptive Field Properties

	SIZE	TYPE	WAVE-LENGTH	CONTRAST SENSITIVITY	SPATIAL RESOLUTION	RESPONSE
Magnocellular	Large	Concentric, antagonistic, center-surround	Insensitive	High	Low, or medium high	Transient
Parvocellular	Small	Concentric, antagonistic, center-surround	Sensitive: red-green blue-yellow opponency	Low	High	Sustained
Koniocellular	Large?	Concentric, antagonistic, center-surround	Sensitive?	?	?	?

PRIMARY VISUAL CORTEX

56. How is retinotopic organization preserved in the visual cortex?

The primary visual cortex, also known as the striate cortex, area 17, or V1, is the recipient of geniculocortical optic radiation fibers and subserves conscious visual perception. There is a precise, retinotopic representation of the contralateral visual field in each hemisphere. The vertical meridian is represented at the border between areas 17 and 18, and the horizontal meridian bisects it midway. Thus, the contralateral upper visual field is "seen" by the lingual gyrus (lower bank of calcarine fissure), while the contralateral lower visual field is represented by the cuneus gyrus (upper bank of calcarine fissure). The central binocular visual field is represented most posteriorly, and the peripheral monocular visual field most anteriorly. The retinotopic organization is quite skewed because a much larger proportion of the cortex represents the fovea than the peripheral visual field (cortical magnification; see Question 57).

57. What is the magnification factor?

The magnification factor is the number of millimeters of cortex (e.g., primary visual cortex) devoted to the representation of 1° of the visual field. The magnification decreases as the representation moves from the central to the peripheral visual field. For example, the magnification changes from about 4 mm per degree to about 0.5 mm per degree as the representation moves from 1° to 25° away from the center of gaze in the macaque V1. This means that one square degree of the central visual field is represented by 64 times the area of the cortex as is devoted to one square degree of the peripheral visual field.

58. What is so special about the laminar organization of the primary visual cortex?

The visual cortex is a multilayered structure, with six major layers (I to VI) and a number of sublayers. Geniculocortical fibers terminate primarily within layers IVA, IVC, and II/III puffs (see Question 62) and less so in layers I and VI.

As a sensory cortex par excellence, the primary visual cortex has a greatly expanded layer IV, which is subdivided in to IVA, IVB, and IVC (IVCα and IVCβ). Layer IVCα receives input from the magnocellular layers, while layers IVCβ and IVA receive input from the parvocellular layers of the LGN (the koniocellular LGN layers project to II/III puffs). Layer IVB also is known as the stripe of Gennari (named after an enterprising Italian medical student who discovered it) and is visible by eye. It contains cortical fibers rather than geniculate projections. As a whole, layer IV is rich in granule (stellate) cells and is devoid of pyramidal cells.

Signals from layer IV are modified and relayed above and below to supragranular and infragranular layers. This vertical connection forms the basis for functional columns (see Question 61). Supragranular pyramidal cells then project to other cortical areas (such as the secondary visual cortex), while infragranular pyramidal cells project to subcortical visual centers (layer V to the superior colliculus and layer VI to the LGN). The supra- and infra-granular layers contain granule cells mixed in with pyramidal cells that are larger in deeper layers (V and VI) than in superficial (II and III) layers.

59. How do receptive field properties of cortical cells differ from subcortical neurons?

Whereas the receptive fields of retinal ganglion cells and LGN neurons are circular with concentric, center-surround antagonism, only the first-stage cortical neurons in layer IVC have a similar arrangement. The receptive fields of most cortical neurons (about 70–80% in the monkey) are elongated, and they respond best to lines, bars, slits, borders, and edges that have a specific orientation. The elongated receptive center is antagonized by its flanking periphery (on one or both sides). The cells typically respond better to a moving or flickering light than to a stationary line.

Layer IVB cells have direction selectivity—they respond to an oriented stimulus moving across their receptive fields in a particular direction.

60. What are the major physiologic cell types in the visual cortex?

There are two major physiologic cell types in the visual cortex (originally described by Hubel and Wiesel in the 1960s). **Simple cells** are found mainly in layers IVA and IVB. They receive input from three or more LGN neurons. Their receptive fields are subdivided into ON and OFF regions with a straight line as the border. They respond best to a bar or edge of light that fills mainly or exclusively the ON region of their receptive field. The orientation and position of the stimulus are critical.

Complex cells are found in the supragranular (interpuff or interblob; see Question 62) and infragranular layers. They respond poorly to stationary spots of light, and their respective fields do not have discrete ON and OFF regions. An optimally oriented line placed anywhere in the receptive field may elicit about the same response. The width of the line is critical, but the length and exact position are not important. Thus, complex cells are specific for orientation but nonspecific for position. These cells are thought to receive input from a number of simple cells with the same orientation preference.

These two major cell types carry other properties, such as preference/lack of preference for color, direction, eye dominance, orientation, high or low spatial frequencies, and contrast sensitivity.

Figure 11.   Major receptive field types. **A,** The circular or annular receptive field type with antagonistic, center-surround organization is characteristic of the retinal ganglion cells, LGN cells, and some small cortical neurons. When the center is excited (E) by certain stimuli, the surround is inhibited (I) by the same stimuli. **B,** Simple cortical cells have elongated receptive fields with antagonistic central and flanking zones. **C,** Complex cortical cells do not have discrete excitatory or inhibitory regions in their receptive fields. They are particular about the orientation, but not the position, of their stimuli. **D,** Some cortical cells show decreased response when a stimulus extends beyond the ends of their receptive field. This is known as "end-stopping." (This property used to describe a "hypercomplex" type of cell until the same property was found in some simple cells.) (Modified from Willis WD, Grossman RG: Medical Neurobiology, 2nd ed. St. Louis, MO, The C.V. Mosby Co., 1977.)

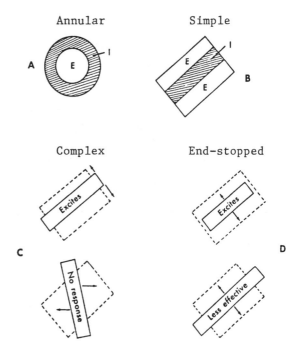

61. What are columns, slabs, and modules?

The primary visual cortex is structurally laminated but functionally columnar. Cells within the same functional column (from laminae I to VI) share similar functions. Hubel and Wiesel (Nobel laureates of 1981) described in both the monkey and the cat visual cortex two major types of **columns**: ocular dominance and orientation.

Within a single *ocular dominance column* (ODC; ~ 0.5 mm wide in humans), lamina IV neurons are strictly monocular, while supra- and infra-granular neurons are binocular but are dominated by the same eye input as lamina IV cells. Left-eye and right-eye columns interdigitate and form zebra-like **slabs** within layer IVC when viewed in a plane tangential to the cortical surface.

Cells within *orientation columns*, which are intermingled within each ODC, respond best to stimuli of a particular orientation (e.g., vertical, horizontal, oblique at 1 o'clock, 2 o'clock). Neighboring columns (each about 50 μm in diameter) have slightly different preferred orientations. As the recording microelectrode advances tangentially through the cortex, orientation preference can be observed to change gradually and progressively.

In addition to eye preference and stimulus orientations, the visual cortex also is concerned with the processing of color, spatial frequencies, and other parameters. Cells involved in such processing are grouped into zones with high or low levels of cytochrome oxidase activity (see Question 62).

A piece of visual cortex with a surface area of 1–2 sq mm probably contains sufficient neural machinery to process visual signals from a particular point in the visual space. It typically includes the minimal and necessary sets of ODCs, orientation columns, and cortical blobs or puffs and is known as a hypercolumn or cortical **module**.

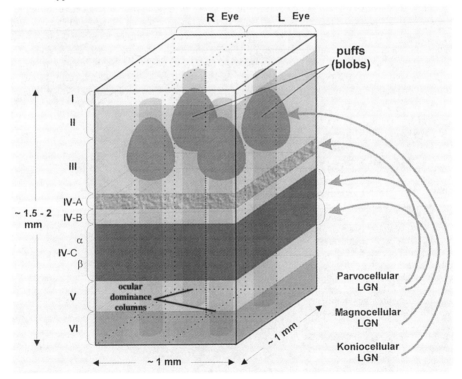

Figure 12.   The primary visual cortex showing cytochrome oxidase-rich and -poor regions. Layers that receive LGN input are moderately to intensely labeled *(light to dark shading)*: IV-A and IV-Cβ from parvocellular LGN; IV-Cα from magnocellular LGN; and II/III puffs (blobs) from koniocellular LGN. Each puff is centered on an ocular dominance column (R = right eye, L = left eye), the centers of which also exhibit slightly higher levels of cytochrome oxidase.

62. What are puffs or blobs?

One of the most striking features of the primate striate cortex is the presence of an extremely regular array of cytochrome oxidase–rich zones in the supragranular layers (II and III). Cytochrome oxidase is a mitochondrial energy–generating enzyme, and so these regions are metabolic "hot spots." They have been given the name puffs or supragranular blobs (also known as dots, patches, or spots). Puffs are laid down before birth in the macaque, but after birth in the human. They receive direct geniculate input from the konio layers and are centered on ocular dominance columns. Cells within puffs have receptive field properties that are distinctly different from those in the interpuffs.

Puffs	*Interpuffs*
Cytochrome oxidase–rich	Cytochrome oxidase–poor
Monocular	Binocular
High spontaneous activity	Low spontaneous activity
Receptive field: mostly circular, color-opponent, center-surround	Receptive field: rectangular; ON- or OFF-center with antagonistic flanks
Orientation-nonspecific	Orientation-specific
Respond to low spatial frequency gratings	Respond to high spatial frequency gratings
Greater color selectivity	Lesser color selectivity
Input: IVCβ and koniocellular LGN layers	Input: IVCβ
Output: thin stripes of V2	Output: interstripes of V2

V2 = secondary visual cortex; see Question 67.

63. What are the known neurotransmitters in the visual cortex?

The major neurotransmitter of cortical projection neurons is glutamate, the universal excitatory transmitter. GABA is the key transmitter of inhibitory interneurons. Other neurochemicals, such as calbindin, calmodulin, neuropeptide Y, parvalbumin, somatostatin, substance P, and nitric oxide, probably serve a modulatory role.

PLASTICITY IN THE VISUAL CORTEX

64. Why is it inadvisable to patch an infant or toddler's eye for long periods of time?

Primates, including humans, are binocular animals. Under normal conditions, the two eyes are equally represented in the visual cortex. If one eye becomes dominant during early stages of development—the critical period—it will command more synaptic space in the cortex. Patching one eye of an infant can result in an imbalance of the two eye–input to the cortex and a subsequent dominance by the open eye. If patching is necessary, alternate patching between the two eyes or patch both eyes to minimize monocular dominance resulting from binocular competition.

65. How plastic is the developing visual cortex?

Even though orientation columns and ocular dominance columns are present in the monkey visual cortex at birth, neurons remain highly plastic during the early stages of postnatal development. Work done in kittens and infant monkeys indicates that a few hours of monocular deprivation during the critical period can alter response properties in the visual cortex. Any type of abnormal visual experience during the critical period of development, such as caused by the deprivation of specific orientational or directional cues, esotropic (convergent) or exotropic (divergent) strabismus, astigmatism, or monocular patching, can lead to irreversible alterations in the functional (and most likely structural) properties of cortical neurons.

66. How plastic is the adult visual cortex?

Although mature neurons have long been regarded as being refractory to change (unless pathology sets in), recent work has demonstrated that they still are capable of responding to altered functional demands. When impulse activity of one eye is blocked in the adult monkey, cortical neurons deprived of their normal input will down-regulate their metabolic enzymes (cytochrome oxidase) as well as other neurotransmitter-related neurochemicals (e.g., GABA, glutamate, NMDA receptors, nitric oxide synthase). Synaptic reorganization also can occur in the mature visual cortex when the input from one eye is perturbed. Changes are reversible when there is no denervation in the adult.

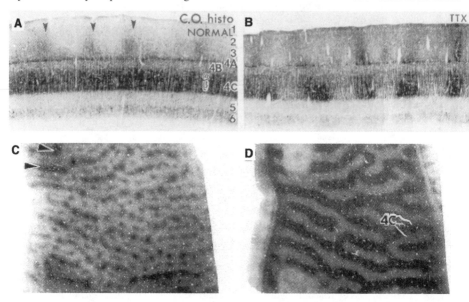

Figure 13. Metabolic plasticity in the mature primate visual cortex. **A**, Cross section of the cortex showing cytochrome oxidase–rich *(dark shading)* and –poor *(light shading)* regions. Note supragranular puffs with high enzyme activity *(arrowheads)*. In **B–D**, the animal was monocularly treated with tetrodotoxin to block retinal ganglion cell activity. **B**, Alternate ocular dominance columns (ODCs) show decreased enzymatic labeling. **C**, Tangential section through layers II/III showing rows of normal puffs *(arrowheads)* interdigitated with rows of shrunken and paler puffs. **D**, Tangential section through layer IVC showing deprived (pale) and nondeprived (dark) ODCs. (Modified from Hevner RF, Wong-Riley MTT: Regulation of cytochrome oxidase protein levels by functional activity in the macaque monkey visual system. J Neurosci 10:1331–1340, 1990.)

SECONDARY VISUAL CORTEX

67. What is the secondary visual cortex?
The secondary visual cortex, known as prestriate cortex, area 18, or area V2 (V2 is only about half the size of Brodmann's area 18 in Old World monkeys and humans), completely surrounds V1 and has its own retinotopic map. Unlike V1, which has a greatly expanded layer IV, the laminar organization of V2 is relatively unremarkable on Nissl stain. However, the metabolic map revealed by cytochrome oxidase is striking. Globular zones of high cytochrome oxidase activity extend from lower layer II to upper layer IV. In tangential sections, these zones form stripes that alternate in thickness.

Thin Stripes	*Thick Stripes*	*Interstripes*
Cytochrome oxidase–rich	Cytochrome oxidase–rich	Cytochrome oxidase–poor
Orientation-nonspecific	Orientation-specific	Orientation-selective
Wavelength-selective	Disparity-selective	——
	Direction-selective	
Respond to:		
Low spatial frequency gratings	Low spatial frequency gratings	High spatial frequency gratings

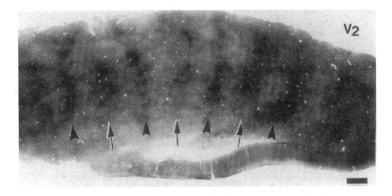

Figure 14. Tangential section through the supragranular layers of the macaque V2, reacted for cytochrome oxidase. Note the enzyme-rich globular zones forming thick *(arrows)* and thin *(arrowheads)* stripes. Scale bar = 1 mm. (From Wong-Riley MTT: Primate visual cortex: Dynamic metabolic organization and plasticity revealed by cytochrome oxidase. In Peters A, Rockland K (eds): Cerebral Cortex, Vol. 10, Primary Visual Cortex in Primates. New York, Plenum Press, 1994, pp 141–200; with permission.)

EXTRASTRIATE VISUAL AREAS BEYOND V2

68. What lies beyond the primary and secondary visual cortical areas?

Beyond area 18, which borders on area 17, Brodmann described an area 19 that surrounds area 18. It initially was regarded as the third visual area, or V3. In reality, area 19 together with several other Brodmann areas can be subdivided into many functional areas, each with is own unique partial visual map. Today, the term area 19 is no longer used, and V3 is only part of the extrastriate cortex that encompass about 30 visual areas in the macaque occipital, parietal, and temporal lobes.

69. What is the middle temporal area?

The middle temporal area, known as **MT** or **V5**, receives direct projections from layer IVB of V1 as well as other cortical areas such as V2 and V3. It is rich in *direction-selective* cells that are organized in functional columns, and it specializes in the processing of *visual motion*. Its input is dominated by influences from the magnocellular LGN projected through V1 to MT. Consequently, its component neurons tend to be highly sensitive to contrast and to dynamic flickering or moving patterns. Activity in MT is altered when a subject attends to movement in the field of view. MT projects heavily to a variety of visual areas in the parietal cortex that are involved in the perception of the spatial arrangement of one's environment. Parietal cortex also is an important component of the system that controls visual attention. A lesion in MT can seriously impair the discrimination of a moving stimulus' direction.

70. What characterizes area V4?

Area V4 in the temporal cortex has been investigated extensively for its color processing property, but it is involved in the spatial perception of both *color* and *shape*. It receives input from the supragranular layers in V1 via V2 and has both orientation-selective and color-selective units. The activity of these units can be altered by changes in the observer's focus of attention.

71. What visual areas lie beyond V4?

Beyond V4 are areas in the **inferotemporal cortex** (IT) that are concerned with visual perception and visual memory. Neurons there often respond well to familiar objects such as faces or food. Lesions in IT can cause selective deficits in restricted portions of vision, such as color or face perception.

72. What is so special about concurrent processing streams?

Much of what we know today about functional streams comes from studies of the macaque monkey, whose visual system resembles ours. Information from the geniculocortical pathway is channeled to different pathways in over 30 extrastriate cortical areas in the occipital, parietal, and temporal lobes. These multiple streams process different attributes of the visual stimuli: color, contrast, form, and movement. The *what* or *ventral* stream for object recognition is channeled to the inferotemporal cortex, and the *where* or *dorsal* stream for spatial localization is channeled to the parietal cortex. The ventral stream is further divided into two parvocellular (P) streams: one for color, form, and movement and the other for color and contrast. The dorsal stream also is known as the magnocellular (M) stream and is concerned with contrast, movement, and stereopsis. Small cells of the LGN (koniocellular) mediate another, less understood pathway. There are, however, crosstalks among the visual centers, especially at the cortical level.

Concurrent Processing Streams

RETINA	LGN	V1	V2	BEYOND V2
		PARVOCELLULAR SYSTEM		
P gang	→ Parvo →	IVCβ → blobs (puffs)	→ thin stripes → V4	→ inferotemporal (color, form, movement)
P gang	→ Parvo →	IVCβ → interblobs (interpuffs)	→ interstripes → V3? V4?	→ inferotemporal (color, contrast)
		MAGNOCELLULAR SYSTEM		
M gang → Magno →	IVCα →	IVB	→ thick stripes → V3 → MT	→ parietal (contrast, movement, stereopsis)
		KONIOCELLULAR: A THIRD CHANNEL?		
? gang	→ Konio →	blobs (puffs)	?	?

73. What is involved in visual perception?

Visual perception is the ability to identify and recognize a stimulus by sight. It requires an intact retino-geniculo-cortical pathway and intact visual cortical areas beyond V1. Within V1, functional modules that are activated by the same visual object are activated at the same time, possibly through horizontal connections that link the cells in layer III (e.g., puff neurons connect to other puff neurons; cells with the same orientation preference are interconnected). Cells in widely separated modules often burst synchronously to the same visual stimulus. Images that span across the vertical meridian are "joined" by callosal fibers representing the vertical midline. A familiar object, such as the face of one's grandmother, may elicit a strong response from a population of neurons in the inferotemporal cortex. In short, neural pathways that started out as separate channels are interconnected at various levels so that the final percept is an integration of various visual attributes (such as color, motion, form, and depth). Moreover, other attributes such as auditory, somatosensory, olfactory, past memory, and emotions often add dimensions to our visual perception. All of these have a neural basis, the details of which are topics of intense investigation.

74. What can functional magnetic resonance imaging (FMRI) tell us about visual processing?

FMRI captures brain signals generated by local changes in blood oxygenation in subjects who respond to sensory (or other) stimuli. This approach has the distinct advantage of being able to investigate the living brain. Results from human studies have been compared with a wealth of information gathered from animal studies. Thus far, borders that are topographically homologous to areas V1, V2, V3, VP (ventroposterior), parts of V3A, V4, and MT (middle temporal/medial superior temporal area complex) of the macaque monkey have been identified in the human visual cortex. Other temporal and parietal visual areas also have been observed.

DeYoe EA, Carman GJ, Bandettini P, et al: Mapping striate and extrastriate visual areas in human cerebral cortex. Proc Natl Acad Sci USA 93:2382–2386, 1996.

Sereno MI: Brain imaging in animals and humans. Curr Opinions Neurobiol 8:188–194, 1998.

Tootell RB, Hadjikhani NK, Vanduffel W, et al: Functional analysis of primary visual cortex (V1) in humans. Proc Natl Acad Sci USA 95:811–817, 1998.

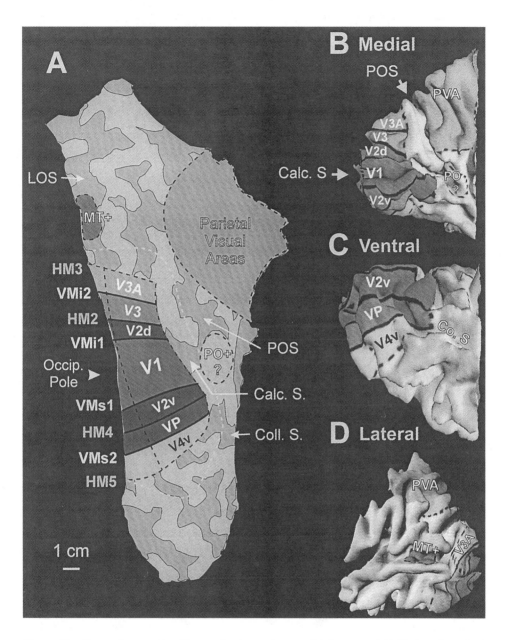

Figure 15. Proposed topography of human visual areas shown on (**A**) flat map and (**B–D**) three-dimensional models of occipital lobe. V1 = primary visual cortex, V2d and V2v = dorsal and ventral divisions of second visual area, V3 = third visual area, VP = ventroposterior visual area, V4v = ventral division of fourth visual area, MT+ = middle temporal area plus neighboring visual areas, Calc. S. = calcarine sulcus, Coll.S. and Co.S. = collateral sulcus, LOS = lateral occipital sulcus, Occip. Pole = occipital pole, POS = parieto-occipital sulcus, PVA = various poorly defined parietal visual areas, HM = retinotopic representations of the horizontal meridian of the visual field, VM = representations of the vertical meridian. (Figure courtesy Dr. Edgar A. DeYoe; visual area nomenclature from reference 16)

75. What are the guiding principles of organization of the visual system?
 • The analysis of change, either spatial or temporal, is the key.
 • Anatomic structures are laminated in the retina, LGN, and the visual cortex.
 • Functional subunits such as columns are present in the retina, LGN, and the visual cortex.
 • Functional modules in the visual cortex can analyze information from discrete areas of the visual field.
 • Signals are modified by interneurons and/or feedback fibers in the retina, LGN, and the visual cortex.
 • Topographic representation of the visual world is maintained, though often skewed in the retina, LGN, and the visual cortex.
 • Visual information is analyzed by many different cortical areas. A single attribute such as shape is analyzed by a subset of these areas. Conversely, single visual areas contribute to more than one function.
 • Concurrent functional streams are specialized in the processing of color, form, contrast, and motion.

76. What are the common visual anomalies involving the central visual pathways?
Tumor, vascular lesion, or head injury can cause visual field deficits. When the lesion is limited in scope, it causes a well-defined scotoma. When the lesion is extensive, partial or entire hemifield blindness can occur.

*Classic Lesion Sites**	*Consequences*
1. Optic nerve	Total blindness in the ipsilateral eye
2. Optic chiasm	Heteronymous bitemporal hemianopsia (tunnel vision)
3. Lateral edge of chiasm	Contralateral hemianopsia in ipsilateral eye
4. Optic tract	Contralateral homonymous hemianopsia
5. Meyer's loop (temporal lobe) or lingual gyrus	Contralateral homonymous superior quadrantanopsia
6. Retrolenticular limb or cuneus gyrus	Contralateral homonymous inferior quadrantanopsia
7. Optic radiation or area 17	Contralateral homonymous hemianopsia, often with macular sparing

* See Figure 16. Numbers correspond.

77. What is cerebral achromatopsia?
Cerebral achromatopsia is a perceptual disorder in which the individual's ability to distinguish objects by their hue (color) is lost after the extrastriate cortex is damaged. Patients are unable to arrange colors in chromatic sequence, and they fail most conventional tests of color blindness. This condition, however, is not to be confused with congenital color blindness, which is caused by genetic mutations. Cerebral achromatopsia often is caused by a vascular lesion involving the ventromedial occipital cortex, either unilaterally or bilaterally. It probably destroys part or all of the color-opponent parvocellular channel in a region of the visual cortex that is rostral to area V4.

78. What is blindsight?
Blindsight is a phenomenon reported in some patients with severe striate cortical lesions. While these patients are unable to consciously see objects in their blind visual field, they are able to detect and discriminate unseen stimuli when subjected to a forced-choice paradigm. They reportedly can look at unseen objects, point to them, and detect movement, wavelength, and flicker even though they deny any visual sensation of their visual tracking. The anatomic basis for blindsight is not entirely clear, but may involve retinal signals reaching the extrastriate cortex via one or more relay stations (such as the superior colliculus, accessory optic nuclei in the brainstem, the lateral geniculate nucleus, or the pulvinar by way of the superior colliculus).

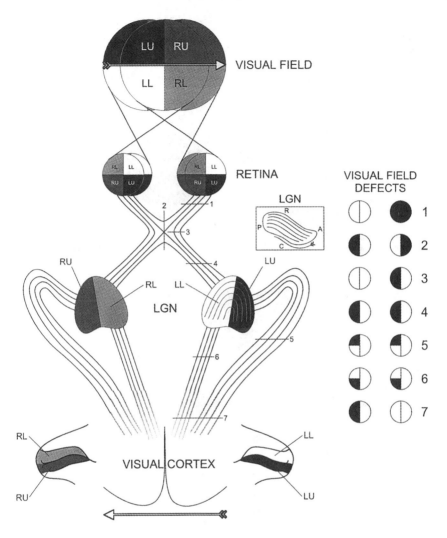

Figure 16.   The retino-geniculo-cortical pathway, showing visuotopic organization. Possible lesions at various sites are marked by numbered lines; numbers correspond to Visual Field Defects chart.

BIBLIOGRAPHY

Non-Neuronal Tissue of the Eye
1. Christen WG, Glynn RJ, Hennekens CH: Antioxidants and age-related eye disease: Current and future perspectives. Ann Epidemiol 6:60–66, 1996.
2. Flanagan JG: Glaucoma update: Epidemiology and new approaches to medical management. Ophthal and Physiol Optics 18:133–139, 1998.
3. Graw J: The crystallins: Genes, proteins, and diseases. Biol Chem 378:1331–1348, 1997.
4. Hersch PS, Scher KS, Irani R: Corneal topography of photorefractive keratectomy versus laser in situ keratomileusis. Summit PRK-LASIK Study Group. Ophthalmol 105:612–619, 1998.
5. Hodge WG, Whitcher JP, Satariano W: Risk factors for age-related cataracts. Epidemiol Rev 17:336–346, 1995.
6. Hook DW, Harding JJ: Protection of enzymes by α-crystallin acting as a molecular chaperone. Int J Biol Macromol 22:295–306, 1998.

7. Safarazi M: Recent advances in molecular genetics of glaucomas. Hum Mol Gen 6:1667–1677, 1997.
8. Silvestri G: Age-related macular degeneration: Genetics and implications for detection and treatment. Mol Med Today 3:84–91, 1997.

Retina
9. Rodieck RW: The First Steps in Seeing. Sunderland, Massachusetts, Sinauer Associates, Inc., 1998.

Subcortical and Cortical Visual Centers
10. Bear MF, Connors BW, Paradiso MA: Neuroscience: Exploring the Brain. Baltimore, Williams and Wilkins, 1996.
11. Cowey A, Heywood CA: There's more to colour than meets the eye. Behav Brain Res 71:89–100, 1995.
12. Cowey A, Stoerig P: The neurobiology of blindsight. Trends Neurosci 14:140–145, 1991.
13. DeYoe EA, Carman G, Bandettini P, et al: Mapping striate and extrastriate visual areas in human cerebral cortex. Proc Natl Acad Sci USA 93(6):2382–2386, 1996.
14. DeYoe EA, Van Essen DC: Concurrent processing streams in monkey visual cortex. Trends Neurosci 11:219–226, 1988.
15. Engel SA, Glover GH, Wandell BA: Retinotopic organization in human visual cortex and the spatial precision of functional MRI. Cerebral Cortex 7:181–192, 1997.
16. Felleman DJ, Van Essen DC: Distributed hierarchical processing in primate cerebral cortex. Cerebral Cortex 1:1–47, 1991.
17. Hendry SHC, Calkins DJ: Neuronal chemistry and functional organization in the primate visual system. Trends Neurosci 21:344–349, 1998.
18. Hevner RF, Wong-Riley MTT: Regulation of cytochrome oxidase protein levels by functional activity in the macaque monkey visual system. J Neurosci 10:1331–1340, 1990.
19. Horton JC, Hedley-Whyte ET: Mapping of cytochrome oxidase patches and ocular dominance columns in human visual cortex. Phil Trans R Soc Lond B 304:255–272, 1984.
20. Hubel DH, Wiesel TN: Receptive field and functional architecture of monkey striate cortex. J Physiol 195:215–243, 1968.
21. Kaas JH: Human visual cortex: Progress and puzzles. Current Biol 5:1126–1128, 1995.
22. Livingstone MS, Hubel DH: Anatomy and physiology of a color system in the primate visual cortex. J Neurosci 4:309–356, 1984.
23. Merigan WH, Maunsell JHR: How parallel are the primate visual pathways? Annu Rev Neurosci 16:369–402, 1993.
24. Tootell RBH, Hamilton SL: Functional anatomy of the second visual area (V2) in the macaque. J Neurosci 9:2620–2644, 1989.
25. Tootell RBH, Silverman MS, Hamilton SL, et al: Functional anatomy of macaque striate cortex. V. Spatial frequency. J Neurosci 8:1610–1624, 1988.
26. Ungerleider LG, Haxby JV: "What" and "where" in the human brain. Curr Opinion in Neurobiol 4:157–165, 1994.
27. Van Essen DC, Gallant JL: Neural mechanisms of form and motion processing in the primate visual system. Neuron 13:1–10, 1994.
28. Wong-Riley MTT: Primate visual cortex: Dynamic metabolic organization and plasticity revealed by cytochrome oxidase. In Peters A, Rockland K (eds): Cerebral Cortex. Vol. 10, Primary Visual Cortex in Primates. New York, Plenum Press, 1994, pp 141–200.

ACKNOWLEDGMENT

The critical reading of the "Central Visual Pathways" portion of the chapter by Dr. E. DeYoe is greatly appreciated. Thanks also go to John Kusch for his computerized artwork.

6. THE AUDITORY SYSTEM

Jon H. Kaas, Ph.D., and Troy A. Hackett, Ph.D.

1. What is the auditory system?

The auditory system is a network of receptors and associated pathways, nuclei, and cortical areas that are used for auditory reflexes and the perception of sounds (Fig. 1). The system is unusual in the number of brainstem nuclei that are involved in the processing of sounds before auditory cortex is reached. The auditory nervous system depends on the ear and associated structures that transform vibratory changes in air pressure to effective stimulations of auditory receptors.

2. How does the ear function in hearing?

The ear is commonly divided into three major divisions: the external ear, the middle ear, and the internal ear (Fig. 2). Each has different functions. The external ear also is called the **pinna**. The pinna is a feature of mammals and is not found in reptiles and birds, although some birds, such as the owl, have ruffs of feathers that serve much the same purpose. The pinna can improve sensitivity to sound by reflecting and directing sound toward the opening of the ear canal, or **external auditory meatus**. The pinna aids in sound localization, especially in mammals that can move it, because its shape allows sounds from some directions to be more effectively reflected than others. Sounds from below are altered differently than sounds from above, providing some information about sound direction.

The acoustic resonance properties of the pinna enhance the intensity of some sounds, so that certain acoustic frequencies reach the tympanic membrane at an increased intensity. The human ear can detect acoustic frequencies from about 20–20,000 hertz (Hz,) but is most sensitive at 250–8000 Hz, which is the frequency range of the most important sounds of communication (e.g., speech). In terms of intensity, the weakest sound detectable by the human auditory system averages 0 decibels (dB). Zero (0) dB does not refer to the absence of sound, but to the average threshold for sound pressure, which is 0.0002 dyne/cm^2, or 20 µPa. At the other end of the intensity range, sound becomes uncomfortably loud at approximately 100–120 dB, and painfully loud above that.

3. Does the ear canal or external auditory meatus have function?

The external auditory canal, or meatus, is part of the external ear. It leaves the pinna and extends into the head to the middle ear. A major function is to protect the eardrum or **tympanic membrane** at its internal end from damage. In many mammals, such as cats, this function is aided by complex folds and turns in the tissue of the pinna near the meatus, so that insects find it difficult to enter the meatus. Also, cells excrete a waxy substance to discourage insects. The meatus has rather complex resonance properties, which increase the sensitivity of the ear in the middle frequency range. Pressure fluctuations in air are reflected by the pinna and propagated through the meatus to vibrate the tympanic membrane. The meatus in humans is about 2.6 cm long and 0.7 cm wide.

4. What is the middle ear?

The middle ear is a small cavity bounded on the outside by the tympanic membrane and the inside by the **temporal bone**, which houses the internal ear. The middle ear contains the three small bones or ossicles that transmit vibrations of the tympanic membrane to the inner ear. The air space around the ossicles is connected to the pharynx by the Eustachian tube, so that the pressure differences between the outer and inner ear can be equalized. Extreme pressure differences displace the tympanic membrane and cause pain. The narrowness of the Eustachian tube means that it can be blocked by secretions during infections and not function properly.

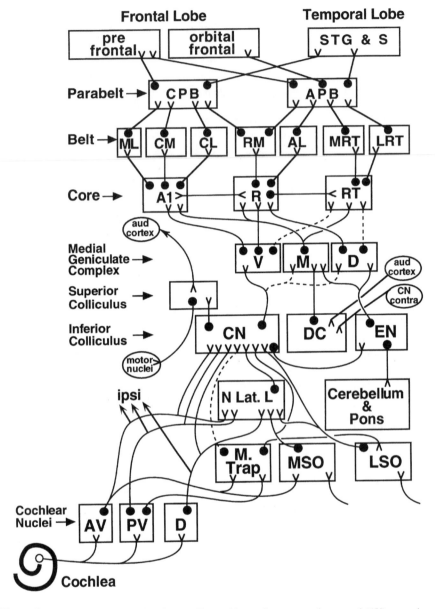

Figure 1. The auditory system in primates. The cochlea projects to anterior ventral (AV), posterior ventral (PV) and dorsal (D) cochlear nuclei. These nuclei project to the lateral superior olive (LSO), the medial superior olive (MSO), the medial nucleus of the trapezoid body (M. Trap), the nucleus of the lateral lemniscus (N Lat. L), and the central nucleus of the inferior colliculus. Other divisions of the inferior colliculus include the dorsal cortex (DC) and the external nucleus (EN). The inferior colliculus projects to the ventral (V), medial (M), and dorsal (D) nuclei of the medial geniculate complex, which relays to auditory cortex, including the core areas of primary auditory cortex (AI), the rostral area (R), and the rostrotemporal area (RT). Proposed belt areas of auditory cortex, with inputs from the core, are named by position as middle lateral (ML), caudomedial (CM), caudolateral (CL), rostromedial (RM), anterior lateral (AL), medial rostrotemporal (MRT), and lateral rostrotemporal (LRT). Belt areas project to the caudal (CPB) and rostral (RPB) divisions of the parabelt region, as well as other cortex. The parabelt projects to the superior temporal gyrus (STG) and sulcus (S), and to the frontal lobe.

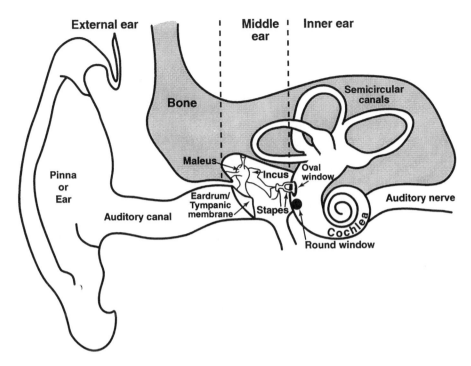

Figure 2.   The external, middle, and internal parts of the ear. The semicircular canals, part of the vestibular system, also are indicated.

5. How do the bones of the middle ear function in hearing?

The middle ear has three small bones (transformed from skull and jawbones of fish) that bridge the space from tympanic membrane to oval window of the inner ear: the **malleus** or hammer, the **incus** or anvil, and the **stapes** or stirrup. The bones are suspended in the middle ear space by ligaments and interconnect so that movement of the malleus, which is attached to the tympanic membrane, moves the incus, which in turn moves the stapes. The footplate of the stapes exactly fills the oval window of the cochlea. Movements of the stapes are transferred to the fluid-filled cochlea by this interface. The large surface area of the tympanic membrane relative to that of the stapes footplate and oval window, and the mechanical advantage introduced by the configuration of the ossicular chain, create a mechanical advantage. The net result is that small movements of the tympanic are transformed into a more forceful movement of the stapes at a ratio of about 17:1. This mechanical advantage is necessary to overcome the impedance mismatch in the transduction of acoustico-mechanical energy into hydraulic energy within the cochlea. Thus, the middle ear bones function as an acoustic transformer that effectively *transforms* the sound energy of moving air to the motions of fluid in the inner ear.

6. The middle ear contains two small muscles. What do they do?

The two muscles of the inner ear are the **tensor tympani** and the **stapedius**. The tensor tympani attaches to the malleus, and the stapedius to the stapes. These muscles contract reflexively to intense sounds with latencies of 150 and 60 msec, respectively, and thereby protect the ear from acoustic trauma by restricting ossicular movements. They also help keep the ossicular chain in position.

7. What is the internal ear?

The internal ear is known as the **cochlea**, or snail, because the structure is coiled like the shell of a snail to save space. It is completely embedded in the temporal bone. The cochlear spiral begins in a fluid-filled chamber, the vestibule, where movements of the oval window displace fluid. The fluid-filled cochlea coils from the vestibule to terminate in a third turn and contains three parallel canals: the scala tympani, scala vestibuli, and scala media. The scala media contains the organ of Corti and the auditory receptors.

8. How does the cochlea work?

The cochlea is a structure designed to transform hydraulic sound energy into the mechanical stimulation of a long row of hair cells, which initiate neural transmission of the signal (Fig. 3). The site of maximal stimulation varies in place with sound frequency and in magnitude with sound intensity. Inward movements of the stapes displace fluid in the scala vestibuli portion of the cochlea, which is compensated for by an outward movement into the middle ear of the round window at the end of the scala tympani. The pressure changes displace the support structure for the auditory receptors, the basilar membrane, so that the receptors move relative to a more stable cover, the **tectorial membrane** in the middle of the scala media. The auditory receptor cells have bundles of "hairs" or **stereocilia** that extend from their apical surface to contact the gelatinous tectorial membrane, which is fixed along its internal margin, but free elsewhere. The movement of the basilar membrane supporting the hair cells produces a shearing motion that bends the stereocilia, leading to a chemo-electrical event in the hair cell. This event triggers action potentials (signals) in the axons of the auditory nerve.

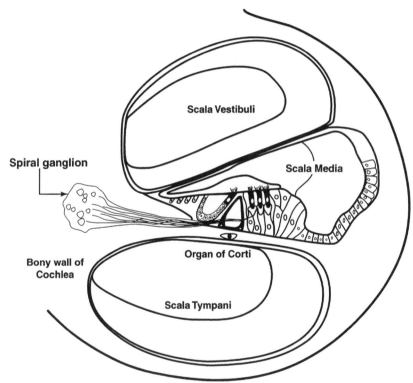

Figure 3. A section of the coiled cochlea showing innervation of the single row of inner hair cells and the three rows of outer hair cells by afferents with their cell bodies (ganglion cells) in the spiral ganglion. Efferents to the outer hair cells have their cell bodies in the brain stem. The tectorial membrane lies over the hair cells, which rest, along with supporting cells, on the basilar membrane. The hair cells, supporting cells, and associated membranes make up the organ of Corti. Fluids are contained within the three channels or ducts: scala vestibuli, scala media, and scala tympani.

9. How are hair cells stimulated by tones of different frequencies and intensities?

Movements of the stapes produce pressure changes in the cochlear fluids, which displace the basilar membrane to bend the stereocilia of the hair cells. The **basilar membrane** is a long, narrow structure with mechanical properties that result in a traveling wave of displacement of the basilar membrane for each displacement of the stapes. Displacements at high frequencies reach a peak only a short way from the stapes, while displacements for low tones peak farther away, largely due to a great change in the stiffness and width of the basilar membrane along its length. Thus, different locations along the basilar membrane, and different hair cells, are maximally stimulated by different frequencies from high to low. More intense tones produce greater displacements and more intense stimulation of hair cells. In addition, more hair cells are activated. Complicated sounds with a number of frequencies distort the basilar membrane in more complex ways, but largely (not completely) as a summation of the effects of the component frequencies and their relative amplitudes.

10. What is the organ of Corti?

The structures resting on the basilar membrane, including the hair cells, the supporting cells, the nerve terminals, and the tectorial membrane, are called the organ of Corti.

11. How are the receptor hair cells arranged in the organ of Corti?

The hair cells are arranged in long rows along the length of the basilar membrane. One group of hair cells is inner, being nearer to the inner part of the organ where the tectorial membrane attaches. Another group of hair cells is outer, closer to the free margin of the tectorial membrane. The inner hair cells form a single long row, while the outer hair cells form three or more rows. In humans, there are about 3500 inner hair cells in a single row and 12,000 outer hair cells, initially in three rows but increasing to four or five rows.

12. What are the functions of the inner and outer hair cells?

Remarkably, all, or nearly all, of the auditory information sent to the brain is from the single row of inner hair cells. Thus, the auditory sensory surface is truly a one-dimensional surface, in contrast to the skin and retina. The much more numerous outer hair cells are effector organs. When stimulated by efferent fibers from the brain stem, the mechanical properties of the outer hair cells are changed, altering the tuning properties and sensitivity of the organ of Corti. The functions of the few afferents arising from the outer hair cells are not known.

13. Are there efferents in the auditory nerve?

Yes. Neurons in the superior olivary complex send axons to the cochlea to make up the **olivo-cochlear bundle** or pathway. Neurons in the lateral superior olive project to the cochlea to terminate on the ends (terminal dendrites) of nerve VIII afferents as these afferents contact the inner hair cells. This neuron-to-neuron synapse modifies the transmission of information in afferents from the inner hair cells to the cochlear nuclei. Medial superior olive neurons project to the outer hair cells, rather than neurons. These projections are bilateral, with most going to the contralateral organ of Corti. These efferents may modify the shape of the outer hair cell, thereby altering the mechanical properties of the organ of Corti.

14. What do the stereocilia on the hair cells do?

The bundles of stereocilia on the apical surface of each hair cell are arranged in a broad V or W formation from shortest to tallest. In the vestibular portion of the inner ear, hair cells have a single, tall **kinocilium** in addition to the bundle of stereocilia, but the kinocilium is absent in the cochlea. In both the vestibular and cochlear systems, the bending of the stereocilia in one direction (i.e., toward the tallest stereocilia/kinocilium) opens ion channels, so that the ion exchange between the inside and outside of the cell increases. Influx of K+ into the hair cell rapidly depolarizes (deactivates) the nerve terminals on the hair cells, so that signals are sent to the brain. Movement of the hair cells in the opposite direction, toward the shortest stereocilia, results in closure of the ion channels and hyperpolarization of the hair cell. Thus, the periodic movements of the basilar membrane generate alternating cycles of hyperpolarization and depolarization of the hair cells that follow the waveform of the acoustic stimulus. The resulting cyclic changes in electrical activity can be measured along with other auditory evoked potentials. This particular electrical potential is commonly called the **cochlear microphonic**, because it faithfully reproduces the acoustic waveform.

15. How do nerve fibers conduct information from the cochlea?

Almost all of the afferents of the cochlea are remarkably alike in how they respond to sounds. Because of the mechanical properties of the organ of Corti, afferents are activated with each displacement of the basilar membrane at low frequencies. At higher frequencies, the afferents cannot respond to every displacement, but fire (discharge) on some of them. Depending on their locations along the basilar membrane, they respond to different ranges of frequencies and have different best frequencies.

The **best frequency** is the tone at which afferents are most sensitive and can respond to the least intense sound. As sounds increase in intensity, the neuron is activated over a greater and greater range of frequencies, and the response may increase in number of action potentials or spikes per stimulus. Neurons typically are characterized by **frequency-amplitude response** curves, which plot the minimum intensity for a response (action potential) as a tone varies in frequency. The response area within the curve is where stimuli effectively activate the afferent.

Afferents are similar in that they have a *single* best frequency, *rapidly* become less sensitive at higher frequencies (the high frequency cut-off), and *gradually* become less sensitive at lower frequencies. Five percent of afferents come from the outer hair cells. These afferents are thin and difficult to record from. It is not known what they do or how they respond to auditory stimuli, if at all.

16. Where are the somata (cell bodies) of auditory afferent neurons located?

The afferent neurons, which constitute 95% of the auditory nerve, are bipolar (two-process) neurons with cell bodies or ganglion cells in the spiral ganglion, which parallels the organ of Corti in a canal in the bone. One process of each ganglion usually innervates a single inner hair cell, and each inner hair cell is innervated by many afferents. The proximal processes of the bipolar cells run together to form the auditory nerve (cranial nerve VIII), which travels through the skull over a 5-mm course to enter the medulla of the brainstem at the level of the cochlear nucleus.

17. What do first-order (nerve VIII) auditory afferents innervate?

Each cochlear nerve fiber enters the brain stem and bifurcates to terminate in the dorsal and ventral cochlear nuclei. The ventral nucleus commonly is divided into anteroventral and posteroventral nuclei. These nuclei have different cell types, and transformations take place at this level to change a rather uniform type of input into several distinct types of output.

18. What do the cochlear nuclei do?

Different synaptic mechanisms and neuron types in these nuclei result in neurons of quite different response properties. Properties of nerve VIII afferents, such as phase-locking (following tone displacement cycles or phases), are preserved and enhanced in the anteroventral cochlear nucleus (AVCN), in part due to large and specialized synaptic endings (the end-bulbs of Held) that secure synaptic transmission. These neurons in the AVCN preserve the information of the auditory nerve for transmission and analysis by neurons in higher centers. In contrast, the neurons of the dorsal cochlear nucleus (DCN) start to analyze the auditory inputs with, of course, a loss of information. Thus, the outputs of these neurons differ from the inputs, and several different types of output are created. Their functions are not well understood.

Afferents terminate in the AVCN and DCN in orderly patterns, so each has a **tonotopic organization**. Thus, neurons across these structures systematically vary in best frequency, the tone for which they are most sensitive.

The role of the posteroventral cochlear nucleus (PVCN) is not well understood.

19. Where do the outputs of the cochlear nuclei go?

The outputs of the cochlear nuclei form three major tracts. The dorsal auditory tract, or **stria**, from the DCN crosses the midline of the brain stem and terminates in contralateral nuclei of the lateral lemniscus and the inferior colliculus. The intermediate auditory stria from the PVCN and DCN supplies neurons around and in the superior and lateral superior olives of both sides. The axons of neurons in the AVCN innervate the trapezoid body, the medial superior olive bilaterally, and the lateral superior olive ipsilaterally. Thus, outputs from different sources reach different targets.

20. How do the medial and lateral nuclei of the superior olive function in sound localization?

Sounds are localized largely by differences in the timing and sound intensity of input; sounds typically reach one ear first and are more intense in the ear nearest the source. Other cues come from head and ear movements that alter loudness ("scanning").

Neurons in the lateral superior olive (LSO) receive ipsilateral excitatory connections from the AVCN and inhibitory inputs indirectly from the contralateral AVCN via a relay in the trapezoid body (Fig. 4). These inputs make LSO neurons extremely sensitive to relative sound intensity differences in the two ears. Further, since the dampening of sound intensities by the head (the "acoustic shadow") is most effective for sounds of higher frequencies, the majority of LSO neurons have high best frequencies.

In contrast, neurons of the medial superior olive (MSO) receive excitatory inputs from the AVCN of both ears, and these neurons tend to respond in a phase-locked manner to the frequency cycle of a tone. Since cycle phase differences increase for low tones as they successively reach the nearer and further ear, MSO neurons tend to have low best frequencies and are very sensitive to phase differences in the two ears. MSO neurons also are extremely sensitive to internal delay, because of the additive effects of precisely concurrent inputs.

Thus, the superior olive codes for stimulus location via different populations of neurons that are sensitive to sound intensity and delay in the two ears. Delays are best detected for low frequency sounds, while intensity differences are best detected for high frequency sounds.

21. What is the lateral lemniscus?

Afferents from the cochlear nuclei and the superior olive ascend to the auditory midbrain (inferior colliculus) in a fiber pathway known as the lateral lemniscus. The pathway also contains descending auditory fibers. By comparison, the medial lemniscus is composed of somatosensory afferents to the thalamus.

The lateral lemniscus includes three groups of auditory neurons: the dorsal, intermediate, and ventral nuclei. These nuclei receive auditory inputs from axons in the pathway and project to the inferior colliculus. Their functions are not well understood.

22. What is the inferior colliculus?

The inferior colliculus (IC) is the major *auditory* structure of the midbrain. The major *visual* structure is the superior colliculus (SC) (see Question 24). The IC features a large, central nucleus where auditory inputs terminate in a precise pattern (or map) that maintains tonotopic order. Neurons preserve information about sound frequency and intensity. Sound localization information in the binaural signals from the superior olive also is preserved, but there is no systematic map of sound location. The central nucleus outputs to the auditory thalamus.

The IC is capped by a **dorsal cortex**, which receives descending inputs from auditory cortex and projects to dorsal cortex of the other side of the brainstem and the auditory thalamus of the same side. More laterally, an external nucleus has connections with the brainstem and auditory thalamus.

23. What are the functions of the components of the inferior colliculus?

The **central nucleus** is regarded as a relay nucleus with purely auditory functions; projections are to the auditory thalamus and then to auditory cortex. The **external nucleus** is thought to have multimodal (auditory and somatosensory) functions and to relay via pontine nuclei to the cerebellum and to midbrain structures having motor functions. Outputs to the auditory thalamus are relayed to widespread regions of auditory cortex to modulate nerve activity. The dorsal cortex, also called the pericentral nucleus, receives descending inputs from the auditory cortex, which probably modulate and influence descending and intercollicular pathways.

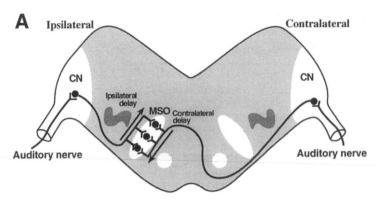

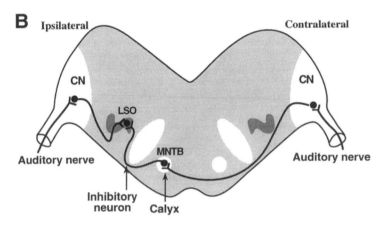

Figure 4. Inputs to the medial superior olive (MSO) and lateral superior olive (LSO) of the auditory brain-stem. **A,** The MSO receives inputs from the cochlear nucleus (CN) of both sides. Because the lengths of axons subserving neurons along the MSO differ, and impulses require more time to travel longer distances, the axons function as **delay lines**, with signals converging at the same or slightly different times on individual neurons in the nucleus. The delay initially is encoded by phase differences in the cochlea based on the arrival time of sound in each ear (remember that neuronal spikes are locked to a phase in the cycle). Thus, phase differences based on sound location are converted to a spatial map in the MSO. **B,** Neurons in the LSO receive excitatory inputs from the ipsilateral CN and inhibitory inputs slightly later from the contralateral CN via a relay in the medial nucleus of the trapezoid body (MNTB). Differences in sound intensity in the two ears are translated into differences of excitation and inhibition as well as LSO output magnitude.

24. Are there other auditory structures in the midbrain?

The superior colliculus, which is primarily a visual structure, also has auditory functions. The superior colliculus is layered, and the superficial (external) layers form a visual map of the retina. Deeper layers form a visuomotor map, so that electrical stimulation of any site in the deeper layers causes the eye and gaze to shift to a location corresponding to the retinal or visual receptive field for neurons just above, in the superficial layer. The deep layers also receive auditory inputs from the brainstem and auditory cortex, and these inputs may form a **map of auditory space**. The visuomotor neurons of the superior colliculus may be employed to move the head and eyes so that sounds of interest are visually inspected.

25. Does a map of auditory space also exist in the inferior colliculus?

In owls and possibly other birds a nucleus homologous to the external nucleus of the inferior colliculus provides a map of auditory space. Owls hunt in the dark using sounds to locate mice and other prey. Such a map has not been found in mammals, and may be a specialization in owls.

26. How is the auditory thalamus organized?

The **medial geniculate nucleus**, the major auditory structure of the thalamus, is more properly called the medial geniculate *complex* (of nuclei) (Fig. 5). The largest component of the complex is the principal or ventral nucleus, MGv. The MGv receives projections from the tonotopically organized central nucleus of the inferior colliculus, and the MGv in turn is tonotopically organized. Neurons have best frequencies, and as they diverge from the best frequencies they respond less well. Neurons are systematically arranged from those having low best frequencies to those having high best frequencies. The MGv provides auditory information to primary auditory cortex and other fields.

A more medial or magnocellular (larger-celled) nucleus, MGm, receives inputs from the central, dorsal, and external nuclei of the inferior colliculus and projects widely to subdivisions of auditory cortex. The MGm is less precisely tonotopically organized; neurons are more broadly tuned to tone frequency, and they may respond to somatosensory stimuli, as well. The dorsal nucleus of the medial geniculate complex, MGd, has widespread projections to auditory cortex and receives input from the dorsal cortex of the inferior colliculus.

Finally, other thalamic nuclei including the suprageniculate (Sg) nucleus, nucleus limitans, and the medial pulvinar have connections with higher-order auditory fields in cortex, but the significance of these connections is not known.

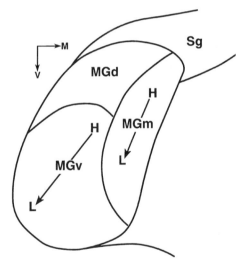

Figure 5. The three main nuclei of the medial geniculate complex in the auditory thalamus: the large ventral (or principal) nucleus, MGv, which represents tonal frequencies from high (H) to low (L) in a dorsomedial to ventrolateral sequence; the medial (or magnocellular) nucleus, MGm, which also is tonotopically organized, but neurons respond more broadly to tones of different frequencies, and the dorsal nucleus, MGd, about which less is known. The suprageniculate (Sg) nucleus is less directly involved in auditory functions.

27. How is auditory cortex organized?

Much of the early research on auditory cortex was conducted on cats, but recently a greater understanding has been obtained from monkeys, which probably have an organization much like that in humans (Fig. 6). In brief, the evidence indicates that there is a core of two or three primary and primary-like areas surrounded by a belt of seven or eight second-level areas, bordered on the lateral side by a parabelt of at least two fields. The belt and parabelt areas are interconnected by additional fields in the temporal, parietal, and frontal lobes. Thus, the processing of auditory information in the cortex involves many fields and several levels of processing. Processing occurs via **parallel channels** or pathways, so that components of auditory stimuli can be processed independently at the same time, and in **serial steps**, so that complexities can be added step-by-step.

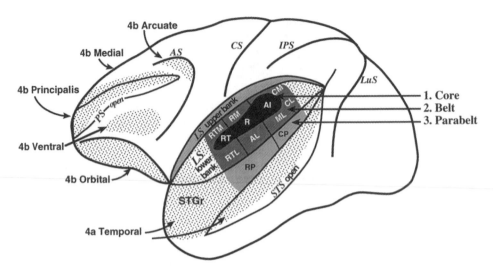

Figure 6. Auditory processing regions in the macaque monkey brain (lateral view). Similar regions are expected in the human brain. The auditory core of primary (A1) and primary-like areas (rostral, R; rostrotemporal, RT) is surrounded by a belt of secondary fields (caudomedial, CM; caudolateral, CL; middle lateral, ML; anterior lateral, AL; rostromedial, RM; medial rostrotemporal, RTM; lateral rostrotemporal, RTL). These areas are located in the lower bank of the lateral sulcus (LS). The rostral (RP) and caudal (CP) divisions of the parabelt constitute a third level of cortical processing. Other parts of the temporal lobe, including rostral superior temporal gyrus (STGr) and cortex in the superior temporal sulcus (STS) constitute a fourth level (4a) of auditory processing, along with auditory regions of the frontal lobe (4b). The lateral sulcus (LS), principal sulcus (PS), superior temporal sulcus (STS) are shown open. The arcuate sulcus (AS), intraparietal sulcus (IPS), and lunate sulcus (LuS) are indicated for reference.

28. What are the three main areas of the auditory core?

About half of the core is occupied by **primary auditory cortex, A1**, which has been identified in a wide range of mammalian species. A1 is tonotopically organized and it has the basic anatomic features of sensory cortex. Just rostral to A1, on the lower or ventral bank of the lateral nucleus, a second field was discovered with characteristics almost identical to A1. It is termed rostrolateral (RL) or **rostral (R)**. Both fields receive inputs from MGv, have tonotopic organizations, and have anatomic features of primary sensory cortex. However, the fields differ in their patterns of tonotopic organization, with low frequencies represented at their common border and high frequencies represented elsewhere. More recently, a **rostrotemporal tip (RT)** of the R region has been discovered to contain a third pattern of tonotopic representation. The core areas represent the **first stage of cortical processing**.

29. How is primary auditory cortex tonotopically organized?

As in the primary-like subcortical subdivisions of the auditory system, A1 neurons have best frequencies—tone frequencies at which they respond to the lowest sound intensities—and as sound levels increase, these neurons respond to an increasingly wider range of frequencies. Neurons may have different best frequencies, and the arrangement of neurons in A1 according to best frequency is orderly. Neurons across the thickness of cortex traditionally are grouped into six layers. Recordings from individual neurons in any electrode penetration through the thickness of cortex reveal that each successive neuron has approximately the same best frequency, although sharpness of tuning varies with depth. Thus, neurons across the *depth* of cortex form **isofrequency** (same frequency) rows or columns. Neurons across the *width* (one dimension) of the cortex surface also do not change in best frequency. Thus, A1 has strips of neurons across its depth and width that have the same best frequency (isofrequency bands).

Across the other dimension (length) of the surface, neurons progressively change in best frequency. In monkeys, the posteromedial corner of A1 represents the highest frequencies, with tones of over 20 kHz (20,000 cycles per second), while best frequencies become progressively lower toward the anterolateral corner of A1, where tones of 1 kHz or less are represented.

30. How are the rostral and rostrotemporal areas tonotopically organized?
R has a mirror-image or reversed organization of that in A1, and RT mirrors that of R.

31. What are the anatomic features of core areas?
Core areas are sensory in appearance. Primary sensory areas have a well-developed layer IV of small, densely packed neurons. Layer IV is the layer that receives sensory information from the thalamus. Primary sensory areas also have other architectonic and histochemical features, including those reflecting a high level of metabolic activity. All three areas, A1, R, and RT, have the characteristic features of primary sensory cortex and receive direct inputs from the MGv. Thus, we refer to these core areas as primary or primary-like.

32. Why are there three main areas rather than one?
The reasons for this are not clear. Visual cortex in primates has only one primary area, and nearly all of the visual information in cortex is distributed from this single field. The auditory system, in contrast, distributes almost identical or very similar types of information from three cortical centers. This must speed up auditory processing, since the same information can be transformed in different ways by the differing target fields of the three distributing centers.

33. Are there other types of organization, in addition to tonotopic, in the neurons of primary auditory cortex?
Recordings from single neurons throughout A1 in cats and more recently in monkeys indicate that neuronal response to several parameters of auditory stimuli varies with **location**. Typically, the neurons with the lowest thresholds for tones and the narrowest tuning curves are centered in A1. In terms of binaural responses, neurons fall into three broad classes: (1) excited by either ear (these neurons respond more when both ears are stimulated); (2) responsive only to the contralateral ear; and (3) excited by the contralateral ear and inhibited by the ipsilateral ear. These classes of neurons tend to be grouped in A1 in bands or patches of tissue that may relate in a systematic way to patches of corpus callosum connections between A1 of the two hemispheres. The binaural neurons have large spatial receptive fields, and they do not represent auditory space in any systematic way, but they may contribute to population (group) coding for auditory space. Neuronal response latencies also vary across A1. Thus, A1 represents complex sounds in a spectrally distributed, spatially dispersed manner that varies with the parameters of the stimulus.

34. What is the auditory belt?
The auditory belt surrounds the three core fields and receives input from the core. Although some thalamic input exists, the belt neurons largely require core inputs for activation. Thus, they represent a **second stage of cortical processing** (see question 28).The eight or so belt fields receive inputs from different core fields or different combinations of core fields, suggesting that they are receiving slightly different types of information. Although little is known about the functions of belt fields, each field likely is specialized for a subset of auditory functions. Neurons in belt fields respond better to complex sounds than to tones.

35. Where does information in the auditory belt go?
The main projections of the belt are to a band of cortex in the temporal lobe just ventrolateral to the core and belt. This parabelt region has rostral (anterior) and caudal (posterior) subdivisions, with rostral belt areas projecting largely to the rostral parabelt and vice versa. The parabelt represents a **third stage of cortical processing**, where neurons have even more complex response properties than those in the belt.

36. What are the cortical connections of the parabelt?
Projections of the parabelt further distribute auditory information to other parts of the temporal lobe, adjoining parts of the parietal lobe, and regions of the frontal lobe.

37. What are the functions of these regions with parabelt auditory inputs?

The functions are not clear, but the posterior parietal cortex may have a special role in locating objects in space. The auditory projections to the parietal lobe may interact with visual and somatosensory inputs so that multimodal information can be used in analyzing spatial aspects of stimuli. The widespread projections to the temporal lobe may be to subdivisions of cortex that are involved in the further analysis and identification of sounds. Projections to the frontal lobe involve several regions. Those to cortex near the frontal eye fields are thought to be important in directing attention and gaze toward sounds. Those to adjacent parts of dorsolateral prefrontal cortex probably function in short-term or "working" memory for auditory stimuli (auditory information is retained for a short period of time after a sound stops). Other projections are to orbitofrontal cortex, which is part of a reward system where stimuli are associated with behavioral consequences. This cortex has emotive and motivational functions.

38. What are the behavioral and perceptual consequences of bilateral damage to auditory cortex?

According to reports, effects vary for several reasons. First, simple auditory detection tasks, such as responding to the onset of a sound, do not depend on auditory cortex and can be mediated by subcortical auditory structure. Second, lesions of the auditory core often are incomplete. Note that the auditory core is a long, narrow strip of cortex where three different areas seem to have highly overlapping functions. In addition, each area is activated by either ear. Thus, the unaffected portion of any core area of either hemisphere is a substrate for considerable auditory performance.

Nevertheless, given the dependence of the belt and parabelt areas on the core, complete bilateral lesions of the core should have a major impact on hearing. In fact, monkeys with large, bilateral lesions affecting the core region are totally unresponsive to sound for a period of days-to-weeks, and they remain unable to discriminate between complex sounds such as vocalizations, or even simple patterns of tones. In addition, sounds are not localized. In humans, this severe impairment of auditory perception after bilateral lesions has been classically referred to as "cortical deafness."

39. How does artificial stimulation of the auditory system work?

In recent years, it has become more common to implant an electrical stimulator in the cochlea of patients that have a severe hearing loss as a result of hair cell receptor loss. If nerve VIII is intact, it can be electrically stimulated at its source in the cochlea to produce auditory sensations. Typically, a row of electrodes are placed along the organ of Corti in the first turn of the cochlea so that sites related to different sound frequencies can be stimulated. A microphone attached to a processor transforms speech and other sounds into a pattern of electrical stimulation that is delivered to the electrode array, and this unnatural input activates the auditory pathways. Because of the great plasticity of the auditory system, especially auditory cortex, a type of learning occurs, and a high level of speech recognition can be achieved.

40. How do sounds acquire emotional significance?

Projections of auditory cortex to orbitofrontal cortex are important in aspects of emotional behavior. The amygdala, a subcortical structure deep to cortex in the tip of the temporal lobe, also is important. The amygdala receives thalamic and cortical auditory inputs. Bilateral damage to the amygdala reduces acoustic startle and avoidance conditioning in animals, and impairs the perception of anger and fear in voices in humans.

41. What types of auditory deficits are associated with auditory pathology?

Auditory pathologies can be divided into two basic categories: conductive (~5%) and sensory-neural (~95%). Many forms of conductive and sensory-neural hearing loss are related to congenital malformations and syndromes, but the majority of auditory deficits are acquired.

Conductive hearing losses are caused by reduced transmission of auditory signals to the inner ear resulting from an abnormal condition in the external or middle ear. Most conditions that produce a conductive hearing loss are totally, or at least partially, reversible given appropriate intervention.

Sensory-neural hearing losses result from a lesion or degeneration in the cochlea (sensory) or higher auditory pathways (neural). Sensory-neural impairments generally are permanent and often are progressive.

A **mixed** hearing loss results from conditions that introduce conductive *and* sensory-neural components. Mixed hearing losses often are associated with congenital malformations that affect development of the auditory system, but also may result from the pathologies that independently affect conductive and sensory-neural components of the system.

42. What are the most common causes of conductive hearing loss?

Conductive hearing losses typically are caused by an obstruction of the external auditory meatus. Accumulation of excess cerumen or water and the insertion of objects in the ear canal are the most common causes when the *external* ear is involved. Otitis externa (external ear infection or "swimmer's ear") and congenital atresia of the external auditory meatus also can cause a significant conductive hearing loss.

In the *middle* ear, otitis media (middle ear infection) is particularly common in children through age twelve. Disarticulation of the ossicles, otosclerosis, perforated tympanic membrane, space-occupying lesion of the middle ear (e.g., cholesteatoma, glomus jugularis), and congenital malformation are other causes of conductive hearing loss involving the middle ear.

43. What are the most common causes of sensory-neural hearing loss?

Sensory-neural hearing loss most often is related to aging (presbycusis) and noise exposure (chronic or acute). The incidence of sensory-neural hearing loss increases with age (> 50% over age 70). A smaller percentage of impairments are related to ototoxicity, congenital anomalies, or the development of pathological conditions such as a tumor, cardiovascular disruption, or degenerative disease.

- The vestibular schwannoma (acoustic neuroma) is the most prevalent type of tumor affecting the central auditory pathways; incidence is about 1 per 100,000 per year. It typically is located in the cerebello-pontine angle where cranial nerve VIII exits the temporal bone and enters the medulla.
- Disruption of the blood supply to the cochlea, auditory cortex, or any of the intermediate pathways may produce an ischemic condition that compromises neural function. Primary examples are obstruction of the internal auditory artery and its branches, anterior-inferior cerebellar artery, posterior-inferior cerebellar artery, vertebral and/or basilar arteries, and middle cerebral artery.
- Degenerative disorders that may cause hearing loss are presbycusis, multiple sclerosis, diabetes mellitus, kernicterus, and Meniere's disease (endolymphatic hydrops).
- A number of drugs and chemical substances induce pharmacologic effects that can cause permanent sensory-neural hearing loss. Several aminoglycoside antibiotics are known to be ototoxic (e.g., streptomycin, kanamycin, neomycin, gentamicin) to variable degrees.
- Among the syndromes associated with sensory-neural hearing loss are: Waardenburg's, Alport's, Usher's, and Down's.
- Infectious disorders that may affect the inner ear and central pathways include: bacterial or viral infection of the labyrinth (inner ear), labyrinthitis, syphilis, meningitis, and cytomegalovirus.

44. What are the conditions most often associated with hearing loss in neonates and young children?

A number of conditions place neonates at risk for hearing loss, including: hypoxia, kernicterus, meningitis, labyrinthitis, Rh incompatibility, maternal rubella, congenital syphilis, perinatal cytomegalovirus, hypothyroidism, closed head injury, skull fracture, otitis media, Waardenburg's syndrome, Alport's syndrome, Usher's syndrome, and Down's syndrome. Also at risk are children who have been treated with ototoxic drugs for other disorders and those with chronic or acute exposure to excessively loud sounds. The presence of any of these conditions may indicate the need for a hearing screening to improve the chances of early identification of a hearing loss.

45. What are the principal sequelae of conductive hearing loss?

In conductive hearing impairments there is a global attenuation of sounds due to the obstruction, which affects higher acoustic frequencies more than lower frequencies. Thus, the overall **volume** of sound is reduced, and the disproportionate reduction of the higher frequencies makes speech sound "muffled" because the consonant sounds are attenuated more than the vowel sounds. A unilateral conductive loss results in unbalanced hearing sensitivity and acuity, but the net effect is nominal. A bilateral conductive loss is less common, but has a more pronounced effect on overall sensitivity and acuity. Conductive hearing deficits are easily offset by an increase in volume; thus, amplification is very effective when the conductive blockade can not be easily resolved.

46. What are the principal sequelae of sensory-neural hearing loss?

In sensory-neural hearing impairments, the hearing loss is due to a reduction in the **neural transmission** of auditory information, rather than an attenuation of acoustic energy. Often, the patient complains of difficulty in understanding speech, even though it is audible, and has tremendous difficulty in noisy listening environments. Sensory-neural losses may be unilateral or bilateral, but usually are bilateral and related to aging or chronic noise exposure. Unilateral losses are more commonly associated with acute acoustic trauma, tumors, stroke, or other pathology (e.g., Meniere's disease or endolymphatic hydrops) affecting one side.

Sensory-neural deficits can be offset by amplification (e.g., hearing aids; increased volume), but the effectiveness of amplification depends on the number of intact components in the pathway; that is, residual hearing. Amplification, per se, has no known regenerative effects on damaged hair cells or neurons and their processes. Consequently, sensory-neural hearing impairments generally are permanent, but a mild sensory-neural hearing loss has a better prognosis in terms of the rehabilitative benefits of amplification than a severe loss. This is because the number of functional neural inputs to the central auditory system is greater in sensory-neural hearing losses that express themselves diagnostically as "mild" in degree. The benefits of amplification diminish with increasing severity of the hearing impairment.

In cases of congenital or acquired deafness, if there is no input from the cochlea to the brainstem, the prognosis is poor for rehabilitation based on amplification. In these patients, direct electrical stimulation of the system (e.g., cochlear implant) has a better prognosis, because at least some type of stimulus-related input is delivered to the central auditory pathways.

47. What is tinnitus, and how is it related to hearing loss?

Tinnitus, commonly referred to as "head noise," is an auditory perception (e.g., ringing, buzzing, crackling) that has no external source. The source of the input that leads to the perception lies somewhere within the auditory system. Tinnitus frequently is associated with hearing loss, but also is reported by patients whose hearing is within normal limits as determined by clinical audiologic criteria. Tinnitus can have an identifiable etiology (e.g., pressure on the tympanic membrane, vestibular schwannoma, acoustic trauma, pharmacologic or dietary effect), but it often is idiopathic. The prognosis is highly variable and generally poor when the specific cause cannot be identified and eliminated.

Chronic tinnitus is commonly reported in cases of sensory-neural hearing loss, but the neural mechanisms contributing to its development are not known. There is experimental evidence for both cortical and subcortical origins of certain types of tinnitus. Some of these models have attempted to relate injury-induced plasticity of central auditory structures to the development of tinnitus, analogous to the development of "phantom-limb" pain/sensations in amputees.

48. What tools are available for diagnosis and assessment of hearing loss?

Aside from the wealth of information that can be obtained from a proper case history and neurologic examination: otoscopy, audiometry, evoked potential, and structural imaging. Each of these tools is designed to contribute to the process of diagnosis and assessment in a particular way. None of the tools alone can give the examiner a complete picture of auditory integrity.

49. What can be learned from an otoscopic examination?

A wide range of conductive hearing problems can be identified by visual inspection of the external auditory meatus, tympanic membrane, and visible portions of the middle ear. Obstructions of the external auditory canal, including foreign objects, polyps, tumors, and evidence of infection, are easily seen with an otoscope or surgical microscope. The most common obstruction is excessive cerumen accumulation. To the trained observer, the appearance of the tympanic membrane can reveal much about the health of the middle ear. A perforated tympanic membrane is clearly visible, as are many forms of otitis media. Tumors of the middle ear (e.g., cholesteatoma) often can be easily seen behind the intact tympanic membrane. A sensory-neural hearing disorder is unlikely to be identified visually, however; nor can the degree to which a conductive or sensory-neural hearing loss affects hearing sensitivity or acuity be assessed by this type of evaluation.

50. What is an audiological examination?

The routine audiological evaluation consists of audiometry and tympanometry and is usually conducted by an audiologist. **Audiometry** is used to assess hearing sensitivity and acuity. Hearing *sensitivity* for air-conducted and bone-conducted sound is indexed by measuring behavioral thresholds for pure tones ranging from 250 to 8000 Hz. Air-conducted stimulation utilizes the external, middle, and inner ears. Bone-conducted stimulation excites the cochlear hair cell system directly, bypassing the external and middle ear mechanisms. Thus, when air- and bone-conduction scores are the same, a sensory-neural hearing loss is indicated. When air-conduction thresholds are poorer than bone-conduction, a conductive hearing loss is indicated.

Hearing *acuity* commonly is assessed by tests that require identification of words or speech sounds presented at a comfortable listening level, rather than at threshold. These tests index the ability to understand audible speech. The results of these tests are recorded on an audiogram.

Tympanometry provides objective measures of middle-ear integrity and is a routine part of a complete audiological evaluation. The tympanometer is the instrument used to measure ear canal volume, pressure on the tympanic membrane, and acoustic reflexes. Taken together, the audiogram and tympanogram can be used to determine if the hearing loss is conductive, sensory-neural, or mixed, and also can indicate the degree of associated hearing loss.

51. What is the auditory brainstem response?

The auditory brainstem response (ABR) refers to a series of auditory evoked potentials that can be recorded noninvasively from the scalp using surface electrodes. The ABR is considered to be an objective measure of auditory brainstem function, as the source generators of the five consecutive waveforms are believed to be associated with auditory brainstem nuclei. However, the source generators have not been precisely identified. The first peak (wave I) most commonly is associated with the auditory nerve. The fifth peak (wave V) often is attributed to the inferior colliculus or lateral lemniscus. A significant increase in the latency of wave V relative to wave I frequently is found in patients with tumors affecting cranial nerve VIII and the lower brainstem. The ABR also is used as an objective estimate of hearing sensitivity in infants and other populations who are difficult to test using conventional audiometric techniques.

52. What are otoacoustic emissions?

Low-level acoustic emissions (sounds) emanating from the cochlea can be recorded in the external auditory meatus using specialized equipment. The source of these emissions usually is attributed to normal mechanisms in the cochlea, especially the outer hair cells. The absence of these emissions is correlated with a loss of sensitivity as measured by the pure tone audiogram. Therefore, the measurement of these emissions can be used as an objective screening of outer hair cell function and an index of the integrity of the cochlea.

Recently, a number of hospitals and clinics have started to use otoacoustic emissions and/or ABR to screen high-risk infants for hearing loss.

53. How can structural imaging be used to diagnose or assess hearing disorders?

Computed tomography and magnetic resonance imaging techniques are widely used to rule out or identify hemorrhage and space-occupying lesions in neural structures. Although very small lesions and tumors affecting the auditory system can be difficult to identify (i.e., cerebellopontine angle tumor, middle ear cholesteatoma), imaging techniques still are helpful in the diagnosis of such pathologies. Assessment of cochlear damage and the degree of impairment is not within the scope of current imaging technology; therefore, the examiner must rely on additional techniques (see Questions 50–52) for a more complete picture of auditory system integrity.

BIBLIOGRAPHY

1. Aitkin A: The Auditory Midbrain. Clifton, New Jersey, Humana Press, 1985.
2. Aitkin A: The Auditory Cortex. New York, Chapman and Hall, 1990.
3. Kaas JH, Hackett TA: Subdivisions of auditory cortex and levels of processing in primates. Audiol Neuro-otol 3:73-85, 1998.
4. Kaas JH, Hackett TA, Tramo MJ: Auditory processing in primate cerebral cortex. Curr Opinion Neurobiol 9:164–170, 1999.
5. National Institutes of Health: Early identification of hearing impairment in infants and young children. NIH Consensus Statement 11(1):1-25, 1993.
6. Webster WA, Garey LJ: Auditory system. In Paxinos G (ed): The Human Nervous System. New York, Academic Press, 1990, pp 889–944.

7. THE CENTRAL VESTIBULAR SYSTEM

Neal H. Barmack, Ph.D.

The central vestibular system encompasses the two regions of the brain to which the vestibular nerve projects—the vestibular nuclei and the cerebellum—and the thalamocortical areas to which vestibular information is relayed. These structures are involved in a host of physiologic and behavioral responses that challenge our understanding: How do we maintain our balance? How do sensory systems, often carrying contradictory information, combine to model the world in which we navigate? How do vestibular and other sensory signals contribute to the regulation of autonomic functions such as blood flow to skeletal musculature? How do mixed vestibular messages contribute to motion sickness and space sickness? How do we adapt to repeated vestibular stimulation, or more generally, how does the central vestibular system learn? How does the vestibular system recover or compensate following damage to the peripheral vestibular system?

In uncovering the secrets of the vestibular system I am reminded of the stern advice offered by my fifth-grade science teacher. Whenever she was asked a question to which she did not know the answer, she would reply, "God does not want us prying into his private secrets." This chapter includes only a fraction of the many secrets worth sharing about the vestibular system. However, I do not plead divine intervention but, rather, space limitations.

1. Describe the receptors of the peripheral vestibular apparatus.

There are two classes of peripheral vestibular receptors: semicircular canals and otoliths. Each labyrinth is endowed with three **semicircular canals**, which are oriented nearly orthogonally with respect to each other, and two different **otoliths**. All five endorgans are encased in membranous ducts filled with fluid (endolymph) and suspended in the bony cavity of the temporal bone. The space between the membranous and bony walls of the labyrinth is filled with perilymph (Fig. 1).

2. How is head movement encoded by the peripheral vestibular apparatus?

The semicircular canals encode angular acceleration of the head in a three-dimensional space, with each dimension provided by a canal's plane: oriented horizontally; at roughly 45 degrees with respect to the sagittal plane; or at roughly 135 degrees with respect to the sagittal plane. Each semicircular canal is paired with a reciprocal counterpart in the opposite labyrinth. For example, the left and right horizontal semicircular canals form a functional pair, as do the left anterior and right posterior semicircular canals and the left posterior and right anterior semicircular canals.

Each canal contains a specialized sensory region, the **ampulla**, that converts hydraulic displacement of the endolymph into a small movement of a gelatinous structure, the **cupula**. The cupula is lined with hair cells with a common polarization vector. These hair cells convert small displacements of the cupula into an electrical signal that controls synaptic release by the hair cell. When the head is moved in the plane of one of the semicircular canals, the endolymph is dragged only partially by the moving walls of the canal. Since the cupula is fixed relative to the wall of the canal, there is an increased force acting against the cupula by the endolymph.

Horizontal angular acceleration of the head, say to the left, causes cupular deflection in the ampullae of the horizontal semicircular canals. The stereocilia of hair cells in the left ampulla are deflected *toward* the kinocilium, causing depolarization of the hair cells and an increased release of synaptic transmitter. At the same time, the stereocilia of hair cells in the ampulla of the right horizontal semicircular canal are deflected *away* from the kinocilium, causing hyperpolarization of these hair cells and a decreased release of transmitter.

3. How do the otoliths contribute to encoding of head movement?

The utricular and saccular otoliths contain hair cells embedded in a sheet of polysaccharide matrix of calcite crystals. When the attitude of the head shifts, this sheet of calcite crystals causes a

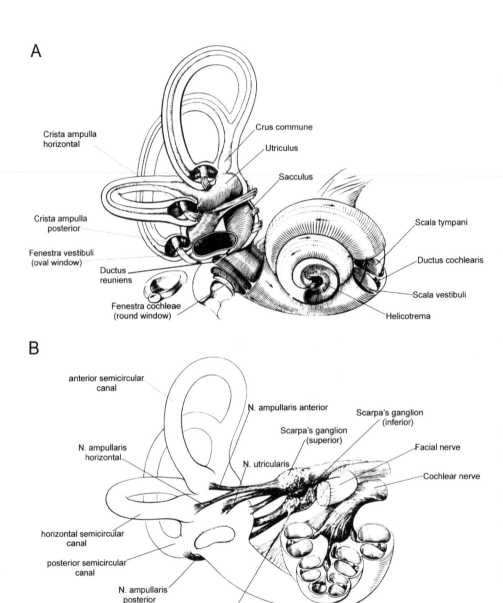

A

Crista ampulla horizontal

Crus commune

Utriculus

Sacculus

Crista ampulla posterior

Fenestra vestibuli (oval window)

Ductus reuniens

Fenestra cochleae (round window)

Scala tympani

Ductus cochlearis

Scala vestibuli

Helicotrema

B

anterior semicircular canal

N. ampullaris anterior

Scarpa's ganglion (inferior)

Scarpa's ganglion (superior)

Facial nerve

N. ampullaris horizontal

N. utricularis

Cochlear nerve

horizontal semicircular canal

posterior semicircular canal

N. ampullaris posterior

Ramus vestibulocochlearis

Figure 1.   Labyrinth and vestibular nerve origins. **A,** Peripheral labyrinth. **B,** The peripheral vestibular nerve is divided into two parts: the superior division consists of vestibular primary afferents originating from the ampullae of the horizontal and anterior semicircular canals and the macula of the utricle; the inferior division consists of afferents originating from the ampulla of the posterior semicircular canal and the macula of the saccule. (Modified from Goldstein MJ: The auditory periphery. In Mountcastle VB (ed): Medical Physiology. Saint Louis, C.V. Mosby Co., 1968, pp 1465–1498; with permission.)

deflection of the stereocilia of these hair cells, which then modulate transmitter release. Unlike the semicircular canal ampullae that contain hair cells with the same polarization, the utricular and saccular maculae contain hair cells with a variety of different spatial polarizations. Both the saccular and utricular maculae are divided into two areas, pars interna and externa. On either side of the dividing line, hair cells have opposite spatial polarizations (Fig. 2).

Functional polarization vectors of utricular and saccular primary afferents have been characterized most completely in the squirrel monkey, using behavioral and electrophysiologic techniques. The preponderance of hair cells in the utricular maculae have a medio-lateral polarization vector, and they respond to head tilt about the longitudinal axis. The left and right utricular maculae behave reciprocally. When the output of one increases, the output of the other decreases. Conversely, the preponderance of saccular hair cells have a down-up polarization vector. This means that for most head movements the two saccular maculae do not behave reciprocally; rather, they are coactivated. As we shall see, this leads to a different *wiring diagram* of secondary neurons in the vestibular nuclei.

Fernandez C, Goldberg JM: Physiology of peripheral neurons innervating otolith organs of the squirrel monkey. III. Response dynamics. J Neurophysiol 39:996–1008, 1976.

Flock A: Structure of the macula utriculi with special reference to directional interplay of sensory responses as revealed by morphological polarization. J Cell Biol 22:413–431, 1964.

Lindeman HH: Anatomy of the otolith organs. Adv Otorhinolaryngol 20:405–433, 1973.

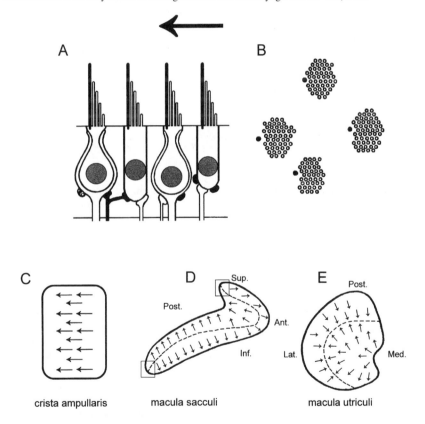

Figure 2. Hair cell polarization in vestibular endorgans. **A,** Polarization of kinocilia and stereocilia in two different types of hair cells. **B,** Cross section through the cilia of hair cells showing that each bundle has a single kinocilium *(black dots)* and a large number of stereocilia. The two-dimensional polarization of these hair cell bundles are characterized for **C,** the crista ampullaris of a semicircular canal, **D,** the macula sacculi, and **E,** the macula utriculi. (Modified from Lindeman HH: Anatomy of the otolith organs. Adv Otorhinolaryngol 20:405–433, 1973; with permission.)

4. What are the origins of the vestibular nerve?

It is no secret that vestibular primary afferents (VPAs) comprise the largest afferent input to the vestibular complex. The distal bundles of the five separate branches of the vestibular nerve are combined into two divisions as they leave the labyrinth. The superior division of the vestibular nerve contains afferents from the horizontal and anterior semicircular canal ampullae as well as the utricular macula. The inferior division contains afferents from the saccular macula and posterior semicircular canal ampulla (see Fig. 1B).

5. Where does the vestibular nerve terminate?

After the central branch of the vestibular nerve exits Scarpa's ganglion, it enters the lateral brainstem and bifurcates into two fiber bundles containing axons of unequal thickness (Fig. 3). The bundle containing the thicker axons enters the medulla between the ventral aspect of the inferior cerebellar peduncle and the dorsal aspect of the spinal tract of the trigeminal nucleus. This bundle turns caudally and passes through the vestibular complex. VPAs synapse upon neurons in each of the vestibular nuclei.

The bundle of thin nerve fibers ascends to the cerebellum through the superior vestibular nucleus (SVN). The thin collateral branches of the vestibular nerve ascend through the lateral vestibular nucleus and SVN to the ipsilateral cerebellum, where they terminate as mossy fibers in the granule cell layer. Although several cerebellar folia receive scattered projections from VPAs, more than 90% of these afferents are restricted to the ipsilateral uvula-nodulus. So the **vestibular complex** and the **uvula-nodulus** are the central sites of termination for VPAs. In both the vestibular complex and the cerebellum, the synaptic transmitter released by VPAs is glutamate.

Barmack NH, Baughman RW, Errico P, Shojaku H: Vestibular primary afferent projection to the cerebellum of the rabbit. J Comp Neurol 327:521–534, 1993.

Korte G, Mugnaini E: The cerebellar projection of the vestibular nerve in the cat. J Comp Neurol 184:265–278, 1979.

Raymond J, Nieoullon A, Dememes D, Sans A: Evidence for glutamate as a neurotransmitter in the cat vestibular nerve: Radioautographic and biochemical studies. Exp Brain Res 56:523–531, 1984.

Yamanaka T, Sasa M, Matsunaga T: Glutamate as a primary afferent neurotransmitter in the medial vestibular nucleus as detected by in vivo microdialysis. Brain Res 762:243–246, 1997.

6. Describe the locations of the vestibular complex and nuclei.

The vestibular complex is located along the floor of the fourth ventricle on the dorsal surface of the brainstem. From its most caudal aspect, approximately 1 mm in front of the obex, it extends rostrally to the dorsal cochlear nucleus. The vestibular complex typically is divided into five separate nuclear groups:

1. Medial vestibular nucleus (MVN)
2. Descending (or spinal) vestibular nucleus (DVN)
3. Lateral (Deiter's) vestibular nucleus (LVN)
4. Superior vestibular nucleus (SVN)
5. Parasolitarius nucleus (Psol).

The fifth vestibular nucleus' name is partially misleading; this nucleus is found at the most caudal part of the vestibular complex, wedged between the MVN and DVN. It consists of a compact cluster of small-diameter neurons extending from the solitary nucleus to the surface of the fourth ventricle (see Fig. 4H).

7. How are the vestibular nuclei identified?

Each of the vestibular nuclei receives a VPA projection, which distinguishes it from the nucleus prepositus hypoglossi (NPH). The NPH shares many of the same afferent and efferent connections with vestibular nuclei, with the exception of VPAs. As it name implies, the NPH lies just rostral to the hypoglossal cranial motor nucleus and extends rostrally along the medial border of the MVN (Fig. 4).

The borders of the individual vestibular nuclei are difficult to distinguish based on cytological characteristics. The giant cells in Deiter's nucleus make the LVN easy to recognize. However, these cells are outnumbered by a mixture of intermediate-sized cells and do not clearly define the spatial extent of the LVN. The borders of other vestibular nuclei are even less distinct. The MVN contains a

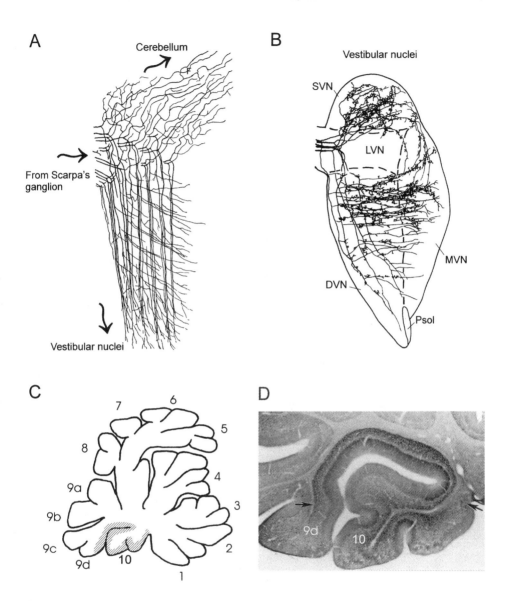

Figure 3. Projection of vestibular primary afferent to the vestibular complex and to the cerebellum. **A,** Bifurcation of VPAs as they enter the brainstem. (Modified from Cajal S Ramon y: Histology of the Nervous System. Vol. 1. [English translation of 1911 text] New York, Oxford University Press, 1995; with permission.) **B,** Distribution of five horizontal semicircular canal afferents to the vestibular complex of the cat. The terminals are mapped onto a horizontal section through the vestibular complex. (Modified from Sato F, Sasaki H: Morphological correlations between spontaneously discharging primary vestibular afferents and vestibular nucleus neurons in the cat. J Comp Neurol 333:554–556, 1993; with permission.) **C,** Cerebellum of the rabbit, showing the location of the uvula nodulus *(shaded area),* the region of the cerebellum that is the termination site for most VPAs. **D,** VPAs labeled by the c-fragment of tetanus toxin previously injected into the endolymph of a rabbit's labyrinth. VPAs terminate as mossy fibers in the granule cell layer. (Modified from Barmack NH, Baughman RW, Errico P, Shojaku H: Vestibular primary afferent projection to the cerebellum of the rabbit. J Comp Neurol 327:521–534, 1993; with permission.)

full range of cell types and is, in total volume, the largest of the vestibular nuclei. The DVN is characterized by longitudinally running fiber bundles that give it the appearance of being less densely populated by neurons. The SVN has a more uniform distribution of medium-sized cells, making its boundaries more easily recognized.

The Psol is identifiable using either cytoarchitectonic or immunohistochemical criteria. It is composed of uniformly small cells that are labeled by an antiserum to glutamic acid decarboxylase (GAD), a synthetic enzyme for the neurotransmitter gamma amino butyric acid (GABA).

Elsewhere within the vestibular complex, the MVN often is divided into a dorsal cluster of small (parvocellular) neurons and a ventral cluster of larger (magnocellular) neurons. These two different divisions also have a different pattern of intrinsic connections.

Barmack NH, Fredette BJ, Mugnaini E: The parasolitary nucleus: A source of GABAergic vestibular information to the inferior olive of rat and rabbit. J Comp Neurol 392:352–372, 1998.

Brodal A: Anatomy of the vestibular nuclei and their connections. In Kornhuber HH (ed): Handbook of Sensory Physiology: Vestibular System, Morphology. Vol. 6. Berlin-Heidelberg-New York, Springer Verlag, 1974.

Brodal A, Pompeiano O: The vestibular nuclei in the cat. J Anat 91:438–454, 1957.

8. Are there topographically-specific termination patterns of primary vestibular afferents within the vestibular complex?

If the various subdivisions of the vestibular complex represented termination sites that were uniquely devoted to a single class of afferent, say from the horizontal semicircular canal, then one would expect to see the restriction of afferent terminals to a single nuclear site. Quite the contrary is observed. The pattern of VPA termination on secondary vestibular neurons has been reconstructed in the cat (see Fig. 3B). Synaptic terminals were found in all of the vestibular nuclei with the exception of the LVN.

Based on electrical simulation of the sacculus, it appears that the saccular afferents terminate primarily, but not exclusively, in the LVN. In contrast to the reciprocally organized responses of left and right pairs of semicircular canals and the left and right utricular otoliths, the two saccular maculae are not reciprocally activated by head movement. The termination of saccular afferents in the LVN suggests that this is the one vestibular nucleus that also is not reciprocally organized through the interconnections of a commissural system.

The fact that single VPAs branch to innervate several vestibular nuclei does not necessarily reflect the absence of topographic projections. Rather, the patterns of afferent projections suggest other possibilities: a precise topography exists, but it does not conform to the cytoarchitecturally defined boundaries of the vestibular nuclei; there is a negative topography, which reflects the absence rather than the presence of VPA projections; or the topography of the vestibular nuclei is more related to the efferent rather than afferent connections. In partial support of the latter two propositions is the observation that the termination of afferents from the horizontal semicircular canal includes all vestibular nuclei except the LVN and Psol. Physiological recordings from Psol neurons indicate that they are driven exclusively by stimulation of the ipsilateral *vertical* semicircular canals and *utricular* otoliths, but not the ipsilateral *horizontal* semicircular canal or *sacculus*.

Sasto F, Sasaki H: Morphological correlations between spontaneously discharging primary vestibular afferents and vestibular nucleus neurons in the cat. J Comp Neurol 333:554–556, 1993.

Sato H, Imagawa M, Isu N, Uchino Y: Properties of saccular nerve-activated vestibulospinal neurons in cats. Exp Brain Res 116:381–388, 1997.

Uchino Y, Sato H, Suwa H: Excitatory and inhibitory inputs from saccular afferents to single vestibular neurons in the cat. J Neurophysiol 78:2186–2192, 1997.

Wilson VJ, Gacek RR, Uchino Y, Susswein AJ: Properties of central vestibular neurons fired by stimulation of the saccular nerve. Brain Res 143:251–261, 1978.

Figure 4 *(facing page).*   Vestibular nuclei of the cat. Transverse sections extending from the rostral *(A)* to caudal *(J)* poles of the vestibular complex illustrate the spatial extent of each of the vestibular nuclei. DVN = descending vestibular nucleus, Ecu = external cuneate nucleus, Icp = inferior cerebellar peduncle, IO = inferior olive, LVN = lateral vestibular nucleus, MVN = medial vestibular nucleus, NPH = nucleus prepositus hypoglossi, Nsol = solitary nucleus, Psol = parasolitary nucleus, Pyr = pyramidal tract, SO = superior olive, sol = solitary tract, Sp5 = spinal trigeminal nucleus, tz = trapezoid nucleus. (Modified from Brodal A, Pompeiano O: The vestibular nuclei in the cat. J Anat 91:438–454, 1957; with permission.)

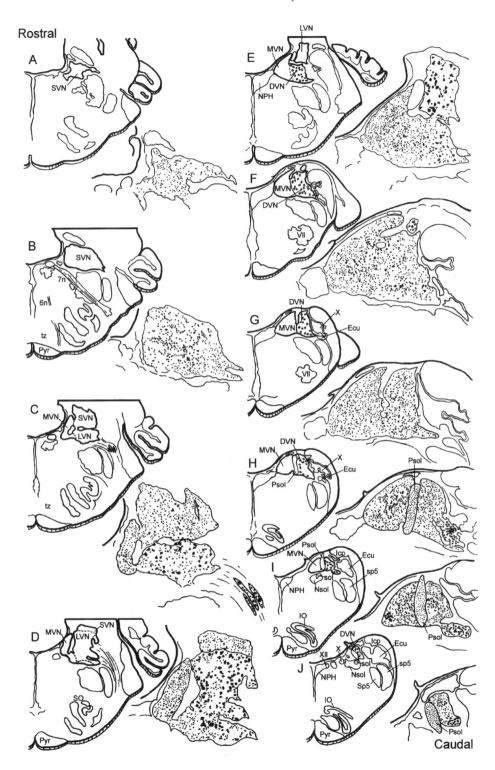

9. How are individual vestibular nuclei interconnected?

The vestibular nuclei, with the exception of the LVN, are connected through a **commissural system**. This system has been studied by injecting ortho- and retrograde tracers into various regions of the vestibular complex. The distribution of labeled cell bodies in the ipsilateral vestibular nuclei reveals *intrinsic* connections (Fig. 5) and in the contralateral vestibular nuclei reveals *extrinsic* (commissural) connections (Fig. 6).

The pattern of interconnections between vestibular nuclei on the same side of the brainstem is complicated. There are two essential points: (1) Interconnections between the SVN, DVN, and MVN are reciprocal, and (2) based upon its intrinsic connections and differences in cell size, the MVN can be subdivided into separate parvocellular (small cell) and magnocellular (large cell) divisions.

Unlike the commissural pathways of the cerebral cortex, the commissural pathways of the vestibular nuclei are not restricted to connections between homologous nuclei. Rather, cells within a nucleus on one side of the brainstem, say the left MVN, have intrinsic connections to cells in other vestibular nuclei on the same side and extrinsic connections to groups of cells within the contralateral MVN, SVN, and DVN. Note that once again the LVN is unique—it lacks commissural connections.

Epema AH, Gerrits NM, Voogd J: Commissural and intrinsic connections of the vestibular nuclei in the rabbit: A retrograde labeling study. Exp Brain Res 71:129–146, 1988.

Gacek RR: Location of commissural neurons in the vestibular nuclei of the cat. Exp Neurol 59:479–491, 1978.

Ito JI, Matsuoka I, Sasa M, Takaori S: Commissural and ipsilateral internuclear connection of vestibular nuclear complex of the cat. Brain Res 341:73–81, 1985.

Newlands SD, Kevetter GA, Perachio AA: A quantitative study of the vestibular commissures in the gerbil. Brain Res 487:152–157, 1989.

10. Is it really necessary to understand these interconnections in such detail?

The purpose of mentioning this seemingly abstruse information about microcircuitry is to emphasize that, as in real estate sales, *location, location, location* is important in the vestibular complex. A lack of appreciation of these anatomic distinctions may impede our discovery of different functional subdivisions with the vestibular complex.

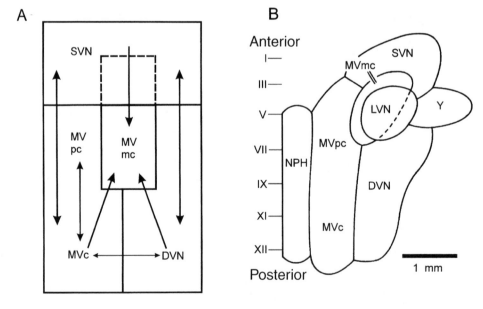

Figure 5. Intrinsic nuclear projections within the vestibular complex of the rabbit. **A,** Schematic of intrinsic projection pattern corresponds approximately to a horizontal slice. **B,** Horizontal slice through vestibular complex. (Modified from Epema AH, Gerrits NM, Voogd J: Commissural and intrinsic connections of the vestibular nuclei in the rabbit: A retrograde labeling study. Exp Brain Res 71:129–146, 1988; with permission.)

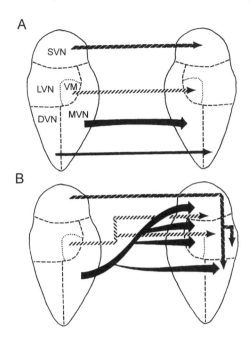

Figure 6. Pattern of commissural (extrinsic) projections within the vestibular nuclei of the gerbil. **A,** Three of the vestibular nuclei (SVN, MVN, and DVN) have homologous and reciprocal connections. The LVN does not. **B,** The vestibular nuclei also have divergent connections to nonhomologous contralateral vestibular nuclei. (Modified from Newlands SD, Kevetter GA, Perachio AA: A quantitative study of the vestibular commissures in the gerbil. Brain Res 487:152–157, 1989; with permission.)

11. Are there other areas providing information to the vestibular complex?

VPAs comprise only one of the sensory inputs to the vestibular complex. Another major source of sensory information originates from the visual system. In particular, visual signals concerning self-motion originate from a specialized part of the visual system termed the accessory optic system (Fig. 7).

Electrophysiologic single-neuron recordings from the vestibular complex demonstrate that most, but not all, vestibular neurons are driven by optokinetic as well as vestibular stimulation. The relative contributions of each of these optokinetic-vestibular pathways have not been determined. Some or all of them may be responsible for the optokinetically-driven activity of *secondary* vestibular neurons.

12. How do visual signals reach vestibular nuclei?

The accessory optic system, which comprises the medial, dorsal, and lateral terminal nuclei (MTN, DTN, LTN) and the nucleus of the optic tract (NOT), is perhaps the best understood of any part of the central visual system. The accessory optic system receives projections from specialized ganglion cells in the retina. Neurons in each of the accessory system's nuclei have receptive fields that are 10 to 100 times larger than the receptive fields of neurons in the striate complex. Neurons within each of the nuclear subgroups of the accessory system evince directional selectivity to large, contour-rich stimuli that move across their receptive fields. For example, neurons in the NOT respond to temporal-to-nasal stimulation of the contralateral eye. The range of stimulus velocities over which this response occurs is 0.1–30.0 deg/sec. These receptive field characteristics suggest that NOT neurons are tuned to detect self-motion rather than the motion of small moving objects, such as the flight of a bird or a baseball. The detection of external moving objects is the province of the geniculo-striate system.

The NOT, MTN, DTN, and LTN have different directional selectivities. Each nucleus represents a preferred stimulation vector. Combined with the spatial information provided by VPAs, these visual nuclei provide an alternative spatial map. At least part of this spatial map is provided to several brainstem nuclei, including the dorsal cap of the inferior olive, the nucleus prepositus hypoglossi, the nucleus reticularis tegmenti pontis, the dorsolateral pontine nuclei, and an area surrounding the terminal region of the fasciculus retroflexus called the parafascicular complex. Each of the target nuclei for the accessory optic system and NOT also projects to the vestibular complex. Direct projections from the accessory optic system to parts of the vestibular complex may exist, as well.

Collewijn H: Direction-selective units in the rabbit's nucleus of the optic tract. Brain Res 100:489–508, 1975.

Schmidt M, Schiff D, Bentivoglio M: Independent efferent populations in the nucleus of the optic tract: An anatomical and physiological study in rat and cat. J Comp Neurol 360:271–285, 1995.

Watanabe S, Kato I, Sato S, Norita M: Direct projection from the nucleus of the optic tract to the medial vestibular nucleus in the cat. Neurosci Res 17:325–329, 1993.

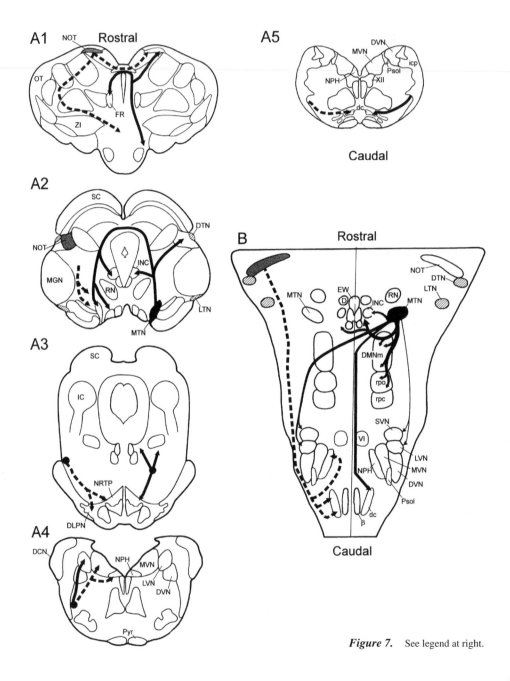

Figure 7. See legend at right.

13. What is the significance of prestriate cortex to the accessory optic system?

While the anatomy and physiology of the accessory optic system have been described most extensively in experiments performed on lower mammals, such as the rabbit, the same fundamental details have been confirmed in primates. In all mammals there is a descending projection from the visual cortex to the accessory optic system and NOT. In primates this projection originates from the prestriate cortex (areas OAa and PGa). Selective stimulation or inactivation of this region can modify the directional selectivity of neurons in the accessory optic system.

Ilg UJ, Hoffmann K-P: Responses of neurons of the nucleus of the optic tract and dorsal terminal nucleus of the accessory optic tract in the awake monkey. Eur J Neurosci 8:92–105, 1996.

Maekawa K, Takeda T, Kimura M: Responses of the nucleus of the optic tract neurons projecting to the nucleus reticularis tegmenti pontis upon optokinetic stimulation in the rabbit. Neurosci Res 1:1–25, 1984.

14. How are neck proprioceptive signals generated? How do they reach the vestibular nuclei?

Movements of the head activate neck proprioceptors that are embedded in the small inter-transverse muscles at the base of the C2 and C3 cervical vertebrae. These muscles rank with eye muscles and finger muscles in the density of muscle spindles. Proprioceptor activation causes changes in length of the inter-transverse muscles, stimulating their muscle spindles. This signal is conveyed to the vestibular nuclei and other brainstem nuclei. If you doubt the importance of a neck proprioceptive contribution to balance, you should read the account of what happens to monkeys whose neck proprioceptors have been silenced by local injections of procaine (see Cohen below).

The extent of the projection from neck proprioceptors to the vestibular complex is less well understood than the projection patterns of either VPAs or optokinetic afferents. However, when horseradish peroxidase is injected into the caudal third of the MVN, it retrogradely labels neurons in the ipsilateral, C2–C3 spinal ganglia. Injections into the DVN, SVN, LVN, and rostral MVN do *not* label neurons in the spinal ganglia. It is possible that neurons in the vestibular complex also receive secondary cervical afferents relayed from the external cuneate nuclei.

Bankoul S, Neuhuber WL: A cervical primary afferent input to vestibular nuclei as demonstrated by retrograde transport of wheat germ agglutinin-horseradish peroxidase in the rat. Exp Brain Res 79:405–411, 1990.

Cohen LA: Role of eye and neck proprioceptive mechanisms in body orientation and motor coordination. J Neurophysiol 24:1–11, 1961.

15. Can movements be evoked and measured by stimulation of vestibular, optokinetic, and neck-proprioceptive systems?

Yes. Each of these sensory systems, when activated, evokes reflexive movements. These movements include those of the eyes, ears, head, and trunk as well as reflexive contractions of gut smooth muscle and reflexive changes in heart rate, blood pressure, and respiration. The most sensitive indication of activity of sensory inputs to the vestibular system are the ocular reflexes: the vestibulo-ocular reflex (VOR), the optokinetic reflex (OKR), and the cervico-ocular reflex (COR). Normally a head movement jointly activates all three; however, each can be evoked separately in the laboratory (Fig. 8).

Figure 7 *(previous page).* Pathways by which optokinetic information reaches the vestibular system. **A,** Transverse sections through the brainstem of the rabbit. Note the descending connections of the nucleus of the optic tract (NOT) *(dashed lines)* and ascending and descending connections of the medial terminal nucleus (MTN) *(solid black lines)*. These transverse sections correspond to different rostral-caudal levels of the brainstem. **B,** Horizontal section through the brainstem showing the caudal paths taken by the descending projections originating from the NOT *(dashed lines)* and MTN *(solid black lines)*. β = β-nucleus, D = nucleus of Darkschewitsch, dc = dorsal cap of Kooy, DCN = dorsal cochlear nucleus, DLPN = dorsolateral pontine nucleus, DMNm = deep mesencephalic nucleus, DTN = dorsal terminal nucleus, DVN = descending vestibular nucleus, EW = Edinger-Westphal nucleus, FR = fasciculus retroflexus, IC = inferior colliculus, icp = inferior cerebellar peduncle, INC = interstitial nucleus of Cajal, LTN = lateral terminal nucleus, LVN = lateral vestibular nucleus, MGN = medial geniculate nucleus, MTN = medial terminal nucleus, MVN = medial vestibular nucleus, NOT = nucleus of the optic tract, NPH = nucleus prepositus hypoglossi, NRTP = nucleus reticularis tegmenti pontis, OT = optic tract, Psol = parasolitary nucleus, Pyr = pyramidal tract, RN = red nucleus, rpc = nucleus reticularis pontis caudalis, rpo = nucleus reticularis pontis oralis, SC = superior colliculus, SVN = superior vestibular nucleus, ZI = zona incerta, XII = hypoglossal nucleus. (Modified from Giolli RA, Blanks RHI, Torigoe Y, Williams DD: Projections of medial terminal accessory optic nucleus, ventral tegmental nuclei, and substantia nigra of rabbit and rat as studied by retrograde axonal transport of horseradish peroxidase. J Comp Neurol 232:99–116, 1985).

Each ocular reflex has a unique gain (response amplitude/stimulus amplitude) and range over which it operates. For example, the vestibulo-ocular reflex evoked by stimulation of the semicircular canals operates over a frequency range of 0.08–5.00 Hz, with a peak gain of 0.90 at a frequency of 0.40 Hz. The frequency range of the vestibulo-ocular reflex for which otoliths are responsible is 0.005–0.10 Hz, with a peak gain of about 0.50 at a frequency of 0.02 Hz. The frequency range of the optokinetic reflex is comparable to that of the otoliths, with a peak gain of 0.90 at about 0.10 Hz. The frequency range of the horizontal cervico-ocular reflex also is comparable to that of the otoliths, with a peak gain of only 0.25 at a frequency of 0.02 Hz.

Movement of the head in the horizontal plane potentially activates three different types of ocular reflex: (1) the horizontal vestibulo-ocular reflex, (2) the horizontal optokinetic reflex, and (3) the horizontal cervico-ocular reflex. For example, movement of the head to the left stimulates the hair cells in the ampulla of the left horizontal semicircular canal. If the eyes are open during the leftward head movement, directionally-selective neurons in the right NOT also are stimulated as the visual field drifts across the left retina in the temporal-nasal direction. Finally, neck proprioceptors in the right cervical vertebrae are stretched. Each of these signals acts synergistically and causes a rightward, conjugate, horizontal movement of the eyes.

16. Do the vestibular nuclei *know* when their neurons are being stimulated by vestibular, optokinetic, or cervical proprioceptive inputs?

No. This is the basis for vestibular-related illusions, such as *linear vection*, the sensation of self-motion experienced by a person seated on a train when an adjacent train, viewed from a side window, pulls out of the station. Illusions of self-motion in their mildest form can be amusing parlor games or even psychophysical experiments. In their extreme form they can lead to spatial disorientation and motion sickness. The point to be made here is that the vestibular system is *hard-wired*. Whenever any of the sensory pathways to the vestibular nuclei are activated, the *default interpretation* of the brain is that the head is moving. The identify of the stimulus that produced this sensation is lost. This default most often, but not always, is true.

17. What are some of the synaptic transmitters associated with the circuitry linking the vestibular system with the cerebellum?

Vestibular primary afferents (VPAs) project directly to the ipsilateral cerebellar nodulus, where they terminate in the granule cell layer as mossy fiber terminals (Fig. 9). The transmitter for VPAs has not been identified conclusively, but it probably is glutamate. Secondary vestibular neurons and cerebellar granule cells express ionotropic glutamate receptors. Granule cells also express muscarinic m2 receptors.

Vestibular secondary afferents (VSAs) originate from the caudal MVN, DVN, and NPH and project *bilaterally* as mossy fibers onto granule cells in the cerebellar nodulus and flocculus. The transmitter for this mossy fiber pathway is acetylcholine. This cholinergic pathway synapses upon granule cells expressing m2 receptors. VSA pathways also include ipsilateral projections from Psol onto neurons in the β-nucleus and dorsal medial cell column of the inferior olive. These descending vestibular

---

Figure 8 (facing page). Comparison of reflexive eye movements evoked by vestibular, optokinetic, and neck proprioceptive stimulation. **A,** The horizontal vestibulo-ocular reflex (HVOR) is evoked by rotation of the rabbit about the vertical axis stimulation (yaw), stimulating the horizontal semicircular canals. Note that the gain of the HVOR increases with stimulus frequency. **B,** The vertical vestibulo-ocular reflex (VVOR) is evoked by rotation of the rabbit about a longitudinal axis (roll). Note that the gain of the VVOR is relatively high even at lower frequencies due to the contribution of the utricular otoliths. At higher frequencies the VVOR can be attributed to stimulation of the posterior and anterior semicircular canals. **C,** The horizontal cervico-ocular reflex (HCOR) is evoked by rotation of the body of the rabbit in the horizontal plane about the fixed head. This is done in total darkness. Note that the gain of the HCOR even at the optimal frequency of 0.02 Hz is only about 0.25. **D,** The horizontal optokinetic reflex (HOKR) is evoked by unidirectional movement of a contour-rich stimulus at a constant velocity. The moving image subtended 70 degrees of visual angle. Note that stimulation in the posterior-anterior direction (P→A) evokes eye movements of higher velocity compared to stimulation in the anterior-posterior direction (A→P). (Modified from Barmack NH: A comparison of the horizontal and vertical vestibulo-ocular reflexes of the rabbit. J Physiol (Lond) 314:547–564, 1981.)

projections are GABAergic and include collateral fibers to the nucleus reticularis gigantocellularis. The distribution of GABAergic receptor subtypes within the inferior olive is unknown.

Vestibular tertiary afferents (VTAs) originate from the β-nucleus and dorsal medial cell column and synapse as climbing fibers on Purkinje cells in the contralateral uvula-nodulus. The transmitter for this pathway probably is glutamate. Climbing fibers also express corticotropin releasing factor. Purkinje cells are endowed with both ionotropic and metabotropic glutamate receptors.

(*Answer continues on following page.*)

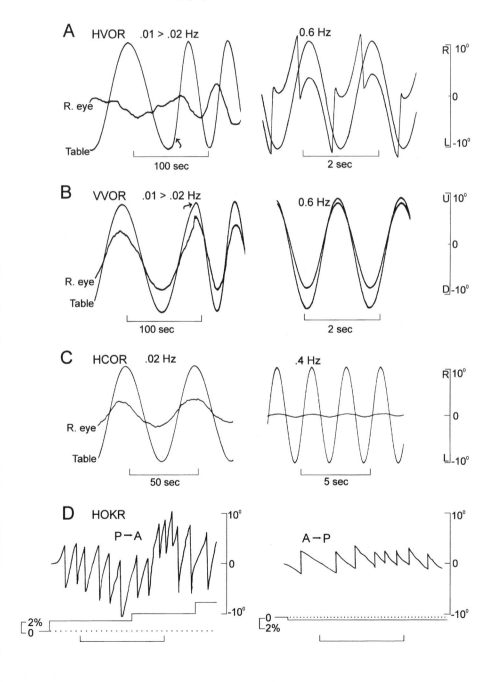

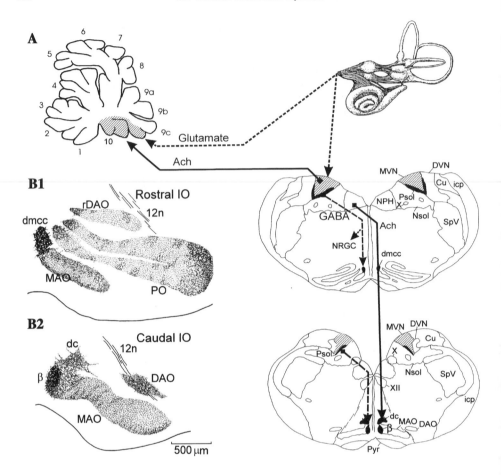

Figure 9.   Projection of primary and secondary vestibular afferents and their transmitter content in the rabbit. **A**, Glutamatergic VPAs project to both the vestibular complex and the cerebellar uvula-nodulus (folia 9d and 10). Cholinergic VSAs leave the MVN, DVN, and NPH and synapse as mossy fibers in the granule cell layer of the uvula-nodulus. GABAergic VSAs convey vestibular inputs to the ipsilateral nucleus reticularis gigantocellularis (NRGC) and inferior olive (β-nucleus and dorsal medial cell column [dmcc]). A cholinergic descending projection from the NPH to the contralateral dorsal cap of the inferior olive synapses upon the same cells that receive directionally specific optokinetic inputs from the contralateral retina. **B**, GABAergic terminals in the β-nucleus *(B1)* and dmcc *(B2)* that originate from the ipsilateral Psol and are immunolabeled with an antibody to glutamic acid decarboxylase Ach = acetylcholine, Cu = cuneate nucleus, DAO = dorsal accessory olive, MAO = medial accessory olive, Nsol = solitary nucleus, rDAO = rostral dorsal accessory olive, SpV = spinal trigeminal nucleus, X = dorsal motor nucleus of vagus, XII = hypoglossal nucleus, 12n = hypoglossal nerve. (Modified from Barmack NH: Cholinergic pathways and functions related to the vestibulo-cerebellum. In Anderson JH, Beitz AJ (eds): Neurochemistry of the Vestibular System. New York, CRC Press, 1999—in press.)

Another VTA is the projection from the NPH onto the contralateral dorsal cap of the inferior olive. This projection contains optokinetic information from the NOT and MTN of the accessory optic system. In the rat the transmitters for this pathway are GABA and acetylcholine. In the rabbit the projection from the NPH onto the dorsal cap primarily is mediated by GABA. This raises the interesting possibility that the same anatomic projection in the rat and rabbit is mediated by different neurotransmitters. It is possible that these transmitters are coexpressed in the NPH of both species. Such coexpression of acetylcholine and GABA has been described in amacrine cells of the retina.

18. What are some of the major transmitter receptors associated with the vestibular system?

Three of the major transmitters in the central vestibular system are glutamate, GABA, and acetylcholine. Both N-methyl-D-aspartate (NMDA) and non-NMDA glutamate receptors are found in secondary vestibular neurons, although there may be regional differences within the vestibular complex for their relative expression (Fig. 10).

Neurons in the vestibular nuclei express both $GABA_A$ and $GABA_B$ receptors. Vestibulo-ocular reflexes, particularly those involving the otoliths, are reduced by administration of the $GABA_A$ agonist benzodiazepine, at concentrations that are 100 times lower than are generally used for analgesia.

The VSA projection to the cerebellum is cholinergic. Granule cells in the cerebellum express muscarinic cholinergic receptors of the m2 subtype. Cells in the dorsal cap of the inferior olive that receive a cholinergic projection from the NPH also express m2 muscarinic receptors.

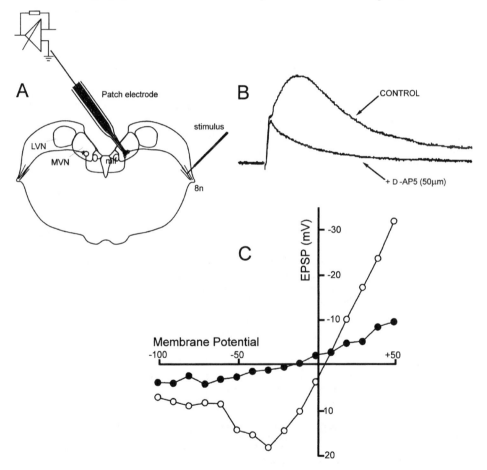

Figure 10. Demonstration of differing classes of glutamate receptors by stimulation of the vestibular nerve. **A,** Slice preparation for patch recording from vestibular neurons. **B,** Excitatory postsynaptic potentials (EPSPs) evoked by stimulation of the vestibular nerve under control conditions and during bath application of D-2-amino-5-phosphonovalerate (D-AP5), an antagonist of NMDA receptors. **C,** Voltage dependence of the peak EPSP amplitude before *(white circles)* and after *(black circles)* bath-applied D-AP5. The D-AP5 eliminated the rectification of the peak EPSP at hyperpolarized potentials by blocking NMDA receptors. (Modified from Kinney GA, Peterson BW, Slater NT: The synaptic activation of N-methyl-D-aspartate receptors in the rat medial vestibular nucleus. J Neurophysiol 72:1588–1595, 1994; with permission.)

19. How does the cerebellum feed back onto the vestibular nuclei?

Cerebellar projections onto the vestibular complex have been studied with orthograde and retrograde tracer techniques. However, a more complete picture can be obtained by using antibodies that recognize the expression of proteins that are unique to Purkinje cells or, better yet, unique to Purkinje cells in specific regions of the cerebellum. For example, Purkinje cells express isozymes of the subcellular signaling enzyme, protein kinase C (PKC). All Purkinje cells express PKC-γ, whereas only Purkinje cells in the posterior vermis express PKC-δ. These isoenzymes of PKC are not expressed in neurons in the vestibular complex, nor are they expressed by VPAs. Therefore, antibodies to these isoenzymes can be used to map the distribution of Purkinje cell terminals within the vestibular complex (Fig. 11).

The picture that emerges from the use of these mapping techniques is that virtually every cell in the LVN, SVN, and rostral MVN receives a projection from "non-nodular" Purkinje cells. The synaptic terminals from Purkinje cells in the uvula-nodulus are restricted to the dorsal aspects of the caudal MVN, DVN, and NPH. *However, large regions of the caudal vestibular complex receive no direct synaptic inputs from Purkinje cells.*

20. What does the cerebellum add to vestibular information processing?

The cerebellum is *not* needed for the elaboration of any of the reflexes discussed thus far. If the cerebellum is removed surgically, these reflexes persist. They might not be of appropriate amplitude, but they are present. The cerebellum may help calibrate reflexive movements and establish a sensory hierarchy for movement guidance. When the brain is provided conflicting sensory signals, the cerebellum may help establish a hierarchy of signal reliability. Then, one sensory system can be used either to suppress or recalibrate signals from another sensory system. There is compelling evidence that part of the cerebellum, the flocculus, may help adjust the gain of the horizontal vestibulo-ocular reflex based on optokinetic information derived from the NOT and inferior olive.

Another function for the cerebellum is to predict spatial environments. If an animal is oscillated for a long time and then stopped, oscillatory eye movements persist. Information about such oscillations arrives at the cerebellum encoded by vestibular climbing fibers (Fig. 12), and the predictive function already may be occurring at the level of either the inferior olive or the vestibular nuclei.

Finally, the cerebellum contains a topographic map of vestibular space conveyed by climbing fiber projections. This map may provide an anatomic substrate for specific modulation of postural reflexes evoked by vestibular and optokinetic stimulation.

Fushiki H, Barmack NH: Topography and reciprocal activity of cerebellar Purkinje cells in the uvula-nodulus modulated by vestibular stimulation. J Neurophysiol 78:3083–3094, 1997.

Ito M: The Cerebellum and Neural Control. New York, Raven Press, 1984.

Kleinschmidt HJ, Collewijn H: A search for habituation of vestibulo-ocular reactions to rotatory and linear sinusoidal accelerations in the rabbit. Exp Neurol 47:257–267, 1975.

21. Are the precise neural circuits that form the substrate for vestibular reflexes understood?

First, the good news: Much of the microcircuitry has been worked out (Fig. 13). For example, the classic **three-neuron arc**, in which the VPAs synapse on secondary neurons in the MVN, is

---

Figure 11 (facing page). Mapping of Purkinje cell terminals in the vestibular complex and cerebellar nuclei of the rat. **A–F**, Transverse sections from the caudal to rostral poles. Regions containing axons and axon terminals are immunolabeled by an antiserum to PKC-γ *(gray areas)*. Note that all of the cerebellar nuclei as well as the LVN, SVN, and parts of the DVN, MVN, and NPH are represented. Bundles of axons and axon terminals are immunolabeled by the antiserum to PKC-δ in the DVN, MVN, NPH, and caudal-medial aspect of the interpositus nucleus *(black marks)*. **D–F**, A separate group of axons, comprising the descending branch of the acoustic stria, are immunolabeled for PKC-δ *(dots)*. The numbers at the top of each section indicate the distance from the caudal pole of the vestibular complex. Amb = nucleus ambiguus, AS = acoustic stria, Cu = cuneate nucleus, DCN = dorsal cochlear nucleus, ECu = external cuneate nucleus, FVe = F cell group vestibular, Gi = nucleus reticularis gigantocellularis, icp = inferior cerebellar peduncle, IntP = interpositus cerebellar nucleus, jx = juxta restiform body, Lat = lateral cerebellar nucleus, LC = locus caeruleus, LPG = nucleus lateral paragigantocellularis, LRN = lateral reticular nucleus, Nsol = solitary nucleus, sg = Scarpa's ganglion, sol = solitary tract, sp5 = spinal trigeminal tract, VCN = ventral cochlear nucleus, 7n = facial nerve.

understood. Excitatory secondary neurons cross the midline to synapse on motoneurons in the abducens (VI) nucleus, which in turn cause contraction of the lateral rectus muscle.

The bad news is that our understanding of the *functionality* of reflexes is vastly overstated by such simplified schematics. In rabbits, it is possible to induce a horizontal optokinetic nystagmus by prolonged optokinetic stimulation. The nystagmus may last for a few days after the optokinetic stimulation has been discontinued; this is termed optokinetic afternystagmus. Following the induction of optokinetic afternystagmus, if the head of the rabbit is maintained in different pitch positions about the interaural axis, the plane of the nystagmus shifts to exactly compensate for the change in the pitch

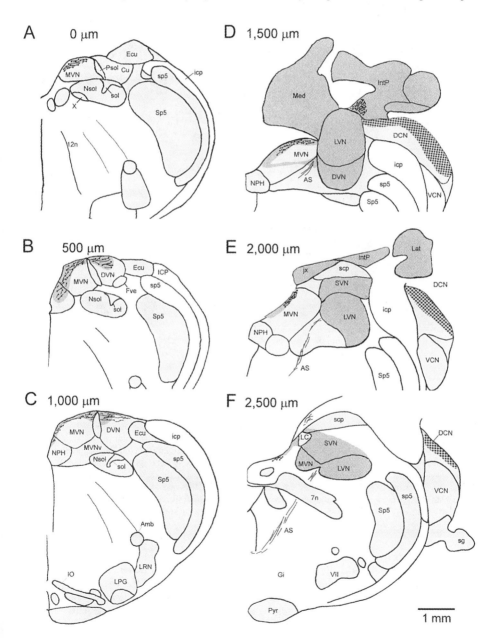

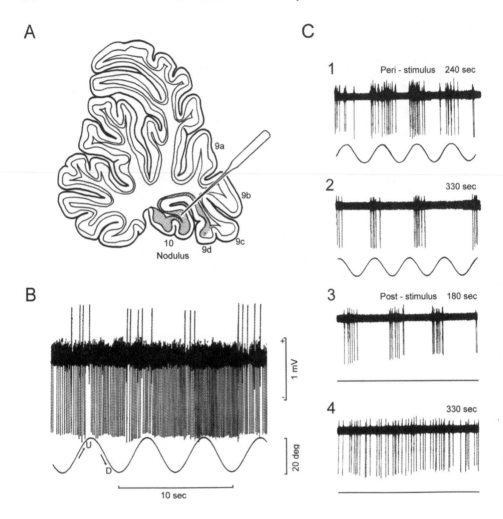

FIGURE 12.   Vestibular-induced oscillation of climbing fiber input to the uvula-nodulus. **A**, Extracellular recording arrangement from the rabbit nodulus. **B**, Example of both climbing fiber responses (CFRs; positive) and simple spikes (negative) recorded from a Purkinje cell in the right nodulus during oscillation about the longitudinal axis. The lower trace indicates table position. When the trace is positive, the rabbit is rotated onto its right side. **C**, Extracellular recording of only CFRs from a Purkinje cell in the right uvula during oscillation about the longitudinal axis *(1, 2)* and at different times after the vestibular oscillation was stopped *(3, 4)*. Note that repeated oscillations about the longitudinal axis decreased CFR modulation. More than 180 seconds after the vestibular stimulation was terminated *(3)*, the stimulus-induced oscillation of CFRs persisted. After 330 seconds, the oscillatory CFRs disappeared in the spontaneous background activity. (Modified from Barmack NH, Shojaku H: Vestibularly induced slow oscillations in climbing fiber responses of Purkinje cells in the cerebellar nodulus of the rabbit. Neuroscience 50:1–5, 1992.)

angle of the head (Fig. 14). A vestibular signal, indicating static head position with respect to gravity, organizes the nystagmus so that appropriate combinations of extraocular motor nuclei are engaged to maintain the plane of the nystagmus in an earth-horizontal orientation. Such a fantastic motor organization does not emerge from a three-neuron arc. It also does not depend on an intact cerebellum, since the reorientation of the nystagmus occurs following near total lesions of the uvula-nodulus.

Leigh RJ: Human vestibular cortex. Ann Neurol 35:383–384, 1994.

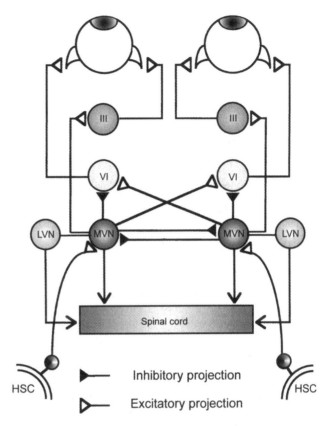

FIGURE 13. Three-neuron arc for the horizontal vestibulo-ocular reflex. Each MVN excites the ipsilateral medial rectus subdivision of the oculomotor nucleus and inhibits the ipsilateral abducens nucleus. In addition, the two MVN are mutually inhibitory through the vestibular commissure HSC = horizontal semicircular canal. (Modified from Smith PF, De Waele C, Vidal P-P, Darlington CL: Excitatory amino acid receptors in normal and abnormal vestibular function. Mol Neurobiol 5:369–387, 1991; with permission.)

22. Is there any evidence for the involvement of the cerebral cortex in central vestibular functions?

When we are the recipients of vestibular stimulation without confirming visual stimulation, as in the case of the parlor game Pin the Tail on the Donkey (in which the player is blindfolded and spun in place), we make incorrect judgments about spatial location of objects. We perceive things to be where they are not. By contrast, have you ever wondered why figure skaters usually do not fall after executing spins that are much faster than those in Pin the Tail on the Donkey? Figure skaters train themselves to use visual cues to overcome the misinformation provided by their vestibular systems. After training, they not only stay virtually upright, but they also significantly reduce the eye nystagmus caused by their high-acceleration spins.

These simple observations suggest that we can use our brains to over-ride information from a sensory system that we choose to ignore. There are other salient examples of this ability. Humans with misalignment of the eyes sometimes learn to suppress the information from one eye because it conflicts with spatial information provided by the other eye. This is one of the cases of **amblyopia**. With regard to the vestibular system, the neural basis for the temporary suppression of vestibular information may reside in the reciprocal pathways between the vestibular cortex and the vestibular nuclei.

Both anatomic and physiologic studies of the thalamus and cortex have delineated several ascending projections from the rostral part of the vestibular complex to the ventrobasal thalamus (VPL, VPM, VPI, and VPL; Fig. 15). Neurons in the ventrobasal complex are driven by stimulation of deep proprioceptors and joint receptors as well as vestibular inputs.

The descending connections from the cerebral cortex onto the vestibular complex have been studied anatomically with retrograde tracer techniques. Interestingly, cortical areas that project to the vestibular complex are known to participate in spatial orientation. The prefrontal motor cortex

(6pa) is linked to the cortical control of eye movements. Areas 3aV and T3 and the posterior insula (PIVC) receive optokinetic and somatosensory as well as vestibular inputs.

Humans with damage to the PIVC do not recognize true vertical. Deprived of surrounding visual cues, they cannot correctly align a disk with a line on it so that the line has a true vertical orientation. Possibly, in certain pathologic cases, dizziness (vertigo) is due to cortical, not peripheral, vestibular dysfunction.

23. How does the vestibular system influence autonomic function?

As everyone knows from personal experience, certain patterns of optokinetic or vestibular stimulation have unpleasant autonomic consequences. The caudal vestibular nuclei (DVN, MVN, and Psol) send axons to the solitary nucleus (Nsol). In the Nsol a variety of autonomic afferents, carried chiefly by branches of the IX and X cranial nerves, terminate. Stimulation of the central vestibular system has normal functional autonomic consequences. The vestibular system causes orthostatic reflex adjustments, such as increases in blood flow, to be targeted to skeletal muscles. The orthostatic reflex controls vascular resistances, so that appropriate blood pressure can be maintained independent of head orientation. This maintenance allows most of us to arise from an easy chair without getting too dizzy.

In the cat, movement of the head about a pitch axis modulates the activity of abdominal and phrenic nerves. These autonomic effects are abolished by lesions of the caudal MVN, DVN, and Psol. Single neuron recordings from the fastigial nucleus have characterized neurons whose firing rates encode cardiorespiratory parameters. Moreover, electrical stimulation of the cerebellar uvula or fastigial nucleus modifies blood pressure, heart rate, and respiration. The fastigial nucleus also appears to have reciprocal connections with a subset of hypothalamic nuclei, some of which, in turn, project to the Nsol.

Haines DE, May PJ, Dietrichs E: Neuronal connections between the cerebellar nuclei and hypothalamus in *Macaca fascicularis:* Cerebello-visceral circuits. J Comp Neurol 299:106–122, 1990.

Moruzzi G: Paleocerebellar inhibition of vasomotor and respiratory carotid sinus reflexes. J Neurophysiol 3:20–32, 1940.

24. What is motion sickness?

Motion sickness is the autonomic consequence of sensory stimulation that induces spatial disorientation. In humans and many mammals, acute motion sickness reaches a climax with retching. This rather ballistic event is heralded by subthreshold peristaltic contractions that can be recorded from either the esophagus or from the lower intestines. Motion sickness also seems to be preceded, in monkeys, by an increase (10–20 fold) in arginine vasopressin, possibly secreted by the hypothalamus.

A popular view of motion sickness is that it is produced by **sensory conflict**—different sensory systems reporting conflicting information about the spatial world. This view must be extended to include conflicts within the same sense. For example, a very compelling nauseogenic stimulus occurs when a subject is pitched continuously, head-over-heals, about an interaural axis. Such a stimulus produces conflict between the information provided by the otoliths and the vertical semicircular canals.

For many people, exposure to just a few minutes of unidirectional optokinetic stimulation is sufficient to induce nausea. Individuals who have bilateral loss of labyrinthine function tend not to experience motion sickness. Interestingly, the nodulus may be contributory: dogs who have had a nodulectomy have a lower likelihood of vomiting. To many people in the throes (pardon the expression) of motion sickness, even a nodulectomy might be considered an acceptable therapeutic procedure.

Figure 14 *(facing page).* Shift in rotation axis of optokinetic afternystagmus induced by change in head pitch angle. **A**, Eye position recordings obtained from a rabbit during optokinetic afternystagmus. When the rabbit was in the first position *(1)*, the nystagmus was purely horizontal. When the rabbit was pitched up *(2)*, the angle of the nystagmus plane changed in the orbit by 45°, so that the nystagmus plane remained horizontal. **B**, Example of horizontal and vertical eye movements as a function of time. The upper pair of traces represent horizontal and vertical eye position. The lower trace represents head pitch angle. **C**, Angle of optokinetic afternystagmus is plotted as a function of head pitch angle. Over a range of ±80° when the head is pitched forward or backward, the angle of the plane of nystagmus is adjusted appropriately to maintain it in an earth-horizontal orientation. (Modified from Pettorossi VE, Errico P, Ferraresi A, Barmack NH: Optokinetic and vestibular stimulation determines the spatial orientation of negative optokinetic afternystagmus in the rabbit. J Neurosci 19:1524–1531, 1999.)

Spatial disorientation does not necessarily produce motion sickness. Here's an interesting secret in support of this argument: *Rabbits don't barf.* That's right. Continuous optokinetic or vestibular stimulation of rabbits makes them spatially disoriented, but they will not vomit. Nor will they lose their appetite to ingest food.

Hasler WL, Kim MS, Chey WD, et al: Central cholinergic and α-adrenergic mediation of gastric slow wave dysrhythmias evoked during motion sickness. Am J Physiol 268:G539–G547, 1995.

Ruggiero DA, Mtui EP, Otake K, Anwar M: Vestibular afferents to the dorsal vagal complex: Substrate for vestibular-autonomic interactions in the rat. Brain Res 743:294–302, 1996.

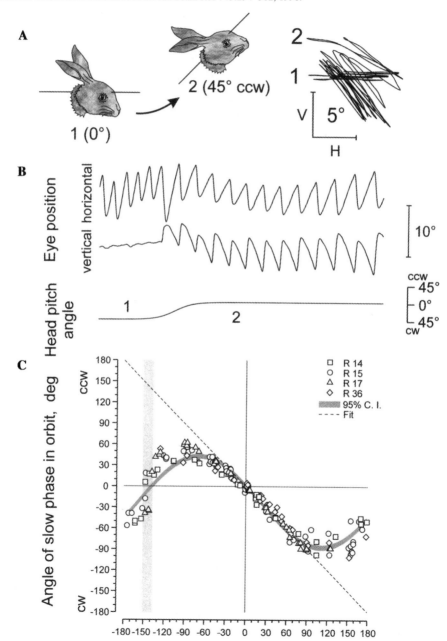

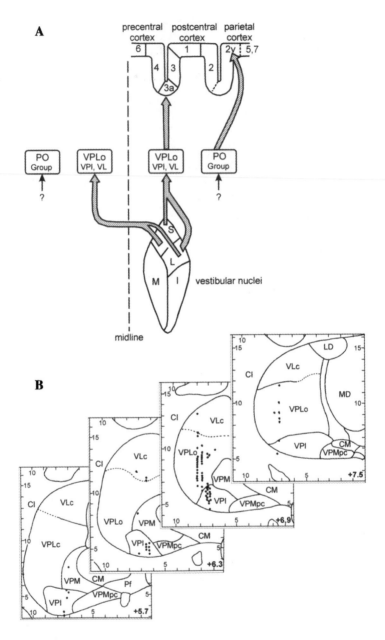

Figure 15. Ascending vestibular input to the cerebral cortex and descending cortical projections to the vestibular complex. **A**, Ascending connections of the vestibular complex with the thalamus and cortex. The vestibular nuclei project to the ventrobasal complex and then to areas of the precentral, postcentral, and parietal cortex. (Modified from Buttner U, Lang W: The vestibulocortical pathway: Neurophysiological and anatomical studies in the monkey. In Granit R, Pompeiano O (eds): Reflex Control of Posture and Movement. Elsevier/North-Holland Biomedical Press, 1979, pp 581–588; with permission.) **B**, Locations in the rhesus monkey thalamus from which vestibular responses can be evoked by electrical stimulation of the labyrinth. (Modified from Deecke L, Schwarz DWF, Fredrickson JM: Vestibular responses in the rhesus monkey ventroposterior thalamus. II. Vestibulo-proprioceptive convergence at thalamic neurons. Exp Brain Res 30:219–232, 1977; with permission). *Figure continues on following page.*

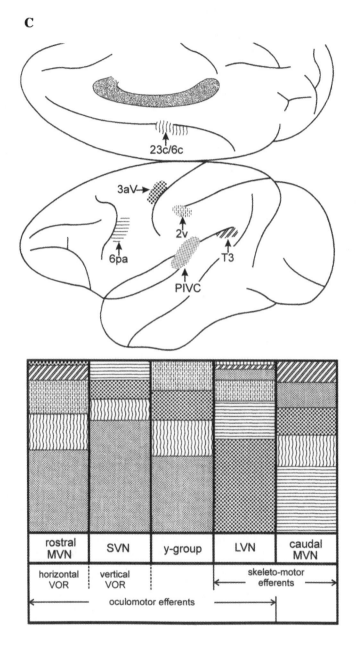

FIGURE 15 (continued).   **C,** Corticofugal projections to the vestibular nuclei determined by retrograde transport of various tracers injected into the vestibular complex of Java monkeys *(top)*. An estimate of the relative size of the projections from different cortical regions *(bottom)*. (Modified from Akbarian S, Grüsser O-J, Guldin WO: Corticofugal connections between the cerebral cortex and brainstem vestibular nuclei in the macaque monkey. J Comp Neurol 339:421–437, 1994; with permission.)

25. Did Astronaut/Senator John Glenn lose his cookies in space? Or, what is the Space Adaptation syndrome?

One of the more loosely guarded secrets of manned space flight is that most astronauts get motion sick when they first encounter microgravity and again when they return to earth. This is known as the Space Adaptation syndrome. In space, otolithic sensations decrease due to reduced gravity, causing an acute sensory conflict.

There is another possibility for why microgravity exposure causes motion sickness. Our genes cannot produce two labyrinths with the exact same sensitivity to vestibular stimulation. During development our central vestibular system must learn to calibrate signals arising from our two labyrinths so that our perception of space corresponds with reality. We rely on gravity, in part, for this calibration. Under conditions of microgravity, differences in signals from our labyrinths must be recalibrated.

The idea of developmental recalibration may be especially pertinent for the gerontological space mission recently completed by Glenn. Glenn suffered a fall in the late 1960s. The prolonged dizziness caused by this fall forced him to abandon his first try for elective office. His recuperation from trauma-induced vertigo might have been a function of vestibular recalibration; thus, he may have been more sensitive than the other astronauts to the transitions to and from microgravity. Only his doctors and his fellow crew members know for sure. Let's assume that Glenn became even more motion sick than his younger crew mates (this is pure speculation) on the recent shuttle mission. Should this difference in severity be attributed to normal gerontological problems or to his earlier vestibular trauma? Interestingly, experienced astronauts adapt to microgravity better than rookies, even when their missions are spaced months and years apart (although not 30 years apart).

26. Are there any effective pharmacologic therapies for motion and space sickness?

There are two separate approaches. The first approach blocks sensory signals whose conflicting information eventually leads to motion sickness. One modestly effective agent is the antimuscarinic compound, **scopolamine**. Scopolamine, administered orally, transdermally, or injected intramuscularly, causes an increased tolerance for sensory stimulation without inducing nausea. The benefit of reduced sensitivity to nauseogenic stimulation is countered by nonspecific muscarinic effects, such as: dry mouth, blurred vision, dizziness, drowsiness, and anxiety. We do not know which neural mechanisms are disrupted by scopolamine. In fact, the effect of scopolamine may be restricted to the periphery, since it has only limited penetration of the blood-brain barrier. Peripherally, it could influence muscarinic receptors located on hair cells in the labyrinth.

Nauseogenic vestibular or optokinetic stimulation causes an increase in blood plasma concentrations of arginine vasopressin (AVP). Sensory stimulation may cause increased activity in the paraventricular nucleus of the hypothalamus, which sends projections to the pituitary controlling the release of AVP. Intravenous administration of vasopressin is sufficient to provoke nausea in otherwise healthy subjects.

A second strategy for preventing motion sickness ignores the sensory conflict and blocks at a more central level the sequence of steps that leads to an overproduction of AVP. Administration of **atropine**, a centrally acting antimuscarinic agent, reduces the release of vasopressin, which in turn reduces gastric dysrhythmias. Vasopressin reduction is not achieved by scopolamine.

Atropine may influence a major cholinergic pathway, the vestibular secondary afferent (VSA) projection to the uvula-nodulus. Since the receptors on cerebellar granule cells for this mossy fiber projection are of the m2 subtype, it is possible that the antinauseogenic effect of atropine might be improved by replacing it with a drug that crosses the blood-brain barrier and has an effect restricted to the m2 receptor. There are, of course, many sites in the brain through which antimuscarinic agents could block the release of AVP.

Antagonists to AVP have met with some treatment success. Presumably AVP antagonists block autoimmune responses evoked by elevated levels of AVP. Exactly how this happens remains a secret.

Cheung BSK, Kohl RL, Money KE, Kinter LB: Etiologic significance of arginine vasopressin in motion sickness. J Clin Pharmacol 34:664–670, 1994.

Kim MS, Chey WD, Owyang C, Hasler WL: Role of plasma vasopressin as a mediator of nausea and gastric slow wave dysrhythmias in motion sickness. Am J Physiol 272:853–862, 1997.

Wood CD, Stewart JJ, Wood MJ, Mims M: Effectiveness and duration of intramuscular antimotion sickness medications. J Clin Pharmacol 32:1008–1012, 1992.

27. What is vestibular compensation?

Unilateral loss of vestibular function creates an imbalance in both postural and oculomotor control. The oculomotor deficit is characterized by a conjugate ocular nystagmus, with the slow phase directed toward the side of the damaged labyrinth. The postural disturbance often includes head and trunk flexion toward the damaged labyrinth (yaw head tilt), with the head twisted so that the ear ipsilateral to the damaged labyrinth is directed down (roll head tilt). In the early postoperative stage, animals frequently roll onto the side of the damaged labyrinth. In humans, similar distortions of posture usually are accompanied by dizziness and severe autonomic distress. Eventually, the spontaneous nystagmus disappears and balance is restored. This *recovery of function* takes hours in rats and weeks in humans. It is termed vestibular compensation.

28. Is function *fully* recovered by compensation?

Certain characteristics of vestibular function *never* return to normal. Although spontaneous nystagmus disappears over a period of hours to days, the gain of the vestibulo-ocular reflex remains depressed at roughly 50% of its preoperative value. Postural changes associated with a unilateral labyrinthectomy appear to be species-dependent. In rabbits and cats, the head tilt that is induced by this surgery is permanent. In rats and primates, symmetry of head posture returns. However, even in human subjects the recovery of vestibular function following a unilateral labyrinthectomy is incomplete, since vestibular reflexes remain impaired. The major behavioral evidence for compensation following a unilateral labyrinthectomy is a decreased ocular nystagmus accompanied by improved postural ability.

29. What are some consequences of unilateral peripheral damage to the vestibular apparatus?

There are at least two major consequences: (1) Loss of VPA activity causes a reduction of synaptic drive to secondary vestibular neurons ipsilateral to the damaged labyrinth, with a consequent loss of spontaneous activity, and (2) loss of stimulus-modulated activity to both the damaged side, by VPAs, and the intact side, through a commissural pathway, reduces the range of stimulus-driven activity of VSAs. This loss of stimulus-modulated activity is particularly severe on the side of peripheral vestibular damage. Consequently, the gain of the vestibulo-ocular reflex is reduced. The decrease of VSA steady-state activity on the side of the unilateral labyrinthectomy appears to be a necessary condition for the expression of the behavioral signs of sensory imbalance, such as oculomotor nystagmus.

30. How does vestibular compensation occur?

Within a few days after a unilateral vestibular neurectomy, there is a loss of nerve terminals in the de-afferented MVN, measured by an immunohistochemical marker for synaptophysin. Over several weeks this relative loss decreases, possibly due to "sprouting" of other inputs. Using ultrasound criteria, there is a loss of synaptic profiles in neurons located in the SVN contralateral to a unilateral neurectomy, when measured 8 weeks after the neurectomy. This implies that vestibular compensation includes **regressive** as sell as **regenerative** mechanisms.

Other possible compensatory mechanisms include: changes in the distribution of synaptic receptors on secondary vestibular neurons; changes in synaptic release mechanisms of neurons that are presynaptic to VSAs; changes in membrane properties of neurons that have suffered a loss in primary afferent innervation; and return of spontaneous activity in surviving VPAs whose cell bodies remain intact in Scarpa's ganglion.

Precht W, Shimazu H, Markham CH: A mechanism of central compensation of vestibular function following hemilabyrinthectomy. J Neurophysiol 29:996–1010, 1966.

31. Please summarize the function of the central vestibular system in 100 words or less.

The central vestibular system consists of the vestibular nuclei, cerebellum, and thalamo-cortical system. It constructs a spatial map from vestibular, visual, and proprioceptive signals to guide postural reflexes and coordinated movements. The central vestibular system regulates autonomic functions related to movement. It is adaptive and capable of recalibration following damage. Conflicting sensory signals to the vestibular system cause spatial disorientation and nausea. Pharmacologic treatments for motion sickness are either targeted at decreasing the sensitivity of the central vestibular system to sensory conflict or preventing the autonomic consequences of vestibular dysfunction.

BIBLIOGRAPHY

1. Akbarian S, Grüsser O-J, Guldin WO: Corticofugal connections between the cerebral cortex and brainstem vestibular nuclei in the macaque monkey. J Comp Neurol 339:421–437, 1994.
2. Barmack NH: A comparison of the horizontal and vertical vestibulo-ocular reflexes of the rabbit. J Physiol (Lond) 314:547–564, 1981.
3. Barmack NH: Cholinergic pathways and functions related to the vestibulo-cerebellum. In Anderson JH, Beitz AJ (eds): Neurochemistry of the Vestibular System. New York, CRC Press, 1999 (in press).
4. Barmack NH, Baughman RW, Errico P, Shojaku H: Vestibular primary afferent projection to the cerebellum of the rabbit. J Comp Neurol 327:521–534, 1993.
5. Barmack NH, Nastos MA, Pettorossi VE: The horizontal and vertical cervico-ocular reflexes of the rabbit. Brain Res 224:261–278, 1981.
5a. Barmack NH, Shojaku H: Vestibularly induced slow oscillations in climbing fiber responses of Purkinje cells in the cerebellar nodulus of the rabbit. Neuroscience 50:1–5, 1992.
6. Brodal A, Pompeiano O: The vestibular nuclei in the cat. J Anat 91:438–454, 1957.
7. Buttner U, Lang W: The vestibulocortical pathway: Neurophysiological and anatomical studies in the monkey. In Granit R, Pompeiano O (eds): Reflex control of posture and movement. Elsevier/North-Holland Biomedical Press, 1979, pp 581–588.
8. Cajal S Ramon y: Histology of the Nervous System. Vol. 1. [English translation of 1911 text] New York, Oxford University Press, 1995.
9. Deecke L, Schwarz DWF, Fredrickson JM: Vestibular responses in the rhesus monkey ventroposterior thalamus. II. Vestibulo-proprioceptive convergence at thalamic neurons. Exp Brain Res 30:219–232, 1977.
10. Epema AH, Gerrits NM, Voogd J: Commissural and intrinsic connections of the vestibular nuclei in the rabbit: A retrograde labeling study. Exp Brain Res 71:129–146, 1988.
11. Giolli RA, Blanks RHI, Torigoe Y, Williams DD: Projections of medial terminal accessory optic nucleus, ventral tegmental nuclei, and substantia nigra of rabbit and rat as studied by retrograde axonal transport of horseradish peroxidase. J Comp Neurol 232:99–116, 1985.
12. Goldstein MJ: The auditory periphery. In Mountcastle VB (ed): Medical Physiology. Saint Louis, C.V. Mosby Co., 1968, pp 1465–1498.
13. Kinney GA, Peterson BW, Slater NT: The synaptic activation of N-methyl-D-aspartate receptors in the rat medial vestibular nucleus. J Neurophysiol 72:1588–1595, 1994.
14. Lindeman HH: Anatomy of the otolith organs. Adv Otorhinolaryngol 20:405–433, 1973.
15. Newlands SD, Kevetter GA, Perachio AA: A quantitative study of the vestibular commissures in the gerbil. Brain Res 487:152–157, 1989.
16. Pettorossi VE, Errico P, Ferraresi A, Barmack NH: Optokinetic and vestibular stimulation determines the spatial orientation of negative optokinetic afternystagmus in the rabbit. J Neurosci 19:1524–1531, 1999.
17. Sato F, Sasaki H: Morphological correlations between spontaneously discharging primary vestibular afferents and vestibular nucleus neurons in the cat. J Comp Neurol 333:554–556, 1993.
18. Smith PF, De Waele C, Vidal P-P, Darlington CL: Excitatory amino acid receptors in normal and abnormal vestibular function. Mol Neurobiol 5:369–387, 1991.

8. CHEMICAL SENSES: OLFACTION AND TASTE

Robert F. Hevner, M.D., Ph.D.

1. Why are olfaction and taste distinguished as "chemical senses"?

These two senses enable us to sample and consciously recognize our chemical environment, unlike vision, hearing, and touch which connect us to our physical environment. Obviously, the chemical composition of our food is vitally important for maintaining energy intake and homeostasis. Unpleasant smells or tastes (which may signify the presence of bacteria or toxic substances) are to be avoided. Also, reproductive behaviors in humans and animals are driven in part by chemical senses (e.g., the smell of a lover). In the modern world, we tend to focus on the esthetics of taste and smell, but these senses have important survival purposes honed by evolution.

2. Are the olfactory and gustatory systems related to each other?

At the level of psychological awareness, olfaction and taste do seem closely related. For example, the smell and taste of a food are both parts of its flavor. People with a deficient sense of smell usually complain that food has lost its taste. However, at the level of neural systems, taste and olfaction are quite distinct in their developmental origins, anatomic pathways, and cellular components. Thus, these systems are probably unrelated in evolutionary terms.

THE OLFACTORY SYSTEM

3. True or false: Peripheral components of the olfactory system derive from neural crest.

False. The paired olfactory placodes (thickenings of cranial ectoderm) are the source of peripheral olfactory neurons.

4. Are humans macrosmatic or microsmatic?

Macrosmatic animals, such as mice and rats, have well-developed olfactory systems both functionally and anatomically. *Microsmatic* species, exemplified by humans, have a less acute sense of smell and poorly laminated olfactory bulbs.

5. What cells transduce odorant stimuli into nerve impulses?

These cells are known as **olfactory receptor neurons**. They are located in the olfactory epithelium, which lines part of the nasal cavity.

6. What cells carry nerve impulses from the olfactory epithelium to the brain?

The olfactory receptor neurons. Note that in this case the same cells that transduce the signal also send axons (collectively forming cranial nerve I, the olfactory nerve) to the brain. This is in contrast to some other systems (e.g., gustatory, auditory, and visual pathways) in which stimuli are transduced and transmitted by distinct receptor and ganglion cells.

7. How many different types of olfactory receptor neurons are there?

Histologically, there is only one type of olfactory receptor neuron. They are bipolar neurons, with a single dendrite that extends into the mucous layer of the olfactory epithelium (where odorant binding occurs) and a single unmyelinated axon that projects to the olfactory bulb.

8. True or false: We are born with all of the olfactory receptor neurons we will ever have.

False. These neurons have a lifespan of only about a month or two, and are replaced continually throughout our lifespans—though this regenerative process may slow with aging. Why do olfactory receptor neurons turn over? Since these neurons are peripherally placed and vulnerable to noxious

141

stimuli within the nose (e.g., viral infection, chemical exposure, heat), it may be important to maintain the capacity for replacing them.

9. How are the terminal nerve and vomeronasal nerve related to the olfactory nerve?

These structures are prominent in some lower animals but rudimentary in humans. Like the main
olfactory nerve, they are derived from the olfactory placodes and project from the nose to the forebrain.

10. What polypeptide hormone is associated with the terminal nerve?

Gonadotropin releasing-hormone (GnRH). The function of the terminal nerve is unclear, but during
development in humans and other species, it is the source of GnRH-containing neurons that migrate
into the hypothalamus and play an important role in sexual development and hormonal regulation.

11. How are pheromones recognized by the olfactory system?

The vomeronasal organ, vomeronasal nerve, and accessory olfactory bulb mediate pheromone
detection and collectively are designated the accessory olfactory system. The vomeronasal organ is
an epithelial structure in the nasal septum; its axons project to the accessory olfactory bulb. The
vomeronasal epithelium and accessory olfactory bulb are related to their counterparts in the main olfactory system, though there are significant structural and biochemical differences. This system is
well-developed in some animals such as rodents, but rudimentary or absent in humans. Thus, contrary to the sales pitch of some fragrance manufacturers, people do not have a well-developed
pheromone system.

12. Where does the accessory olfactory bulb project?

The accessory olfactory bulb projects directly to a discrete nucleus (known as the vomeronasal
nucleus) in the amygdala. From there, pheromone signals are relayed directly to the hypothalamus
where they influence sexual and neuroendocrine responses; cortical centers are not involved.
(Although humans lack a well-developed vomeronasal system, it seems probable that our sexual responses bypass higher cognitive processing as well!)

13. How many different odorant receptor molecules are there?

In the main olfactory system, about 1000! The odorant receptor molecules compose a large family
of G protein–coupled, seven-transmembrane-domain proteins, each encoded by a different gene.

**14. Does the vomeronasal system use the same family of odorant receptor molecules as the
main olfactory system?**

No. Two different families of vomeronasal receptor molecules, designated V1Rs and V2Rs,
have been identified. Neither vomeronasal receptor family is closely related to the other or to olfactory receptors, although the molecules in all three families have seven transmembrane domains. The
V2Rs are related to metabotropic glutamate receptors.

15. How many odorant receptor genes are expressed by each olfactory receptor neuron?

Only one. This situation is similar to that of cone photoceptors in the retina—which each express either the red, green, or blue light receptor—except that the number of odorant receptor molecules greatly exceeds the number of visual pigment molecules. The same one receptor–one neuron
model seems to hold in the vomeronasal system.

16. Do individual olfactory receptor neurons recognize a wide or narrow range of odorants?

Since each olfactory receptor neuron expresses only a single odorant receptor gene, one might
expect that only a narrow range of odorants would be recognized; but this is not the case. Typically,
a wide range of chemically similar odorants are recognized, implying that odorant receptor proteins
have a relatively broad binding specificity. Again, the situation is analogous to cone photoreceptors
in the retina, which are tuned to a rather broad range of wavelengths centered about either red, green,
or blue light.

17. What second-messenger systems are coupled to odorant receptors?

Since odorant receptor molecules belong to the G protein–coupled, seven-transmembrane-domain family of proteins, the reader may have surmised (correctly) that G proteins have a role. Olfactory receptor neurons contain a distinct G protein called G_{olf}, and possibly other G proteins. Some G proteins stimulate adenylate cyclase to synthesize increased cAMP, which opens a cyclic nucleotide-gated ion channel, thus depolarizing the receptor neuron. In other cases, the G protein may stimulate phospholipase C, which catalyzes the production of inositol triphosphate (leading to increased cellular calcium ion concentration) and diacylglycerol (which activates protein kinase C, leading to protein phosphorylation). The full complexities of these systems and their relative contributions to olfactory transduction remain to be elucidated.

18. Describe the course of the olfactory nerve from the nose to the brain.

The axons of olfactory receptor neurons fasciculate into about 20 or 30 bundles (fila) on each side. Each filum passes individually through the cribriform plate of the ethmoid bone to enter the cranial cavity. The olfactory nerve fibers then enter the paired olfactory bulbs, located directly over the cribriform plate.

19. Identify the layers of the olfactory bulb in the cross-section from a newborn mouse shown below.

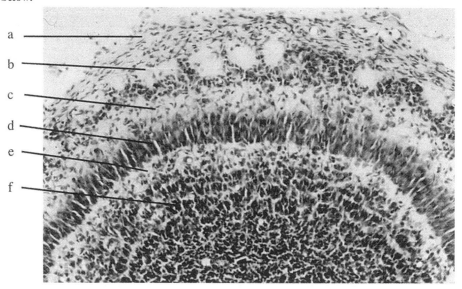

Olfactory bulb histology.

a: olfactory nerve; b: glomerular layer; c: external plexiform layer; d: mitral cell layer; e: internal plexiform layer; f: granule cell layer. Note that the human olfactory bulb does not have these well-formed layers.

20. In which layer of the olfactory bulb do olfactory nerve fibers terminate?

Axons end in the glomerular layer, within the cell-sparse centers of glomeruli. There, they contact the dendrites mainly of mitral cells, though tufted cells also receive olfactory nerve inputs. The glomeruli have a complex synaptic organization also involving interneurons (periglomerular cells). Mitral and tufted cells are the principal relay neurons that relay information from the olfactory bulb to higher processing centers in the telencephalon. The flow of information can be simplified as follows:

Olfactory receptor neurons (olfactory epithelium) → Mitral cells (olfactory bulb) →
Higher olfactory centers (anterior olfactory nucleus, piriform cortex)

21. How many olfactory nerve axons end in each glomerulus?

One thousand or more. The glomerulus is a neuropil structure that contains many axodendritic synapses.

22. True or false: All of the olfactory receptor neurons that project to a particular glomerulus express the same odorant receptor protein.

True. Thus, each glomerulus processes information concerning the activation of only one of the 1000 or so different odorant receptors, and the convergence of receptor axons may result in tremendous signal amplification.

23. True or false: All of the olfactory receptor neurons that express a particular odorant receptor gene project to one glomerulus.

False. In known examples, two glomeruli in each bulb receive projections representing a particular odorant receptor gene. Thus, for each nostril, olfactory receptor neurons project to one of two glomeruli specific for the appropriate odorant receptor gene. The mechanism of this precise mapping of inputs onto the olfactory bulb is unknown.

24. How many mitral cells have dendrites within each glomerulus?

On average, about 25. On the other hand, each mitral cell sends its primary dendrite to only one glomerulus, and therefore receives information mainly concerning activation of a single odorant receptor type. Tufted cells have similar connections, as do mitral cells.

25. Where do mitral cells send their outputs?

The glomerular inputs received via dendrites are processed by the mitral cells and relayed by them through the **lateral olfactory tract** mainly to the **piriform cortex** (also known as the pyriform or prepyriform cortex) in the medial temporal lobe. Piriform cortex is regarded as the primary sensory cortex for the olfactory system. Mitral and tufted cells also send axons to the anterior olfactory nucleus (AON), olfactory tubercle, amygdala, and entorhinal cortex. Fibers from the AON cross through the anterior commissure and project to the contralateral olfactory bulb.

26. Is piriform cortex regarded as archicortex, paleocortex, or neocortex?

Piriform cortex is made up of only three layers, and is traditionally regarded as paleocortex. Archicortex likewise contains three layers, but is part of the hippocampal complex. Neocortex contains six layers.

27. Which thalamic nucleus relays olfactory information from the bulbs to the olfactory cortex?

Sorry, trick question! Olfaction is the only sense that does not pass directly through a thalamic relay en route to cortex. The olfactory bulbs (themselves closely related to the cerebral cortex in molecular and histologic properties) relay information directly to the olfactory paleocortex (i.e., piriform cortex) and entorhinal cortex. The bulbs also send projections to the olfactory tubercle, which relays signals to the medial dorsal (MD) thalamic nucleus. The MD nucleus in turn projects to orbitofrontal cortex. Thus, a thalamic nucleus is involved in relay of olfaction to the neocortex, but only indirectly.

28. How are odors represented in the olfactory bulb?

Obviously this is a complex question, and any answer must account for the capabilities of the olfactory system that allow us to discriminate among thousands of odors. Current evidence indicates that for any given smell (whether comprised of one or many odorants), a combination of glomeruli is activated. Such a combinatorial code provides for tremendous versatility in the representation of different odors. Again, this system is analogous to color vision, in which three types of cone photoreceptors can encode millions of colors.

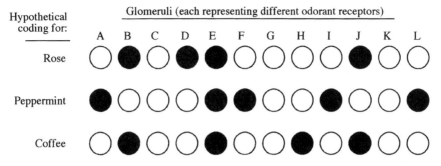

Combinatorial coding of smell by activation of different combinations of glomeruli in the olfactory bulb.

29. Where in the olfactory system does conscious perception of smell occur?

Again, a complex question for which only a provisional answer may be given. As for other perceptions, conscious awareness of smell presumably is confined to the cortex. The piriform and entorhinal cortex may be involved, or (perhaps more likely) the orbitofrontal neocortex.

THE GUSTATORY SYSTEM

30. What are the sensory organs of taste? Where are they located?

In mammals, **taste buds** are the organs of taste sensation. They are scattered mainly over the tongue, but also on the palate, in the pharynx, and on the epiglottis and esophagus. Each taste bud is embedded within the epithelial lining of the mouth or pharynx and has a narrow opening to the surface known as the **taste pore**.

31. What cell types make up the taste bud?

Three types of cells are contained within the taste bud: dark (type I) and light (type II) cells, so designated according to their relative density as observed by electron microscopy, and basal cells. Recent evidence suggests that the light (type II) cells are gustatory receptor cells, whereas dark (type I) cells probably are supportive. Basal cells are a reserve population, which divides and gives rise to new receptor cells. The receptor cells constantly turn over, at the rate of about once every 10 days. Note that this property of constant replacement is shared by olfactory receptor neurons.

32. True or false: Taste receptor cells contribute axons to cranial nerves and thus innervate the brainstem.

False. The taste receptor cells remain entirely within the taste bud. Afferent neurons located in cranial nerve ganglia send peripheral processes to innervate the taste buds and central processes to innervate the brainstem. The peripheral tips of afferent neurons are found within the taste buds, in close association with the dark (type I) and light (type II) cells. Note that the taste receptors differ in this respect from the olfactory receptors, which do send axons into the brain (specifically, the olfactory bulb).

33. Do taste receptor cells develop from neural crest, epibranchial placodes, or oropharyngeal epithelium?

Unlike most types of sensory receptors, taste receptor cells do not originate from placodal or neural crest cells, but instead differentiate directly from the oropharyngeal epithelium in which they are embedded. Recent evidence even suggests that their differentiation is genetically programmed and independent of induction by developing nerves (although their subsequent trophic support is innervation-dependent).

34. Taste buds reside within specialized epithelial structures known as papillae. Name the three different types of papillae.

Name	Location	Major Innervation	Taste Buds Per Papilla
Fungiform	Anterior ⅔ of tongue	Facial	1–5
Foliate	Posterior lateral tongue	Glossopharyngeal	Thousands
Circumvallate	Posterior ⅓ of tongue	Glossopharyngeal	Thousands

35. Which three cranial nerves carry taste sensation?

The facial (VII), glossopharyngeal (IX), and vagus (X) nerves carry taste fibers. The anterior two-thirds of the tongue are innervated by the facial nerve (chorda tympani branch); the posterior one-third of the tongue and palate by the glossopharyngeal nerve; and the epiglottis, pharynx, and esophagus by the vagus nerve.

36. Where are the cell bodies of taste nerve fibers located?

Cranial Nerves	Ganglion Containing Cell Bodies
Facial	Geniculate
Glossopharyngeal	Inferior glossopharyngeal (petrosal)
Vagus	Inferior vagal (nodose)

Note that the cell bodies of glossopharyngeal and vagal taste fibers (special *visceral* afferent) are located in the *inferior* ganglia of those nerves, whereas the cell bodies of *somatic* sensory neurons are located in the *superior* ganglia (mnemonic: somatic and superior both start with "s").

37. Name the five "primary" taste qualities.

Sweet, salt, sour, and *bitter* were identified in the 1920s as four primary sensations that, in combination, could seemingly account for all other flavors—no matter how apparently complex. More recent studies identified a fifth primary quality, known as *umami*—the flavor of glutamate. Taste buds in different parts of the mouth are differentially sensitive to each of these qualities, such that sweet taste is best detected at the anterior tip of the tongue; salt in the anterior half of the tongue; sour in the lateral part of the tongue; and bitter on the soft palate and posterior tongue. (Note that the present list of primary taste qualities may be incomplete.)

38. What types of molecules elicit specific taste sensations?

Taste Quality	Molecular Properties
Sweet	Stereochemical resemblance to glucose
Salt	Sodium ions
Sour	Hydrogen ions
Bitter	Alkaloids
Umami	Glutamate

Note that the receptors for these properties may exhibit a wide range of molecular specificity (i.e., broad "tuning"). For example, the synthetic sweeteners aspartame and saccharin are very effective at stimulating sweet receptor cells.

39. Which taste receptors are stimulated by spicy-hot flavors?

None of them! Spicy-hot foods activate a distinct receptor present on general somatic afferent endings, which belong to trigeminal nerve fibers. This receptor is not specific to the gustatory system, but instead is associated with the pain and temperature system. In fact, the full taste of food is really a combination of gustatory, olfactory, and somatic sensations.

40. How many different gustatory receptor molecules are there?

Unknown. With regard to identification and characterization of receptor molecules, our progress in understanding the gustatory system lags behind that of the olfactory system. This is one reason it may be premature to enumerate a specific number of primary taste qualities.

41. What types of receptor proteins and second messengers transduce gustatory stimuli?

Multiple ligand-binding receptors, ion channels, and second messenger systems contribute to the transduction of different taste stimuli.

Taste Quality	Receptor Protein	Second Messengers
Sweet	TR1 (GPCR)	Gustducin, CNGC, other
Salt	Ion channel	None (direct depolarization by Na^+)
Sour	Ion channel	None (direct depolarization by H^+)
Bitter	TR2 (GPCR)	Gustducin, CNGC, other
Umami	mGluR4	G protein

TR = taste receptor; GPCR = G protein–coupled seven-transmembrane receptor protein; mGluR4 = metabotropic glutamate receptor 4; CNGC = cyclic nucleotide-gated ion channel.

Gustducin is closely related to the photoreceptor G protein, transducin, and both regulate cyclic nucleotides that gate membrane ion channels. Other second messenger systems, including inositol triphosphate and calcium, also play a role. Of the receptor proteins listed above, only TR1, TR2, and MGluR4 have been cloned. Since salt and sour sensations are elicited by ions (sodium and hydrogen, respectively), they are able to depolarize receptor cells directly by passing through ion channels.

42. What brainstem nucleus receives primary afferent taste stimuli?

Regardless of which nerve (facial, glossopharyngeal, or vagal) transmits the taste stimuli, the primary afferent fibers end on second-order neurons in the rostral portion of the solitary nucleus. This rostral subdivision also is known as the **gustatory nucleus**.

43. True or false: The gustatory nucleus is located in the pons.

True. The gustatory nucleus is in the caudal pons and is continuous with the solitary nucleus, located mainly in the medulla.

44. Which thalamic nucleus relays taste sensation to the cerebral cortex?

From the solitary nucleus, fibers travel in the central tegmental tract to the ventral posteromedial (VPM) thalamic nucleus, which transmits impulses via the internal capsule to cortex. Note that the VPM nucleus also relays general somatic sensation from the face to the cortex.

45. True or false: Gustatory cortex is located in the parietal lobe.

False. Unlike general somatic afferent information from VPM to the parietal lobe, taste sensation is relayed to primary gustatory cortex ("area G") in the insula and frontal operculum. This area actually is adjacent to cortical areas 3, 1, and 2—which together comprise the primary somatosensory cortex of the parietal lobe.

46. Name three brain areas that mediate the pleasurable or displeasurable aspects of taste.

The three nuclei that figure most prominently in the involuntary response to taste stimuli are the **parabrachial nucleus**, the **amygdala**, and the **hypothalamus**. From the gustatory nucleus, fibers relay information to the parabrachial nucleus located in the lateral pons, which in turn relays signals to the amygdala and hypothalamus. These limbic regions participate in the autonomic response to taste and its association with other stimuli.

CLINICAL ASPECTS

47. What is an uncinate seizure?

In uncinate seizures, olfactory hallucinations occur in association with other features of epilepsy, such as involuntary movements, altered consciousness, or subsequent loss of consciousness. They are called uncinate seizures because abnormal electrical activity involves the uncus, the part of the medial temporal lobe where piriform and entorhinal cortices are located.

48. What is anosmia?

This the clinical term for loss of the sense of smell. **Hyposmia** is decreased sense of smell.

49. Which forebrain neurons are lacking in Kallmann syndrome?

Clinically, Kallmann syndrome is defined as the association of anosmia or hyposmia (usually due to agenesis of the olfactory bulbs) with hypogonadotropic hypogonadism (impaired gonadal function due to decreased secretion of gonadotropic hormones from the pituitary gland). With this information, can you now guess which forebrain neurons might be missing? In addition to the absent olfactory bulbs, hypothalamic neurons containing GnRH also are missing. Recall that these neurons, like the olfactory receptor neurons, are derived from the olfactory placode.The GnRH-positive neurons migrate from the terminal nerve into the hypothalamus. Olfactory bulb agenesis is likely secondary to a failure of innervation from the olfactory receptor neurons.

50. What is the inheritance pattern of Kallmann syndrome?

Familial cases of Kallmann syndrome have led to the identification of several genes that, when mutated, cause the disease. Some are X-linked and some are autosomal.

BIBLIOGRAPHY

1. Boughter JD Jr, Pumplin DW, Yu C, et al: Differential expression of α-gustducin in taste bud populations of the rat and hamster. J Neurosci 17:2852–2858, 1997.
2. Brennan PA, Friedrich RW: Something in the air: New vistas on olfaction. Trends Neurosci 21:1–2, 1998.
3. Buck L, Axel R: A novel multigene family may encode odorant receptors: A molecular basis for odor recognition. Cell 65:175–187, 1991.
4. Dulac C: How does the brain smell? Neuron 19:477–480, 1997.
4a. Hoon MA, Adler E, Lindemeier J, et al: Putative mammalian taste receptors: A class of taste-specific GPCRs with distinct topographic selectivity. Cell 96:541–551, 1999.
5. Ito S, Ogawa H: Cytochrome oxidase staining facilitates unequivocal visualization of the primary gustatory area in the fronto-operculo-insular cortex of macaque monkeys. Neurosci Lett 130:61–64, 1991.
6. Kinnamon SC, Margolskee RF: Mechanisms of taste transduction. Curr Opin Neurobiol 6:506–513, 1996.
7. Ming D, Ruiz-Avila L, Margolskee RF: Characterization and solubilization of bitter-responsive receptors that couple to gustducin. Proc Natl Acad Sci USA 95:8933–8938, 1998.
8. Nolte J: The Human Brain: An Introduction to its Functional Anatomy, 4th ed. St. Louis, Mosby, 1999.
9. Northcutt RG, Barlow LA: Amphibians provide new insights into taste-bud development. Trends Neurosci 21:38–43, 1998.
10. Shepherd GM: Synaptic organization of the mammalian olfactory bulb. Physiol Rev 52:864–917, 1972.
11. Shepherd GM: Discrimination of molecular signals by the olfactory receptor neuron. Neuron 13:771–790. 1994.
12. Stewart RE, DeSimone JA, Hill DL: New perspectives in gustatory physiology: Transduction, development, and plasticity. Am J Physiol 272(Cell Physiol 41):C1–C26, 1997.
13. Wilson-Pauwels L, Akesson EJ, Stewart PA: Cranial Nerves: Anatomy and Clinical Comments. Toronto, B.C. Decker, 1988.
14. Wong GT, Gannon KS, Margolskee RF: Transduction of bitter and sweet taste by gustducin. Nature 381:796–800, 1996.

9. CRANIAL NERVES AND NUCLEI

Robert F. Hevner, M.D., Ph.D.

1. What is a cranial nerve?

A cranial nerve is any nerve that exits the brain within the skull, i.e., above the foramen magnum.

2. What is a cranial nerve nucleus?

A cranial nerve nucleus is a collection of cells in the brainstem (none are located in the forebrain) that either sends efferent axons into a cranial nerve, or receives synaptic input directly from a cranial nerve primary afferent fiber. For the student, memorizing the names, locations, and functions of the various cranial nerve nuclei can be one of the most challenging exercises in neuroanatomy.

3. How do cranial nerves differ from spinal nerves?

The cranial nerves have more variable structure (including exit from the ventral, dorsal, or lateral part of the brain); more diverse composition (motor, sensory, autonomic, and/or special sensory); and more complex development (from neural tube, neural crest, and/or ectodermal placode).

4. How many cranial nerves are there?

The standard answer is 12 (numbered 1–12, aptly enough). However, after the original 12 were identified, a 13th cranial nerve was discovered, first in the dogfish shark and later in other species. It is known as the nervus terminalis (terminal nerve), or cranial nerve 0 (zero). It is extremely small, but present in humans. For more about it, see Chapter 8.

5. Name the cranial nerves.

Nerve #	Name	Major Function(s)
I	Olfactory	Smell
II	Optic	Vision
III	Oculomotor	Eye movement, pupillary constriction
IV	Trochlear	Eye movement
V	Trigeminal	Facial sensation, mastication (chewing)
VI	Abducens	Eye movement
VII	Facial	Facial expression, taste, lacrimation, salivation
VIII	Acoustic (Vestibulocochlear)	Hearing, balance
IX	Glossopharyngeal	Taste, salivation, swallowing, visceral sensation
X	Vagus	Taste, swallowing, autonomic, visceral sensation
XI	Accessory	Neck and shoulder movement
XII	Hypoglossal	Tongue movement

For those who find mnemonics helpful, the following bit of apocrypha may be useful: "On old Olympus' towering top a Finn and German viewed a hop." (See figure at top of following page.)

6. List the five special senses of the cranial nerves.

Smell, vision, taste, hearing, and balance. These senses, of course, are unique to the cranial nerves. They further classified as either *visceral* (smell, taste) or *somatic* (vision, hearing, balance).

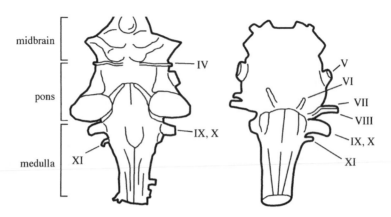

Dorsal *(left)* and ventral *(right)* views of the brainstem and some cranial nerves.

7. Which cranial nerve has no peripheral component?

The **optic nerve** and retina are, in fact, extensions of the central nervous system into the eye. Thus, the glial cells associated with the optic nerve are astrocytes and oligodendroglia, rather than Schwann cells.

8. Which is the only cranial nerve that entirely crosses the midline within the brain?

The **trochlear nerve**. Fibers of this nerve decussate within the midbrain before exiting the brainstem. The significance of this unique trajectory is unclear.

9. Which is the only cranial nerve that exits the dorsal aspect of the brain?

The trochlear nerve. Again, the reason for this singular pathway is unknown. However, some insight into the developmental mechanism that drives trochlear fibers dorsally has come from studies of the **netrins**, molecules related to laminin that act as diffusible chemoattractants or chemorepellents in the developing brain. Trochlear axons ares repelled by netrin-1, which is secreted from the ventral midline.

10. List the three cranial nerves that control eye movements.

Nerve #	Name	Muscle(s) Innervated
III	Oculomotor	Medial rectus, superior rectus, inferior rectus, inferior oblique
IV	Trochlear	Superior oblique
VI	Abducens	Lateral rectus

Some people find the chemical pseudo-formula "SO_4Lr_6" to be a helpful mnemonic for remembering which muscles are innervated by the trochlear and abducens nerves. The oculomotor nerve innervates all the rest.

11. Taste sensation is mediated by which three cranial nerves?

The facial (VII), glossopharyngeal (IX), and vagus (X) nerves.

12. Continual regeneration is a feature of which cranial nerve?

The olfactory (I) nerve. It is the only nerve in the body that continually regenerates. The olfactory receptor neurons undergo continual turnover and replacement throughout life.

13. List the seven columnar components of cranial nerves.

Component	Comments
General somatic efferent (GSE)	Motor to somite-derived muscles
Special visceral efferent (SVE)	Motor to branchial arch–derived muscles
General visceral efferent (GVE)	Autonomic (sympathetic, parasympathetic)
General visceral afferent (GVA)	Sensory from gut, heart, etc.
Special visceral afferent (SVA)	Olfaction, taste
General somatic afferent (GSA)	Sensory from skin, voluntary muscle, etc.
Special somatic afferent (SSA)	Vision, hearing, balance

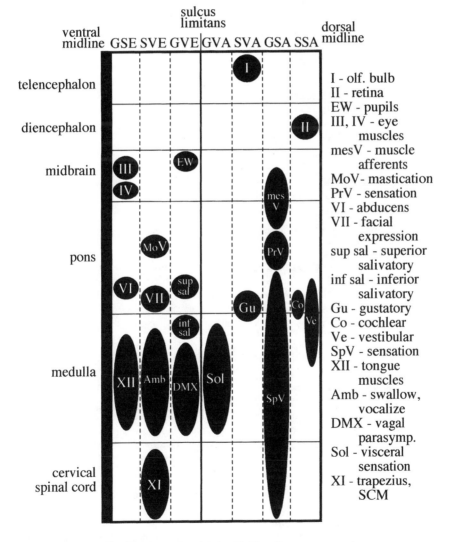

Cranial nerves and nuclei classified by columnar components.

14. Why are the components listed above regarded as columnar?

The central neurons associated with each component are organized in a roughly columnar fashion throughout the neuraxis. An understanding of this columnar organization is useful for memorizing the locations of the cranial nerve nuclei and their developmental origins. Recall that in the spinal cord, motor neurons and their roots develop in the **basal plate**, while sensory neurons and their afferents develop in the **alar plate**. The same is essentially true in the brainstem. The alar plate develops from the more lateral portion of the primitive neural plate, and tends to assume a dorsal position during neural tube closure (especially in the spinal cord), though alar plate derivatives remain lateral in most of the brainstem. The basal plate develops from medial portions of the neural plate and assumes a ventral position in the spinal cord. The dividing line between alar and basal plates is approximated by the **sulcus limitans**, visible in the developing spinal cord and much of the brainstem.

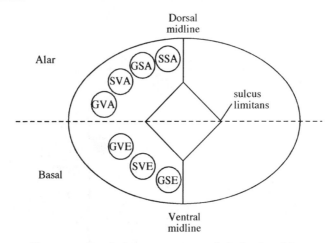

The arrangement of columnar components of spinal and cranial nerves.

15. Identify the one cranial nerve that has primary sensory neurons located within the brain.

The cranial nerves are full of oddities, and one peculiarity is that trigeminal muscle afferents somehow end up in the brainstem and form the **mesencephalic trigeminal nucleus**. These neurons send peripheral processes out to the muscles of mastication and, in that respect, are equivalent to sensory ganglion neurons (dorsal root ganglion neurons in the spinal column; cranial nerve ganglion cells in the head).

CRANIAL NERVE 0: THE TERMINAL NERVE

16. Where is the terminal nerve located?

The terminal nerve (nervus terminalis, cranial nerve zero) consists of a plexus of nerve fibers with peripheral processes in the nasal septum, cell bodies in the region of the cribriform plate, and central processes terminating in the medial forebrain (septum and preoptic nuclei). It is prominent in some lower species, but rudimentary in adult humans. For additional information on the terminal nerve, see Chapter 8.

CRANIAL NERVE I: THE OLFACTORY NERVE

17. What columnar components comprise cranial nerve I?

Special *visceral* afferents. Both "chemical senses" (olfaction and taste) are classified as special visceral afferents.

18. True or false: Cranial nerve I also is known as the olfactory tract.

False. The olfactory *tract* is distinct from the olfactory *nerve*. The nerve is located in the periphery, whereas the tract is composed mainly of second-order axons from mitral cells to the piriform cortex.

19. Where are the cell bodies of cranial nerve I located?

In the olfactory epithelium of the nasal cavity. The cell bodies of cranial nerve I are, in fact, the same cells that function as olfactory receptor neurons and transduce odorant stimuli.

20. Where do the peripheral processes of cranial nerve I terminate?

The peripheral processes consist of short dendrites with terminal cilia that extend into the mucus layer of the nasal cavity. Odorant transduction occurs on the cilia.

21. Where do the central processes of cranial nerve I terminate?

The central processes terminate in the olfactory bulb, in specialized neuropil structures known as **glomeruli**. There, they synapse with the dendrites of mitral cells, the main projection neurons that relay signals from the olfactory bulb to the cortex and other higher-order centers.

22. Through what bone do the olfactory nerve fibers pass to enter the cranial cavity?

The olfactory nerve fibers fasciculate into about 20 bundles (fila) that penetrate the cribriform plate of the **ethmoid bone**. The cribriform plate is so named because of its resemblance to a sieve.

23. What is the clinical consequence of olfactory nerve transection?

Transection (complete cutting or disruption) of the olfactory nerve fibers causes complete loss of the sense of smell, a condition known as **anosmia**.

CRANIAL NERVE II: THE OPTIC NERVE

24. What are the columnar components of cranial nerve II?

Special *somatic* afferents. The senses associated with physical stimuli (light, sound, motion, position) are classified as somatic.

25. Where are the cell bodies of cranial nerve II located?

In the retina. The optic nerve carries the axons of retinal ganglion cells, the innermost neurons of the retina.

26. True or false: Retinal ganglion cells also function as light receptors.

False. Rods and cones are the photoreceptors of the retina. Since their signals are relayed by bipolar cells to retinal ganglion cells and modified by other retinal neurons such as amacrine cells, there is substantial processing of light information before it is transmitted through the optic nerve to the brain.

27. What are the central targets of cranial nerve II?

Target	Location	Functional Importance
Lateral geniculate nucleus	Thalamus	Relay to cortex for visual awareness
Pretectal nuclei	Pretectum	Pupillary reflexes
Superior colliculus	Midbrain	Visual tracking movements
Suprachiasmatic nucleus	Hypothalamus	Circadian rhythms

28. True or false: Cranial nerve II also is known as the optic tract.

False. Each optic *nerve* extends from the eye to optic chiasm, where retinal axons redistribute (some crossing the midline, some not). The optic *tract* extends from the optic chiasm to the lateral geniculate nucleus.

29. What is the clinical consequence of transection of one optic nerve?
Loss of vision from one eye.

30. What is the clinical consequence of transection of one optic tract?
Loss of vision from one visual hemifield. All of the fibers receiving input from one hemifield (left or right) redistribute at the optic chiasm, to innervate the lateral geniculate nucleus contralateral to the hemifield.

31. Which cortical lobe contains the primary visual cortex?
The occipital lobe. The primary visual cortex (area 17, striate cortex) receives its projections from the lateral geniculate nucleus.

CRANIAL NERVE III: THE OCULOMOTOR NERVE

32. What columnar components are in cranial nerve III?
General somatic efferent (GSE) and general visceral efferent (GVE). All motor fibers to extraocular muscles are GSE, since the extraocular muscles are derived from somites. The GVE component functions in pupillary constriction and lens accommodation (shape adjustment for near or distant focus).

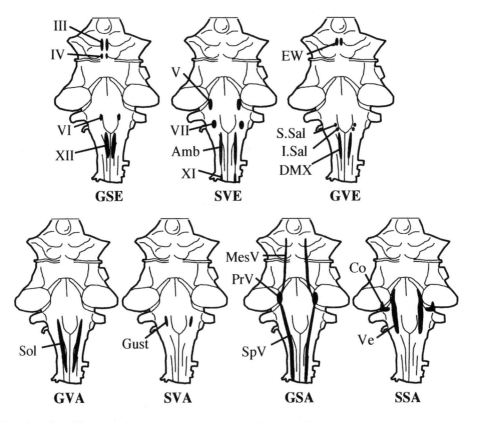

Locations of cranial nerve nuclei and columnar components. GSE = general somatic efferent, SVE = special visceral efferent, GVE = general visceral efferent, GVA = general visceral afferent, SVA = special visceral afferent, GSA = general somatic afferent, SSA = special somatic afferent.

33. Cranial nerve III innervates four external ocular muscles. Name them.

Medial rectus, superior rectus, inferior rectus, and inferior oblique.

34. Cranial nerve III also helps control pupillary size via autonomic fibers. Are these fibers sympathetic or parasympathetic?

Parasympathetic. All cranial nerve autonomic fibers are parasympathetic. Sympathetic fibers arise only from the thoracolumbar spinal cord.

35. What eponymous cranial nerve III nucleus contains neurons that control pupillary size and lens accommodation?

The **Edinger-Westphal nucleus,** located in the midbrain, contains the preganglionic parasympathetic neurons that control these autonomic functions. Note that this control is indirect, since the Edinger-Westphal nucleus innervates a peripheral ganglion, which in turn projects to the muscles.

36. What peripheral autonomic ganglion is innervated by cranial nerve III?

The **ciliary ganglion.** This ganglion receives its innervation from the Edinger-Westphal nucleus and sends projections to the ciliary muscle (which controls accommodation) and sphincter pupillae (which control pupillary size).

37. Define miosis.

This is not a form of cell division! (That would be meiosis.) Miosis is excessive pupillary constriction. The opposite condition, excessive pupillary dilatation, is called *mydriasis*. These conditions may be caused by toxin poisoning, pharmacological treatment (e.g., dilatation by an ophthalmologist), or nerve damage.

38. What brainstem nucleus contains the cranial nerve III motor neurons that innervate external ocular muscles?

The oculomotor nucleus.

39. True or false: The oculomotor nucleus is located in the pons.

False. Both the Edinger-Westphal nucleus and the oculomotor nucleus reside in the midbrain tegmentum. (The midbrain is divided into the *tectum*, consisting of structures dorsal to the cerebral aqueduct—mainly the superior and inferior colliculi; and the *tegmentum*, consisting of structures ventral to the aqueduct of Sylvius.)

40. Does voluntary control over the oculomotor nucleus arise in ipsilateral, contralateral, or bilateral cortical regions?

Bilateral. Cortical upper motor neurons (e.g., from the frontal eye fields) generally control complex movements of both eyes—such as lateral gaze—rather than unilateral eye muscles.

CRANIAL NERVE IV: THE TROCHLEAR NERVE

41. What columnar components comprise cranial nerve IV?

General somatic efferent.

42. Is the trochlear nucleus an alar or basal plate derivative?

Like all motor nuclei, it is considered a basal plate derivative.

43. What external ocular muscle is innervated by the trochlear nerve?

The superior oblique muscle. Recall the pseudo-chemical formula: SO_4Lr_6 (superior oblique innervated by cranial nerve IV, lateral rectus by cranial nerve VI).

44. Why is cranial nerve IV called the trochlear nerve?

The superior oblique muscle pulls its tendon over a small strap of connective tissue that acts like a pulley, which is the root meaning of the word "trochlear."

45. True or false: The trochlear nucleus is located in the pons.

False. The trochlear nucleus resides in the midbrain, ventral to the periaqueductal gray.

46. Describe the course of trochlear nerve fibers within the brainstem.

Trochlear nerve fibers exit the nucleus dorsally and decussate in the posterior midbrain tectum prior to exiting the brainstem just caudal to the inferior colliculi. IV is the only cranial nerve in which all fibers cross the midline and the only cranial nerve to exit the dorsal aspect of the brainstem. These characteristics are atypical of motor nerve fibers.

CRANIAL NERVE V: THE TRIGEMINAL NERVE

47. What columnar components does cranial nerve V include?

Component	Targets
Special visceral efferent	Temporalis, masseter, and other muscles
General somatic afferent	Sensation from face, scalp, conjunctiva, nasal and oral cavities, and meninges

Although cranial nerve V has only two components, it has four major nuclei within the brainstem. This complex nuclear organization reflects the unique development and innervation of the head region.

48. Why is cranial nerve V called the trigeminal nerve?

Maybe the reader can deduce the answer to this question from the astrological sign Gemini, which means twins—signifying the good and evil sides of people born under this sign. "Trigeminal" means three twins, in this case the three large branches of the nerve, which arise just peripheral to the trigeminal ganglion.

49. Name the three branches of the trigeminal nerve.

The ophthalmic (V_1), maxillary (V_2), and mandibular (V_3). Although the "V" of each branch is meant to denote the Roman numeral five, the branches are commonly pronounced "vee" (e.g., the abbreviated name for the ophthalmic branch is pronounced "vee-one"). Each branch innervates the region of the face corresponding to its name.

50. True or false: The motor nucleus of cranial nerve V is located in the pons.

True. The trigeminal motor nucleus, also known as the **masticator nucleus**, is located in the pontine tegmentum, near the exit point of the trigeminal nerve. (The pons is divided into the ventrally situated *basis pontis*, where the pontine nuclei are located; and the *tegmentum*, immediately ventral and lateral to the fourth ventricle.)

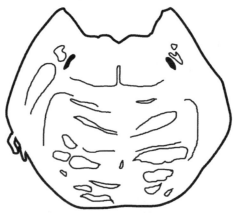

The trigeminal motor nucleus (pons).

51. True or false: Trigeminal motor neurons are categorized as special visceral efferent rather than general somatic efferent because they innervate smooth muscle.

False! SVE neurons are categorized on the basis of innervating branchial arch–derived muscle, which is striated. Somite-derived muscle (innervated by GSE neurons) also is striated and indistinguishable histologically from branchial arch–derived muscle.

52. Name the three major sensory nuclei associated with cranial nerve V.

Sensory Nucleus	Major Function
Mesencephalic nucleus of V	Proprioception from muscles innervated by cranial nerve V
Principal nucleus of V	Tactile information from face
Spinal nucleus of V	Pain and temperature sensation from face

Note that these three sensory nuclei all transmit the same category of information: general somatic afferent. The sensory information is segregated according to modality (proprioception, touch, pain, and temperature) and distributed to different nuclei. However, the principal nucleus of V and the spinal nucleus of V are in reality continuous with each other, with no boundary to clearly separate them.

53. True or false: The sensory nuclei of cranial nerve V are located in the pons.

Trick question! The correct answer is that *some* of the sensory nuclei of cranial nerve V are located in the pons. The principal sensory nucleus of V is located entirely within the pons; the mesencephalic nucleus is located mainly in the midbrain (as its name suggests), but continues into the upper pons; and the spinal trigeminal nucleus forms a column stretching from the pons, through the full rostrocaudal extent of the medulla, into the upper cervical spinal cord.

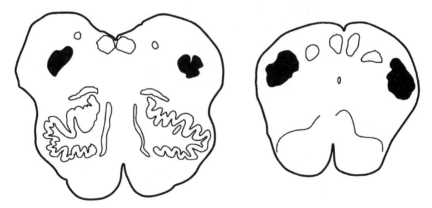

The spinal trigeminal nucleus at the level of the upper medulla *(left)* and lower medulla *(right)*.

54. Fill in the blank: Cranial nerve V innervates muscles of _____.

Mastication (i.e., chewing). A few other muscles also are innervated by cranial nerve V—such as the tensor tympani, which has no involvement in chewing—but it is easier to remember functions than muscles.

55. What eponym is given to the trigeminal ganglion?

The **Gasserian ganglion**. (It sometimes seems to be a general rule that all structures in neuroanatomy have at least two names. The trigeminal ganglion is so important that it even has a third name: the **semilunar ganglion**.)

56. Which central nucleus of cranial nerve V is developmentally derived from neural crest cells?

The mesencephalic nucleus of V. This is the only known example of a central nucleus that originates from neural crest. Of course, like most peripheral ganglia, the trigeminal *ganglion* derives mainly from neural crest cells (though cranial placode cells may contribute too).

57. Which sensory nucleus of cranial nerve V contains *primary* sensory neurons?

The mesencephalic nucleus of V (MesV). Most central sensory nuclei are comprised of secondary sensory neurons, which receive their inputs from the central processes of neurons located in the peripheral ganglia. In contrast, MesV is comprised of primary sensory neurons that directly innervate muscles of mastication, where they collect proprioceptive input. In fact, MesV is essentially equivalent to a peripheral ganglion that has been displaced into the central nervous system (CNS), because it develops from neural crest and is made up of primary sensory neurons.

CRANIAL NERVE VI: THE ABDUCENS NERVE

58. What columnar components are in cranial nerve VI?

General somatic efferent only. The nerve innervates the lateral rectus muscle, which is developmentally derived from somitic mesoderm.

59. Why is cranial nerve VI called the abducens nerve?

Because the lateral rectus muscle (innervated by cranial nerve VI) abducts the eye (i.e., turns it away from the anterior midline).

60. True or false: The abducens nucleus is located in the pons.

True. The abducens nucleus is located at the caudal end of the pons, near the pontomedullary junction.

61. Which peripheral ganglion is associated with cranial nerve VI?

None. (Sorry, another trick question.) The abducens nerve is purely somatic motor, and requires no peripheral ganglion. Only afferent nerves and visceral efferent (autonomic) nerves have peripheral ganglia.

62. What are internuclear neurons? Why are they important?

Internuclear neurons are a population of cells in the abducens nucleus that project across the midline and ascend to the contralateral oculomotor nucleus, where they synapse on medial rectus muscles innervating the contralateral eye. Thus, these neurons coordinate lateral gaze so that abduction of one eye drives adduction of the other eye, and both eyes remain pointed in the same direction during movement.

63. What is the medial longitudinal fasciculus (MLF)?

The MLF is the myelinated longitudinal tract that carries the axons of internuclear neurons from the abducens nucleus to the (contralateral) oculomotor nucleus. (The MLF carries several other fiber tracts that coordinate eye movement, as well). The MLF is heavily myelinated, and indeed is the first central tract to be myelinated in human brain development.

64. Why does damage to one abducens *nucleus* cause a more severe deficit of eye movements than does damage to one abducens *nerve*?

Because internuclear neurons are involved in damage to the abducens nucleus, but not in damage to the abducens nerve.

CRANIAL NERVE VII: THE FACIAL NERVE

65. What columnar components make up cranial nerve VII?

Component	Target/Function
SVE	Facial musculature
GVE	Autonomic fibers to pterygopalatine and submandibular ganglia; then to lacrimal, submandibular, and sublingual glands
GSA	Sensation from small area around external ear
SVA	Taste fibers from anterior two-thirds of tongue

66. Which branch of the facial nerve carries taste sensation?

The **chorda tympani**. This branch merits special mention because of its particular importance for the sense of taste. It also carries GVE fibers to the submandibular ganglion.

67. Name the three peripheral ganglia associated with cranial nerve VII.

The facial (or geniculate), pterygopalatine, and submandibular ganglia. The geniculate ganglion is sensory (GSA and SVA), whereas the pterygopalatine and submandibular ganglia are autonomic.

68. Are the autonomic fibers of cranial nerve VII sympathetic or parasympathetic?

Parasympathetic. (If you are not getting tired of being reminded that all cranial autonomic fibers are parasympathetic, then something is wrong!)

69. What functions are performed by the glands innervated by GVE fibers of cranial nerve VII?

Gland	Peripheral Ganglion	Product
Lacrimal	Pterygopalatine	Tears
Submandibular	Submandibular	Saliva
Sublingual	Submandibular	Saliva

70. Name the one CNS nucleus in which all of the preganglionic autonomic fibers of cranial nerve VII originate.

The superior salivatory (or lacrimal) nucleus. This nucleus does not form a discrete structure, but consists of scattered neurons in the pontine tegmentum.

71. Fill in the blank: Cranial nerve VII generally innervates muscles of _____.

Facial expression. (Pop quiz: which cranial nerve innervates muscles of mastication? Answer: V.)

72. True or false: The facial motor nucleus is located in the pons.

True. This is the nucleus that gives rise to SVE fibers of cranial nerve VII and innervates the muscles of facial expression. It is located in the caudal pons, near the pontomedullary junction.

73. Describe the course of cranial nerve VII motor fibers within the brainstem.

These fibers are notable for first coursing dorsally, then rostrally, and finally ventrolaterally, thus forming an acute angle or *internal genu* near the abducens nucleus. The fibers exit from the ventrolateral aspect of the pontomedullary junction.

74. What is the nervus intermedius?

This is the smaller root of cranial nerve VII. It emerges from the brainstem between the larger root of VII and nearby cranial nerve VIII. The nervus intermedius carries fibers mediating the non-SVE functions of cranial nerve VII. These include GVE fibers destined for the pterygopalatine ganglion (which in turn projects to the lacrimal gland) and submandibular ganglion (which projects to the submandibular and sublingual salivary glands); GSA fibers from the external ear area; and SVA (taste) fibers from the anterior two-thirds of the tongue.

75. General somatic afferent fibers of cranial nerve VII innervate what region of the head?
An area including part of the external ear and adjacent skin. The cell bodies of these fibers are located in the geniculate ganglion.

76. Where do the central processes of facial nerve GSA fibers project?
This is almost a trick question. These fibers from cranial nerve VII project to the spinal trigeminal nucleus, which (as you recall) receives sensory information from the face, primarily from the trigeminal nerve, but also smaller inputs from the facial, glossopharyngeal, and vagus nerves.

CRANIAL NERVE VIII: THE VESTIBULOCOCHLEAR (ACOUSTIC) NERVE

77. What columnar components are found in cranial nerve VIII?
Special somatic afferent (SSA). These fibers carry auditory and vestibular inputs. These systems are covered at length in Chapters 6 and 7.

78. Name the two peripheral ganglia associated with cranial nerve VIII.
The cochlear (or spiral) and vestibular ganglia.

CRANIAL NERVE IX: THE GLOSSOPHARYNGEAL NERVE

79. Name all of the columnar components associated with cranial nerve IX.

Component	Target/Function
SVE	Stylopharyngeus muscle
GVE	Autonomic fibers to otic ganglion, then to parotid gland
GSA	Sensation from posterior one-third of tongue, and part of external ear
SVA	Taste fibers from posterior one-third of tongue
GVA	Receptor input from carotid body and carotid sinus

80. How many peripheral ganglia are associated with cranial nerve IX?
Three. They are the otic, superior glossopharyngeal (or jugular IX), and inferior glossopharyngeal (or petrosal) ganglia.

81. What central nucleus contains the SVE motor neurons of cranial nerve IX?
The **nucleus ambiguus**. Although this nucleus typically is considered in relation to the vagus nerve, it also contains motor neurons that send fibers through the glossopharyngeal nerve.

82. What central nucleus contains the GVE motor neurons of cranial nerve IX?
The **inferior salivatory nucleus**. The preganglionic parasympathetic fibers that arise from this nucleus innervate the otic ganglion, which sends postganglionic parasympathetic fibers to the parotid gland. Neurons of the inferior salivatory nucleus are located in the upper medulla.

83. What types of sensory input are carried by the GVA fibers of cranial nerve IX?
The carotid *body* has chemoreceptors that detect oxygen tension. The carotid *sinus* has baroreceptors that detect arterial blood pressure.

84. Where do GSA fibers of cranial nerve IX project in the brainstem?

To the **spinal trigeminal nucleus**. Recall that essentially all GSA information from the face and scalp is transmitted to the trigeminal sensory nuclei, whether it is carried from the periphery by the trigeminal, facial, glossopharyngeal, or vagus nerve.

85. Where do SVA (taste) fibers of cranial nerve IX project in the brainstem?

To the **nucleus solitarius**. Like the nucleus ambiguus, the nucleus solitarius mainly is associated with the vagus nerve. However, the anterior portion of the nucleus solitarius (sometimes called the gustatory nucleus) receives all taste inputs from the tongue, whether they arrive via cranial nerves VII, IX, or X. The remainder of the nucleus solitarius receives GVA input from cranial nerves IX and X.

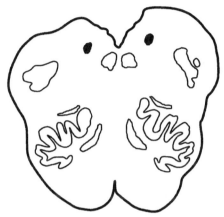

The nucleus solitarius in the medulla.

CRANIAL NERVE X: THE VAGUS NERVE

86. Name all the columnar components associated with cranial nerve X.

Component	Target/Function
SVE	Striated muscle of pharynx and larynx
GVE	Autonomic fibers to viscera of the neck, thorax, and abdomen
GSA	Sensation from back of the ear and pharynx
SVA	A few taste fibers from the epiglottis
GVA	Sensation from viscera of the neck, thorax, and abdomen

Note that the vagus nerve has the same set of columnar components as the glossopharyngeal nerve, and that these two cranial nerves project to and from some of the same brainstem centers (the solitary, ambiguus, and spinal trigeminal nuclei).

87. Why is cranial nerve X called the vagus nerve?

The root of "vagus" means wandering, and this nerve wanders throughout the body all the way from the head to the abdomen (specifically, the colon).

88. How many peripheral ganglia are associated with cranial nerve X?

Three. They are the superior vagal (or jugular X), inferior vagal (or nodose), and enteric ganglia (parasympathetic ganglia which are, in fact, scattered throughout many visceral organs).

89. True or false: Autonomic fibers of cranial nerve X are entirely parasympathetic.
True. All cranial nerve autonomic fibers are entirely parasympathetic.

90. Which brainstem nucleus contains preganglionic parasympathetic neurons of cranial nerve X?
The dorsal motor nucleus of cranial nerve X, located in the medulla.

91. Name the brainstem nucleus that contains SVE motor neurons of cranial nerve X.
The nucleus ambiguus. This nucleus also is located in the medulla and contains some motor neurons that send fibers through the glossopharyngeal nerve.

92. What are the main functions of the muscles innervated by SVE fibers of cranial nerve X?
Swallowing (the pharynx) and vocalization (the larynx).

93. What effect do vagal autonomic fibers have on gastric secretions?
The vagus nerve stimulates secretion of acidic gastric fluid. Thus, hyperactivity of the vagus nerve may be associated with gastric ulceration. Prior to the advent of highly effective medications that block gastric acid secretion, and before it was known that gastric ulcerations are associated with bacterial infection, one treatment of gastric ulceration was vagotomy (surgical transection of a branch of the vagus nerve).

94. What effect do vagal autonomic fibers have on heart rate?
The vagus nerve decreases heart rate. Recall that parasympathetic fibers tend to have effects opposite to the "fight or flight" response associated with sympathetic activation. Thus, decreased heart rate and increased digestive activity are typical parasympathetic functions of the vagus nerve.

CRANIAL NERVE XI: THE ACCESSORY NERVE

95. Name all the columnar components carried by cranial nerve XI.
Special visceral efferent only. These SVE fibers innervate the trapezius and sternocleidomastoid muscles, both branchial arch derivatives.

96. Why is cranial nerve XI called the accessory nerve?
Although it is a cranial nerve, all of the roots arise from the spinal cord. Thus it may be considered a spinal nerve that has been recruited to become a cranial nerve.

97. Which spinal cord levels contain the SVE motor neurons of cranial nerve XI?
Levels C1–C5. These motor neurons reside in a lateral motor column, similar to position to the nucleus ambiguus (the SVE motor nucleus of cranial nerves IX and X).

98. Describe the course of cranial nerve XI fibers as they exit the spinal cord.
The fibers exit the cord laterally, forming intermediate rootlets positioned between the dorsal and ventral roots. These rootlets join together, pass rostrally into the cranium through the foramen magnum, and then turn caudally to pass through the jugular foramen and out of the cranium.

99. Why is cranial nerve XI defined as a branchial rather than somatic motor nerve?
Because the sternocleidomastoid and trapezius muscles are derived from the branchial arch rather than somitic mesoderm. Furthermore, the motor neurons of cranial nerve XI are not located in the usual ventral position of spinal cord GSE nuclei, but in the more lateral SVE position.

CRANIAL NERVE XII: THE HYPOGLOSSAL NERVE

100. What columnar components make up cranial nerve XII?
General somatic efferent. This nerve innervates striated muscle that develops from somitic mesoderm.

101. What muscles does cranial nerve XII innervate?
Intrinsic and extrinsic muscles of the tongue.

102. True or false: The hypoglossal nucleus is an alar plate derivative.
False. Like all motor nuclei, the hypoglossal nucleus is derived from basal plate. It is medially located within the medulla.

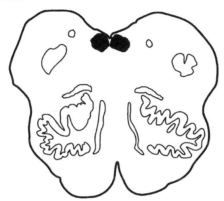

The hypoglossal nucleus (medulla).

103. Describe the course of hypoglossal fibers within the brainstem.
Fibers exit the nucleus ventrally and continue on a direct ventrolateral course to exit the brainstem as rootlets between the pyramid and inferior olive. These rootlets join to form the hypoglossal nerve, which then exits the cranium through the hypoglossal foramen.

CRANIAL NERVE NEUROLOGIC EXAMINATION

104. How is cranial nerve I tested clinically?
The patient is tested for his or her ability to identify different odorants (with closed eyes), such as coffee or peppermint. Since the olfactory nerve or bulb may be damaged on either the left or right side, each nostril must be tested separately. Impairment of olfactory nerve function is a common finding in old age, or may be observed after trauma involving the face or skull.

105. A light shined into one eye normally elicits constriction of both pupils (ipsilateral or *direct* response, and contralateral or *consensual* response); this is the pupillary light reflex. Which cranial nerves and nuclei are tested by this procedure?
Like any reflex, this involves an afferent limb (carried by cranial nerve II from the retina) and efferent limbs (carried by cranial nerve III from the Edinger-Westphal nucleus to the sphincter pupillae). In addition, there is some central processing, mainly through the pretectal nuclei.

106. Which cranial nerves and nuclei mediate the near (or accommodation) reflex?
The *near reflex* consists of pupillary constriction in response to convergence of the two eyes. This reflex is accompanied by *accommodation*, or contraction of the ciliary muscle to relax tension

on the lens and allow it to thicken, thus focusing closer objects on the retina. This complex pathway involves alignment of the visual images (a cortical function based on retinal input from cranial nerve II); further processing in the superior colliculus and pretectal area; efferent output to the medial rectus muscle bilaterally (originating from the oculomotor nuclei and carried by cranial nerve III); and efferent output to the sphincter pupillae bilaterally (originating from the Edinger-Westphal nuclei, also carried by cranial nerve III). Since the medial rectus muscles rarely act alone, all of the cranial nerves and nuclei that control eye movements may participate in this reflex—including the trochlear and abducens nuclei and nerves.

107. What is strabismus?

Strabismus (or **squint**) is failure of the eyes to align along the same axis. When severe, this misalignment may give the unfortunate patient a "cross-eyed" appearance. Since the two eyes do not focus on the same points, there may be **diplopia** (double vision), although the image from one of the eyes may be suppressed by the visual system so that no diplopia is reported by the patient. Surgical treatment by tightening of one external ocular muscle often is helpful.

108. What is gaze palsy?

This is the clinical term for inability to move one or both eyes in a particular direction (e.g., right lateral gaze palsy). It may indicate problems with cranial nerves or nuclei, or with extraocular muscles.

109. In comatose patients who have suffered brain trauma, one or both pupils may be "blown" (dilated and unresponsive to light). What are the usual anatomical cause and clinical significance of this sign?

Following trauma, there frequently is brain swelling (edema) with consequent pressure of medial temporal lobe structures on one or both oculomotor nerves. The parasympathetic fibers that help maintain pupillary constriction are particularly sensitive to this pressure, and their malfunction is an early indicator of increasing intracranial pressure requiring medical intervention. A unilaterally blown pupil may be associated with increased pressure ipsilaterally, contralaterally, or bilaterally.

110. The jaw jerk reflex tests which cranial nerves?

In the jaw jerk reflex, contraction of muscles that close the jaw (i.e., muscles of mastication) is elicited by rapid downward movement of the lower jaw (usually caused by a neurologist's hammer). The afferent limb of this reflex consists of muscle stretch proprioceptor fibers (from the temporalis and masseter muscles), carried by cranial nerve V through the mesencephalic trigeminal nucleus. The efferent limb consists of trigeminal motor fibers to the muscles of mastication, also carried by cranial nerve V. Thus, this monosynaptic reflex involves only the trigeminal nerve.

111. The corneal (or blink) reflex tests which cranial nerve(s)?

The afferent limb consists of touch receptors innervating the cornea and carried by cranial nerve V (division V_1). The efferent limb consists of bilateral facial motor fibers carried by cranial nerve VII to the muscle that close the eyelids (orbicularis oculi). The blink reflex also can be activated by visual (objects approaching the eyes) or acoustic (loud noises) stimuli. Thus, cranial nerves II or VIII also may form the afferent limb of the reflex.

112. How does an upper motor neuron (UMN) lesion of cranial nerve VII differ clinically from a lower motor neuron (LMN) lesion?

Facial LMNs that innervate the upper quadrant muscles of facial expression (e.g., frontalis) receive bilateral UMN innervation, whereas facial LMNs that innervate lower quadrant muscles of facial expression (e.g., orbicularis oris) receive unilateral (contralateral) UMN innervation. Thus, unilateral UMN lesions (e.g., due to stroke) cause paralysis of only the lower facial muscles on the contralateral side. Unilateral LMN lesions (e.g., Bell's palsy; see Question 116) cause paralysis of all (upper and lower quadrant) muscles of facial expression on the ipsilateral side.

113. The gag reflex involves which cranial nerve(s)?

Sensory stimulation of the back of the oropharynx (e.g., by stroking with a tongue depressor) activates afferent fibers carried by cranial nerve IX to the spinal trigeminal nucleus. The efferent limb of this reflex is carried by cranial nerves IX and X to pharyngeal muscles.

114. A lesion affecting cranial nerve XI causes what clinical signs?

Damage to the accessory nerve (e.g., due to trauma) causes paralysis of the sternocleidomastoid and/or trapezius muscles, resulting in decreased ability to turn the head (sternocleidomastoid) and/or shrug the shoulders (trapezius).

115. True or false: The tongue deviates toward the side of a lesion affecting cranial nerve XII.

It depends on whether the lesion affects the UMN or LMN. Muscles innervated by the hypoglossal nerve push the tongue forward and medially, mainly by action of the genioglossus muscle. When one hypoglossal nerve or nucleus (LMN) is impaired, the genioglossus on the opposite side acts without opposition, so the tongue is pushed across the midline towards the affected side. Since UMN innervation is crossed, lesions affecting the UMN cause the tongue to deviate *away* from the side of the lesion.

DISEASES OF THE CRANIAL NERVES

116. What is Bell's palsy? Which cranial nerve does it affect?

Bell's palsy is a clinical syndrome mainly affecting SVE fibers of the facial nerve (VII) and paralyzing the muscles of facial expression. The cause of the disease usually is a flare-up of infection with the herpes simplex virus, more commonly associated with common cold sores. Bell's palsy may strike at any age and usually resolves completely after a period of weeks to months. The paralysis is of the lower motor neuron type, and thus affects the entire face (upper and lower quadrant muscles). The muscular paralysis may lead to atrophy over time. Since the eyelids and lips droop, the tears and saliva leak on the affected side, resulting in "crocodile tears" and drooling. Other facial nerve fibers also may be affected, causing such symptoms as decreased taste sensation.

117. What is tic douloureux? Which cranial nerve does it affect?

Tic douloureux, also known as **trigeminal neuralgia**, is a pain syndrome affecting the trigeminal sensory fibers. It usually occurs in patients over 50, more often women. The attacks of pain are sudden and severe, and usually are described as shock-like or lancinating. They last for several seconds and may be triggered by various stimuli such as chewing. The cause is unknown, but is suspected to be viral. The disease is treatable, with anticonvulsant medications usually providing the best relief. The course is relapsing and remitting.

118. What is shingles? Which cranial nerve is most commonly affected?

Shingles—also known as **herpes zoster**—is a skin rash that can affect the sensory distribution of any sensory nerve; among cranial nerves, the trigeminal nerve most commonly is affected. The disease usually affects adults and consists of vesicular lesions that crust and resolve over a period of days to weeks. It is caused by reactivation of latent infection by varicella-zoster virus (VZV), a member of the herpesvirus family that causes chickenpox (varicella) during primary infection. After a patient has had chickenpox, the VZV virus persists in latent form in neurons of the sensory ganglia. Reactivation occurs sporadically by unknown mechanisms. The rash usually conforms to a dermatomal pattern, most often involving the V_1 branch of cranial nerve V. There is no cure, and treatment is symptomatic.

119. What is postherpetic neuralgia? Which cranial nerve most commonly is affected?

This condition is a sequela of shingles usually seen in elderly patients. After resolution of the shingles rash, pain and paresthesias (abnormal sensations in the affected region) may persist for a prolonged period of weeks to months. As for shingles, the trigeminal nerve most often is affected.

120. What is an Argyll Robertson pupil?

This eponym designates a pupil that constricts in response to eye convergence (the near reflex, associated with accommodation), but not in response to light. (The favored mnemonic for the Argyll Robertson pupil is: *a*ccommodates but does not *r*eact.) The condition is usually bilateral. It most commonly was seen in the context of neurosyphilis, but with the advent of effective treatments for syphilis, the Argyll Robertson pupil is much less common nowadays.

121. What is the cerebellopontine angle syndrome? Which cranial nerve(s) does it affect?

This is a clinical syndrome affecting nerves that emerge from the brainstem at the cerebello-pontine angle near the pontomedullary junction, i.e., the facial and acoustic nerves. The initial symptoms are usually related to the vestibular branch of cranial nerve VIII; they include vertigo and impaired sense of balance. With involvement of the cochlear branch of cranial nerve VIII, there may be tinnitus (ringing in the ears) and decreased auditory acuity. Ipsilateral facial paralysis of the lower motor neuron type occurs once the facial nerve is involved. The most common cause of the cerebellopontine angle syndrome is a benign tumor (schwannoma) arising from the vestibular branch of the vestibulocochlear (acoustic) nerve.

122. What is internuclear ophthalmoplegia?

Internuclear ophthalmoplegia (INO) refers to a specific pattern of gaze palsy, caused by lesions in the medial longitudinal fasciculus (MLF). Recall that the MLF contains the axons of internuclear neurons that project from the abducens nucleus to the contralateral oculomotor nucleus, and thus coordinate lateral gaze by linking lateral rectus contraction on one side to medial rectus contraction on the other side. With INO, attempted lateral gaze to the side opposite the lesion results in normal lateral movement of the abducting eye, but impaired medial movement of the adducting eye. INO is a common finding in multiple sclerosis, a neurologic disease affecting myelinated tracts in the CNS.

BIBLIOGRAPHY

1. Fuller GN, Burger PC: Nervus terminalis (cranial nerve zero) in the adult human. Clin Neuropathol 9:279–283, 1990.
2. Kandel ER, Schwartz JH, Jessell TM: Principles of Neural Science, 3rd ed. New York, Elsevier, 1991.
3. Martin JH: Neuroanatomy: Text and Atlas. 2nd ed. New York, Elsevier, 1996.
4. Nolte J: The Human Brain: An Introduction To Its Functional Anatomy, 4th ed. St.Louis, Mosby, 1999.
5. Romer AS, Parsons TS: The Vertebrate Body, 6th ed. Philadelphia, W.B. Saunders, 1986.
6. Schwanzel-Fukuda M, Pfaff DW: Origin of luteinizing hormone-releasing hormone neurons. Nature 338: 161–164, 1989.
7. Wilson-Pauwels L, Akesson EJ, Stewart PA: Cranial Nerves: Anatomy and Clinical Comments. 2nd ed. Toronto, B.C. Decker, 1998.

10. MOTOR SYSTEMS: SPINAL CORD AND SPINAL REFLEXES

Patrick R. Walsh, M.D., Ph.D.

1. What is meant by the terms motor system and motor unit?

Motor activity is expressed through movement. All movement in the mammal, from a whisper to the most vigorous physical activity, is the result of electrochemical activation of striated muscle. The *motor system* includes those neurons at multiple hierarchal levels operant in effecting movement. The *motor unit* is comprised of a single alpha (largest of category) motor neuron ("final common pathway") and the extrafusal muscle fibers with which it establishes direct synaptic contact. Alpha motor neurons are located in the ventral horn of the spinal cord in a cellular column that extends longitudinally from coccygeal to cranial segments on a more or less continuous basis, with segmental representation a function of the relative commitment of the segment to motor activity.

The population of alpha motor neurons is greater at segments associated with appendicular innervation than in those limited to truncal configuration. Disposition of alpha motor neurons in the ventral horn of the spinal cord is **somatotopic**, with more distally projecting motor neurons, which subserve appendicular musculature, situated laterally. Axial musculature is represented by a medially situated motor neuronal column. Physiologic flexors are dorsally disposed in ventral spinal gray matter with respect to extensors.

The ultimate expression of activity of a given motor unit is the result of the interplay of segmental neuronal activity and connectivity with extrasegmental mechanisms, which arise from both spinal and cranial sources. Collectively, the motor unit and the neuronal elements that modulate its activity are considered the motor system. Sophistication of motor control is intuitively and factually dependent upon sensory input for visual, postural, and proprioceptive quantification; however, afferent mechanisms are considered elsewhere in this text and will be explored here only in specific aspects that directly impact motor systems.

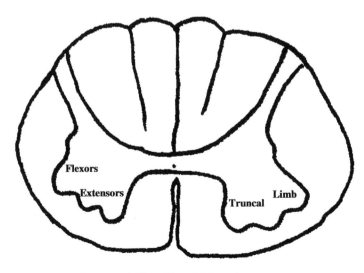

Somatotropic disposition of alpha motoneurons.

2. Which descending tracts from cranial sources subserve motor functions?

Descending tracts which subserve motor function originate in the cerebrum, the brainstem, and the cerebellum. The structure and function of these tracts have generated intense investigative efforts and clinical interest, but the mechanisms of their intracranial integration are beyond the scope of this section. Specific contributions of these tracts to spinal motor control will be briefly addressed.

Germane to consideration of motor function are the corticospinal (pyramidal), reticulospinal, tectospinal, rubrospinal, vestibulospinal, interstitiospinal, and olivospinal tracts; the ceruleospinal system (noradrenergic); the raphe-spinal system (serotonergic); and the medial longitudinal fasciculus. Kuypers divided extrapyramidal tracts into two functionally and anatomically disparate groups: group A comprises the medial reticulospinal, vestibulospinal, tectospinal, and interstitiospinal tracts; rubrospinal and pontospinal tracts constitute group B. Group A tracts course in the spinal anterior funiculus, collateralize extensively, and tend to subserve axial and proximal appendicular functions of posture and synergistic global appendicular movement. In contrast to tracts in group A, rubrospinal descent is identified in the dorsolateral funiculus, and termination involves primarily distal limb musculature with flexor dominance. Of equal interest are intersegmental intrinsic spinal fiber systems, which provide for intersegmental connectivity and integration of reflex circuitry; short bundles generally are unnamed, and the fasciculus proprius and fasciculus interfascicularis are constituted of fibers that may span multiple segments.

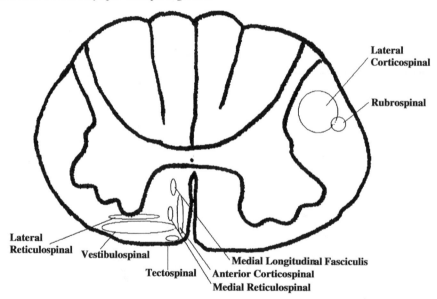

Localization of descending tracts.

3. What is a reflex?

In general terms, reflexes are reactions. A reflex is a nonvolitional, relatively fixed, but potentially graded biologic response evoked by a specific stimulus. The reader with a Skinnerian belief system may substitute the term "on command" for the term "volitional" without disservice to the discussion.

4. How are reflexes beneficial?

Reflexes are demonstrable at all levels of phylogeny. Chemotaxis provides a reflexive mechanism for directed locomotion of unicellular organisms, and phototactic behavior of the botanical kingdom may be considered a reflex. The potential biologic benefits of these patterns of activity are clear. In segmented organisms, segmental reflexes provide behavioral fragments of greater complexity than displayed by motor units in isolation. Therefore, these reflexes may be seen to constitute an order of targets that is more complex than motor units for extrasegmental systems to modulate as components of complex behavior.

Consider the neuronal circuitry in the isolated spinal cord of the chicken with its head cut off: reflexive mechanisms therein generate coordinated, complex, and appendicular locomotor and postural behavior in the absence of influence of cranial systems. Such reflexive mechanisms promote efficiency in cranial control systems, because far fewer cephalic neurons are required to direct behavior with interneurons and related reflex arcs as substrates for termination than if motor units required individual and solitary connectivity. Indeed, in the subhuman primate only digital intrinsic musculature of the hand, involved in fine control, receives direct monosynaptic input from the corticospinal system, which demonstrates predominately internuncial termination. In the human, corticospinal monosynaptic connectivity to motor neurons beyond distal limb motor units is relatively sparse; however, it provides a mechanism for delicate control of axial and proximal appendicular integrated movement.

Reflexes can provide the clinician valuable information about the segmental status of the nervous system and the function of extrasegmental tracts (primarily descending) that modulate graded reflex activity.

5. What are the components of a reflex?

A reflex is a biologic response to a specific stimulus; as such, a method of stimulus recognition is required. In mammalian systems other than hollow viscera and vascular trunks, in which a local plexus provides for integrated regional reflex responses similar to those of the annelid, stimuli are identified, categorized, and transduced to graded, nonpropagated, electrochemical potentials by specialized nerve end structures of afferent neurons (see Chapters 1 and 2). Afferent impulses generated by these structures are conveyed to the spinal segment as saltatory action potentials along the processes of unipolar primary afferent neurons with somata located in dorsal root ganglia. The central axonal processes of these sensory neurons find access to the spinal segment at the dorsal root entry zone and direct collateral processes to various segmental and extrasegmental terminations.

Afferent fibers are grouped by size: largest diameters constitute group 1. Afferent axons of large diameter tend to be segregated to the medial aspect of the dorsal root entry zone and divide to direct axonal processes to segmental alpha motor neurons (class 1a afferent fibers), to gamma motor neurons (in lower vertebrates), to segmental interneurons, to projectional neurons, to extrasegmental sites in great measure through the fasciculi proprii (a thin penumbra of ascending and descending processes that envelops spinal gray matter; long projections for axial motor neuronal columns and short systems for appendicular columns), to the fasciculus interfascicularis, and to medullary relay nuclei through the dorsal columnar system (see figure on following page). Each of these branches plays a specific role in control of posture and movement through processes of facilitation and inhibition. Autonomic reflexes typically are afferently driven by fibers of smaller diameter that enter the lateral aspect of the dorsal root entry zone.

The reflex arc is completed through coupling of the afferent limb to an effector or efferent circuit; in the most elementary, monosynaptic, myotatic reflex the motor unit is recruited by direct synaptic excitation of the alpha motor neuron, and muscular contraction is elicited by muscle stretch. In more complex reflexes, a variable number of segmental and extrasegmental interneurons may be interposed between primary afferent and efferent neural elements. In any form of reflex, collateral branches of the afferent limb may terminate on additional neurons that facilitate or inhibit expression of the reflex directly or through influence on antagonistic factors. Recurrent inhibition of the motor unit efferent output is provided by the Renshaw neuron.

6. What is grading of a reflex?

Gradation of reflexes refers to intensity of reflexive expression related to the magnitude of the stimulus or to modulation by subject-specific neural mechanisms outside of the reflex arc.

7. What does grading of reflexes accomplish?

Were reflexes to function without modulation or grading, fluid and delicate movement would be impossible. Flaccidity would be the anticipated state of muscle tone (resistance to stretch) in the absence of reflex activation and rigidity or oscillatory hypertonia would be expected with uninhibited reflex activity.

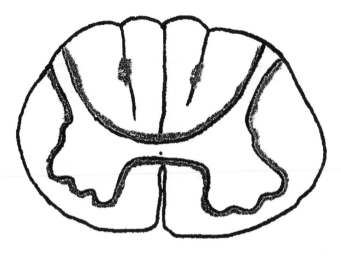

Fasciculus proprius *(shaded margin of spinal gray matter)* and fasciculus interfascicularis *(shaded area in dorsal columns).*

8. How is grading of the myotatic reflex achieved?

The monosynaptic tendon stretch reflex provides an excellent model for the study of gradation of reflex activity. Ultimate expression of the reflex is a function of the interplay of descending cranial tracts, the state of muscular contraction and tone, sensory transduction, afferent parameters, segmental and extrasegmental neuronal circuitry, and the motor unit's excitation status. Extensive evaluation of this reflex in feline subjects rendered decerebrate or decorticate through transection of the brainstem (as initially described by Sherrington) and clinical examination of humans with spinal, cerebral, and brainstem injuries has provided a wealth of information. In addition to the transient muscular contraction elicited by stretch, a sustained or tonic muscular contraction upon activation of the myotatic reflex—not observed outside of pathologic states—has been demonstrated. These reflexes are tonically inhibited by supraspinal systems in the intact organism.

Additional tracts of import in maintenance of posture and control of movement (both dependent upon gradation of reflex activity) include the vestibulospinal and reticulospinal tracts, which facilitate physiologic extensor musculature (antigravity groups) seen fully expressed in the decerebrate state,

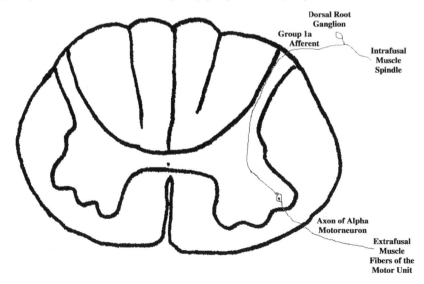

Schematized myotatic reflex.

and the rubrospinal tract, which facilitates flexors (withdrawal) in the upper extremity and is fully expressed in the decorticate state.

9. What mechanisms are involved in gradation of the myotatic reflex with respect to intensity of the applied stimulus?

The adequate stimulus for activation of the myotatic reflex is stretch of the homonymous muscle. The intrafusal muscle-spindle apparatus includes the annulospiral nerve ending that transduces this stimulus; spindles are distributed throughout the muscle. Although the action potential conducted centrally by the group 1a (largest of category) fiber arising from the spindle is an all-or-nothing event, gradation of the reflex may be accomplished by alteration in resting musculotendinous and related receptor spindle tension or length. This alteration affects the "perceived" intensity of the stimulus, which may dictate the absolute number of afferent fibers activated.

Magnitude of stretch correlates with the amplitude of the annulospiral end-organ graded generator potentials, which must achieve threshold to elicit centrally directed action potentials. (Nerve endings tend to form a helix, similar to a coil spring, around the meridian of the intrafusal fiber; thus, the term annulospiral.) The muscle spindle is specifically configured for muscle length gradation and is composed of specialized intrafusal muscle cells that structurally parallel extrafusal fibers forming the bulk of the muscle. These extrafusal cells are solely responsible for contraction of muscle (intrafusal fibers of spindles make essentially no contribution to contractile force).

Contractile elements are isolated to polar regions of intrafusal fibers. The annulospiral nerve ending is confined to the cell's central zone, which is devoid of actin and myosin and provides the basis for division of these cells into two types in reflection of nuclear configuration (bag and chain). Afferent innervation is provided to the central zone of both nuclear chain and nuclear bag fibers in primary form by axons of group 1a and in secondary form by group 2 axons. The length of the nerve ending is obligately coupled to the length of the intrafusal muscle cell's central segment.

On physiologic grounds, nuclear bag fibers are categorized as either static (unchanging or plastic) or dynamic (phasic or transient with units of velocity). Capsular enclosure of the nuclear segment of fibers within the spindle is the norm. Length and tension of the innervated central nuclear zone may be maintained by contraction or relaxation of the polarly situated contractile elements independent of overall muscular length, despite obligate parallel coupling of spindle length to extrafusal muscle length. This process provides for relative anatomic stability of end-organ configuration

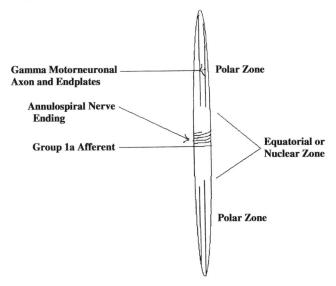

Intrafusal muscle-spindle fiber.

and of afferent output at virtually any muscle length. The process is directed by activity of gamma motor neurons that terminate on the polar, contractile regions of intrafusal fibers.

The muscle-spindle apparatus is sensitive to static and dynamic parameters of muscle (spindle) length that dictate the pattern of afferent discharge. Proportionality of afferent response to intensity of stimulus is primarily a function of the number of spindles recruited to threshold at inframaximal levels of muscular stretch. For any fixed level of fusimotor tone (intensity of gamma activation; see Question 11), group 1a primary spindle afferent activity is most clearly augmented by small changes in muscular length, as witnessed at the onset of stretch. Activity also varies directly with velocity of stretch. Secondary group 2 axons innervate only nuclear chain and static nuclear bag fibers. Group 1a primary axons innervate each of the intrafusal fiber variants. This distinction provides explanation for the relative insensitivity of group 2 afferents to rapid changes in muscular length of low magnitude and categorization as tonic elements.

10. What mechanisms operate to effect gradation of the myotatic reflex *independent* of stimulus level?

The membrane potential of the axon hillock reflects somatodendritic level of excitation and is the ultimate determinate of axonal output. The alpha motor neuron of myotatic reflex receives facilitory and inhibitory input from tracts, segmental and extrasegmental internuncials, and afferent branches, in addition to group 1a afferent direct termination. Interplay of these inputs determines the state of alpha motor neuronal excitation. Elimination of input of descending tracts through cranial ablative procedures and of intraspinal connectivity through section of the spinal cord in investigative studies has generated disconnection syndromes in which the influence of specific fiber populations on the reflex arc have been examined in some detail. Clinical counterparts can be seen in various craniospinal disease states; these states are properly considered disconnection syndromes in which "release" phenomena are generated by neural circuits liberated from influences specific to the lesion. With mature lesions of the corticospinal system, hypertonia (increased resistance to stretch of various types) is witnessed, in addition to hyperreflexia as a component of spasticity. Various clinical signs such as clonus (sustained oscillatory movement across a joint elicited by stretch) may be seen to represent unmodulated myotatic reflexes.

In the acute phase, after disconnection of input of descending tracts, a state of atonic neural "shock" occurs; the reflex arc is essentially unresponsive to activation of the afferent limb. With passage of time and repopulation of afferent terminal sites through neuroplastic phenomena, expression of the myotatic reflex once again becomes apparent. The hyporeflexia of the acute phase is replaced by a state of hyperreflexia, which supports the concept that descending tracts generally tonically inhibit the myotatic reflex and facilitate or reduce inhibition only in behaviors that may employ the reflex as a component of more complex activity or posture. A mechanism for gradation of the reflex through activity of descending tracts, independent of stimulation intensity, is immediately evident in the neurologically intact subject. A number of clinical and investigative studies have confirmed this pattern for the corticospinal tract, in contrast to the vestibulospinal and reticulospinal tracts, which selectively facilitate physiologic extensors (antigravity musculature) and account for the motor expression of the decerebrate state. Facilitation of physiologic flexor-withdrawal groups in the upper extremity by the rubrospinal tract generates the characteristic findings of the decorticate state.

In addition to mechanisms operative on the efferent limb of the myotatic reflex, direct modulation of afferent sensitivity and activation are subject to control of the central nervous system through the gamma efferent motor system or "loop."

11. What is the gamma loop?

The gamma loop comprises the spindle, the group 1a afferent, and the alpha and gamma efferents. It provides a mechanism for maintenance of the length-related sensitivity of the intrafusal spindle central segment—independent of muscular length, tension, and the active or passive nature of muscular shortening. Absent the loop, muscular shortening (which attends contraction of extrafusal fibers) would shorten the central section of the intrafusal fiber and render the spindle unresponsive.

The group 1a fiber and the muscle-spindle apparatus provide the afferent limb of the myotatic reflex. The end-organ of the afferent fiber is manifest in the equatorial section of nuclear bag and chain intrafusal fibers, which is essentially devoid of contractile elements. Afferent discharge is generated by elongation of the afferently innervated segment of the intrafusal fiber either through muscle stretch, which globally lengthens the "parallel" spindle, or through contraction of the intrafusal fiber's polar regions, which effectively lengthens the central segment directly. Efferent innervation of the contractile polar segments of the intrafusal fiber is provided by the gamma efferent neuron. Activation of this motor neuron evokes a response in the group 1a afferent through lengthening of the intrafusal central segment, which elicits activity in the alpha motor neuron of the motor unit and thereby closes the gamma loop.

In less complex vertebrates, the loop is fully closed by termination of the group 1a afferent on the gamma motor neuron; this 1a afferent coactivation of both alpha and gamma motor neurons is not in evidence in more complex vertebrates, including humans. Because the gamma motor neuron is not a terminal site of the group 1a afferent in higher vertebrates, the amplitude of the afferent volley in the group 1a fibers that attends muscular contraction depends on integrated coactivation of alpha and gamma motor neurons by supraspinal neural mechanisms.

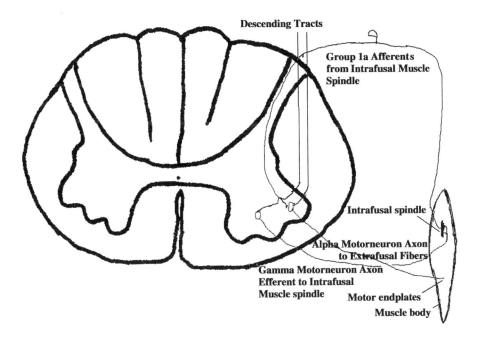

Gamma loop.

12. How is the gamma loop controlled if the group 1a afferent does not terminate on the gamma motor neuron in the human?

Both alpha and gamma motor neurons receive extensive input from descending tracts. Dissociation of gamma motor neuronal activation from primary afferent coactivation dictates that gamma activation strictly depend on descending influences and permits substantial suprasegmental variability in control of movement. The relative level of preactivation of gamma systems has been termed **fusimotor set**. Fusimotor set reaches a zenith in complex motor activity with high levels of static and dynamic gamma activation. No clinical or investigative model of isolated gamma dysfunction is currently accessible for consideration.

13. What effects do radicular lesions have on the segmental myotatic reflex?

The myotatic reflex in isolation is essentially a segmental phenomenon. Radicular dysfunction, which may involve afferent or efferent limbs in isolation or combination, dictates hyporeflexia (**lower motor neuron lesion**), which in clinical practice may be of value in localization.

14. How are the segmental characteristics of the myotatic reflex valuable in clinical practice?

The segmental nature of the myotatic reflex dictates obligate coupling to appropriate segmental radicular expression. In the vertebrate, the myotome typically extends over multiple spinal segments; corresponding afferent input of the myotatic reflex is to be found in the dorsal divisions of the segmental roots. In clinical injury of the spinal cord, the level of the lesion is defined by the most caudal zone of sensory preservation (dermatome) and by the most caudal myotomal segment spared disconnection from descending tracts. Although myotomes are multisegmental, in practical terms a dominant or indicator root may be considered operative with respect to assignation of level of spinal injury reflex findings. Recall the expectation of hyporeflexia with radicular dysfunction and of hyperreflexia with disconnection from descending tracts (**upper motor neuron lesion**).

Spinal Segments of Particular Import in Localization

SPINAL SEGMENT	INDICATOR OF MYOTOME	MYOTATIC REFLEX	LIMITED DERMATOMAL EXPRESSION
C5	Deltoid	Deltoid	
C6	Biceps brachii	Bicipital	Thumb, index digit
C7	Triceps	Tricipital	Long digit
C8–T1	Intrinsic hand musculature	Hoffmann's digital flexor	Ring, fifth digits
L4	Quadriceps femoris	Patellar	Anterior medial thigh
L5	Pedal extensors		Great toe
S1	Gastrocnemius-soleus	Achille's	Lateral toes

15. The myotatic reflex obviously generates *stretch* of antagonistic muscles, for example of the triceps with activation of the bicipital myotatic reflex; why is the myotatic reflex of the antagonistic muscle not activated?

Oscillatory activation of antagonistic myotatic reflexes across a joint provides physiologic explanation for the phenomenon of clonus. In the intact subject, an inhibitory interneuron (1a), demonstrated physiologically by Sherrington in segmental spinal grey matter, inhibits activation of antagonistic myotatic reflexes. This circuit may be considered a **disynaptic inhibitory reflex**. (See figure on facing page.)

16. Is group 1a afferent activity linked to reflex activity other than the myotatic reflex?

Afferent Group 1 fibers have myriad terminations (see Question 5). Specific connectivity of import in motor function, in addition to interneuronal and intersegmental pools, includes the spinocerebellar projectional systems and medullary relay nuclei of the medial lemniscal system, which provide proprioceptive and postural information to supraspinal levels.

Unlike the annulospiral muscle-spindle endings of Group 1a afferents, which *parallel* extrafusal muscular fibers, the Golgi tendon organs of Group 1b afferents demonstrate *serial* disposition with respect to muscle. This arrangement makes them sensitive to muscle tension, rather than length. Sensitivity to tension of the Golgi tendon receptor protects the muscle from excessive force of contraction, as the 1b afferent fiber inhibits homonymous motor units in the clasp-knife and contact inhibitory disynaptic reflexes.

17. What reflexes exist beyond the myotatic reflex?

In contrast to the monosynpatic myotatic reflex, all other spinal reflexes appear to involve internuncials and are therefore polysynaptic. **Polysynaptic spinal reflexes** are classified on the basis of segmental disposition, nature of activation, or mode of expression. The myotatic reflex affords reflex

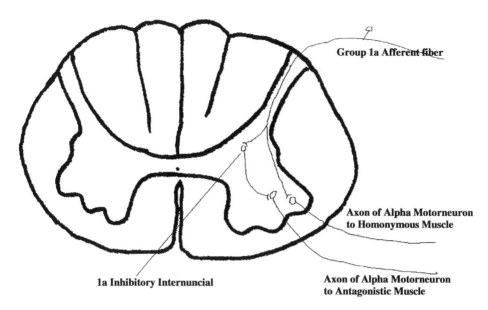

Antagonistic inhibition in the myotatic reflex.

control only of homonymous muscular length and tension and antagonistic muscular inhibition; works through a single internuncial; and is expressed across a single joint. Polysynaptic reflexes can generate far more complex movement, such as fragments of postural states and of integrated behavior (e.g., locomotion), with expression beyond the myotome. Certain polysynaptic spinal reflexes manifest autonomic phenomena. The connectivity of internuncials dictates the specific temporal and spatial nature of expression of polysynaptically mediated spinal reflexes. Connectivity has been inferred by physiologic observations, such as delay attributed to synaptic transmission. Anatomic localization of internuncials has been accomplished through ablative and microelectrode studies and by using agents that reflect neuronal metabolic response to activation. Polysynaptic spinal reflexes generally are tonically inhibited by supraspinal influences in the neurologically intact adult, and are seen as fragments of more complex behavior. Specific demonstration of these reflexes may vary substantially between experimental preparations and between individuals with similar neurologic lesions.

18. What forms of connectivity are seen in internuncial pools?

Inhibition (1a, internuncial, and Renshaw or alpha motor neuron recurrent; presynaptic and postsynaptic), facilitation (presynaptic), convergence, divergence, gating, reinforcement, reverberation, rhythmicity, feedback, commissural, and intersegmental physiologic mechanisms and forms of connectivity are operant alone and in combination in the internuncial pools of polysynaptic spinal reflexes; clinical expression of each reflex is seen to be a function of this connectivity. Intersegmental connectivity is provided by the fasciculus proprius. This system is fundamental in reflex integration that extends beyond the segmental level, and commissural or crossing interneurons permit coordinated, bilateral reflex responses. Presynaptic processes entail local changes in membrane potential that either approach, or diverge from, threshold level to augment or reduce the net potential change of the action potential. Postsynaptic inhibition generates hyperpolarization, which moves the membrane potential further from threshold. (See Chapter 2 for detailed information on mechanisms of presynaptic and postsynaptic inhibition and of presynaptic facilitation.) Convergence and divergence provide mechanisms for amplification and diminution of descending signals and of internuncial processing: a single descending impulse volley may elicit an amplified, multisegmental, integrated, and crossed response, or a number of descending tracts may generate an extremely focused response.

19. What are the appropriate stimuli for and motor expression of spinal polysynaptic reflexes?

Polysynaptic spinal reflexes elicited by **proprioceptive input** include the tonic neck reflex and a variety of crossed and uncrossed flexor-adductor reflexes. **Cutaneous stimulation** evokes the abdominal, cremasteric, anal, palmar and plantar reflexes. **Nociceptive input** can adequately stimulate either group of reflexes, as well as autonomic reflexes. Several polysynaptic reflexes can be induced by either cutaneous or proprioceptive stimulation.

Proprioceptively induced polysynaptic spinal reflexes are of special interest, because they allow coordinated movements of limbs; myotatic reflexes allow only single joint expression.

20. How are polysegmental spinal reflexes demonstrated?

Polysynaptic spinal reflexes may be prominently displayed by the neonate prior to maturation of supraspinal systems; by the adult with spinal or supraspinal neural injury after an initial, acute phase of hyporeflexia; and by experimental preparations with spinal or supraspinal lesions. Palmar, plantar, and unsustained and incomplete tonic neck reflexes are commonly seen in the neonate until approximately 4 months of age and are essentially invariable in the premature infant because normal neonatal posture entails appendicular flexion. These reflexes and posture also are seen in the adult with paraplegia in flexion due to spinal cord injury. Palmar stroking in these states elicits a grasp reflex; plantar pedal stroking may elicit an "extensor" toe sign of Babinski, with upward movement of the great toe and flaring of the remaining digits. In physiologic terms, pedal digital dorsiflexion is a component of a flexor-withdrawal reflex (recall that physiologic extensor activity is specifically antigravity), and in certain hyperreflexive states the plantar stimulus may evoke ipsilateral flexion-withdrawal and crossed adduction or extension of the lower limbs.

Reflexively induced appendicular flexion with crossed extension constitutes a substantial component of locomotor activity and has been extensively studied in feline and other animal models. Adequate stimuli include cervical rotation through various arcs, nociceptive input, and cutaneous stimulation. "Spinal" gait has been demonstrated in the feline model of mature spinal supralumbar cord transection: alternating flexion with crossed extension reflexes generated fairly functional hindlimb gait. The reflexes appear to be triggered by both cutaneous and proprioceptive afferents of the disconnected caudal lumbar segments. Unfortunately, this purely reflexive gait has been misconstrued as a sign of recovery of descending tract connectivity in experimental studies of spinal cord injury and has generated false hope in the clinically afflicted. Polysynaptic spinal reflexes may manifest extrasegmental, coordinated, and global appendicular movements ipsilaterally in addition to crossed (contralateral segmental) findings. Both upper and lower limb reflexes can be elicited by a single stimulus of tonic neck movement and by other proprioceptive and cutaneous stimuli in various clinical and experimental situations.

21. Are hyperreflexive states potentially harmful?

Polysynaptic spinal reflexes, unmodulated in pathologic states of the nervous system, may constitute specific risks beyond loss of mobility. A state of hyperreflexia (dysreflexia) can develop in clinical spinal cord injury in which stimuli such as distension of the urinary bladder may reflexively evoke severe hyperhidrosis, hyperpyrexia, and change in blood pressure through autonomic mechanisms.

BIBLIOGRAPHY

1. Brazis PW, Masdeu JC, Biller J: Localization in Clinical Neurology, 2nd ed. Boston, Little Brown and Co., 1990.
2. Granit R (ed): Muscular Afferents and Motor Control. Nobel Symposium I. New York, John Wiley and Sons, 1966.
3. Granit R: The Basis of Motor Control. London, Academic Press, 1970.
4. Haymaker W: Bing's Local Diagnosis in Neurological Diseases, 15th ed. St. Louis, C.V. Mosby, 1969.
5. Kandel ER, Schwarz JH, Jessell TM (eds): Principles of Neural Science. New York, Elsevier Science Publishing, 1991 (please refer especially to chapters 37–39).
6. Kuypers HG: Anatomy of the descending pathways. In Field J, Magoun HW, Hall VE (eds): Handbook of Physiology, Vol 11. Washington Physiology Society. Baltimore, Waverly Press, 1981, pp 597–665.
7. Menkes JH: Textbook of Child Neurology, 2nd ed. Philadelphia, Lea and Febiger, 1980.
8. Parent A: Carpenter's Human Neuroanatomy, 9th ed. Baltimore, Williams and Wilkins, 1996.
9. Paxinos G: The Human Nervous System. San Diego, Academic Press, 1990.
10. Sherrington CS: The Integrative Action of the Nervous System. New York, Scribner, 1906 (reprinted).

11. MOTOR CORTEX

Jon H. Kaas, Ph.D., and Iwona Stepniewska, Ph.D.

1. What is motor cortex?

In humans and other primates, motor cortex is the posterior portion of the frontal lobe where electrical stimulation of sites in cortex produces movements at low to moderate levels of current.

2. Where did the concept of a motor cortex come from?

In the 1860s, after Broca proposed a center for motor speech in the frontal lobe, Jackson proposed that an orderly representation of body movements exists in the frontal lobe. He based his idea on observations of how movements induced by an epileptic convulsion progress from an initial movement of some part, such as a toe, to increasingly distant parts of the body. Jackson noted that the sites of brain damage that resulted in such epileptic focus of movements were in the frontal lobe. Because it was possible to electrically stimulate the brain long before we could amplify signals and record them, Fritsch and Hitzig (1870) soon tested this idea by stimulating the frontal cortex and evoking movements. Electrical stimulation has remained the primary way of exploring and defining motor cortex.

3. Sometimes the term sensorimotor cortex is used instead of sensory or motor cortex. Why?

Early investigators were uncertain if motor cortex was sensory, motor, or both, and the sensorimotor view, although not clearly established, was widely held. In addition, electrical stimulation is capable of evoking movements from wide regions of cortex, including sensory areas posterior to the central sulcus. Under light anesthesia, it also is possible to record evoked sensory responses in motor areas of the frontal lobe. Thus, some continue to use the term sensorimotor cortex for areas of sensory and motor cortex bordering the central sulcus. However, precentral cortex is clearly more motor than sensory in function, and postcentral cortex is more sensory. In the 1950s, Woolsey suggested the terms MsI and SmI for primary motor and sensory areas so that the less pronounced sensory and motor components of motor and sensory would be remembered. Now it is more common to simply refer to sensory and motor fields.

4. What is the architectonic difference between motor and somatosensory cortex?

Postcentral (behind central fissure) somatosensory cortex has a well-developed layer 4 with small granular cells that receive sensory input. Therefore, this cortex is called *granular*. In contrast, the precentral motor cortex has a poorly developed or missing layer 4, but a well-developed layer 5 with large pyramidal cells. The motor cortex is called *agranular*. These large pyramidal cells are the source of corticospinal projections.

5. Does motor cortex contain functionally distinct subdivisions?

Yes. The largest subdivision is **primary motor cortex, M1**, which is located just anterior to somatosensory cortex on the anterior bank of the central sulcus and the precentral gyrus (Figs. 1 and 2). Movements can be evoked from M1 at the lowest levels of stimulating current. Since movements also can be evoked from cortex anterior to M1, but at higher levels of current, this cortex has long been known as **premotor cortex**. Recent research has led to the current view that premotor cortex contains three major subdivisions: the supplementary motor area and the dorsal and ventral premotor areas. In addition, two or more subdivisions of **cingulate cortex** on the medial wall of the cerebral hemisphere have motor functions.

6. What do the motor areas do?

The common feature of all motor cortical areas is that their electrical stimulation elicits movements and tonic contractions of muscles on the opposite side of the body, and sometimes also on the ipsilateral side. Motor areas control the planning, programming, initiation, and execution of movements.

7. What are characteristic features of M1?

Actually, the precise location of the border between M1 and premotor cortex is still somewhat uncertain, especially in humans. However, M1 has several distinguishing characteristics: (1) It represents the body from the foot medially to the tongue laterally. (2) Movement of these body parts are evoked at relatively low levels of current. The lowest levels are obtained when microelectrodes are used to penetrate cortex so that the electrode tip is near the large pyramidal cells of layer 5, which project to motor neurons of the brain stem and spinal cord. With intracortical microstimulation, pulses of 30 μ amperes (amps) or less of cathodal current typically evoke movements, while higher levels of 50–60 μ amps are needed in premotor fields. (3) Most or all of M1 has a distinctive cytoarchitectonic appearance. M1 is called **agranular cortex**, or **area 4 of Brodmann**. (4) M1 has connections with other structures, especially the dense corticospinal projections, that differ from premotor fields.

8. What are Betz cells?

The largest of the layer V pyramidal cells in M1 are called Betz cells. These cells are larger than those in other cortical areas, and they help identify M1, which closely corresponds to area 4 of Brodmann. M1 also includes part of the lateral area 6.

9. What is Penfield's motor homunculus?

In the 1930s, the neurosurgeon Penfield electrically stimulated the brain of patients during brain surgery and found an orderly arrangement of movements in M1, from toes in the medial wall of the cerebral hemisphere to tongue most laterally in cortex. Penfield depicted these findings by drawing a distorted little man, the homunculus, draped across the mediolateral extent of M1. The distortion of the homunculus was the result of more cortex being devoted to hand, lips, and tongue movement and little cortex being devoted to trunk and leg movement. The homunculus commonly was included in textbook illustrations, because it nicely summarized the overall organization of MI. However, the homunculus suggests a detailed pattern of representation that does not exist. Instead, local regions of M1 have a mosaic arrangement of groups of cells related to different movements.

10. How is M1 functionally organized?

In a gross overall pattern, M1 represents body movements on the opposite side from foot, leg, trunk, arm, digits, face, and mouth in a medial to lateral sequence in the strip-like field. Locally, within specific sectors of M1, the organization is a bit more complex. Within a hand region, for example, a number of scattered sites for electrical stimulation will evoke movements in a specific finger or that finger and several adjacent fingers. Other nearby sites may relate to wrist, elbow, or even arm movements, as well as movements of other digits. Thus, locally M1 seems to consist of a mosaic of small regions or modules, each representing movements of a restricted part of the body, with multiple modules for each type of movement. Adjacent modules tend to be, but are not always, related to adjacent body parts. This **mosaic of efferent zones** may allow more flexibility in the ways movements are combined.

11. Are distal and proximal movements evoked from M1 segregated?

There is no rigid segregation of joint representations. Proximal segments tend to be represented rostrally and distal caudally, as described by Woolsey in 1958. Most authors now agree that territories representing distal and proximal movements are intermingled within M1, although there is some tendency for distal forelimb segments to be represented caudally and proximal segments to be represented rostrally.

Figure 1 *(facing page).* Some proposed subdivisions of motor cortex in lateral views of the frontal lobe. **A,** New World owl monkey. **B,** Old World macaque monkey. Electrical stimulation of cortex produces orofacial (OF) movements, and movements of the hindlimb (HL) and forelimb (FL). Upper (U) axial (arm) movements also are indicated. Sulci: CS = central sulcus, LS = lateral sulcus, AS = arcuate sulcus. Motor areas: M1 = primary motor cortex (rostral = M1r, caudal = M1c), SMA = supplementary motor area (with medial and dorsal divisions), PMD = dorsal premotor area (with rostral and caudal divisions), PMV = ventral premotor area, Pre-SMA = presupplementary motor area, FEF = frontal eye field, SEF = supplementary eye field, OMD = dorsal oculomotor field. (Modified from Preuss TM, Stepniewska I, Kaas JH: Movement representation in the dorsal and ventral premotor areas of owl monkeys: A microstimulation study. J Comp Neurol 371:649–676, 1996.)

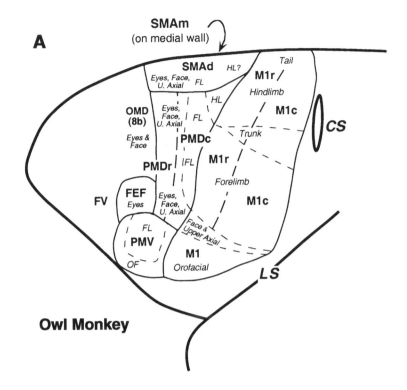

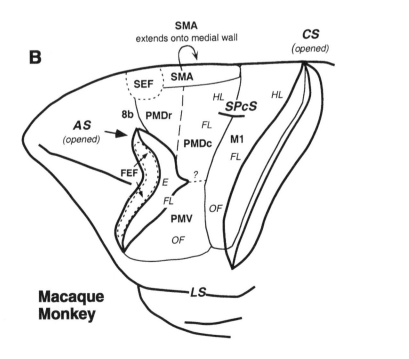

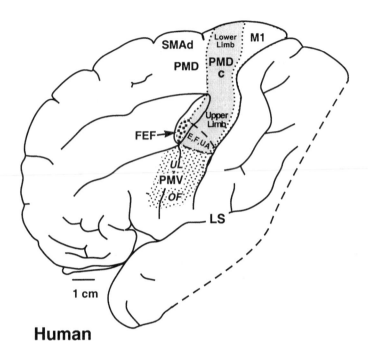

Figure 2. Proposed motor fields of the human frontal lobe. (Modified from Preuss TM, Stepniewska I, Kaas JH: Movement representation in the dorsal and ventral premotor areas of owl monkeys: A microstimulation study. J Comp Neurol 371:649–676, 1996.)

12. What do single corticospinal neurons in M1 do?

Each corticospinal neuron generally projects somewhat broadly to several sets of motor neurons controlling different muscles. For example, terminations of a single cortical neuron may involve spinal neurons that activate wrist muscles and finger muscles. Cortical neurons thus control synergistic sets of muscles, and muscles are controlled by multiple sets of cortical neurons.

13. How do the different groups of neurons in M1, related to different movements and combinations of neurons, become coordinated?

The factors important in such coordinations are uncertain. The spread of inputs from premotor cortex to M1 could be important. In addition, each major portion of M1 has an extensive system of intrinsic connections that connect and probably coordinate the different neuronal groups.

14. How does damage to M1 alter motor behavior?

Motor behavior in humans is altered by lesions of motor cortex in several ways. Patients demonstrate a weakness of contralateral muscles, spasticity with increased muscle tone, exaggerated reflexes, and impaired dexterity. A large lesion may result in the inability to move a part. Impairments typically decrease over time, and they are less pronounced in mammals with less cerebral cortex. Movement control is more dependent on motor cortex in humans than other mammals. In humans and monkeys, lesions of the motor cortex (or corticospinal tract) produce profound and long-lasting deficits in the ability to individuate movements. Although the ability to use all fingers together may recover, the ability to move them individually remains permanently defective. The motor cortex thus appears necessary for **movement individuation**.

15. Is motor cortex under sensory control?

Sensory inputs to M1 are critical in guiding motor acts. Important but sparse inputs come from subdivisions of anterior parietal cortex, especially area 3a which is activated by muscle spindle receptors. Areas of anterior parietal cortex project to the second somatosensory area, S2, and posterior parietal cortex (area 5), which in turn project to motor cortex. M1 also receives somatosensory and other inputs from the cerebellum via a relay in the ventrolateral thalamus.

16. What does the output of M1 do?

Pyramidal neurons in M1 provide outputs to cortical and subcortical targets. M1 projections to somatosensory cortex provide feedback and modify the responses of somatosensory neurons. Projections to premotor areas provide feedback to the neurons that project to and influence M1. Other feedback projections are to regions of the ventrolateral thalamus that relay cerebellar inputs to M1. Important subcortical projections are to the putamen, which is the input nucleus of the basal ganglia. This input is part of a circuit from motor cortex through the basal ganglia and back to motor cortex, especially premotor areas, so that the activities of cortical motor areas are integrated and reinforced. Most importantly, M1 provides the major component of the corticospinal and corticobulbar motor tracts that directly and indirectly control the motor neurons projecting to muscles.

17. What activates neurons in M1?

Inputs signaling plans for movements probably initiate neural responses in M1. A large body of evidence supports the conclusion that neurons in M1 are involved in computations for the control of voluntary movements. Neural activity in M1 strongly correlates with the force and directions of arm movement, for example. Some neurons responds strongly for arm movement in one direction, while others respond strongly for movements in other directions. Many neurons are involved in any one movement, collectively contributing to what is termed a **population code** for the movement. Many M1 neurons also respond to sensory events or cues, suggesting a role in sensory or sensorimotor processing as well. However, neurons do not seem to code the metrics of sensory stimuli as they do in sensory cortex.

18. Are there subdivisions of M1?

Current evidence suggests that M1 is not a homogenous cortical area (Fig. 1). Studies of the cytoarchitecture, histochemistry, and connectivity of M1 in nonhuman primates suggest that M1 consists of at least two subdivisions: **caudal (M1c)** and **rostral (M1r)**. Results from recent studies in humans support this conclusion.

19. What are the main differences between the caudal and rostral subdivisions?

The rostral subdivision, M1r, has smaller pyramidal cells in layer 5, but larger pyramidal cells in layer 3. M1r also is less excitable and receives stronger projections from premotor cortex than M1c, which receives diverse somatosensory inputs.

20. What does M1 represent?

Microstimulation at any site in M1 causes a body part to move or muscles to contract. The current level can be decreased until just a muscle or a few muscles twitch, without any body part moving. As the stimulation level is increased, more and more muscles contract; movements emerge, become greater, and involve more body parts and joints. Each cortical site, which involves the outputs of a limited number of neurons, relates to a number of muscles rather than a single muscle, but some muscles are activated more easily than others. While nearby cortical sites may evoke different movements at threshold, they have partially or largely overlapping muscle targets at suprathreshold levels of current. Thus, during natural movement of discrete body parts, neurons are active over large portions of M1. M1 represents movements, but the representation of each movement is distributed.

21. What factors can affect motor responses resulting from intracortical microstimulation?

The general state of the animal, the kind and depth of anesthesia, as well as the parameters of stimulation all greatly affect the results of brain stimulation. Thresholds or levels of current needed to evoke movements change with the variables, as well as the magnitude and complexity of the movement.

22. Is M1 the only motor area that has direct access to the spinal cord?

No. Anatomic and physiologic studies based on intracortical microstimulation show that areas in premotor cortex, supplementary motor cortex, and cingulate cortex also have direct access to the spinal cord. Somatosensory areas provide some projections, too.

23. Can movements be evoked from cortical areas other than motor areas?

Yes. Movements can be evoked from other cortical areas outside the frontal cortex closely connected to M1, such as the postcentral and posterior parietal cortex. The neurons of these areas, like motor cortical neurons, can respond during movement execution. In fact, some prefrontal cortex neurons display changes of activity during limb movements, suggesting an involvement in motor control.

24. What is the difference between the corticospinal tract and the pyramidal tract?

There is no difference. The corticospinal tract, known also as the pyramidal tract, refers to that part of the motor system arising from specific areas of the cerebral cortex and descending through the fiber bundles in the ventral medulla (pyramids) to end on motor neurons. The corticospinal tract is a direct link from cerebral cortex to the spinal cord.

25. What are the "nonprimary" motor areas?

Some researchers consider motor-related areas, such as postcentral somatosensory areas or posterior parietal sensorimotor areas, as nonprimary, in contrast to premotor areas that have strong connections with M1 and project densely to the spinal cord. However, most agree that all areas outside of M1 are nonprimary motor areas.

26. How can the primary motor area, M1, be distinguished from nonprimary motor areas?

Nonprimary motor areas have markedly higher thresholds for eliciting movements with intracortical microstimulation. Also, movements elicited from nonprimary motor areas are more complex and often involve coactivation of several muscle groups. Moreover, there are architectonic differences between primary and nonprimary motor cortices. M1 coincides with gigantocellular (huge layer 5 pyramidal cells or Betz cells) cytoarchitectonic area 4. Nonprimary motor cortex in front of M1 is formed by cytoarchitectonic area 6, with smaller layer 5 pyramidal cells.

27. What is the supplementary motor area?

The supplementary motor area (SMA) is a subdivision of premotor cortex that is unusual in that it was first described in humans and only later in monkeys and other mammals. Electrical stimulation of SMA evokes movements of all body parts in an anteroposterior pattern from face to foot. SMA is located just anterior to the foot representation of M1, on the medial wall of the cerebral hemisphere in humans and partly on the dorsomedial surface in monkeys.

28. What are the other names for the supplementary motor area?

SMA is known by many names, including medial premotor cortex (F3, for third frontal field in cytochrome oxidase preparations), SMA-proper, to distinguish it from pre-SMA, and MII or M2 (secondary motor area).

29. What happens when SMA is electrically stimulated in humans?

Stimulation of SMA in awake humans during surgery elicits movements, often of the forelimbs. Patients also report the feeling of the need or urge to move. In contrast, stimulation of M1 evokes movements without this feeling.

30. What are the functions of SMA?

SMA was thought to "supplement" the motor role of M1; currently, it is considered a major factor in motor planning. The area is active when sequences of movements are thought about, before the movements start and even if the movements do not occur. When a monkey is instructed to perform a certain movement but delay the movement for a few seconds, many neurons in SMA are vigorously active during the delay, and activity often increases or decreases as the movement starts. This pre-movement activity indicates that the area helps to prepare for the movement.

Other functions also are likely. Although electrical stimulation of SMA generally produces contralateral movements, as in M1, SMA has dense callosal connections with SMA of the other cerebral hemisphere. In addition, lesions of SMA can alter motor performance bilaterally. Thus, one of the functions of SMA may be to let one hand know what the other hand is doing or will do. Finally, some investigators divide SMA into two parallel fields, one more dorsal than the other. These two fields may have somewhat different functions.

31. Does SMA have a role in motor learning?

Yes. When monkeys learn a simple motor task, neurons in SMA are active during the learning period. However, the premovement activity is reduced or absent after the monkeys are overtrained and the task becomes automatic. Thus, SMA may be important in programming and guiding *new* sequences of movement, but only until these sequences become programmed in M1.

32. Does SMA directly participate in the control of single movements?

Probably most of the motor control elicited by SMA comes indirectly via its dense projections to M1. SMA does contribute somewhat to the corticospinal tract, and crude movements can be evoked from SMA after lesions of M1. However, microstimulation of sites in SMA produce much less facilitation of muscle activity than sites in M1. Thus, SMA does have a direct role in evoking *simple* movements, but the role is modest and limited.

33. How do lesions of SMA affect motor behavior?

In contrast to the marked impairments of motor behavior observed after M1 lesions, damage restricted to SMA has surprisingly little effect. Monkeys seem little altered in their normal motor activity, although finger movements may be uncoordinated. Humans may show greater impairments, but lesions generally are larger and involve other motor areas as well. As for M1 lesions, impairments are reduced or disappear with time.

34. What are the major connections of SMA?

SMA receives somatosensory information from anterior and posterior parietal cortex and thalamic inputs from parts of the ventrolateral thalamus that receive basal ganglia inputs. It has access to sensory information and is part of a cortical-basal-ganglia-thalamic-cortical loop that is subject to the effects of activity in motor and premotor areas of cortex. Direct cortical interconnections also relate SMA to M1 and to adjacent premotor areas, including the dorsal premotor area, the cingulate motor areas, and the presupplementary motor area.

35. Is SMA a single area?

For a long time SMA was considered as a single area, architectonically distinguished from the laterally adjacent premotor cortex by prominent, densely packed neurons in layers 3 and 5. Recently, SMA has been divided into two areas that differ slightly in cytoarchitecture and the distribution of the metabolic enzyme, cytochrome oxidase. The two separate areas within the cortex traditionally defined as SMA also differ physiologically. The term **pre-SMA** is now used for the rostral part, to distinguish it from caudal **SMA-proper** (see Fig. 1). SMA-proper sometimes is divided into dorsal and medial fields (see Fig. 1A).

36. What are the main differences between SMA and pre-SMA?

SMA-proper can be activated with low-intensity stimuli, and it is somatotopically organized. Pre-SMA is difficult to electrically stimulate, responds less frequently to somatosensory stimuli but more frequently to visual stimuli, and contains fewer movement-related cells but more cells responsive to the pre-movement phase. Unlike most agranular motor areas, pre-SMA is not connected with M1, but with prefrontal cortex, ventral premotor cortex, and cingulate cortex. Additionally, pre-SMA sends only weak, if any, projections to the spinal cord. Functionally, SMA is more directly linked to movement execution, whereas pre-SMA has been implicated in more cognitive aspects of motor behavior.

37. What is the supplementary eye field, and how is it distinguished from SMA and pre-SMA?

The supplementary eye field (SEF) is a small area located with pre-SMA and SMA in the dorsomedial frontal cortex. SEF is distinguished by its role in eye movements, architecture, and anatomic connections to cortical and subcortical oculomotor centers. SEF is connected to the frontal eye field and the brainstem oculomotor center (or superior colliculus). It also shares common terminal fields of corticostriatal projections with the frontal eye field. The SMA and pre-SMA areas do not exhibit these features.

38. Are there motor areas in cingulate cortex?

Yes. Cingulate cortex of the medial wall of the frontal lobe (Brodmann's areas 23 and 24) has long been associated with limbic functions. Recent studies have implicated the cortex of the cingulate sulcus in motor functions. In monkeys, electrical stimulation of cingulate cortex evokes movements, although the levels of current needed are higher than in M1 and SMA. In addition, tracer injections into arm or leg regions of M1 label portions of cingulate cortex. Finally, cingulate cortex sends sparse projections to the spinal cord and brain stem, suggesting a direct role in motor control.

39. Is there more than one motor area in cingulate cortex? What is the evidence?

Since the access to cingulate motor areas buried in the cingulate sulcus is difficult, there are not many systematic microstimulation studies of this region, and existing data are not consistent. Recording neuronal activity during performance of a motor task demonstrates two or even three movement-related foci in the cingulate cortex of monkeys. Cytoarchitectonically, the cingulate motor cortex is formed by two clearly distinct areas: posterior area 23c and anterior area 24c, both located ventral to the agranular frontal cortex (SMA and M1), in the depths and on the ventral bank of the cingulate sulcus. Area 23c has a well developed layer 4, whereas area 24c has an agranular structure and a thicker layer 5 with densely packed pyramidal cells. The agranular cingulate cortex described as cytoarchitectonic area 24c is not homogeneous, and investigators now divide area 24c into two areas, 24c and 24d.

40. What types of movements are evoked from cingulate cortex?

Stimulation of cingulate cortex in nonhuman primates gives rise to complex and integrated somatic movements that include motor activity in the head, neck, and contralateral upper extremity.

41. Is cingulate cortex also involved in vocalization?

Yes. Vocalizations can be elicited by electrical stimulation of a more anterior portion of cingulate cortex in monkeys.

42. Is cingulate motor cortex somatotopically organized?

It is likely that at least three somatotopically organized motor fields exist in cingulate cortex. Early studies of the connections of cingulate cortex with area M1 in monkeys demonstrated a topographic pattern. The anterior portion of the cortex in the lower bank of the cingulate sulcus projects to the face representation in M1, middle levels to the forelimb, and posterior levels to the hindlimb M1 representations. Later studies, however, showed that not one but three motor areas exist in the anterior cingulate cortex. Their topography has been established mainly on the basis of the distribution of corticospinal projections and connections with somatotopic sectors of M1 or M2.

Area 24d is easily excitable and contains an arm and a leg and possibly a face motor field. It has a dense projection to all segments of spinal cord. Area 24c is less excitable and relates mainly to arm movements. It has relatively weak spinal projections, mostly to the cervical and thoracic segments. Area 23, which is virtually unexcitable, shows the weakest corticospinal projections, and it projects mainly to the lumbar spinal cord, so it represents a leg field. The anterior part of area 23c projects to forelimb areas of M1 and SMA.

Despite this evidence, more documentation is needed about the somatotopy of this region.

43. How can somatotopic organization of nonprimary motor areas, which are less excitable than M1, be defined?

Since representations of each major body segment in the various motor areas are interconnected, the somatotopic organizations of less-excitable motor areas can be defined on the basis of patterns of connections with well-delineated somatotopic sectors of M1 or SMA. The arrangements of corticospinal cells also can be used in determining the somatotopy of less-excitable motor areas. The corticospinal neurons are somatotopically organized in such a way that the neurons projecting to lumbar spinal levels originate from different parts of the cortex than those with axonal projections to the cervical spinal cord.

44. What is the dorsal premotor area?

Premotor cortex traditionally has been subdivided into the SMA and dorsolateral premotor cortex. Now there is good evidence for distinguishing dorsal (PMD) and ventral premotor areas within dorsolateral cortex. Although the exact boundaries are uncertain, the PMD includes cortex just lateral to SMA and just rostral to the leg and arm portions of M1. Movements can be evoked by electrical stimulation in PMD at thresholds that are higher than those in M1. PMD represents the leg most medially in cortex, and the arm more laterally. PMD corresponds to part of Brodmann's area 6.

45. Are there subdivisions of dorsal premotor cortex?

Yes. The PMD is not a homogeneous structure. Experimental studies in nonhuman primates indicate that it consists of at least two parts: a caudal zone, which mainly represents movements of the upper and lower limbs, and a rostral zone, which may represent head and eye movements, or complex movement synergies that involve the head, eyes, and limbs. In both humans and nonhuman primates, caudal PMD is quite responsive to electrical stimulation. In humans, caudal PMD occupies much of the convexity of the precentral gyrus (see Fig. 2), and its responsiveness to electrical stimulation led early workers to erroneously conclude that this region was part of M1.

46. What does PMD do?

Recordings from PMD neurons in monkeys suggest that PMD is involved in the preparation or planning of motor movements more than the direct control of motor movements. A basic feature of preparing for a motor movement is to form a "motor set" or a state of readiness. Certain PMD neurons, called motor set neurons, respond after a monkey is signaled to get ready for a learned movement, but before any activity in the muscles can be observed. Although sensory stimuli are used to signal that a motor act will soon be expected, the neural activity in PMD reflects the preparation for the motor act rather than any aspect of the sensory signal.

Neural activity in PMD is largely confined to the planning phase and is over before movement onset. Injections of substances into PMD that temporarily block the activity of neurons increase errors in a visually cued task requiring a delayed response. Thus, PMD is a motor area that seems to be specialized for planning motor acts.

47. What are set-related neurons?

Set-related neurons are those neurons in premotor cortex that are active after the animal receives an instruction to make a particular movement. An instructional stimulus signals the type of movement, but the movement must be withheld for a 2- to 5-second period that is terminated by a trigger stimulus. Set-related neurons fire vigorously during the delay period and often either cease or increase their activity just before movement. The activity does not depend on the modality of the instruction stimulus and can vary among neurons according to the type of movement. Evidently, set-related neurons are active for the planning of some movements, but not others.

48. How does PMD get information about visual and tactile signals for motor acts?

PMD gets input from areas of posterior parietal cortex that are involved in the higher-order processing of somatosensory data, visual information, or both. Some inputs may be from higher-order auditory cortex of the temporal lobe, as well.

49. What are the other cortical connections of PMD?

The major cortical connections of PMD are in the frontal lobe. They include many interconnections with M1, and PMD is thought to have a strong influence on M1. Other interconnections are with the SMA, cingulate motor fields, presupplementary motor area, and ventral premotor area. Premotor fields are strongly interrelated, and form an interacting network. Callosal connections are with PMD of the opposite hemisphere and adjoining premotor fields.

50. What are the subcortical connections of PMD?

Important projections are to motor neurons of the spinal cord and brain stem; PMD has a direct influence on muscle control. PMD also projects back to the same portion of the ventrolateral thalamus that receives inputs from the globus pallidus of the basal ganglia and cerebellum and projects to PMD. Other outputs are to the basal ganglia and brain stem.

51. What is the ventral premotor area?

Investigators have discovered a third movement map in premotor cortex (area 6). In addition to the more extensively studied supplementary motor area and the dorsal premotor area, a ventral premotor area (PMV) is located immediately anterior to the representation of the face and mouth in M1.

52. Can PMV be identified by cytoarchitecture?

Yes. PMV can be distinguished from PMD more medially and M1 more caudally by a thin but often distinct layer IV of granular cells. Layer V pyramidal cells are generally smaller than the large pyramidal cells of M1 (area 4). Cortex ventral to PMV has a more developed layer IV.

53. What movements are evoked from PMV?

Electrical stimulation of PMV evokes movements of the forelimb, face, and mouth. The forelimb representation is clearly more ventral and separate from the forelimb representation in PMD. Within the forelimb region of PMV, both simple digit and arm movements can be elicited, but the complex reaching movements are common. Other movements evoked from the area include those of the tongue and jaw. Hindlimb movements generally are not evoked from PMV.

54. Does PMV have functionally distinct subdivisions?

There have been several proposals to divide PMV into anterior and posterior subdivisions based on differences in histologic appearance, cortical connectivity, and response properties of neurons. These proposals deserve further study.

55. Do PMV neurons respond to sensory stimuli?

Yes. Neurons in PMV typically respond to visual stimuli within large receptive fields. Most of the visual neurons also respond to touch on the face or arms. The visual receptive fields tend to extend outward into space related to the tactile receptive field. Compared to the small tactile receptive fields of M1 neurons, the neurons in PMV have large receptive fields, often involving much of the face and arm.

56. How do PMV neurons respond to sensory stimuli?

The receptive fields of neurons in PMV have remarkable properties. In most visual areas, receptive fields for neurons are based on inputs from restricted portions of the retina, and receptive fields move with the eyes. In contrast, visual receptive fields for neurons in PMV relate to the body. Neurons with tactile receptive fields on the side of the face, for example, may be activated by visual stimuli approaching the side of the face, but only within a certain distance, regardless of direction of gaze. Other neurons with tactile receptive fields on the arm encode visual space around or near the arm, so when the arm moves, the visual receptive field moves.

Although tactile receptive fields are in the contralateral body surface, and visual receptive fields are generally in contralateral space, a visual receptive field may extend into ipsilateral visual space if the contralateral hand is extended into that space. In addition, neurons that respond as a monkey reaches for a small bit of food near his face also may respond when an investigator reaches for that food. Finally, some of the neurons that respond to visual stimuli relative to the head or arm continue even after the lights have been turned off and the object is no longer visible. These neurons seem to code for a memory of an object.

57. Where does the sensory information in PMV come from?

PMV receives visual and somatosensory information from higher-order visual and somatosensory fields of posterior parietal cortex. PMV also receives more direct inputs from somatosensory areas of the lateral sulcus. Visuomotor signals arise from both the frontal eye field and the supplementary eye field of the frontal lobe.

58. What does PMV do?

PMV appears to play a critical role in guiding arm, hand, head, and mouth movements toward objects of interest and in guiding hand movements toward the mouth. The guidance can be based on either tactile data, visual information, or both. Objects too far away to be grasped are not of interest. The guidance depends on the location of objects relative to the hand and face, rather than where the eyes are directed.

The neurons in PMV appear to maintain a memory for the location of objects, even when the objects disappear from gaze for a short period of time. Thus, you can reach for your cup while looking elsewhere, and reach for a light switch in the dark. Lesions of PMV produce visual neglect. Large lesions of premotor cortex that include PMV impair the ability of monkeys to reach for food around a transparent obstacle.

59. How are the effects of PMV computations mediated?

PMV is strongly interconnected with M1 and the cingulate and supplementary motor fields. Weaker connections exist with PMD. Thus, the premotor fields interact, and they all influence primary motor cortex. PMV also projects to brain stem and spinal cord motor centers and therefore has a more direct effect than other premotor areas on movement control.

60. How is PMV related to Broca's motor area for speech in humans?

Broca's speech area in the left ventral frontal lobe corresponds in part to Brodmann's area 44, which has long been believed to be unique to humans. Present evidence now suggests that Broca's area is a specialization of the ventral premotor area, so that linguistic functions have been acquired in addition to the original sensorimotor functions. The role of PMV in controlling head and arm movements may be related to the reason why humans use manual and facial gestures in language as well as speech.

61. How are eye movements controlled by cortex?

Eye movements are controlled by an extensive network of cortical and subcortical centers, especially the superior colliculus. In frontal cortex, two visuomotor areas have important roles: the frontal eye field and the supplementary eye field. In addition, eye movements can be evoked from portions of the dorsal premotor area. These visuomotor fields receive visual inputs from higher-order visual areas of the temporal, occipital, and parietal lobes. They interact through connections with each other, and they project to the superior colliculus and other brain stem structures.

62. What is the extrapyramidal system? How does it influence the motor cortex?

The *extra*pyramidal system is composed of all tracts other than pyramidal pathways, including nuclei and feedback circuits, that influence somatic motor activity of voluntary muscles. Extrapyramidal structures exert their influences on behavior through their projections back to the cortex. They do not project directly to the cortex, but they influence it via relays in the thalamus. For example, the M1 is influenced by the cerebellum and basal ganglia via projections from the ventrolateral thalamic nucleus and from intralaminar nuclei. Premotor cortex is influenced by cerebellum, basal ganglia, and superior colliculus via projections from ventral thalamus, the mediodorsal thalamic nucleus, and the intralaminar nuclei.

63. Are cerebellar and pallidal inputs segregated within the motor cortex?

Whereas there is considerable agreement about the nearly complete segregation of cerebellar and pallidal inputs in the thalamus, the distribution of projections from motor thalamus to frontal motor areas remains incompletely understood. In general, the globus pallidus influences mostly non-primary motor areas through anterior divisions of motor thalamus, whereas the cerebellum projects mostly to primary motor area through the posterior divisions of motor thalamus. However, the segregation of these inputs within the cortex is not complete and they overlap to some extent.

BIBLIOGRAPHY

1. Dum RP, Strick PL: Medial wall motor areas and skeletomotor control. Curr Opin Neurobiol 2:836–839, 1992.
2. Fink GR, Frackowiak RSJ, Pietrzyk U, Passingham RE: Multiple nonprimary motor area in the human cortex. J Neurophysiol 77:2164–2174, 1997.
3. Jackson SR, Husain M: Visuomotor functions of the lateral premotor cortex. Curr Opin Neurobiol 6:788–795, 1996.
4. Preuss TM, Stepniewska I, Kaas JH: Movement representation in the dorsal and ventral premotor areas of owl monkeys: A microstimulation study. J Comp Neurol 371:649–676, 1996.
5. Rizzolatti G, Fadiga L, Gallese V, Fogassi L: Premotor cortex and the recognition of motor actions. Cognit Brain Research 3:131–141, 1996.
6. Sakai ST, Inase M, Tanji J: Pallidal and cerebellar inputs to thalamocortical neurons projecting to the supplementary motor area in *Macaca tuscata*: A triple-labeling light microscopic study. Anat Embryol 199:9–19, 1999.
7. Stepniewska I, Preuss TM, Kaas JH: Architectonics, somatotopic organization, and ipsilateral cortical connections of the primary motor area (M1) of owl monkeys. J Comp Neurol 330:238–271, 1993.
8. Tanji J: The supplementary motor area in the cerebral cortex. Neurosci Research 19:251–268, 1994.
9. Wise SP: The primate premotor cortex: Past, present, and preparatory. Ann Rev Neurosci 8:1–19, 1985.
10. Wise SP: Premotor and parietal cortex: Corticocortical connectivity and combinatorial computations. Ann Rev Neurosci 20:25–42, 1997.

12. PYRAMIDAL AND EXTRAPYRAMIDAL SYSTEMS

Diane Daly Ralston, Ph.D.

The motor systems that control our interactions with our environment are highly ordered, carefully regulated, and integrated to aggregates by neuronal pathways and connections. They function simultaneously—in cooperation and in parallel—to allow the simplest or the most complex of movements. Consider a baseball batter with a narrow piece of wood, who must, under the high pressure of the game, hit an object less than 4 inches in diameter hurtling at him at 90–100 miles per hour. His stance must be secure, his arms poised for a powerful swing, his hands tightly gripped around the bat. His eyes must be fixed on that tiny object, all muscles of his body ready to respond into a sprint. He needs alert visual and auditory systems and an immediately responsive motor system. He needs good balance, planning, and initiation of movement; accurate body position; and knowledge of where his limbs are in his three-dimensional space and how much force he needs to swing the bat into exact position for contact with the ball.

The same complex needs are required to walk across the room, to go up and down the stairs, or to sit down, pick up a pen, and write. All of these movements require planning, initiation, and execution; accurate range of motion; target achievement; appropriate force and velocity; and coordination. Sensory feedback is critical so that muscle length and position sense are known by the brain in advance.

This chapter explores how the pyramidal and extrapyramidal systems inter-relate and how they work in parallel to other motor pathways, all critical to normal functioning of the motor system. These neuronal aggregates and tracts control motor output for the body, head structures, and targeted eye movements and enable us to maintain posture and equilibrium in a three-dimensional, gravitational field.

THE PYRAMIDAL SYSTEM

1. What is the pyramidal system?

The pyramidal system is defined by all the cortical fibers, both motor and sensory, that descend to synapse upon spinal motor neurons and interneurons. During the descent, 90–95% of the fibers cross in the medulla, forming the pyramidal decussation as can be seen grossly on the ventral surface of the medullary brainstem. This is the pyramidal tract. More rostrally, cortical fibers influence brainstem neurons, creating the corticobulbar system ("bulb" refers to the brainstem).

2. How long have we known about the existence of the pyramidal system?

The pyramidal system or tract is recorded in ancient literature beginning with Hippocrates in the 3rd century B.C. and early Italian, German, and British neuroanatomists, many of whom observed the decussation of the fiber tracts in the medulla. This decussation was confirmed by Von Haller in 1754 and Vicq d'Azir in 1786. Concomitant with the advent of better and more sophisticated experimental techniques, other famous anatomists and physiologists added their names to the list, providing us with functional as well as anatomic knowledge of this elegant and complex system. More recent studies elucidate the development, synaptic organization, and contribution of each of the cortical areas involved in the system.

Armand J: The origin, course, and terminations of corticospinal fibers in various mammals. In Kuypers HGJM, Martin GF (eds): Descending Pathways to the Spinal Cord, Progress in Brain Research. Amsterdam, Elsevier, 1982, pp 329–360.

3. What does the pyramidal tract do?

The pyramidal tract arises from many diverse motor and sensory regions of the cortex. It comprises a major component of the internal capsule, creates the cerebral peduncles and the descending fibers through the base of the pons, and then forms the medullary pyramids, from whence the origin of its name. The pyramids then decussate in the medulla to occupy the contralateral dorsolateral portion of the spinal cord, where the fibers from somatosensory cortex descend to synapse on dorsal horn neurons and interneurons. Fibers from motor cortices synapse on interneurons and spinal motoneurons.

The pyramidal tract is involved in innervation of motoneurons that control primarily distal musculature, such as those that subserve finely controlled movements involving the opposable thumb. For example, painting miniatures, handwriting, and picking up small objects all involve the use of the pyramidal tract. Although the pyramidal tract exists in many mammalian species, it is highly developed in primates—both in cortical origin and spinal terminations—and therefore primates have been used extensively as models for study.

Brösamle C, Schwab ME: Cells of origin, course, and termination patterns of the ventral, uncrossed component of the mature rat corticospinal tract. J Comp Neurol 386:293–303, 1997.

Diener PS, Bregman BS: Fetal spinal cord transplants support growth of supraspinal and segmental projections after cervical spinal cord hemisection in the neonatal rat. J Neurosci 18:779–793, 1998.

Giehl KM, Schacht CM, Yan Q, Mestres P: GDNF is a trophic factor for adult rat corticospinal neurons and promotes their long-term survival after axotomy in vivo. Eur J Neurosci 9:2479–2488, 1997.

Joosten EAJ: Corticospinal tract regrowth. Prog Neurobiol 53:1–25, 1997.

Pauvert V, Pierrot-Deseilligny E, Rothwell JC: Role of spinal premotoneurones in mediating corticospinal input to forearm motoneurones in man. J Physiol (Lond) 508:301–312, 1998.

Maier MA, Olivier E, Baker SN, et al: Direct and indirect corticospinal control of arm and hand motoneurons in the squirrel monkey *(Saimiri sciureus).* J Neurophysiol 78:721–733, 1997.

Morecraft RJ, Louie JL, Schroeder CM, Avramov K: Segregated parallel inputs to the brachial spinal cord from the cingulate motor cortex in the monkey. Neuroreport 8:3933–3938, 1997.

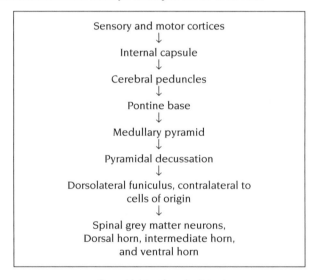

Sensory and motor cortices
↓
Internal capsule
↓
Cerebral peduncles
↓
Pontine base
↓
Medullary pyramid
↓
Pyramidal decussation
↓
Dorsolateral funiculus, contralateral to
cells of origin
↓
Spinal grey matter neurons,
Dorsal horn, intermediate horn,
and ventral horn

Pyramidal (corticospinal) tract.

THE EXTRAPYRAMIDAL SYSTEM

4. What is the extrapyramidal system?

All nonpyramidal motor systems, such as rubrospinal, vestibulospinal, tectospinal, reticulospinal, cerebellar, and basal ganglia circuitry, are called extrapyramidal. This term is used most often in the clinical neurologic and pharmacologic literature when describing motor abnormalities in relation to the administration of drugs. One common reference to disorders of the extrapyramidal system is to the side effects of therapeutic drug administration for the psychiatric illness called schizophrenia. Many of these motor abnormalities involve basal ganglia. This aside, we shall deal with the extrapyramidal system in the sense of motor systems that are not pertaining to the pyramidal tract.

5. What does the term extrapyramidal mean?

This term is rather imprecise, encompassing the many motor systems working in parallel that are not part of the pyramidal tract.

6. What are the medial and lateral motor pathways?

Pyramidal and extrapyramidal motor systems are part of either a medial or lateral pathway. Medial and lateral motor pathways control proximal or distal musculature innervated by these descending systems. The lateral system comprises the pyramidal tract and the rubrospinal tract, which also innervates spinal motoneurons involved in the control of distal musculature. These two tracts work in parallel. Those motor systems that control our proximal muscles—posture and ability to stand or sit upright in a three-dimensional, gravitational field—and control our righting reflexes, such as the vestibulospinal system, are components of the medial motor system.

The separation of medial and lateral systems is best demonstrated by the studies of Lawrence and Kuypers in 1968, in which they found that animals deprived of their descending pyramidal tract were unable to retrieve small pieces of food using independent finger movement; instead the animals had to use a grasping movement of the whole hand. Interrupting the rubrospinal system compounded the deficit, leaving primarily the medial postural and proximal muscles to accomplish these tasks, resulting in a less efficient performance.

Lawrence DG, Kuypers HGJM: The functional organization of the motor system in the monkey. I. The effects of bilateral pyramidal lesions. Brain 91:1–14, 1968.

Lawrence DG, Kuypers HGJM: The functional organization of the motor system in the monkey. II. The effects of lesions of the descending brain-stem pathways. Brain 91:15–36, 1968.

7. What neurotransmitters are associated with the extrapyramidal system?

Many of these systems arise from brainstem neurons that synapse on spinal neurons. These brainstem neurons secrete serotonin, amino acids, or catecholamines as their neurotransmitters (just to name a few). For example, catecholaminergic neurons have been reported to be diminished in cases of muscular dystrophy called myotonic dystrophy, a relatively common, autosomal-dominant disease producing distal muscular weakness.

Ono S, Takahashi K, Jinnai K, et al: Loss of catecholaminergic neurons in the medullary reticular formation in myotonic dystrophy. Neurology 51:1121–1124, 1998.

DESCENDING EXTRAPYRAMIDAL MOTOR SYSTEMS

8. What is the red nucleus?

The red nucleus is a prominent oval- to round-shaped structure that is present bilaterally in the midbrain above the substantia nigra. It first appeared in phylogeny when limbs appeared. There are two major parts to its structure: a parvicellular or small-celled portion that is important for communicating cerebral cortical information to the cerebellum via the inferior olivary nucleus; and a magnocellular or large-celled portion that receives information from both cerebral cortical neurons and neurons of the deep cerebellar nuclei.

The red nucleus appears to integrate cerebral cortical and cerebellar processing.

Ralston DD: Red nucleus of *Macaca fascicularis*: An electron microscopic study of its synaptic organization in relation to afferent and efferent connectivity and proposals for the role of the red nucleus in motor mechanisms. Proefschrift, Rijksuniversiteit Groningen, 1994.

9. What is the function of the magnocellular portion of the red nucleus?

The magnocellular portion that is the origin of the rubrospinal tract projects to spinal interneurons and motoneurons that subserve the function of distal musculature. It is a prominent tract in the nonhuman primate, but humans rely more on the pyramidal (corticospinal tract) for distal musculature control and function.

10. What is the function of the parvicellular portion of the red nucleus?

Control of Purkinje cells may occur through the parvicellular portion's influence on the electrically coupled oscillations of the inferior olivary nucleus. These oscillatory olivary neurons give rise to the climbing fibers that surround Purkinje cell dendrites in a one-to-one relationship. Their oscillations are present in particular in relation to step-cycles (one foot in front of the other in locomotion) of certain species. The inferior olivary nucleus is important in motor system function not only because of its sensory and motor input but also because of its influence on the cerebellar Purkinje cells.

McCormick DA: The cerebellar symphony. Nature 374(6521):412–413, 1995.

Smith SS: Step-cycle–related oscillatory properties of inferior olivary neurons recorded in ensembles. Neuroscience 82:69–81, 1997.

11. Describe the rubrospinal system.

Axons of the magnocellular portion of the red nucleus cross in the mesencephalon and descend in the dorsolateral funiculus of the spinal cord, overlapping the descent of the corticospinal tract. Depending upon the species, the axons enter the spinal cord at appropriate topographical levels to synapse on interneurons or motoneurons for innervation of distal musculature. Cats do not have opposable thumbs, and they possess rubrospinal connections to interneurons. Nonhuman primates, for whom the opposable thumb is a characteristic, possess direct connections to spinal motoneurons. In humans the rubrospinal tract does not appear to be as prominent; the corticospinal tract has occupied an increasingly more prominent role phylogenetically.

Holstege G, Blok BF, Ralston DD: Anatomical evidence for red nucleus projections to motoneuronal cell groups in the spinal cord of the monkey. Neurosci Lett 95:97–101, 1988.

Ralston DD, Milroy AM: Red nucleus of *Macaca fascicularis*: An electron microscopic study of its organization. J Comp Neurol 284:602–620, 1989.

Ralston DD, Ralston HJ III: The terminations of corticospinal tract axons in the Macaque monkey. J Comp Neurol 242:325–337, 1985.

Red nucleus in midbrain
↓
Decussation at level of red nucleus
↓
Pontine and medullary levels
↓
Spinal grey matter neurons,
Intermediate horn and
ventral horn

Rubrospinal tract.

12. Describe the vestibulospinal system.

The vestibulospinal system is somatotopically organized and arises from the vestibular nuclei located in the dorsolateral portion of the rostral medulla. Prominent features of these nuclei include input from the vestibular regions of the cerebellum and information from the vestibular apparatus and semicircular canals in the labyrinth. Vestibular nuclei possess many component parts and project both rostrally to control eye movements and caudally to the spinal cord for posture and righting reflexes. (See Chapter 7, The Vestibular System.)

Cerebellum, vestibular apparatus and vestibular nuclei
↓
Spinal grey motoneurons innervating axial and postural muscles

Vestibulospinal tract.

13. What are the functions of the vestibular system's rostral projections?

Most of the rostrally projecting vestibular fibers are involved with eye movements and special reflexes called the vestibulo-ocular reflex and the optokinetic reflex. Many components of the vestibulospinal system form connections to cervical motoneurons so that we can turn our head a precise amount of rotation, allowing us to maintain our horizontal gaze on a target.

14. What is the vestibulo-ocular reflex?

The vestibulo-ocular reflex (VOR) is critical for us to be able to fixate our eyes on a target when our head moves. The vestibulo-ocular fibers that subserve this reflex ascend via the medial longitudinal fasciculus to the horizontal and vertical gaze centers so that the eyes move together with exquisite precision to keep our retinae on target. The VOR controls the contraction of agonists and antagonists simultaneously in both eyes to achieve this precision. It is part of our own personal gyroscope. The VOR is now a model for studying motor learning. Also under examination are the role and involvement of the cerebellum in conjunction with this reflex.

Lisberger SG, Pavelko TA, Broussard DM: Neural basis for motor learning in the vestibulo-ocular reflex of primates. I. Changes in the responses of brain stem neurons. J Neurophysiol 72:928–953, 1994.

Lisberger SG, Pavelko TA, Bronte-Stewart HM, Stone LS: Neural basis for motor learning in the vestibulo-ocular reflex of primates. II. Changes in the responses of horizontal gaze velocity Purkinje cells in the cerebellar flocculus and ventral paraflocculus. J Neurophysiol 72:954–973, 1994.

Lisberger SG: Neural basis for motor learning in the vestibulo-ocular reflex of primates. III. Computational and behavioral analysis of the sites of learning. J Neurophysiol 72:974–998, 1994.

Raymond JL, Lisberger SG: Neural learning rules for the vestibulo-ocular reflex. J Neurosci 18:9112–9129, 1998.

15. What is the "doll's eye" maneuver, and how does it relate to the VOR?

The doll's eye maneuver also is called the oculocephalic maneuver. Normally, when a patient's head is rotated side to side and the eyes are fixed on a target, the eyes move in a conjugate fashion equal and opposite to the direction of the head movement. This is a normal oculocephalic or positive doll's eye response. It means that the brainstem with its vestibular connections is intact, boding well for the patient. However, when there is a disturbance or interruption in the pathway of the VOR, the eyes move with the head instead of in an equal and opposite fashion. This occurs in the presence of brainstem lesions.

There also are asymmetric responses of the VOR following damage to the medial longitudinal fasciculus. Such damage is demonstrated by abnormal eye movements that only *partially* effect the positive response of the doll's eye maneuver.

Dysfunction of the VOR can produce an uncontrolled, repeated nystagmus, which results in a smooth pursuit movement followed by a rapid resetting saccade. These eye movements can be elicited by gently turning the patient's head.

16. What is the optokinetic reflex?

The optokinetic reflex is quite different from the VOR in that it allows us to follow a target with smooth pursuit eye movements and then fixate on the next target with a saccadic movement. The best example of this is watching passing telephone poles from the window of a moving train.

17. What are the functions of the vestibular system's caudal projections?

These nuclei are separated into medial and lateral systems, with the lateral arising from Deiter's (lateral vestibular) nucleus. Both systems project via the anterolateral funiculus to spinal neurons in the ventral horn for postural, gravitational, and righting reflexive controls.The vestibulospinal tract is under the influence of the cerebellum and is important for our ability to stand or sit upright, make adjustments for gravitational shifts, and prevent a fall. In case of a fall, the vestibulospinal system allows us to reflexively protect the head and upper body by extension the upper extremities.

18. What is the structure and function of the tectospinal system?

The tectospinal tract arises from the neurons in the superior colliculi, where visual and sensory information is processed, and the inferior colliculi, where auditory information is processed. These are not primary visual or auditory areas of the brain, but they process visual and auditory reflexes by synapsing uopon cervical spinal motoneurons. These reflexes allow us to turn our heads in the direction of a visual or auditory stimulus. (See figure next page.)

> Superior and inferior colliculi in midbrain
> ↓
> Descent of tract adjacent to medial longitudinal fasciculus
> ↓
> Cervical spinal motoneurons to
> allow turning of the head in response to
> visual or auditory stimuli

Tectospinal tract.

19. What is the contribution of the reticulospinal system?

The neurons of the reticulospinal system are located in the medulla, pons, and midbrain and are composed of a reticulum of loosely interwoven neurons. These neurons are important facilitators of movements by attending to gamma motoneurons for muscle spindle function, phasic functions such as respiration, and inhibition or excitation of pyramidal tract influences on voluntary movement.

Parent A: Carpenter's Human Neuroanatomy, 9th ed. Baltimore, Williams and Wilkins, 1996.

THE EMOTIONAL MOTOR SYSTEM

20. Are there other motor systems that are critical for our motor function?

Yes. In recent years, Holstege and his colleagues have given important recognition and emphasis to the **limbic system's contribution** to motor system function. This contribution is called the "emotional motor system." Emotional expression is a normal part of our behavioral interaction with our environment. This system is considered to work in parallel with the other motor systems—not as an "override," but as a separate entity of its own. It allows those who are afflicted with motor system deficits to produce normal emotional motor output. For example, a young person with a motor cortical lesion resulting in facial paralysis is unable to show her teeth on command. However, when told a funny story she will smile relatively symmetrically. Thus, the voluntary control is absent but the emotional motor system is intact. Holstege, et al. describe extensive contributions from the somatic, endocrine, and autonomic nervous systems that facilitate the initial sensory input involving limbic processing as well as the emotional behavioral motor output.

The limbic system's involvement in motor function is complex and extensive, with a vast number of component parts from cortex to hypothalamus and brainstem as well as a myriad of neurotransmitters that are incorporated in transmission in the emotional motor system. The role of the hippocampal formation, amygdala, and anterior thalamus are critical in the processing of expressions of memory, fear, and motivation. Cortical areas such as the cingulate gyrus have come under greater scrutiny by basic scientists, psychologists, and clinical researchers. Imaging with positron emission tomography to identify areas of the brain involved with emotion (e.g., pain) has assisted in furthering our knowledge.

Holstege G, Bandler R, Saper CB (eds): The emotional motor system. In Progress in Brain Research. Amsterdam, Elsevier, 1996, pp 3–6.

Rainville P, Duncan GH, Price DD, et al: Pain affect encoded in human anterior cingulate but not somatosensory cortex. Science 277:968–971, 1997.

Talbot JD, Marrett S, Evans AC, et al: Multiple representations of pain in human cerebral cortex. Science 251:1355–1360, 1991.

DISORDERS OF THE PYRAMIDAL OR EXTRAPYRAMIDAL SYSTEMS

21. What are the signs in a patient when there is a disorder of the pyramidal system?

The loss of the ability to use distal musculature for fine movements is most prominent (as noted in monkey studies by Lawrence and Kuypers in 1968). If, however, the damage is great, such as that seen in stroke involving the descending fibers of the internal capsule, serious contralateral paralysis may ensue. If the dominant hemisphere is involved, then loss of communication skills may be added to the patient's disability.

In humans the clinical effects are similar, with the addition of what we call an upper motor neuron (UMN) syndrome. This is characterized by an initial hypotonia that is replaced by a spastic paresis, increased deep tendon reflexes, and possibly the presence of a Babinski sign. This sign, in which the toes curl up and splay out when the outer sole of the foot is stroked with a firm object, such as the handle of a reflex hammer, is not always present. It is considered normal in infants whose pyramidal tract is not yet fully myelinated.

UMN syndromes are in direct contrast to lower motor neuron (LMN) syndromes. By definition, the LMN is that neuron which projects directly to skeletal muscle. The LMN can be either a spinal motoneuron or a cranial nerve nucleus motoneuron. Loss of the LMN, such as that seen in poliomyelitis or the neurodegenerative disease called amyotrophic lateral sclerosis, leads to hypotonia, decreased deep tendon reflexes, and muscle wasting due to deprivation of neuromuscular trophic factors.

22. What is meant by "decerebrate" or "decorticate" rigidity?

In animals, bilateral brainstem lesions that remove descending influences above the level of the colliculi induce a condition called decerebrate rigidity. In humans, this condition usually is due to diffuse, bilateral lesions at the level of the midbrain. Under these circumstances all four extremities are under tonic excitatory influence, such that alpha motoneurons continue to fire, maintaining contraction in the flexor and extensor muscles. Decerebrate rigidity also can be seen in humans following stroke or trauma in this same region or higher up in the neuraxis.

Decerebrate posture, in which the upper extremities are in a state of spastic flexion and the lower extremities are in a state of spastic extension, is due to a bilateral brainstem lesion. Decorticate posture, in which all four extremities are in a state of spastic extension, is due to a lesion above the level of the brainstem. Both situations are a serious prognostic sign of the loss of normal descending control of spinal motoneurons.

DISEASES OF THE PYRAMIDAL AND EXTRAPYRAMIDAL SYSTEMS

23. What are the most prominent diseases of the pyramidal system?

These are mainly diseases that affect the upper or lower motoneurons. Examples are poliomyelitis, in which the polio enteric virus enters the neurons by retrograde transport, or amyotrophic lateral sclerosis, a motor system disease whose cause is unknown at present.

A major contribution to disability in the category of pyramidal tract dysfunction is stroke related to hypertension. Humans suffering these pyramidal tract disabilities following stroke can receive much benefit from physical therapy. In a study of the nonhuman primate in which stroke-like lesions were induced in the hand region of the cortex, resulting in the typical deficit of an inability to retrieve small objects using fine movements of the hand, many of the monkeys eventually developed either a return towards normalcy or compensatory movements to accomplish the task. The authors of this study concluded that the degree of recovery was related to the extent of the damage, which may be true in humans as well.

Friel KM, Nudo RJ: Recovery of motor function after focal cortical injury in primates: compensatory movement patterns used during rehabilitative training. Somatosens Mot Res 15:173–189, 1998.

24. What are the most prominent diseases of the extrapyramidal system?

These diseases usually involve the basal ganglia. Signs include dyskinesias, tremors, and involuntary movements, many of which may be related to therapeutic drugs.

Most of the diseases associated with the extrapyramidal system involve vascular strokes, trauma, tumors, or neurodegenerative diseases, most involving basal ganglia or structures that are involved in innervation of eye muscles. There also are specific stroke- or lesion-associated deficits, such as Weber's or Benedikt's syndrome, that involve the red nucleus or the cerebellar fibers that course through the red nucleus en route to the motor thalamus.

- **Weber's syndrome** is located at the level of the midbrain and involves a third nerve palsy and a contralateral paralysis. The proximity of the red nucleus and its crossing fibers may lead to involvement of the extrapyramidal system.
- **Benedikt's syndrome**, which is similar to Weber's syndrome, also is located at the level of the midbrain. It features a third nerve palsy and contralateral paralysis involving cerebellar fibers and the red nucleus and its crossing fibers. Patients may demonstrate ataxia or tremor due to possible involvement of the cerebellar fibers in transit.
- **Multiple sclerosis**, which causes central nervous system demyelination, may effect the conduction of impulses in the medial longitudinal fasciculus and disturb normal eye movements, causing patients to complain of double vision (diplopia). Multiple sclerosis also may affect the function of the vestibulo-ocular reflex.

BIBLIOGRAPHY

1. Bradley WG, Daroff RB, Fenichel GM, Marsden CD (eds): Neurology in Clinical Practice, Vol. II. Boston, Butterworth-Heinemann, 1991.
2. Brodal P: The Central Nervous System, 2nd ed. New York, Oxford University Press, 1998.
3. Gilman S, Newman SW: Manter and Gatz's Essentials of Clinical Neuroanatomy and Neurophysiology, 9th ed. Philadelphia, FA Davis Co., 1996.
4. Holstege G, Bandler R, Saper CB (eds): The emotional motor system. In Progress in Brain Research. Amsterdam, Elsevier, 1996.
5. Kandel ER, Schwartz JH, Jessel TM (eds): Essentials of Neural Science and Behavior. Norwalk, Connecticut, Appleton & Lange, 1995.
6. Kuypers HJGM, Martin GE (eds): Descending Pathways to the Spinal Cord: Progress in Brain Research. Amsterdam, Elsevier, 1982.
7. Parent A: Carpenter's Human Neuroanatomy, 9th ed. Baltimore, Williams and Wilkins, 1996.
8. Stedman TL: Stedman's Medical Dictionary, 24th ed. Baltimore, Williams & Wilkins, 1982.

13. BASAL GANGLIA

Diane Daly Ralston, Ph.D.

Much of what we know of motor systems arises from clinical observations of disease processes, war-associated head wounds, and basic animal research. However, newer and more sophisticated methods are providing us with incredible knowledge about neurotransmitters, pathways, and local and projection circuits associated with the basal ganglia. Computational and theoretical models (Houk, et al., 1995; Wichman and DeLong, 1996) based on current functional anatomy and physiology, can predict circuitry and resultant behavioral manifestations in the normal versus the diseased state by projecting function based on overall mechanisms or at biomolecular levels. These helpful models are constantly being reviewed and revised to account for the living, dynamic system.

This chapter explores the interesting neuronal aggregates of the basal ganglia, which not only control motor output for the body, head, and eyes, but also are thought to affect motor cognitive functions since they project to association and limbic motor cortices.

COMPONENTS OF THE BASAL GANGLIA

1. What does the term "basal ganglia" mean?

It is an old term referring to several aggregates of neurons that function together under cortical command to produce and maintain motor control. This chapter describes five component parts of the basal ganglia and how they are interconnected, although some authors and neuroanatomists consider the basal ganglia in a broader sense. There is current evidence to show that the basal ganglia exist in ancestral tetrapods that are regulated by homeobox genes, demonstrating that these structures are well conserved in phylogeny and thus long represented in motor function. An important feature of the basal ganglia circuitry is that it forms loops originating from and returning to multiple motor, sensory, and association cortical areas.

2. What are the components of the basal ganglia?

There are five major components to the basal ganglia:

1. The **caudate** (Latin, tail) nucleus, which forms part of the lateral walls of the lateral ventricles
2. The **putamen** (Latin, pruned off), located lateral to the internal capsule
3. Two divisions of the **globus pallidus** (Latin, pale globe), which are located medial to the putamen
4. The **subthalamus**, which is located ventral and inferior to the thalamus
5. The **substantia nigra** pars compacta (neuromelanin- and dopamine-producing neurons; thus, dark substance) and pars reticulata (gamma-aminobutyric acid [GABA]-producing neurons), both of which are located in the ventral portion of the midbrain.

The caudate and putamen are called the striatum because of the striped appearance that results from bundles of myelinated axons traversing the structures, the dorsal portion having motor thalamic and cortical connections and the ventral striatum (nucleus accumbens) having limbic cortical connections. The putamen and globus pallidus together are referred to as the lentiform nucleus because of its combined shape.

The caudate and putamen (the striatum), receive a topographically organized glutamatergic projection from many areas of the cerebral cortex primarily via n-methyl-D-aspartate (NMDA) receptors, and project to the globus pallidus via GABAergic inhibition. The striatum also is interconnected with the substantia nigra and the centromedian nucleus of the thalamus. The inner division of the globus pallidus (GPi) sends a large number of GABA-containing fibers to a component of the ventrolateral (VL) thalamic nucleus, which in turn projects to the primary motor cortex, to the supplementary motor area, and to other motor cortical areas of the frontal lobe. Thus, there is a feedback loop from wide areas of cortex to basal ganglia, an inhibitory GABAergic projection from globus pallidus to thalamus, and then an excitatory projection from thalamus to cortical motor areas of the frontal lobe. The basal ganglia do not project caudalward to the spinal cord. Recent evidence shows that particular subsets of GPi neurons project to zones of VL that, in turn, project to individual cortical motor areas such as primary motor cortex or supplementary motor cortex, each of which contributes to the corticospinal tract. Thus, the multiple projections from GPi back to cortex influence different cortical zones with different motor functions.

The substantia nigra and subthalamic nucleus also are considered integral parts of this system. The substantia nigra pars compacta receives a projection from striatum (caudate and putamen), and in turn sends fine dopaminergic fibers back to the striatum to bind with D_1 and D_2 receptors. Lesions of this latter fiber system have been implicated in Parkinsonism and other basal ganglia disorders. The substantia nigra also projects to a region of the ventroanterior thalamus, which then projects to various motor cortical areas.

The subthalamic nucleus has substantial interconnections with the external division of the globus pallidus. Subthalamic lesions result in uncontrolled ballistic movements, a motor disorder called hemiballismus. The subthalamic nucleus does not project to the thalamus, but instead to the globus pallidus, substantia nigra pars reticulata, and striatum.

These cerebello-thalamo-cortical loops and the chemoarchitecture of the basal ganglia system offer a good example of parallel processing in the central nervous system (see Questions 7–13).

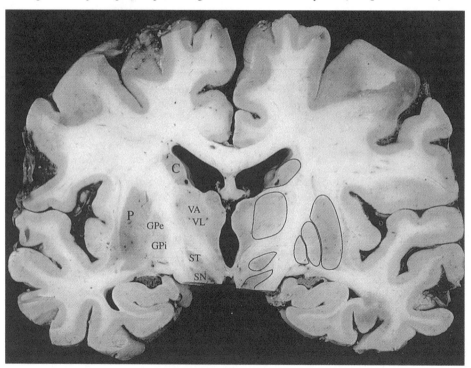

A coronal section through the brain demonstrating the component parts of the basal ganglia. *Left side:* C = caudate nucleus, VA/VL = ventroanterior and venterolateral nuclei of the motor thalamus, P = putamen, Gpe and Gpi = globus pallidus externa and interna, ST = subthalamus, SN = substantia nigra. *Right side:* Outline drawings of nuclear boundaries.

3. What is the embryologic origin of each of the basal ganglia components?

Each basal ganglia region has its own embryologic origin arising from the rostral portion of the developing neural tube:

- The caudate, putamen, and outer division of the globus pallidus are derived from the telencephalon that creates the cerebral hemispheres.
- The inner division of the globus pallidus and the subthalamic nuclei arise from the developing diencephalic vesicle.
- The substantia nigra arises from the developing mesencephalon.

4. The basal ganglia have been described as possessing a "mosaic." Please explain.

A mosaic pattern is formed by **compartmentalization** within the striatum. The compartments are determined by how the striatum receives and processes cortical information, based on projections from areas of the cortex and overlapping biochemical compartments of neurotransmitters and receptors. It was proposed that this compartmentalization created a greater complexity to allow a multilevel, hierarchical structure and to refine motor processing while preserving topography. The intriguing puzzle of matching up mosaic patterns, neuroanatomic structures, chemoarchitecture, and function presently is being researched in animal models. In addition, the compartmentalization of the mosaic relates to the organization and origin of the projecting cortical layers, in that the patches receive projections from the superficial layers of the cortex, and the matrix receives projections from the deep cortical layers (see Question 5). This provides an example of parallel processing within the motor system for the nuances of the control and execution of movement. Extrapolating this information from the basal ganglia of the monkey to the human may provide us with clues to the myriad of movement disorders.

Gerfen CR: The neostriatal mosaic: Multiple levels of compartment organization. Trends Neurosci 15(4):133–139, 1992.

5. What does "patch and matrix" mean in the striatum?

Patch and matrix refers to the unique manner in the primate in which the basal ganglia, particularly the caudate and putamen, are biochemically organized. **Striosomes** are patch-like compartments of tissue embedded within a background matrix of the striatum. These patch-like areas are low in choline acetyltransferase (ChAT) and acetylcholinesterase (AChE), but rich in enkephalin, tyrosine hydroxylase, the calcium-binding protein calbindin, somatostatin, substance P, and opiate and dopamine receptors, to name only a few constituents. Striosomes possess an immunohistochemical profile, and anatomic clusters of neurons correspond to the patches. The boundaries are not totally strict, and overlapping occurs in some areas. While striosomes have low levels of ChAT, the matrix contains high levels. This is not a uniform distribution, however, as the profiles of striosome and matrix change between the dorsal striatum and the more complex ventral striatum, which has limbic connections.

Striosomes also possess rings, or annulae. These rings are rich in enkephalin and substance P, but low in AChE. The neurons associated with the rings appear to overlap the patch-and-matrix arrangement, leading researchers to consider that they might be an interface for integration of these two biochemically and neuroanatomically distinct regions.

Study of the matrix using enzymatic and fluorescent tracers has revealed structures similar to striosomes, called **matrisomes**. These are embedded within the matrix and appear to represent clusters of striatopallidal and striatonigral neurons along with terminations of corticostriatal afferents, although no neurotransmitters have been specifically associated with them. The pathways appear to be maintained in parallel and may integrate their motor information at the cortical level via cortico-cortical connections.

Consider the functional significance of the neurotransmitters present in the specific regions of striatum. Do you think they are responsible for the nuances of function or the parallel processing? Increased understanding of basal ganglia may illuminate the nuances within the functional areas of the striatum that determine the exquisite control of motor output.

Holt DJ, Greybiel AM, Saper CB: Neurochemical architecture of the human striatum. J Comp Neurol 384:1–25, 1997.

Selemon LD, Goldman-Rakic PS: Topographic intermingling of striatonigral and striatopallidal neurons in the rhesus monkey. J Comp Neurol 297:359–376, 1990.

6. How are the structures of the basal ganglia related?

They are related by their embryology, connectivity, and roles in parallel processing of motor output. They are linked to a variety of uncontrolled movement disorders, ranging from the akinesia seen in some forms of Parkinson's disease to the hyperkinesia seen in choreas such as Sydenham's chorea, Huntington's disease, Tourette's syndrome, dystonias, and ballism.

CONNECTIONS OF THE BASAL GANGLIA

7. How are the structures of the basal ganglia connected?

The basal ganglia (caudate, putamen, globus pallidus, subthalamic nucleus, and substantia nigra) are a complex interconnected link of several nuclear groups within the brain and brainstem. They are involved in parallel modular loops that leave and return to the cortex much modulated and processed. They receive afferents from many motor and limbic areas to process motor information, and they modulate the excitement level of the thalamus' motor nuclei that project to motor cortices. In general, the basal ganglia utilize inhibitory GABA as the main neurotransmitter; the subthalamic nucleus uses glutamate.

Basal ganglia circuitry may be described as having two major pathways: the direct and the indirect. The indirect pathway includes a connection via the glutamatergic subthalamic nucleus. Both pathways are "in balance" in the normal brain and both affect the level of excitation of the motor thalamus and its effect on the output of the cerebral cortex. Diminished inhibitory output via the direct pathway of the basal ganglia allows for facilitation of the thalamic neurons. Increased inhibition via the indirect pathway leads to suppression of thalamic neurons. Altered output or imbalance of these inhibitory pathways in the diseased brain can account for the hyperkinesia seen in diseases such as Huntington's chorea and the hypokinesia seen in Parkinson's disease.

Parent A, Hazrati LN: Functional anatomy of the basal ganglia. I. The cortico-basal ganglia-thalamo-cortical loop. Brain Res Revs 20:91–127, 1995.

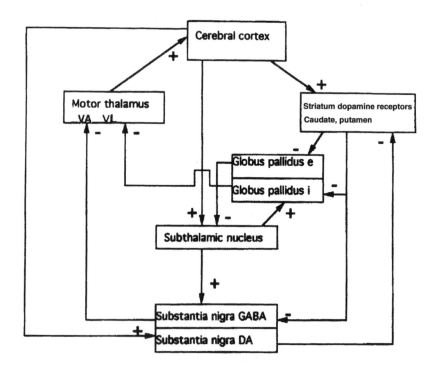

Basal ganglia circuitry. VA = ventroanterior, VL = ventrolateral, e = external, i = interior, DA = dopaminergic.

8. Describe the corticostriatal projections.

Corticostriatal projections influence the function of neurotransmitters by genetic regulation. Neurons of wide areas of the cortex in this corticostriatal pathway project topographically to the striatum and secrete the excitatory amino acid glutamate, which binds primarily to NMDA and non-NMDA (AMPA) receptors in the striatum. This is the beginning of the basal ganglia loop that eventually, via the direct or indirect pathway, will terminate at the cortical level for cortico-cortical processing. These projections participate in a parallel processing adhering to the striasomal, matrix, and matrisomal patterns. The striatum receives many other projections from the substantia nigra pars compacta (dopaminergic pathway) and from the complex of intralaminar nuclei of the thalamus as well as the major motor thalami VA and VL, suggesting these latter as a center for motor integration of converging information.

Holt DJ, Greybiel AM, Saper CB: Neurochemical architecture of the human striatum. J Comp Neurol 384:1–25, 1997.

Parent A: Carpenter's Human Neuroanatomy, 9th ed. Baltimore, Williams and Wilkins, 1996.

9. Are there projections from the cortex to the substantia nigra?

Yes. Corticonigral projections from primary motor cortex are considered to be glutamatergic. The substantia nigra has many component and subcomponent parts. The major divisions are determined by the chemical neurotransmitter: pars compacta melanin-containing neurons produce dopamine and project to the striatum to bind with dopamine receptors: pars reticulata neurons secrete GABA and project to several areas. There also are nigral projections to the superior colliculus and another to the thalamus for control of eye movements and integration in the tectospinal pathway.

10. Does the subthalamus receive input from the cortex as well?

Yes. Corticosubthalamic projections arise primarily from the primary motor cortex, although not exclusively. These topographic projections also are glutamatergic. The subthalamus possesses sensorimotor regions that are topographically organized and associative areas important for oculomotor and behavioral output. The subthalamus is connected to the globus pallidus and brainstem nuclei. It is the only subcortical basal ganglia component that is excitatory, as its neurons are exclusively glutamatergic.

11. Describe the importance of the nigrostriatal pathway.

Nigrostriatal projections originate from the pars compacta dopaminergic pathway. The dopaminergic effect depends upon whether the nigrostriatal axons terminate upon neurons in the striatum that are GABAergic, enkephalinergic, or substance P-containing, as well as the presence of D_1 or D_2 receptors. The receptor determines whether the dopamine produces an excitatory or inhibitory effect. Parallel processing can be maintained on its route back to the cortex.

12. What is the role of the basal ganglia in relation to the motor thalamus?

Thalamocortical projections are critical for the functional output of the motor and sensory cortices. The basal ganglia project to the motor thalamus (VA, VL) with processed inhibitory information; the cerebellum also projects to the thalamus, with information for coordination. The thalamus may be the center for integrating these inputs and informing the cortex what its output should be.

13. Does the thalamus project back to the basal ganglia?

Yes. Thalamostriatal projections arise primarily from centromedian, centrolateral, and parafascicular nuclei as well as limbic thalamus that deal with emotional and behavioral manifestations of motor output. They project to the caudate and nucleus accumbens using glutamate to have an excitatory effect on these regions of striatum.

Parent A: Carpenter's Human Neuroanatomy, 9th ed. Baltimore, Williams and Wilkins, 1996.

NEUROTRANSMITTERS AND RECEPTORS

14. What are the principal neurotransmitters and receptors associated with the basal ganglia?

Structure	Transmitter	Recipient	Receptor	Effect
Cortex	Glutamate	Striatum	NMDA Non-NMDA	Excitation
Cortex	Glutamate	Nigral	NMDA Non-NMDA	Excitation
Cortex	Glutamate	Subthalamus	NMDA Non-NMDA	Excitation
Striatum	GABA	Globus pallidus	———	———
Striatum	GABA Substance P, enkephalin dynorphin	Substantia nigra, pars reticulata	GABA Substance P, enkephalin, dynorphin	Inhibitory Excitatory
Striatum	GABA Substance P, enkephalin, dynorphin	Substantia nigra, pars compacta	GABA Substance P, enkephalin, dynorphin	Inhibitory Excitatory
Globus pallidus externa	GABA	Substantia nigra pars reticulata	GABA	Inhibitory
Globus pallidus interna	GABA	Thalamus, VA, VL, CM	GABA	Inhibitory
Subthalamus	Glutamate	Globus pallidus	NMDA Non-NMDA	Excitatory
Subthalamus	Glutamate	Substantia nigra pars reticulata	NMDA Non-NMDA	Excitatory
Substantia nigra pars compacta	Dopamine	Striatum	D_1 D_2	Excitation or inhibition depending on receptor
Substantia nigra pars reticulata	GABA	Superior colliculus	GABA receptors	Eye movements, tecto- spinal tract function
Thalamus	Glutamate	Striatum	NMDA Non-NMDA	Excitatory
Thalamus	Glutamate	Cortex	NMDA Non-NMDA	Modulated levels of excitation due to basal ganglia loop

VA = ventroanterior, VL = ventrolateral, CM = centromedian nucleus of thalamus.

Some of these neurotransmitters and receptors, such as glutamate and GABA, are considered to be fast and more uninterrupted in projection. Others appear to have a slower action and are therefore considered modulatory to neurons within the circuit.

Di Chiara G, Morelli M, Consolo S: Modulatory functions of neurotransmitters in the striatum: ACH/dopamine/NMDA interactions. Trends Neurosci 17(6):228–233, 1994.
Parent A: Carpenter's Human Neuroanatomy, 9th ed. Baltimore, Williams and Wilkins, 1996.

15. Are the neurons of the basal ganglia different than those seen in other areas of the brain?
Yes. Neurons in the basal ganglia are numerous, unique, and well categorized in the literature. They differ in size, location, absence or presence of spines on their receptive dendritic arbors (called spiny or aspiny neurons), transmitters secreted, and type of receptors residing within their membranes. They may receive thousands of synapses upon each cell.

There are two types of **spiny neurons** in the striatum. The smaller of the two, called Type I, is more numerous and has a spherical dendritic arbor of approximately 200 μm. They possess long axons with many proximal and distal collateral processes, inferring the capability for local interactions as well as projection. Type II spiny neurons are larger, possessing a dendritic field of approximately 600 μm, and they are specifically projection neurons.

In contrast, there are **aspiny neurons** whose sphere of influence is restricted to the area where the neuron is located in the striatum. These local circuit neurons are notable by their lack of spines and by their neurotransmitter profile. Some of these aspiny neurons are governed by GABA and parvalbumin; others are directed by a variety of transmitters, such as nitric oxide and somatostatin.

Parent A: Carpenter's Human Neuroanatomy, 9th ed. Baltimore, Williams and Wilkins, 1996.

DISORDERS OF THE BASAL GANGLIA

16. A disorder of the basal ganglia is indicated by what signs?

Basal ganglia disorders usually present symptoms of three major types:
1. Changes in muscle tone
2. A poverty of voluntary movement (akinesia)
3. Uncontrolled involuntary movements and/or resting tremors

The term "extrapyramidal sign" often is used to describe one or more of these symptoms.

17. How are the involuntary movements associated with disorders of the basal ganglia classified?

A **resting tremor**, resulting from lesions in the basal ganglia, is characterized by a continuous tremor at rest. It is diminished or lost during voluntary movement of the affected part. A resting tremor (characteristic "pill rolling" movements of the fingers on the side opposite of the lesion) often is seen in Parkinson's disease.

Athetosis is a term used to designate slow, writhing, wormlike movements. The extremities typically are involved, but the muscles of the face and neck also may be affected. Athetoid movements of the axial musculature produce torsion of the neck, shoulder, and pelvic girdle. Athetoid movements cannot be correlated with a specific lesion site in the basal ganglia. Athetosis, which may occur due to anoxic ischemic encephalopathy (cerebral palsy), produces uncontrolled gyrational movements involving some or all parts of the body.

Chorea is characterized by a series of brisk, graceful, successive movements. They usually involve the distal portions of the extremity, muscles of facial expression, and the tongue. Most often, the pathologic changes in cases of chorea are found within the striatum.

Ballismus (or hemiballismus if unilateral) is a condition in which large-scale, violent, flail-like or ballistic movements occur, most often as a result of lesions of the subthalamic nucleus.

DISEASES OF THE BASAL GANGLIA

18. What are some of the salient features of Parkinson's disease?

Parkinson's disease is not described in the ancient literature as definitively as many other diseases. It is now considered to be an acquired disease related to environmental toxins that appeared around the time of the Industrial Revolution. Described in an essay by Dr. James Parkinson as the "shaking palsy" in 1817, it is characterized by rigidity, tremor at rest (pill rolling and head bobbing), akinesia or a loss of initiation of movement, a masked face (loss of expression), and slow, monotonous speech. In this disorder there is a loss of the dopamine-containing pigmented cells in the substantia nigra. Parkinson's is widespread throughout the United States, including some juvenile and hereditary cases, and varies greatly in its severity. The form of Parkinson's disease found on the Pacific island of Guam is a more severe form of the illness associated with dementia, other complicating factors, and a high mortality rate.

19. Can administration of dopamine cure Parkinson's disease?

Dopamine does not cross the blood-brain barrier; therefore, administration of L-DOPA, a precursor that is converted by the brain to dopamine, and/or the administration of dopamine receptor agonists or L-DOPA in combination with carbidopa may alleviate the rigidity and tremor. However, these measures do not slow the overall progression of the disease.

Hardman JG, Limbird LE, Malinoff PB, Rudden RW (eds): Goodman and Gilman's The Pharmacological Basis of Therapeutics, 9th ed. New York, McGraw Hill, 1996.

20. How is Parkinson's disease studied?

In 1983, Dr. J.W. Langston of the Santa Clara Valley Medical Center in California treated several young adults for severe symptoms of a Parkinsonian-like syndrome. He was able to ascertain that they had intravenously administered a compound called methyl phenyl tetrahydropyridine whose metabolite methyl phenyl pyridinium is toxic to the dopaminergic neurons of the substantia nigra by interfering with mitochondrial function. These neurons appear to have a selective affinity for this metabolite. The death of these neurons, in particular, leads to the Parkinsonian-like syndrome. Knowledge of this compound and its effects have opened up research possibilities in that there are now animal models that allow investigation into triggering mechanisms of the syndrome, pathogenesis, and pharmacologic and surgical interventions that may be used in the human. The latter of these has encompassed the use of transplants of fetal midbrain tissue into the striatum to return a source of dopamine to the nigrostriatal pathway. Alternatively, the direct or indirect pathways may be interrupted by creating a lesion in the globus pallidus (pallidotomy) or in the motor thalamus (thalamotomy). Some of these procedures have ameliorated the motor disorders associated with Parkinson's disease.

Tasker RR, Lang AE, Lozano AM: Pallidal and thalamic surgery of Parkinson's disease. Exp Neruol 144:35–40, 1997.

21. Are there other diseases similar to Parkinson's disease?

Another disease state, called supranuclear palsy (Steele-Richardson-Olszewski syndrome) mimics Parkinson's disease. Supranuclear palsy involves the basal ganglia, in particular both the reticulata and compacta of the substantia nigra. Dementia, rigidity, akinesia, and gaze palsies are integral signs of this neurodegenerative disease.

Hardman CD, Halliday GM, McRitchie DA, et al: Progressive supranuclear palsy affects both the substantia nigra pars compacta and reticulata. Exp Neurol 144:183–192, 1997.

Valldeoriola F, Tolosa E, Valls-Sole J: Differential diagnosis and clinical diagnostic criteria of progressive supranuclear palsy. In Battisin L, Scarlato G, Caraceni T, Ruggieri S (eds): Advances In Neurology. Philadelphia, Lippincott-Raven, 1996.

22. What is Huntington's disease?

Huntington's disease (or chorea), described by Dr. G. Huntington in 1872, is a Mendelian dominant inherited disorder that typically has its onset at 35–45 years of age. Profound atrophy of the caudate and putamen is a late manifestation of this illness. It progresses with involuntary muscle contractions until almost all muscles in the body are involved. The movements are dance-like; thus, the name chorea. Dementia almost always occurs, presumably due to loss of cortical cells. After 10 years of intense work, an international team under the direction of Dr. Jim Gusella in Boston recently reported the isolation of the responsible gene. The 210 kbase gene is found on the short arm of chromosome 4 and is characterized by 42 to 100 copies of the motif CAG (11 to 34 copies is normal). This trinucleotide repeat expansion also is associated with other human genetic diseases. At present there is no cure for Huntington's disease, but neurotrophic factors and transplants currently are avenues of research.

Critical work on the origin of Huntington's disease was carried out by Dr. Nancy Wexler, who traveled to Lake Maracaibo, Venezuela, a region with one of the highest incidences in the world, to develop the most comprehensive genetic mapping of the disease. This work advanced studies of the disease and attributed its origin to one ancestor many generations earlier. Dr. Wexler has been influential in research, public awareness, and ethical issues associated with hereditary diseases.

Wexler NS: Disease gene identification: ethical considerations. Hospital Practice 26(10):145–152, 1991.

Wexler NS: Molecular approaches to hereditary diseases of the nervous system: Huntington's disease as a paradigm. Annu Rev Neurosci 14:503–529, 1991.

23. Are there other types of chorea?

Yes. Choreas such as Sydenham's chorea usually are restricted to the childhood years and are associated with rheumatic fever of the streptococcal A variety. This type of chorea, which can be quite disabling, typically is reversible but with occasional short relapses. Other choreas are associated with toxins, metabolic diseases, developmental disorders, and heredity (e.g, Huntington's).

24. Is Huntington's chorea the only inherited basal ganglia disease?

No. Tourette's syndrome is an inherited disease first seen in childhood that also is attributed to a malfunction of the basal ganglia. Behavioral manifestations vary dramatically, from uncontrollable mild facial or eyelid tics to outbursts of uncontrolled speech, sometimes including obscenities or repetitive mimicking. These behavioral tics may be complicated by obsessive compulsive behavior and/or hyperactivity. The cause of this disease is presently attributed to disruption of the dopaminergic pathway within the basal ganglia, especially in relationship to D_2 receptors in the striatum. This attribution is based on the pharmacokinetics of D_2 receptor antagonists and their effect on Tourette's syndrome behavioral manifestations.

Robertson MM, Yakely J: Gilles de la Tourette syndrome and obsessive compulsive disorder. In Fogel BS, Schiffer RB, Rao SM (eds): Neuropsychiatry. Baltimore, Williams and Wilkins, 1996.

25. What is the overall effect of the basal ganglia?

There has been much thought and creative speculation about the role of each component of the basal ganglia and the overall effect that this loop has on the motor cortex. For example, neurons of the basal ganglia and the supplementary motor area (SMA) with which it is connected through the thalamus have been shown to be active in the planning of movements, prior to their initiation. Patients with damage of the basal ganglia or SMA have difficulty initiating voluntary movements, as seen in Parkinson's disease, or demonstrate a heterogeneous range of uncontrolled movements, as seen in choreas and dystonias. It appears from movement disorders that each of the components of the basal ganglia is unique, but together they perform as an ensemble via direct or indirect pathways to influence the function of the motor thalamus. The thalamus, in turn, affects the cortex for descending motor control. A recent study by Brown and Marsden suggests an important role in successive or sequential stages of motor processing.

We continue to learn about the precise motor function roles of the individual nuclei of the basal ganglia through patients, animal models, and increasingly sophisticated investigative techniques.

BIBLIOGRAPHY

1. Anderson KD, Panayotatos N, Corcoran TL, et al: Ciliary neurotrophic factor protects striatal output neurons in an animal model of Huntington's disease. Proc Natl Acad Sci 93:7346–7351, 1996.
2. Bradley WG, Daroff RB, Fenichel GM, Marsden CD (eds): Neurology in Clinical Practice, Vol. II. Boston, Butterworth-Heinemann, 1991.
3. Brodal P: The Central Nervous System, 2nd ed. New York, Oxford University Press, 1998.
4. Brown P, Marsden CD: What do the basal gangalia do? Lancet 351:1801–1804, 1998.
5. Gusella JF, MacDonald ME: Huntington's disease: CAG genetics expands neurobiology. Curr Opinions Neurobiol 5:656–662, 1995.
6. Houk JC, Davis JL, Beiser DG (eds): Models of Information Processing in the Basal Ganglia. Cambridge, The MIT Press, 1995.
7. Kandel ER, Schwartz JH, Jessel TM (eds): Essentials of Neural Science and Behavior. Norwalk, Connecticut, Appleton & Lange, 1995.
8. Marin O, Smeets WAJ, Gonzalez A: Evolution of the basal ganglia in tetrapods: A new perspective based on recent studies in amphibians. Trends Neurosci 21(11):487–494, 1998.
9. Parent A, Hazrati LN: Functional anatomy of the basal ganglia. II. The place of subthalamic nucleus and external pallidum in basal ganglia circuitry. Brain Res Rev 20:128–154, 1995.
10. Stedman TL: Stedman's Medical Dictionary, 24th ed. Baltimore, Williams & Wilkins, 1982.
11. Wichman T, DeLong MA: Functional and pathophysiological models of the basal ganglia. Curr Opinion Neurobiol 6:751–758, 1996.

14. CEREBELLUM

Linda J. Larson-Prior, Ph.D.

GROSS STRUCTURAL FEATURES

1. Where is the cerebellum?

The cerebellum occupies the posterior cranial fossa and is covered by the tentorium cerebelli. The largest part of the hindbrain, it lies posterior to the pons and medulla oblongata and is separated from them by the fourth ventricle.

2. What are the external features of the cerebellum?

The cerebellum consists of two prominent hemispheres joined by a median vermis (Fig. 1). The cerebellar cortex is divided anteroposteriorly into three lobes: the anterior lobe, separated from the posterior lobe by the primary fissure; the large posterior lobe; and, separated by the posterolateral fissure, the flocculonodular lobe.

3. Do the lobes have subdivisions?

Yes, there are several named subdivisions with multiple terminologies. While useful experimentally, this complex parcellation has little functional or clinical relevance. Clinically, three major subdivisions are recognized: the flocculonodular lobe (archicerebellum), the anterior lobe (paleocerebellum), and the posterior cerebellum (neocerebellum). While these subdivisions frequently are stated to correspond to the vestibulocerebellum, spinocerebellum, and pontocerebellum respectively, the actual connectivity of these areas is more complex (see section on connectivity, page 215).

4. What was the basis for the lobular subdivisions if it wasn't functional?

The basis was morphologic. The cerebellar surface consists of a series of transversely oriented, parallel ripples known as **folia**. The folia are aggregated into lobules which in turn aggregate to form the named lobes. Individual folia are separated by narrow grooves: the lobules by shallow fissures and the lobes by deep ruts. Thus, by one terminology, the anterior lobe comprises lobules I–IV, the posterior lobe comprises lobules VI–IX, and and the flocculonodular lobe is lobule X plus the flocculus. This morphologic organization is seen clearly in sagittal section, where it produces the appearance of a repeating series of branches.

5. How is the cerebellum connected to the rest of the brain?

The cerebellum is connected to other brain regions by three large fiber bundles known as the **peduncles**: the superior cerebellar peduncle (SCP), the middle cerebellar peduncle (MCP), and the inferior cerebellar peduncle (ICP) (Fig. 2). The peduncles represent the only path by which axons can enter or leave the cerebellum.

6. Where are the peduncles located?

The SCP, or brachium conjunctivum, runs laterally along the upper half of the fourth ventricle to enter the brainstem tegmentum at the level of the pontomesencephalic junction.

The MCP, or brachium pontis, is the largest of the three peduncles and arises from the pontine nuclei. The MCP sweeps into the cerebellum from the posterolateral pons.

The ICP is composed of the juxtarestiform and restiform bodies and is first definable in the caudal medulla as olivocerebellar and spinocerebellar fibers coalesce. The ICP travels in the dorsal medulla and enters the cerebellum at the pontomedullary border.

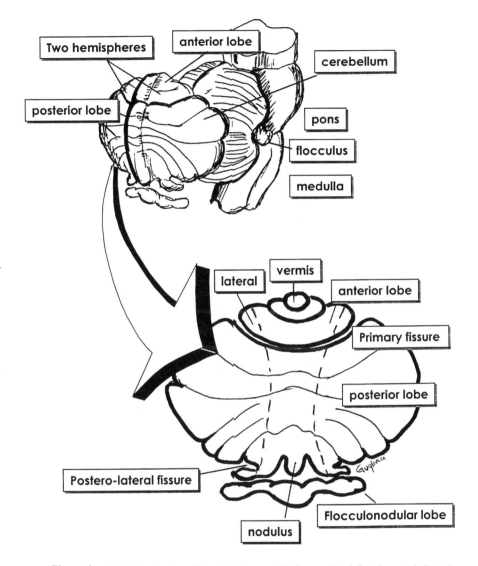

Figure 1. Cerebellar structure. The major lobes and the fissures that define them are indicated.

7. What are the functional components of the cerebellum?

The cerebellum consists of a central core of fiber bundles overlain by a three-layered rind of cortex. The central core of white matter is carried into each of the folia. Buried within the central core lie three deep cerebellar nuclei: the fastigial nuclei medially, the dentate nuclei laterally, and interposed nuclei (which, from medial to lateral, are composed of the globose and emboliform nuclear masses) between.

8. What are the functional components of the cerebellar cortex?

The cerebellar cortex consists of three cellular layers (Fig. 3). Closest to the white matter core lies the densely packed granule cell layer. Sitting on the granule cell layer is a monolayer of large

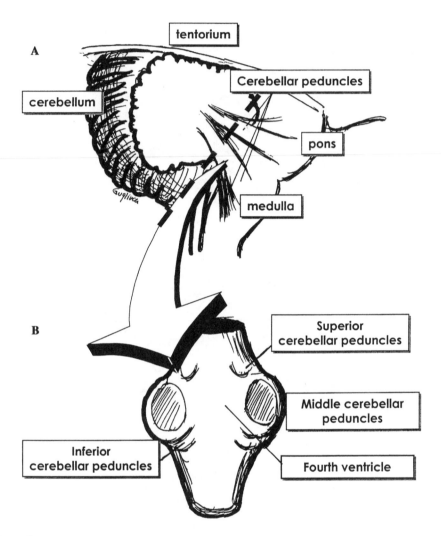

Figure 2. Cerebellar peduncles. **A,** The position of the cerebellum and the relationship of the peduncles to the brainstem. **B,** A dorsal view, in which the cerebellum has been removed to show the arrangement of the peduncles.

neurons, the Purkinje cell layer. The Purkinje cell represents the sole output neuron of the cerebellar cortex. The Purkinje cell layer separates the granule cell and molecular layers of the cortex. The molecular layer contains two major classes of inhibitory interneuron: the large and highly arborized Purkinje cell dendrites and the long axons of the granule cells.

9. What is the vascular supply of the cerebellum?
The cerebellum is supplied by the superior cerebellar and anterior inferior cerebellar arteries arising from the basilar and posterior inferior cerebellar arteries. The latter, in turn, arises from the vertebral artery. The distribution of these arterial systems is not regionally specific, nor do they supply exclusively cerebellar structures.

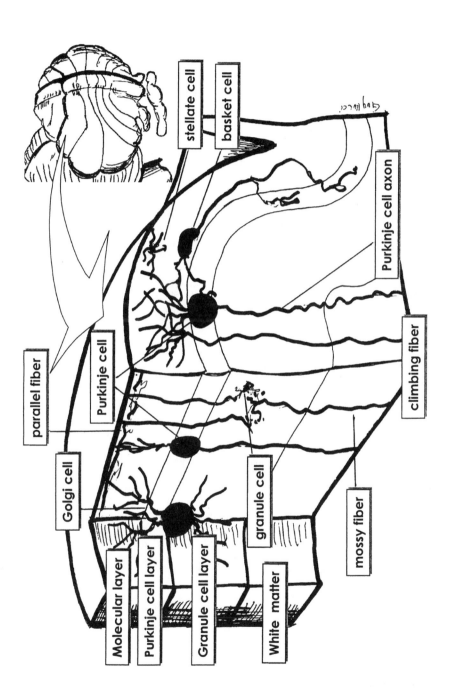

Figure 3.   Internal architecture of the cerebellar cortex.

INTERNAL ARCHITECTURE AND CIRCUITRY

10. What are the cellular elements of the granule cell layer?

The granule cell layer is the thickest and most densely packed of the three cortical layers. The most numerous neuronal cell type in this layer (and, it has been suggested, in the entire brain) is the granule cell. This small cell extends its axon through the Purkinje cell layer and into the molecular layer, where it bifurcates and travels parallel to the pial surface of the cerebellum in the coronal plane (see Fig. 3). The large Golgi cells have extensive dendritic and axonal arbors and are inhibitory to the granule cells. Several other cell types, whose functions currently are not well understood, also are located in the granule cell layer.

11. Does the Purkinje cell layer contain only Purkinje cells?

Yes. The large and elaborately arborized Purkinje cells have an entire layer all to themselves. However, two cell types lie closely adjacent to them: the inhibitory basket cells and the Bergmann glial cells. Basket cell somata are located at the interface of Purkinje cell and molecular layers, and Bergmann glia somata are found at the interface of the granule cell and Purkinje cell layers.

12. Are the Purkinje cells easily differentiated from other cells in the cerebellar cortex?

Yes, the Purkinje cell has a large soma (~ 40 μm in diameter) and an extensive and highly branched dendritic arbor that extends throughout the molecular layer. The Purkinje cell dendritic arbor has a distinct orientation (see Fig. 3), such that the branches fan out in the sagittal plane (perpendicular to the long axis of the folium) in a relatively flat plate 8–10 μm across. The distal dendrites are covered with dendritic spines, specialized synaptic structures that extend from the dendritic membrane and are the main contact site for the parallel fibers.

This unique architecture allows each Purkinje cell to be contacted by a large number of parallel fibers that run orthogonal to the axis of the Purkinje cell dendritic arbor. A single Purkinje cell may receive more than 200,000 parallel fiber synapses.

13. Are there any cells in the molecular layer?

Yes, the molecular layer is home to two inhibitory interneurons, the stellate and basket cells (see Fig. 3). **Basket cells** are highly specialized and named for the "basket" of axons that they form around Purkinje cell somata. A single basket cell axon contacts multiple Purkinje cell somata, as it extends parallel to the Purkinje cell dendritic arbor (perpendicular to the long axis of the folium). **Stellate cells** are found in the outer two-thirds of the molecular layer and send their axons to Purkinje cell dendrites in that region. The deeper the stellate cell lies in the molecular layer, the longer its axons tend to be. Both stellate and basket cells receive their input largely from parallel fibers.

14. If the Purkinje cell is the only output neuron, what are the other cells doing?

Each cellular layer can be thought of as an individual processing network. The granule cell is the output neuron of the granule cell layer, sending information to the Purkinje cells via its long, bifurcated parallel fiber axon. In the molecular layer, information from the granule cell network is modulated and refined for transmission to the Purkinje cells. The Purkinje cell layer accepts information from both granule cell and molecular networks, processes that information, and transmits it to the deep cerebellar and vestibular nuclei.

15. Where do the Purkinje cells project their axons?

The Purkinje cells project their information to the deep cerebellar nuclei and the vestibular nuclei. Remember that the Purkinje cell is inhibitory to its target cells; thus, the output of the cerebellar cortical circuit is inhibitory.

16. Are the deep cerebellar nuclei also inhibitory?

The deep cerebellar nuclei are largely excitatory to their extracerebellar targets, which are widespread in the central nervous system. However, there are inhibitory connections made to inferior olivary neurons by the dentate nuclei as well as some intracerebellar inhibitory connections.

17. Do the deep cerebellar nuclei receive input only from the Purkinje cells?

The deep cerebellar nuclei receive Purkinje cell, mossy fiber, climbing fiber, and multilayer fiber inputs in addition to inputs from other nuclear cells, both projecting and nonprojecting. Although the majority of synaptic contacts are inhibitory, these cells also receive excitatory inputs. If inhibition is reduced, the deep nuclear cells will fire rhythmically and spontaneously, illustrating the importance of inhibitory drive in normal cerebellar neurotransmission.

The vestibular nuclei, while receiving Purkinje cell output, do not receive climbing fiber or mossy fiber inputs. Rather, they are contacted by afferent fibers from other systems (see Chapter 7).

18. Where does the granule cell receive its information?

The granule cell layer receives sensory information from all areas of the brain. This information is carried predominantly by mossy fibers that contact granule cell dendrites in specialized synaptic complexes known as **glomeruli**. These glial-encased glomerular complexes contain mossy fiber terminals, Golgi cell axonal terminals, Golgi cell dendritic contact sites, and granule cell dendritic contact sites.

19. Does the Purkinje cell layer get information only from the granule cell axons?

No, a major input to the Purkinje cell comes from the brainstem inferior olivary nucleus in the form of climbing fibers. This unique input system "climbs" the Purkinje cell dendrite located in the molecular layer and makes strong excitatory contact with the proximal Purkinje cell dendrites. The climbing and parallel fibers terminate on distinctly separate regions of the Purkinje cell dendritic arbor that have been shown to correlate to subcellular domains definable by specific molecular markers.

Oberdick J, Baader SL, Schilling K: From zebra stripes to postal zones: Deciphering patterns of gene expression in the cerebellum. Trends Neurosci 21:383–390, 1998.

20. What kind of information does the inferior olivary nucleus send to the Purkinje cells?

Like the granule cell layer, the inferior olivary nucleus receives sensory information from all major modalities with the exception of olfaction. Each olivary axon contacts only a few Purkinje cells (approximately 10–15), but the activity of the nucleus produces synchronized discharging of all the contacted Purkinje cells. This complex network may act to produce synchronized inputs, which may be important in timing and sequencing, to Purkinje cells.

21. What processing is done in the molecular layer?

In the molecular layer, the stellate and basket cells receive input from the parallel fibers and help to shape Purkinje cell responses to convergent input from multiple parallel fibers (about 200,000/ cell) and individual climbing fibers. Presumably, these interneurons aid in the parcellation of information so that appropriate patterns of Purkinje cell activation are transmitted to the deep cerebellar nuclei.

22. Is there a basic circuit present in the cerebellar cortex?

Although simplified, a basic cortical circuit has been described. Information from peripheral and central sensory systems enters via mossy fiber inputs to the granule cells (modified by the Golgi cell that samples both mossy fiber and granule cell activity). The granule cells send parallel fibers to the molecular layer, where they contact Purkinje cell dendrites and stellate and basket cells. The climbing fibers, arising from the inferior olivary nucleus, also synapse on Purkinje cell dendrites in the molecular layer. Thus, climbing fiber and parallel fiber excitatory inputs, modified by stellate and basket cell interneuronal inhibition, converge on the Purkinje cell. The Purkinje cell transmits inhibitory signals to the deep cerebellar nuclei and the vestibular nuclei, which are the sole output centers of the cerebellum.

23. Does the cerebellum receive any other afferent fiber types?

Yes, a multilayered pathway has been described by several authors. Other afferent fibers include beaded afferent fibers from the raphe and reticular nuclei, the locus coeruleus, and the hypothalamus. These afferent fibers are found in all three cortical layers. Although this system is not well understood, it appears to modulate synaptic transmission mediated through the better known mossy and climbing fiber systems.

Dietrichs E, Haines DE, Roster GK, Roste LS: Hypothalamocerebellar and cerebellohypothalamic projections—Circuits for regulating nonsomatic cerebellar activity? Histol Histopath 9:603–614, 1994.

Ottersen OP: Neurotransmitters in the cerebellum. Rev Neurol (Paris) 149:629–636, 1993.

24. Which neurotransmitters are used by the intrinsic cerebellar neurons?

The cerebellar cortex is largely an inhibitory network. The Purkinje cells, stellate cells, basket cells, and Golgi cells all utilize the inhibitory amino acid neurotransmitter GABA as their primary chemical signal. The granule cell is the only excitatory interneuron in the cerebellar cortex, and it uses glutamate as its neurotransmitter. Although its function is less clearly understood, glycine also may be used as an inhibitory transmitter by the Golgi cells, where it appears to be colocalized with GABA. In addition, glycinergic inhibitory currents have been recorded in Golgi cells, suggesting the presence of glycinergic inhibitory interneurons.

Dieudonne S: Glycinergic synaptic currents in Golgi cells of the rat cerebellum. Proc Natl Acad Sci 92: 1441–1445, 1995.

Otterson OP, Storm-Mathisen J, Somogyi P: Colocalization of glycine-like immunoreactivities in Golgi cell terminals in the rat cerebellum: A postembedding light and electron microscopy study. Brain Res 450:342–353, 1988.

25. Which neurotransmitters are used by the climbing fiber inputs to the cerebellum?

Although there is still some controversy on this subject, it generally is agreed that the climbing fibers primarily use glutamate as their neurotransmitter, although they also express other neuroactive chemicals. Because of the large number of excitatory synaptic connections of climbing fibers to their Purkinje cell targets, Purkinje cells respond to climbing fiber activation with a large and prolonged, all-or-nothing, excitatory discharge.

26. Which neurotransmitters are used by the mossy fiber inputs to the cerebellum?

The mossy fiber inputs are extremely varied in their chemical nature. While glutamate is the principal transmitter of fast, excitatory neurotransmission, afferent fibers in the granule cell layer have been shown to contain several different peptides and acetylcholine.

27. Which neurotransmitters are used by the multilayered inputs to the cerebellum?

The best studied of these systems are the noradrenergic input from the locus ceruleus and the serotonergic input from the raphe and reticular nuclei. It appears that most hypothalamocerebellar fibers utilize histamine as their neurotransmitter. Although it has been suggested that the multilayered inputs also utilize dopamine, glycine, and some peptidergic substances as neurotransmitters, these systems have not been widely investigated and remain more speculative.

Dietrichs E, Haines DE, Roster GK, Roste LS: Hypothalamocerebellar and cerebellohypothalamic projections—Circuits for regulating nonsomatic cerebellar activity? Histol Histopath 9:603–614, 1994.

28. Are these input systems somatotopically mapped?

A rough somatotopic representation is mapped onto the cerebellar cortex by incoming mossy fibers (Fig. 4). Both the anterior and posterior lobes exhibit a somatotopy in which the head is mapped to the dorsal cortex, the hind limbs are mapped to the ventral cortical areas, and the upper limbs lie between. However, careful studies have shown that, as in the cerebral cortices, this is a **fractured mapping** in which adjacent receptive fields are not necessarily topographically contiguous, and multiple representations of a given receptive field exist.

29. Since mossy fiber inputs map with a fractured somatotopy, do the climbing fibers have their own map?

Yes, they do. Axons arising in specific subnuclei of the inferior olivary nucleus terminate as climbing fibers in sagitally oriented zones of varying width. Purkinje cells located in specific zones project their axons to specific, somatotopically organized regions of the deep cerebellar nuclei. Climbing fibers projecting to a Purkinje cell zone also send collateral input to the corresponding deep cerebellar nucleus. The functional relationship between the mossy fiber and climbing fiber mapping patterns currently is unknown.

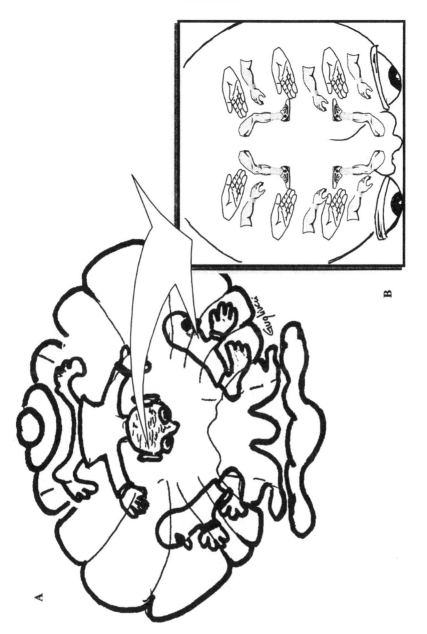

Figure 4. Somatotopy in the cerebellar cortex. **A,** The classic view of cerebellar somatotopic mapping. **B,** The current view, showing a fractured somatotopic map in the anterior lobe.

30. Is there any clear functional mapping in the cerebellar cortex akin to that represented by Brodmann's map of the cerebral cortices?

There is a broad mapping of specific sensory systems in the cerebellar cortex that roughly approximates the designations used clinically. The flocculonodular lobe and most regions of the vermis are concerned with the processing of vestibular information and together closely approximate the vestibulocerebellum. The vermis and intermediate hemispheres from lobules I–IX largely are concerned with the processing of information arising from the spinal cord and are accordingly termed the spinocerebellum. The pontine nuclei, which receive a massive projection from the cerebral cortices, project to all areas of the cerebellar cortex except the flocculus. Classically, the pontocerebellum is defined as the lateral cerebellar hemisphere (most texts continue to use this designation).

31. If the cerebellar cortex has no projections outside of the cerebellum, how is this mapping maintained?

Each of the cortical zones projects its output to a specific deep cerebellar nucleus (Fig. 5). In the coarse mapping noted in Question 30, the vestibulocerebellum maps to the vestibular nuclei and part of the fastigial nucleus, the spinocerebellum maps to the fastigial and interposed nuclei, and the pontocerebellum projects to the dentate nucleus. Thus, the vestibular nuclei of the brainstem act as, and frequently are classed as, deep cerebellar nuclei.

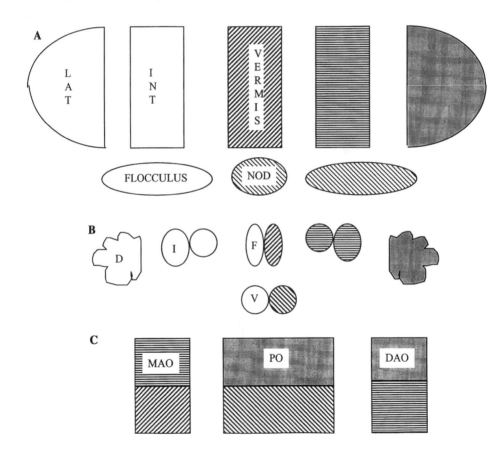

Figure 5. A coarse mapping of the sagittal organization of three major cerebellar zones. **A,** Cerebellar cortical zones are arranged as sagittal strips. **B,** Each sagittal zone projects to a specific region of the deep cerebellar nuclei (DCN), which maintains a reciprocal connection to a specific area of the inferior olivary nucleus (ION). **C,** The ION projects to a specific cerebellar zone and to the DCN connected to that zone. LAT = lateral cerebellar hemispheres, INT = intermediate cerebellar hemispheres, NOD = nodulus, D = dentate nucleus, I = interposed nuclei, F = fastigial nucleus, V = vestibular nuclei, MAO = medial accessory olivary nucleus, PO = principal olivary nucleus, DAO = dorsal accessory olivary nucleus.

32. Are there differences in the basic circuitry of these functional zones?

No, the basic circuitry and the morphology of each cellular element remain the same throughout the cerebellum. Interestingly, there is a growing body of evidence supporting a chemical compartmentalization in the cerebellar cortex. At present, the precise relationship of chemically defined zones to other zonal patterns, such as the sagittal zonation defined by climbing fiber axons, is not well understood. A complete understanding of such compartmental patterns may clarify the functional mapping of information into and out of the cerebellum.

Oberdick J, Baader SL, Schilling K: From zebra stripes to postal zones: Deciphering patterns of gene expression in the cerebellum. Trends Neurosci 21:383–390, 1998.

33. What makes up a cerebellar module or microzone?

Several lines of investigation have indicated that the cerebellum is organized in a series of parallel, longitudinally organized zones of various width. Fundamentally, a microzone or module is defined by the projection of specific subnuclei of the inferior olivary nucleus to one or more longitudinal zones of Purkinje cells, with a collateral projection to the region of the deep cerebellar nuclei to which the Purkinje cell zone projects. These cerebellar modules have a reciprocal linkage to the inferior olivary nucleus via the deep cerebellar target nuclei.

34. What are the internal connections of these modules?

The modules are associated most readily with the deep cerebellar nuclei.

- At their coarsest (see Fig. 5), the modules correspond to projections from the lateral hemispheres (pontocerebellum) to the dentate nucleus, and from the principal and caudal dorsal inferior olivary subnuclei to the pontocerebellum and the dentate nuclei.
- Similarly, the intermediate hemispheres project to the interposed nuclei, while the the the dorsal accessory and dorsal medial accessory subnuclei of the inferior olivary nucleus send input to both the intermediate hemispheres and the interposed nuclei.
- The vermis and fastigial nuclei receive climbing fiber input largely from the medial accessory olive, and the vermal cortex projects to the fastigial nuclei.
- The flocculonodular lobe projects primarily to the vestibular nuclei and receives input from the principal olivary subnucleus.

CONNECTIVITY

35. What are the external connections of the vestibulocerebellum?

- The vestibulocerebellum (Fig. 6) receives mossy fiber input from first- and second-order vestibular afferents that transmit information on the position of the head and body in space. Most primary afferent information (97%) reaches the nodulus.
- In addition, pontocerebellar fibers transmit information concerned with visual function and eye movements to the flocculus.
- Olivocerebellar information is transmitted via climbing fibers and carries both visual and vestibular information.
- Flocculonodular outflow consists of Purkinje cell projections to the ipsilateral vestibular nuclei via the juxtarestiform body. These projections are inhibitory to their target neurons.
- Vermal vestibulocerebellar Purkinje cells make inhibitory synaptic contact on neurons in the fastigial nucleus.
- The fastigial nuclei project bilaterally to the vestibular and reticular nuclei, providing excitatory input. Fastigial efferent fibers also project to the thalamus, hypothalamus, and the inferior olivary nucleus.

36. What is the function of the vestibulocerebellum?

The vestibulocerebellum influences balance and equilibrium through its influence on spinal-projecting vestibular neurons and reticular formation neurons. In addition, the vestibulocerebellum is involved in the modulation of eye motor reflexes via its influences on vestibular nuclei that project to the eye motor nuclei.

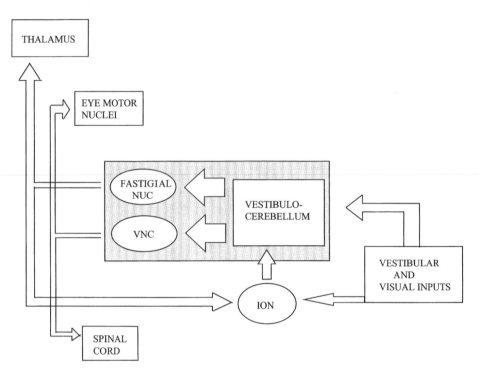

Figure 6.   The major connection patterns of the vestibulocerebellum. NUC = nucleus, VNC = vestibular nuclear complex, ION = inferior olivary nucleus.

37. What dysfunctions result from damage to the vestibulocerebellum?

Damage to the flocculonodular lobe, or to midline cerebellar structures such as the fastigial nucleus, results in an unstable, lurching gait known as **truncal ataxia**. There is a tendency to fall and the head may be tilted to one side. Due to the truncal instability, there may be a widened stance that is carried into the gait pattern. Finally, there frequently is an associated axial tremor (titubation).

38. What are the connections of the spinocerebellum?

- The vermal and intermediate cerebellar cortices receive input largely from the dorsal and ventral spinocerebellar tracts and the cuneocerebellar tract (Fig. 7). These systems provide somatosensory information from the limbs and trunk.
- Additional inputs come from the vestibular system, the contralateral pons, the reticular formation, and the inferior olivary nucleus (ION). The output of the spinocerebellum via the fastigial nucleus is to the vestibular and reticular formation, the thalamus, the ventromedial spinal gray matter, and the ION—with which it makes a reciprocal connection. These efferent pathways are involved in the control of axial musculature.
- Efferent pathways via the interposed nuclei are focused largely on control of limb and musculature. Axons from the interposed nuclei exit the cerebellum via the brachium conjunctivum (SCP) and cross in its decussation to terminate in the magnocellular division of the red nucleus, the ventral lateral thalamic nucleus, the reticular formation, and the ION—with which the axons are reciprocally connected.

39. What are the functions of the spinocerebellum?

The spinocerebellum is involved in the modulation of limb movement and has extensive connections to motor nuclei of the brainstem. Thus, this cerebellar area is involved in the smooth execution of movement.

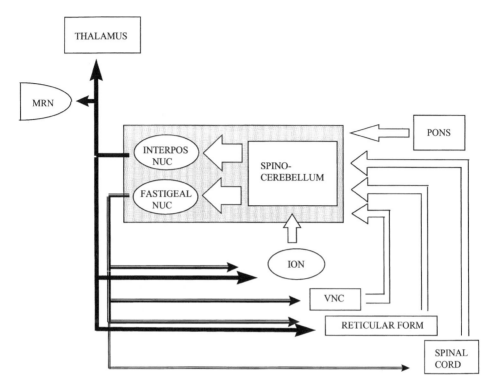

Figure 7.   The major connection patterns of the spinocerebellum. MRN = magnocellular red nucleus, NUC = nucleus, VNC = vestibular nuclear complex.

40. What dysfunctions result from damage to the spinocerebellum?

The spinocerebellum is seldom damaged in isolation, so that the clinical picture tends to be dominated by problems related to damage of either more medial (vestibulocerebellar) or more lateral (pontocerebellar) cortices. The most common clinical picture is that in which spinocerebellar and pontocerebellar structures are both damaged (see Question 43).

41. What are the connections of the pontocerebellum?

- The pontocerebellum is strongly linked to thalamic and cortical structures, receiving its mossy fiber input from the pontine nuclei via the brachium pontis (MCP).
- Climbing fiber input arises in the principal ION and enters the cerebellum via the restiform body (ICP).
- Purkinje cells in the pontocerebellar hemispheres integrate that information with climbing fiber input from the ION and project to the dentate nucleus.
- The dentate projects to the thalamus, which maintains reciprocal connections to the neocortex.
- Both the dentate nucleus and the cerebral cortex provide input to the parvocellular red nucleus, which projects to the principal ION.

In addition to its function in the modulation and control of movement, this loop has been suggested to underlie the cognitive function of the cerebellum.

42. What are the functions of the pontocerebellum?

The pontocerebellum has been hypothesized to represent the circuit that underlies cognitive functions of the cerebellum. These functions include visuospatial processing, sensory discrimination, linguistic processing, attention shifting, and the modulation of emotional state. In addition,

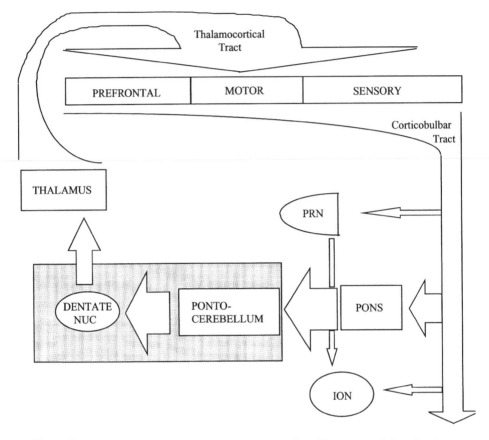

Figure 8.   The major connection patterns of the pontocerebellum. PRN = parvocellular red nucleus.

the pontocerebellar circuitry is likely to play an important role in motor learning. This area is classi-cally defined as the region subserving the planning and execution of multi-joint movement.

Schmahmann JD: The Cerebellum and Cognition. San Diego, Academic Press, 1997.

43. What dysfunctions result from damage to the pontocerebellum?

In general, lesions of the lateral hemispheres result in incoordinated movement. Because the cerebellum has no direct projections to the spinal cord but influences movement via its influence on corticospinal and rubrospinal pathways, the effects are seen ipsilateral to the side of damage. In ad-dition, damage only to the cerebellar cortex rarely results in a permanent motor deficit. Uncoordinated or decomposed movement leads to several well-described signs, including ataxia of gait, dysmetria, intention tremor, and dysdiadochokinesia.

44. What is the source of the multilayered projection fibers in the cerebellum?

The multilayered fibers come from many different brain regions. These include serotonergic fibers from the reticular formation and the raphe, noradrenergic fibers from the locus coeruleus, his-taminergic fibers from the hypothalamus, and dopaminergic fibers from the ventral tegmental area.

45. What are the connections between the hypothalamus and cerebellum?

The lateral, dorsal, and posterior hypothalamic areas are the principal regions that project di-rectly to the cerebellum. Hypothalamic neurons send a diffuse projection through the periventricular gray matter to all three layers of the vermis and flocculonodular lobe. Hypothalamic neurons also send projections to the deep cerebellar nuclei. There are projections from the deep cerebellar nuclei to the hypothalamus as well, although it currently appears that only a small number of these make reciprocal connections with cerebellar-projecting hypothalamic neurons.

Dietrichs E, Haines DE, Roster GK, Roste LS: Hypothalamocerebellar and cerebellohypothalamic projections—Circuits for regulating nonsomatic cerebellar activity? Histol Histopath 9:603–614, 1994.

46. What is the functional role of the hypothalamocerebellar system?

It has been known for some time that stimulation of the deep cerebellar nuclei or adjacent white matter could produce changes in autonomic function. However, until recently this finding inspired little experimental interest. Studies have begun to examine the role of the cerebellum in vasomotor regulation, pupillary responses, and even endocrine regulation. Clinically, such effects generally are overshadowed by the classical somatomotor deficits, which are more readily observable. The cerebellum may, however, coordinate visceral, motor, sensory, and even emotional inputs so as to aid in the evocation of appropriate responses to environmental stimuli. Hypothalamocerebellar projection systems may play a role in that function.

Dietrichs E, Haines DE, Roster GK, Roste LS: Hypothalamocerebellar and cerebellohypothalamic projections—Circuits for regulating nonsomatic cerebellar activity? Histol Histopath 9:603–614, 1994.

Reis DJ, Golanov EV: Autonomic and vasomotor regulation. In Schmahmann JD (ed): The Cerebellum and Cognition. San Diego, Academic Press, 1997, pp 121–149.

CLINICAL FEATURES

47. What are the most common clinical features associated with cerebellar dysfunction?

Cerebellar lesions lead to disturbances in gait and posture and an incoordination of both simple and compound movement, but do not generally prevent the execution of movement. The classic features include ataxia, dysmetria, dysdiadochokinesia, and tremor that is associated either with stance or movement. Dysarthria often is a clinical feature of cerebellar damage, as are oculomotor disturbances. Hypotonia is notable, at least in early stages of cerebellar disease.

48. Is ataxia a feature exclusive to cerebellar dysfunction?

No, ataxia is an umbrella term descriptive of a condition in which there is a reduction in or a lack of normal speed and skill in the smooth coordination of multiple muscle groups. Ataxias can result from immune dysfunction, infection, mass lesions or systemic disorders. In addition, a large number of hereditary ataxias have been identified.

49. How can cerebellar ataxia be differentiated from noncerebellar ataxias?

Sensory ataxias can be difficult to distinguish from cerebellar ataxias, as gait disturbances may be very similar. However, sensory ataxias, unlike the cerebellar variety, are accompanied by a positive Romberg sign (patient cannot maintain posture when eyes are closed), a lack of oculomotor signs, no dysarthria, and an increase in ataxic movement with loss of visual input. Cerebellar ataxia seldom is accompanied by complaints of vertigo.

50. What type of tremor is associated with cerebellar dysfunction?

Cerebellar tremor often is described as "intention tremor," a term that is falling from favor. In fact, both **kinetic** and **static** tremor are associated with cerebellar dysfunction, although kinetic tremor is the classically defined cerebellar tremor.

51. What characterizes cerebellar kinetic tremor?

Tremor is an involuntary, rhythmic, oscillatory movement. Kinetic tremor occurs in conjunction with active movement, and it can be task specific. With lateral cerebellar dysfunction, kinetic tremor of a specific type—terminal tremor—commonly is noted. This means that the tremor occurs at the end of a movement rather than at its initiation or throughout its execution.

52. What type of static tremor is seen with cerebellar dysfunction?

The static tremor characteristic of cerebellar dysfunction is known as **titubation**. It is character-ized by an anteroposterior rhythmic tremor of the head or trunk or both.

53. What are the oculomotor disturbances associated with cerebellar damage?

Damage to vermal cortex and/or the fastigial nuclei, the flocculus, and/or the nodulus can lead to a number of abnormalities in eye movement. These include: saccadic dysmetria leading to deficits in pursuit eye movements, several types of nystagmus, post saccadic drift, and a difficulty in adjust-ing the gain of the vestibulo-ocular reflex.

54. Is there a seminal clinical feature of cerebellar dysfunction?

If there is a seminal problem with cerebellar injury, it might be dysmetria, in which movement either falls short of (hypometria) or exceeds (hypermetria) its target. This fundamental abnormality can be seen to underlie dysdiadochokinesia, in which the sequencing of rhythmic alternating movements is lost due to the inability to adequately terminate each phase of the movement. It also leads to the char-acteristic "check and rebound" phenomenon in which return to position after passive displacement is abnormal. In addition, it could clearly underlie ataxia of gait and dysarthria. Dysmetria could even go some way to explaining kinetic tremor. However, though it may explain many of the overt signs of cerebellar injury, it does not explain them all, and a truly seminal cause awaits further research.

55. Are there any cognitive deficits seen with cerebellar damage?

Yes, although these deficits are not as obvious to the observer as are the motor deficits. Many authors have reported that cerebellar atrophy or agenesis is associated with mental retardation or re-duced intellect; however, these reports tended to be clinical case studies. Recently, functional neuro-imaging studies have served to focus attention on cognitive functions of the cerebellum, showing that the cerebellum is involved in attention, working memory, visuospatial information processing, and verbal learning and memory. The cerebellum also has been hypothesized to play a major role in the expression of infantile autism and may thus have a role in attention.

Courchesne E, Yeung-Courchesne R, Press GTA, et al: Hypoplasia of cerebellar lobules VI and VII in infan-tile autism. N Engl J Med 318:1349–1354, 1988.

Schmahmann JD: The Cerebellum and Cognition. San Diego, Academic Press, 1997.

56. What types of hereditary disorders primarily affect the cerebellum?

This includes a group of inherited neurodegenerative disorders, known as the hereditary ataxias, that are characterized by progressive ataxia. These disorders can be classified as autosomal domi-nant, autosomal recessive, or genetic mutations.

57. What are the most common autosomal dominant disorders?

Autosomal dominant ataxias are generally triplet repeat disorders caused by the inheritance of an unstable, expanded CAG trinucleotide repeat. They are known collectively as spinocerebellar ataxias (SCA), and there are now several known types which are designated by number: SCA1, SCA2, SCA3, and SCA7. A second group of autosomal dominant disorders includes SCA6 and two episodic ataxias (EA-1 and EA-2) that affect genes encoding for ion channels. SCA6 is also a trinu-cleotide repeat disorder, EA-1 is a missense mutation, and EA-2 is a splice mutation.

58. What are the clinical features of the SCA mutations?

Of the SCA mutations, the most common form is SCA1. This is a progressive ataxia with an age of onset between 20 and 40 years. The most prominent sign is gait ataxia, often accompanied by sudden falls. Hyperreflexia often is present initially, but as the disease progresses tendon reflexes generally are reduced, and there may be proprioceptive loss. Nystagmus and ophthalmoparesis are common early signs; there also may be muscle wasting distally, facial fasciculations, and dementia. Severity tends to be inversely related to age of onset, but most patients are wheelchair-bound within 20 years of disease onset.

59. What are the most common autosomal recessive disorders?

The most common type of autosomal recessive ataxia is **Friedreich's ataxia** (frequency of 1–2/100,000). This is an early-onset disorder in which pathologic changes include loss of dorsal root ganglia neurons and degeneration of the spinocerebellar, dorsal column, and pyramidal tracts. This disorder is due to expansion of a GAA repeat in a novel gene *(X25)* on human chromosome 9. **Ataxia telangiectasia** is another autosomal recessive disorder that occurs in childhood (frequency 1/40,000–1/100,000 live births). It results from defective DNA repair and has been localized to chromosome 11.

60. What are the clinical features of Friedreich's ataxia?

Essential clinical features include early onset, usually between 8 and 15 years of age; a progressive ataxia of gait; and absent tendon reflexes and extensor plantar responses. Other neurologic features include dysarthria, clumsiness, abnormal eye movements, and proprioceptive loss in the limbs. Non-neurologic symptoms commonly include skeletal abnormalities such as scoliosis or kyphosis (seen in over 75% of patients), heart disease (seen in about 75% of patients), and diabetes mellitus (seen in 10–20% of patients). The disease course is progressive and, although variable, generally results in an inability to walk 15 years after the age of onset. Death often occurs from infection or cardiac disease when patients are in their 40s or 50s.

61. Are vascular lesions common in the cerebellum?

Vascular lesions are far less common in vessels supplying the cerebellar cortex than in those supplying the cerebral cortex. Due to heavy collateralization, large infarcts are uncommon, and smaller infarcts usually are not clinically apparent. However, branches of the superior cerebellar artery are vulnerable to vascular hypertension. They are of a caliber similar to the lenticulostriate arteries and are the most common source of intracerebellar hematomas.

The typical syndrome usually has an abrupt onset accompanied by vomiting and severe ataxia (sufficient to prevent standing and walking). There is no change in the level of consciousness and no loss of sensation. There is a small margin of time between alertness and coma as the mass enlarges to encompass brainstem structures; therefore, *immediate* surgical intervention is required.

62. Are there specific tumor types associated with cerebellar signs?

Tumors affecting the cerebellum rarely are limited to any single area and usually involve adjacent brain areas by compression or displacement. Cerebellar tumors may be quite extensive by the time that cerebellar signs and symptoms appear. The most common cerebellar tumors include astrocytoma, medulloblastoma, metastatic tumors, ependymoma, and acoustic neuroma (which actually originates outside of the cerebellum).

63. Is acoustic neuroma intrinsic to the cerebellum?

No, but it is a relatively common (accounting for 5–10% of all intracranial tumors) benign tumor that results in the production of many cerebellar signs. Acoustic neuromas usually are derived from Schwann cells of the vestibular portion of cranial nerve VIII. As the tumor grows, it expands through the internal auditory meatus and into the cerebellopontine angle, where it displaces the pons, cerebellum, and cranial nerves VII and VIII. Most acoustic neuromas grow slowly (2–10 mm/year), and they may be quite large and cystic before they become symptomatic.

64. What is posterior fossa syndrome?

In children, medulloblastomas develop preferentially in the vermis and flocculonodular lobes. In about 15% of children who undergo surgical resection of large vermian tumors, mutism develops postoperatively. Transient mutism and neurobehavioral deficits such as eating dysfunction, emotional lability, and impaired eye opening constitute the posterior fossa syndrome. These deficits usually resolve over a few weeks or months. The interconnectivity of cerebellum and higher cortical centers may provide the substrate for this wide range of seemingly disparate clinical signs.

CURRENT CONCEPTS OF CEREBELLAR FUNCTION

65. Does the cerebellum play any role in learning?

Yes, the cerebellum is believed to play a major role in motor learning and in the adaptive control of motor reflexes. At the present time this is an area of intense investigation, because such a role implies that the cerebellum is important in motor memory formation, storage, and/or retrieval.

66. What is meant by motor learning?

In general, this term can be construed to refer to the establishment of a permanent change in a motor process with practice. However, there is disagreement over the precise form of motor learning influenced by the cerebellum. It has been proposed that the cerebellum is involved in associative learning, in the improved performance of skilled movement with practice (adaptive learning), and in the acquisition of novel movement patterns with practice (skill learning). However, others note that there is ample reason to differentiate between adaptation or scaling of movement and the acquisition of new skilled movement patterns. These investigators argue that the cerebellum is involved only in adaptive learning, in which learned movement parameters are fine tuned.

Cordo PJ, Bell CC, Harnard S: Motor Learning and Synaptic Plasticity in the Cerebellum. Cambridge, Cambridge University Press, 1997.

67. Are there other types of learning in which the cerebellum is thought to play a role?

Yes. In classical conditioning studies, the cerebellum has been shown to be involved in "learning" a new, adaptive motor output in response to an imposed perturbation of the original reflex. The two systems for which the most data currently exists are those involving changes in the gain of the vestibulo-ocular reflex and in the conditioning of reflex responses to noxious stimuli.

68. What evidence is there that the cerebellum is involved in learning of skilled movements?

Many studies have pointed to an important role for the cerebellum in skilled volitional movement. One paradigm is a hand-eye coordination task in which human subjects are asked to throw a dart at a target. This is a skilled movement, and practice is required to accurately hit the target. After the skill is learned, subjects put on prism glasses that shift the visual path so that target position is perceptually shifted. With practice, the subjects correct for the distortion in target position and once again reliably hit the target. Subjects with cerebellar damage do not learn to adjust for the prism-mediated shift in target position.

Functional imaging studies also have confirmed the activation of the cerebellum with motor learning. Note, however, that it is not activated in isolation: other motor centers also are active.

69. What are the cellular substrates for cerebellar learning?

Because the Purkinje cell is the output neuron of the cerebellar cortex, the first investigations of cellular events that may underlie associative learning in the cerebellum focused on changes in Purkinje cell output. These investigations found that paired presentations of climbing and parallel fiber inputs to a Purkinje cell resulted in a long-term reduction in Purkinje cell responses, termed **long-term depression**. We now known that **long-term potentiation** of Purkinje cell responses also can be evoked. Having established that it is possible for the Purkinje cell to "learn" new responses to its synaptic inputs, current investigations have broadened their focus to include long-lasting changes in the response of granule cells to both excitatory and inhibitory inputs.

70. So what, exactly, does the cerebellum do?

This is the 64-dollar-question, and the answer is: we don't know. This question centers not on the overt behaviors in which the cerebellum plays an important role, but on the precise information set that cerebellar activity transmits to other brain centers. What is the output signal of the cerebellum? Many interesting hypotheses have been presented in the literature; let's look at a few of them.

71. Is the cerebellum fundamentally a sensory processor?

One of the newest theories of cerebellar function posits that it monitors and adjusts the sensory information received by the central nervous system and provides brain effector systems with information that enables them to do their job more efficiently. This theory suggests that the cerebellum is not necessary for normal brain function, but that it does make normal brain function smoother and more efficient. The theory is entirely consistent with the known inputs to the cerebellum, which include processed sensory information received both as mossy fibers and from a second sensory processing center, the inferior olivary nucleus.

Bower J: Is the cerebellum sensory for motor's sake, or motor for sensory's sake: The view from the whiskers of a rat? Prog Brain Res 114:463–496, 1997.

72. Or, does the cerebellum serve to link context to appropriate response patterns?

Recently Thach has suggested that the cerebellum acts to link a complex movement or response strategy to a specific context. This linkage is important not only for performed movements, but also for mental rehearsal of movement. In mental movement, cerebellar connections to prefrontal cortices are involved in the planning of a movement sequence that need never actually be performed. This theory posits that the apparent role of the cerebellum in cognitive processing comes from errors in movement-associated mentation.

Cordo PJ, Bell CC, Harnard S: Motor Learning and Synaptic Plasticity in the Cerebellum. Cambridge, Cambridge University Press, 1997.

Schmahmann JD: The Cerebellum and Cognition. San Diego, Academic Press, 1997.

73. Or, does the cerebellum provide a timing signal that allows appropriate temporal patterning?

This theory proposes that the cerebellum provides a timing signal that can be used by both motor and nonmotor centers to appropriately sequence their outputs. Recall that a principal deficit noted with cerebellar dysfunction is incoordination of movement. Ivry theorizes that the cerebellum is responsible for establishing the temporal patterning of muscular activation, rather than producing a motor template of the anticipated or controlled movement pattern. This computational function also arises in nonmotor tasks, such as perception and learning, and thus could generalize to cognitive domains while maintaining a fundamental role in motor control.

Schmahmann JD: The Cerebellum and Cognition. San Diego, Academic Press, 1997.

74. Perhaps the cerebellum is not sensory, motor, or cognitive?

Ito has proposed that the cerebellum is a regulator of neural function that acts as an error-driven adaptive control system independent of the specific executive function that it is modulating. In this theory, the cerebellum is suggested to provide an internal model of the dynamic properties of the system to be controlled, whether motor, sensory, or cognitive. In concert with neocortical feedforward control of the overt behavior, cerebellar microcomplexes subserving the stored model receive an error signal that allows recalibration of the model for transmission to those cortical areas. In this manner, new behavioral patterns are learned or fine tuned regardless of their modality.

Schmahmann JD: The Cerebellum and Cognition. San Diego, Academic Press, 1997.

75. Is there any consensus of opinion?

If any consensus can be found, it is in the idea that cerebellar output is both plastic and multimodal. Although some authors contend that the cerebellum remains exclusively a motor control structure, most are willing to acknowledge a broadened definition of its essential function. It certainly could be argued that complex behaviors require the integration of sensory, motor, autonomic and even "cognitive" functions so that, by virtue of its involvement in complex behaviors such as learning and movement, the cerebellum defies categorization. That said, it should be kept in mind that cerebellar damage does result in a degradation of motor performance. Whatever the output signal of the cerebellum, its involvement in motor learning and motor performance is unequivocal.

ACKNOWLEDGMENT

The author gratefully acknowledges the artwork of Dr. A. Gugliucci and the thoughtful comments of Dr. N. Barmack.

BIBLIOGRAPHY

1. Bower J: Is the cerebellum sensory for motor's sake, or motor for sensory's sake: The view from the whiskers of a rat? Prog Brain Res 114:463–496, 1997.
2. Cordo PJ, Bell CC, Harnard S: Motor Learning and Synaptic Plasticity in the Cerebellum. Cambridge, Cambridge University Press, 1997.
3. Courchesne E, Yeung-Courchesne R, Press GTA, et al: Hypoplasia of cerebellar lobules VI and VII in infantile autism. N Engl J Med 318:1349–1354, 1988.
4. Dietrichs E, Haines DE, Roster GK, Roste LS: Hypothalamocerebellar and cerebellohypothalamic projections—Circuits for regulating nonsomatic cerebellar activity? Histol Histopath 9:603–614, 1994.
5. Dieudonne S: Glycinergic synaptic currents in Golgi cells of the rat cerebellum. Proc Natl Acad Sci 92: 1441–1445, 1995.
6. Duus P: Topical Diagnosis in Neurology. Stuttgart, Thieme Medical Publishers, 1998.
7. Haines DE: Fundamental Neuroscience. New York, Churchill Livingstone, 1997.
8. Ito M: The Cerebellum and Neural Control. New York, Raven Press, 1984.
9. Oberdick J, Baader SL, Schilling K: From zebra stripes to postal zones: Deciphering patterns of gene expression in the cerebellum. Trends Neurosci 21:383–390, 1998.
10. Ottersen OP: Neurotransmitters in the cerebellum. Rev Neurol (Paris) 149:629–636, 1993.
11. Otterson OP, Storm-Mathisen J, Somogyi P: Colocalization of glycine-like immunoreactivities in Golgi cell terminals in the rat cerebellum: A postembedding light and electron microscopy study. Brain Res 450:342–353, 1988.
12. Reis DJ, Golanov EV: Autonomic and vasomotor regulation. In Schmahmann JD (ed): The Cerebellum and Cognition. San Diego, Academic Press, 1997, pp 121–149.
13. Schmahmann JD: The Cerebellum and Cognition. San Diego, Academic Press, 1997.

15. THE AUTONOMIC NERVOUS SYSTEM

Linda Rinaman, Ph.D.

OVERVIEW

1. What does the autonomic nervous system (ANS) do?

Working in concert with the endocrine system, the ANS is the fast, neural part of the functional system that is responsible for maintaining physiologic homeostasis (a steady internal environment) in the face of constantly changing external conditions. The ANS controls the contractile activity of cardiac muscle (heart) and visceral smooth muscle (e.g., blood vessels, intestinal wall, piloerectors). The ANS also controls secretion from exocrine glands (e.g., salivary, sweat, and tear glands) and from the endocrine pancreas (islet cells).

2. Why is it called "autonomic"?

Autonomy refers to independence and self-regulation, two unique hallmarks of the ANS. Under normal conditions, physiologic homeostasis is maintained autonomously through ongoing, coordinated actions of the ANS and endocrine system, placing vital body functions beyond the reach of conscious control. (Imagine how distracting and exhausting it would be if your attention was required to initiate appropriate adjustments of cardiovascular, gastrointestinal, and reproductive tissues!)

3. What cells make up the ANS?

Strictly speaking, the ANS is a motor system that comprises two large groups of cells:
1. neurons lying wholly within the periphery (postganglionic autonomic neurons)
2. neurons in the brainstem and spinal cord that directly innervate cells in the first group (preganglionic autonomic neurons).

However, a functionally inclusive view of the ANS also acknowledges the vitally important roles of spinal and cranial sensory pathways and central integrating mechanisms in controlling ANS motor output and, hence, visceral autonomic function.

4. Why do some textbooks state that the ANS has two divisions, while others refer to three?

Classically, the ANS is considered to have two divisions: the sympathetic and the parasympathetic. However, it is appropriate to consider the enteric nervous system as the third division of the ANS because it does not fit simply into either the sympathetic or the parasympathetic classification. The enteric division comprises a highly complex and functionally integrated network of neurons located in intramural plexuses in the wall of the gastrointestinal tract and associated organs (pancreas, liver, gallbladder). Sympathetic and parasympathetic fibers terminate on subsets of enteric neurons, but the enteric system also can perform numerous sensory-motor integrative functions independent of extrinsic neural input.

5. Which body organs are innervated by the ANS?

All of them. Many visceral targets are innervated by both sympathetic and parasympathetic fibers, but some are innervated only by the sympathetic nervous system (i.e., adrenal medulla, sweat glands, piloerectors, spleen, white and brown adipose tissue, most blood vessels). The gastrointestinal tract (from the distal esophagus to the distal colon), pancreas, liver, and gallbladder are innervated by sympathetic, parasympathetic, and enteric divisions.

STRUCTURE AND DEVELOPMENT

6. How does the ANS differ from the somatic motor system?
- Most skeletal muscle movements initiated by the somatic motor system are under voluntary control and are accessible to conscious perception, whereas most autonomic adjustments of visceral targets are not.

- Somatic motor neurons in the CNS have direct (monosynaptic) axonal projections to skeletal muscle. In contrast, a synapse in a peripheral autonomic ganglion is interposed between autonomic motor neurons in the CNS and their visceral target (Fig. 1).
- Somatic motor neurons exert exclusively excitatory (depolarizing) effects on skeletal muscle targets. Conversely, visceral target cells can receive both excitatory and inhibitory synaptic input from autonomic neurons.

A Somatic motor system

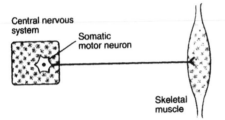

Figure 1. **A,** Organization of the somatic motor system. **B,** Organization of the autonomic motor system. (From Dodd J, Role LW: The autonomic nervous system. In Kandel ER, Schwartz JH, Jessell TM (eds): Principles of Neural Science, 3rd ed. Norwalk, Appleton & Lange, 1991, pp 761–775; with permission.)

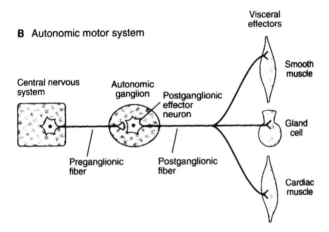

7. What anatomically descriptive terms often are used in referring to the sympathetic and parasympathetic divisions of the ANS?

The **thoracolumbar division** (sympathetic) and the **craniosacral division** (parasympathetic). These terms derive from the anatomic location of preganglionic neurons in the CNS:
- The spinal ventral roots from T1 to L2–3 contain sympathetic preganglionic fibers that arise from neurons in the thoracolumbar spinal cord.
- Parasympathetic preganglionic fibers are found in cranial nerves III, VII, IX, and X in spinal ventral roots S2–S4; these fibers arise from neurons in the associated brainstem nuclei and sacral spinal cord, respectively (Fig. 2).

8. The sympathetic and parasympathetic divisions differ in the general relationship between pre- and postganglionic neurons. Describe this difference.

Characteristically, the axons of parasympathetic preganglionic neurons are considerably longer than those of parasympathetic postganglionic neurons. The converse is true of the sympathetic system. Thus, parasympathetic preganglionic neurons within the brainstem and spinal cord project to postganglionic neurons in ganglia that are close to visceral targets or are actually embedded in

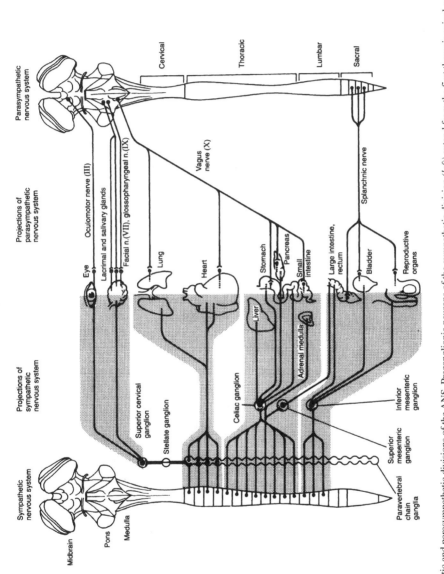

Figure 2.   Sympathetic and parasympathetic divisions of the ANS. Preganglionic neurons of the sympathetic division (*left*) extend from the first thoracic spinal segment to lower lumbar segments. Parasympathetic preganglionic neurons (*right*) are located within the brainstem and in segments S2–S4 of the spinal cord. (From Dodd J, Role LW: The autonomic nervous system. In Kandel ER, Schwartz JH, Jessell TM (eds): Principles of Neural Science, 3rd ed. Norwalk, Appleton & Lange, 1991, pp 761–775; with permission.)

them. In contrast, sympathetic postganglionic neurons, located in para- or prevertebral ganglia, are relatively distant from their targets (Fig. 3).

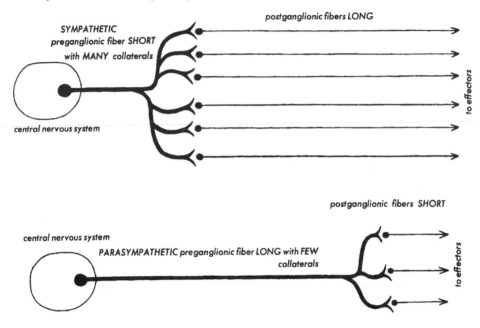

Figure 3. Comparison of the basic arrangements of sympathetic *(top)* and parasympathetic *(bottom)* motor neurons. (From Pick J: The Autonomic Nervous System. Philadelphia, J.B. Lippincott Co., 1970; with permission.)

9. What neurotransmitters are released by pre- and postganglionic sympathetic and parasympathetic neurons? Note any exceptions.

Both sympathetic and parasympathetic preganglionic neurons release acetylcholine (ACh) from their axon terminals in autonomic ganglia. Parasympathetic postganglionic neurons also release ACh from their axon terminals at visceral target tissue, whereas sympathetic postganglionic neurons release norepinephrine (NE). Thus, most visceral targets receive parasympathetic cholinergic innervation and sympathetic noradrenergic innervation.

Exceptions: Sympathetic postganglionic neurons that innervate sweat glands (sudomotor neurons) use ACh as their neurotransmitter, as do certain sympathetic postganglionic vasodilator fibers in skeletal muscle.

10. How do neuroanatomic and chemical differences between the sympathetic and parasympathetic divisions impact their functions?

The sympathetic system is set up to affect many visceral systems simultaneously. Each sympathetic preganglionic fiber synapses with many postganglionic neurons that often are distributed among several paravertebral ganglia. Such divergence permits coordinated activation of sympathetic neurons at several spinal levels. Activation of sympathetic input to the adrenal gland leads to increased circulating levels of epinephrine, which acts on sympathetic targets throughout the body (see Question 25). In addition, some NE released from postganglionic sympathetic nerve terminals at visceral targets escapes reuptake and enters the circulation to ultimately affect more distant targets throughout the body.

Conversely, the parasympathetic system is designed more for precise control of specific visceral targets, and the effects of ACh (released by parasympathetic postganglionic neurons) usually are limited to the site of release.

11. Describe the composition, origin, and destination of splanchnic nerves.

In general, splanchnic nerves contain the axons of preganglionic sympathetic neurons en route to postsynaptic targets in abdominal prevertebral (preaortic) sympathetic ganglia (i.e., the coeliac, aorticorenal, superior mesenteric, and inferior mesenteric ganglia). Preganglionic sympathetic fibers destined for splanchnic nerves traverse the paravertebral ganglia (sympathetic chain) without synapsing. Some of the preganglionic fibers running with the thoracic splanchnic nerve do not synapse in prevertebral ganglia, but instead directly innervate cells in the adrenal medulla. Splanchnic nerves also contain many sensory fibers carrying interoceptive (inner sensory) information from the viscera to the spinal cord (Fig. 4).

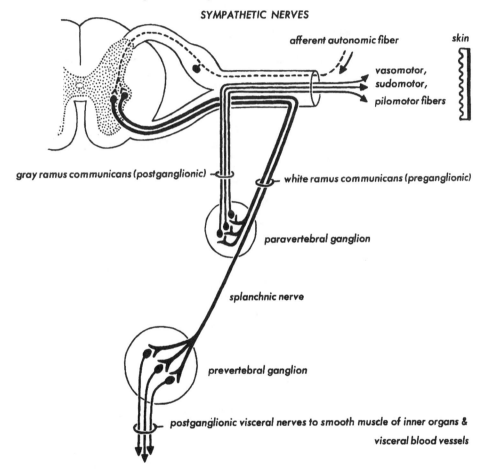

SYMPATHETIC NERVES

Figure 4. Sympathetic outflow from the thoracolumbar spinal cord and the course and distribution of sympathetic fibers, including preganglionic (thick lines) and postganglionic (thin lines) fibers. (From Pick J: The Autonomic Nervous System. Philadelphia, J.B. Lippincott Co., 1970; with permission.)

12. What are white and gray rami?

The rami contain pre- and postganglionic sympathetic nerve fibers entering and leaving the paravertebral sympathetic chain ganglia; the chain ganglia are physically attached to the ventral roots of the thoracic and lumbar segments by these sympathetic fibers. **White rami communicantes** contain mostly myelinated (whitish-looking) preganglionic sympathetic fibers arising from neurons in the intermediolateral (IML) cell column of the thoracolumbar spinal cord. These sympathetic fibers leave the ventral horn, pass through the ventral roots, and then enter the chain ganglia. **Gray rami communicantes** contain mostly unmyelinated (grayish-looking) postganglionic fibers arising from sympathetic chain ganglia neurons, en route to visceral targets.

13. What visceral target structures are innervated by neurons in the prevertebral sympathetic ganglia?

Postganglionic sympathetic neurons in the coeliac and superior mesenteric ganglia innervate the foregut, midgut, and derivatives (e.g., stomach, small intestine, pancreas, liver). Neurons in the aorticorenal ganglion innervate the kidney. Neurons in the inferior mesenteric ganglion innervate the hindgut (colon, rectum), bladder, pelvic organs, and external genitalia.

14. Describe the visceral topography that is evident in the organization of target structures innervated by postganglionic sympathetic chain (paravertebral ganglia) neurons.

Postganglionic sympathetic neurons in the cervical and upper thoracic sympathetic chain ganglia innervate vascular and pilomotor smooth muscle, visceral organs, and glands of the head and neck, as well as visceral organs in the chest. Postganglionic sympathetic neurons in the lower thoracic and lumbar paravertebral ganglia innervate vascular and pilomotor smooth muscle and sweat glands of the limbs and body wall.

15. Summarize the pre- and postganglionic organization of the "cranio" part of the parasympathetic division of the ANS.

See Figure 5.

16. Describe the parasympathetic innervation of the colon and pelvic viscera.

Preganglionic neurons occupy an intermediolateral position in the sacral spinal cord (but not a distinct IML column). Their axons leave through the S2–S4 ventral roots and run with the pelvic splanchnic nerve to reach postganglionic neurons in the pelvic ganglion plexus. Pelvic postganglionic neurons innervate the bladder, descending colon, rectum, reproductive organs, and external genitalia (Fig. 6).

17. Which visceral targets are innervated by the enteric division of the ANS?

The enteric nervous system lies within and innervates the gastrointestinal tract (distal esophagus to rectum), pancreas, and gallbladder. Neurons of the enteric nervous system are arranged in complex interconnected meshworks of ganglia and interconnecting nerve fibers situated between the various layers of muscle and endothelium. The two major intrinsic plexuses are the **myenteric plexus** (Auerbach's plexus) and the **submucosal plexus** (Meissner's plexus). The myenteric plexus lies between the external longitudinal and circular smooth muscle layers. Sympathetic and parasympathetic inputs to the enteric division terminate primarily or exclusively in the myenteric plexus. The submucosal plexus lies within the connective tissue between the circular muscle and the mucosa. The myenteric and submucosal plexuses are richly interconnected through direct and polysynaptic neural circuits, as are enteric neurons in widely-spaced regions of the gastrointestinal system (e.g., stomach and distal colon) (Fig. 7).

18. Are all enteric neurons autonomic motor neurons?

No. The enteric division is composed of local sensory neurons that register alterations in the tension of the gut walls and the chemical environment, as well as interneurons and motor neurons that control the muscles of the gut wall and vasculature and the secretory activity of endocrine and exocrine glands. It has been estimated that the enteric division contains as many intrinsic neurons as are found within the entire spinal cord.

19. What neurotransmitters are used in the enteric division of the ANS?

The enteric division of the ANS is quite complex in its neurochemical coding. Many enteric neurons are cholinergic, but many are nonadrenergic and noncholinergic (NANC neurons). NANC enteric neurons release a wide variety of neurochemical substances, including serotonin, nitric oxide, vasoactive intestinal polypeptide, and substance P.

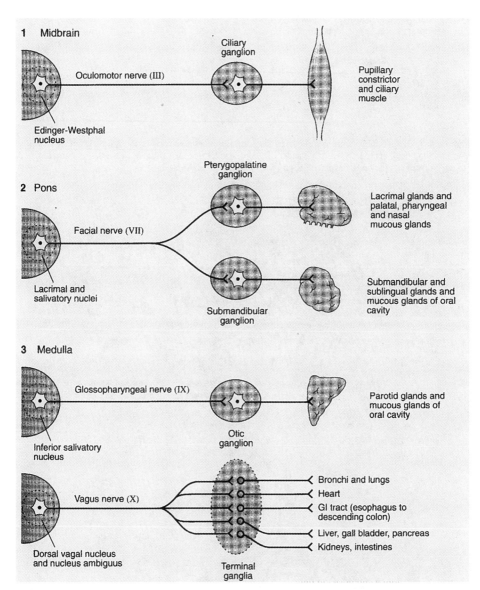

Figure 5. Organization of the cranial part of the parasympathetic division of the ANS, originating from neurons in the midbrain, pons, and medulla. (From Dodd J, Role LW: The autonomic nervous system. In Kandel ER, Schwartz JH, Jessell TM (eds): Principles of Neural Science, 3rd ed. Norwalk, Appleton & Lange, 1991, pp 761–775; with permission.)

20. Does the enteric system receive preganglionic input from neurons in the central nervous system? Why is this significant?

Yes. The enteric system receives parasympathetic innervation from preganglionic neurons in the dorsal motor nucleus of the vagus (via cranial nerve X) and sacral spinal cord (via the pelvic splanchnic nerve). The enteric division also receives input from a subpopulation of postganglionic sympathetic neurons in the coeliac and mesenteric ganglia, which synapse on enteric neurons rather than directly on visceral target tissue.

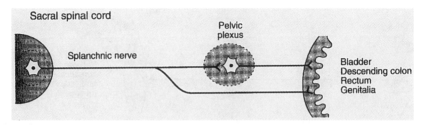

Figure 6. Organization of the sacral part of the parasympathetic division of the ANS. (From Dodd J, Role LW: The autonomic nervous system. In Kandel ER, Schwartz JH, Jessell TM (eds): Principles of Neural Science, 3rd ed. Norwalk, Appleton & Lange, 1991, pp 761–775; with permission.)

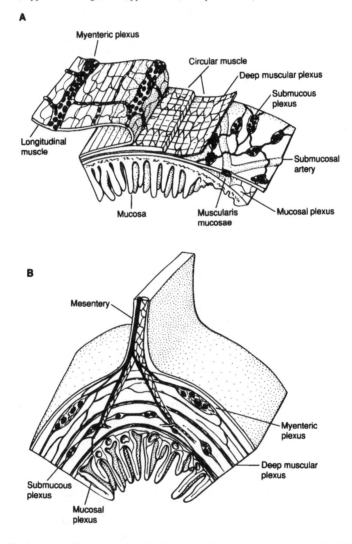

Figure 7. The locations of the myenteric and submucosal plexuses. **A,** A three-dimensional view. **B,** In cross section. (From Dodd J, Role LW: The autonomic nervous system. In Kandel ER, Schwartz JH, Jessell TM (eds): Principles of Neural Science, 3rd ed. Norwalk, Appleton & Lange, 1991, pp 761–775; with permission.)

Although the intrinsic sensory-motor circuits of the enteric nervous system endow it with significant autonomous function, enteric activity normally is precisely regulated by the parasympathetic and, to a lesser extent, the sympathetic divisions. This allows additional CNS control of motility and secretion under normal conditions. For example, anticipation of an expected meal prepares the digestive system for the imminent arrival of food through activation of parasympathetic pathways. This has been called the psychogenic or "cephalic phase" of the digestive response (think of Pavlov's dogs, salivating and secreting gastric acid on cue). The CNS also acts through the sympathetic division to essentially shut down the enteric system in situations of emergency or stress.

21. Describe the developmental origins of sympathetic, parasympathetic, and enteric neurons.
    Preganglionic autonomic neurons in the brainstem and spinal cord derive from the basal (ventral motor) plate, similar to somatic motor neurons. Peripheral autonomic neurons and associated glia derive from cells that migrate out of the neural crest, similar to spinal sensory ganglia neurons.
    Sympathetic: Peripheral sympathetic neurons migrate from the midtrunk level of the spinal neural crest to initially form primitive groupings along the dorsolateral surface of the aorta. Some neurons remain in this location as the prevertebral (preaortic) sympathetic ganglia, while others continue to migrate laterally along segmented branches of the aorta to form the paravertebral sympathetic chain ganglia. Adrenal chromaffin cells also originate from the midtrunk level of the neural crest from the same precursor cells that give rise to postganglionic sympathetic neurons.
    Parasympathetic: Postganglionic parasympathetic ganglia neurons in the walls of the thoracic and abdominal viscera migrate there from the neural crest of the caudal rhombencephalon (for targets in the head, neck, thorax, and upper digestive tract) or lower spinal cord (for targets in the lower digestive tract and pelvic cavity).
    Enteric: Enteric precursor cells first migrate into the walls of the gastrointestinal tract and then continue to proliferate. The myenteric (Auerbach's) plexus is formed first. Later, cells migrate from the myenteric ganglia through the circular muscle layer to the submucosa to form the submucosal (Meissner's) plexus.

FUNCTION

22. Under what conditions does the ANS become activated?
    Contrary to common belief, the ANS is not recruited only for emergency ("fight or flight") or restorative ("rest and digest") purposes. Most components of the sympathetic, parasympathetic, and enteric divisions are **tonically active**. For example, peripheral sympathetic vasomotor fibers provide constant basal tone to arterioles, from which vascular resistance is further mediated up or down according to environmental demand.

23. What are the general functions of the sympathetic and parasympathetic divisions?
    In most cases, the sympathetic and parasympathetic divisions exert antagonistic effects on visceral targets. Sympathetic functions have been described as preparatory for **fight or flight**. For example, catecholaminergic output from the sympathetic division increases heart rate, causes vasodilation in skeletal muscle, promotes glucose utilization, enlarges the pupil, erects body hairs, and inhibits gut vascular flow and motility. Conversely, parasympathetic actions generally are restorative, as captured by the descriptive term **rest and digest**. For example, cholinergic output from the parasympathetic division decreases heart rate, constricts the pupil, and promotes digestion by enhancing gastrointestinal motility and secretion/absorption. (See table on following page).

24. How can monitoring ANS functions provide information about an individual's emotional state?
    The central integration and control of ANS functions make them immediately subject to cortical and limbic influence, as evidenced in the often dramatic relationship between ANS function and emotional state. The polygraph (lie detector) test is founded upon scientific evidence that emotional responses generally are accompanied by measurable, reproducible changes in ANS output.

Effects of Sympathetic and Parasympathetic Stimulation on Visceral Targets

VISCERAL TARGET	SYMPATHETIC STIMULATION		PARASYMPATHETIC STIMULATION	
	Transmitter	*Effect*	*Transmitter*	*Effect*
Eye				
Dilator pupillae muscle	NE	Pupillary dilation	—	—
Constrictor pupillae muscle	—	—	ACh	Pupillary constriction
Ciliary muscle	NE	Slight relaxation	ACh	Contraction
Glands of head				
Salivary and nasopharyngeal	NE	Increased secretion (viscous)	ACh	Increased secretion (watery)
Lacrimal	—	—	ACh	Increased secretion (watery)
Lungs (bronchioles)				
Bronchiolar smooth muscle	NE	Bronchiolar dilation	—	—
Glands	—	—	ACh	Mucous secretion
Heart				
Pacemaker cells	NE	Increased heart rate	ACh	Decreased heart rate
Cardiac myocytes	NE	Increased contractility and conduction velocity	ACh	Decreased contractility (minor) and conduction velocity
Blood vessels				
Head and pelvis	NE	Vasoconstriction	ACh	Vasodilation
Coronary and pulmonary	NE	Vasodilation	—	—
Some skeletal muscle	ACh	Vasodilation	—	—
All other vessels (majority)	NE	Vasoconstriction	—	—
Gastrointestinal tract				
Motility	NE	Decreased motility	ACh	Increased motility
Sphincters	NE	Increased tone	ACh	Decreased tone
Associated glands	—	—	ACh	Increased secretion
Liver	NE	Glycogenolysis, gluco-neogenesis, lipolysis	ACh	Glycogen synthesis
Kidney	NE	Renin secretion	—	—
Bladder				
Detrusor muscle	NE	Relaxation	ACh	Contraction
Sphincters	NE	Increased tone	ACh	Relaxation
Sex organs	NE	Ejaculation	ACh	Erection, glandular secretions
	ACh	Erection	—	—
Skin				
Sweat glands	ACh	Secretion	—	—
Pilomotor muscles	NE	Contraction	—	—
Adrenal medulla	ACh	Secretion of epinephrine	—	—

25. What makes the adrenal medulla unique among visceral targets?

The adrenal medulla receives direct innervation from sympathetic preganglionic neurons in the thoracic spinal cord whose axons terminate on adrenal chromaffin cells. Although chromaffin cells are not neurons, they express nicotinic cholinergic receptors (like all autonomic ganglion neurons) and share a common developmental lineage and catecholaminergic phenotype with postganglionic sympathetic neurons. However, catecholamines released from adrenal chromaffin cells after cholinergic stimulation enter the blood stream to act as hormones at sympathetic targets (adrenergic receptors) throughout the body. The catecholamines released from the adrenal medulla consist of a mixture of about 80% epinephrine and 20% NE. Epinephrine and NE have similar effects at adrenergic receptors, but epinephrine is longer-lived than NE.

26. What is meant by "mass activation"?

The sympathetic division of the ANS has the unique ability to undergo mass activation under emergency conditions of threatened homeostasis (stress). Under such conditions, increased preganglionic sympathetic drive to chromaffin cells in the adrenal medulla causes them to release epinephrine and NE into the general circulation. This property underlies the ability of the sympathetic division to achieve a concerted hormone-like activation of sympathetic targets throughout the body.

27. What advantages are offered by having peripheral autonomic ganglia, rather than direct projections from CNS motor neurons to visceral targets?

Autonomic ganglia extend nervous system capabilities by filtering and integrating information arising from the CNS before it is relayed to visceral targets. Postganglionic neurons typically receive and combine convergent inputs from several preganglionic sources; this is especially true in the sympathetic division. The arrangement of pre- and postganglionic cells allows both diffuse visceral activation and precise end organ–specific control, while using a limited number of CNS neurons and neural circuits.

28. Can an animal survive without a sympathetic nervous system?

Yes, but only if it is not subjected to severe homeostatic challenges. Almost 60 years ago, Walter Cannon demonstrated that sympathectomized animals cannot survive in stressful environments; they cannot work strenuously nor fend for themselves in situations of homeostatic challenge or social confrontation. For example, blood sugar is not mobilized on demand from the liver (leading to hypoglycemia), blood pressure does not increase in response to physical activity (leading to hypotension), and vasoconstriction and piloerection do not occur in response to cold (leading to hypothermia).

29. Why do fear and anxiety often cause a person to "break into a cold sweat"?

Cognitive perceptions of fear and anxiety are transmitted to the hypothalamus and other CNS regions to promote sympathetic activation (e.g., the fight or flight response: sympathetic mass activation). Two results of circulating epinephrine and increased sympathetic drive are vasoconstriction and activation of sweat glands in the skin. The decrease in blood flow makes the skin appear pale, while the sweat production makes the skin feel cold and clammy.

30. How can the forebrain control ANS output?

Many cortical and subcortical forebrain regions exert control over the ANS. Most of these regions produce their actions by way of the hypothalamus, which integrates the information it receives into a coherent pattern of autonomic commands. These commands are then relayed directly to the ANS from the lateral and paraventricular nuclei of the hypothalamus via long descending projections to sympathetic and parasympathetic preganglionic neurons in the spinal cord and brainstem. The hypothalamus also controls the endocrine system, which releases hormones that influence visceral functions on a slower/longer time scale (e.g., minutes to months to years).

31. Describe two major ways that the nucleus of the solitary tract (NTS) influences autonomic outflow.

The NTS, located in the caudal brainstem near the floor of the 4th ventricle, receives first-order sensory information from most major body organs through afferent fibers traveling in cranial nerves VII, IX, and X. It modulates ANS function in two major ways:

- By providing the central link for multiple ANS sensory-motor reflexes (e.g., the carotid sinus baroreceptor reflex, the gastric receptive relaxation reflex). Visceral afferent (sensory) fibers from the heart, lungs, and gastrointestinal tract terminate in specific NTS subnuclei in a viscerotopic manner. Intrinsic NTS neurons that receive visceral sensory information relay it to the ANS via direct and indirect central neural pathways.
- By coordinating more elaborate homeostatic adjustments by transmitting visceral sensory information to the forebrain and other CNS regions involved in complex and integrated autonomic control. Such brain regions include the parabrachial nucleus, hypothalamus, amygdala, and bed nucleus of the stria terminalis. Most of these regions contain neurons that project reciprocally to the NTS and to brainstem and spinal autonomic neurons.

CLINICAL EXAMPLES

32. Why do paramedics and physicians shine a light in the eyes of patients with suspected head injury?

They are testing the pupillary light reflex as a quick assessment of brain and peripheral nerve function. Lack of pupillary constriction after light stimulation is evidence of brain and/or nerve damage. Postganglionic parasympathetic neurons in the ciliary ganglion innervate the circular sphincter muscle to constrict the iris. (Sympathetic postganglionic neurons in the superior cervical ganglion innervate the pupillary radial dilator muscle to enhance dilation of the pupil.) Light stimulates retinal ganglion cells. These cells send the signal to the pretectal nuclei, which project to preganglionic parasympathetic neurons in the Edinger-Westphal nuclei (cranial nerve III); these, in turn, innervate the ciliary ganglion.

33. How can exercise- and stress-induced increases in cardiac output occur in individuals with transplanted (denervated) hearts?

Although deprived of extrinsic neural input, transplanted cardiac pacemaker cells and myocytes possess adrenergic receptors that are responsive to the stimulatory effects of circulating epinephrine and NE released from adrenal and synaptic sources after sympathetic activation. The lack of antagonistic parasympathetic cholinergic innervation significantly prolongs catecholamine-induced increases in cardiac output.

34. Describe the cause and symptoms of Horner's syndrome.

Horner's syndrome is caused by interruption of sympathetic innervation to the head and neck. This could result from damage to central pathways driving upper thoracic sympathetic preganglionic neurons; sympathetic neurons or processes in the upper thoracic spinal cord; fibers in the sympathetic chain; and/or the superior cervical ganglion or its efferent projections.

Symptoms generally are unilateral, and always occur on the same side as the lesion. The most obvious symptoms displayed by individuals with Horner's syndrome include **ptosis** (drooping eyelid; due to loss of sympathetic input to the smooth superior tarsal muscle), **miosis** (constricted pupil), facial **anhidrosis** (absence of sweating), and **redness and warming of the skin** (due to loss of sympathetic vasoconstriction). Less obvious symptoms include changes in the composition of salivary secretions.

35. Why is it important for many elderly individuals to limit physical activity after a meal?

Postprandial hypotension is relatively common in the elderly and in patients with general autonomic failure. Postprandial hypotension is defined as a decrease in systolic blood pressure of 20 mmHg or more. Severe cases are characterized by dizziness, fainting, and even stroke, due to decreased blood flow to the brain. Under normal conditions, blood flow to splanchnic-mesenteric arterial beds in the gut increases following a meal, but sympathetic compensation maintains adequate blood flow to the brain. One likely cause of postprandial hypotension is inadequate sympathetic compensation for meal-induced splanchnic blood pooling.

36. Why does uncontrolled diabetes mellitus often lead to autonomic neuropathy?

Uncontrolled diabetes mellitus is characterized by elevated blood glucose levels (hyperglycemia) as the result of inadequate insulin levels which prevent the movement of glucose into body cells. The persistent hyperglycemia results in damage to peripheral Schwann cells (glia) and axons. Small myelinated and nonmyelinated fibers are most vulnerable to damage. Postganglionic autonomic fibers are almost exclusively nonmyelinated and are, therefore, highly susceptible to damage from high blood glucose levels.

37. Hirschsprung's disease is a congenital disorder characterized by an absence of enteric neurons within the wall of the distal colon. What functional complications are produced by this disease?

Peristaltic intestinal contractions stop upon reaching the aganglionic segment of colon, which is completely denervated and significantly constricted. The colon above the aganglionic region usually is grossly distended due to backup of intestinal contents. When pressure proximal to the denervated segment of colon is sufficiently high, feces are forced through the rectum in explosive bouts of diarrhea. The chronic stasis of feces in the expanded colon allows overgrowth of normal bacteria, resulting in recurring colitis. The enteric rectoanal reflex (which involves sensory-motor circuits in the myenteric plexus of the distal colon) is absent: the anal sphincter does not relax in response to rectal distension, making normal defecation almost impossible. Surgical treatment of Hirschsprung's disease involves removal of the aganglionic bowel segment.

38. What is dysautonomia?

Dysautonomia is a general term that is used to describe many conditions in which the ANS is malfunctioning. Other generally synonymous terms include autonomic dysfunction, autonomic failure, and autonomic neuropathy. Dysautonomia has many causes, including primary disorders (e.g., orthostatic intolerance, multiple system atrophy or Shy-Drager syndrome, Parkinson's disease) and secondary/acquired disorders (e.g., diabetes mellitus, Guillain-Barré syndrome).

BIBLIOGRAPHY

1. Appenzeller O, Oribe E: The Autonomic Nervous System, 5th ed. Amsterdam, Elsevier, 1997.
2. Burnstock G: The Autonomic Nervous System, Vols. 1–7. Chur, Switzerland, Harwood Academic Publishers, 1992–1997.
3. Cannon WB: The Wisdom of the Body. New York, Norton, 1932.
4. Ciriello J, Calaresu FR, Renaud LP, Polosa C (eds): Organization of the Autonomic Nervous System: Central and Peripheral Mechanisms. New York, Liss, 1987.
5. Dodd J, Role LW: The autonomic nervous system. In Kandel ER, Schwartz JH, Jessell TM (eds): Principles of Neural Science, 3rd ed. Norwalk, Appleton & Lange, 1991, pp 761–775.
6. Loewy AD, Spyer KM (eds): Central Regulation of Autonomic Functions. New York, Oxford University Press, 1990.
7. Pick J: The Autonomic Nervous System. Philadelphia, J.B. Lippincott Co., 1970.
8. Powley TL: Central control of autonomic functions. In Zigmond MJ, Bloom FE, Landis SC, Roberts JL, Squire LR (eds): Fundamental Neuroscience. San Diego, Academic Press, 1999, pp 1027–1050.
9. Robertson D, Low PA, Polinsky RJ (eds): Primer on the Autonomic Nervous System. San Diego, Academic Press, 1996.
10. Wilson-Pauwels L, Stewart P, Akesson EJ: Autonomic Nerves. Hamilton, B.C. Decker Inc., 1997.

16. HYPOTHALAMUS—NEUROENDOCRINOLOGY

Hershel Raff, Ph.D., and William E. Cullinan, Ph.D.

ANATOMY OF THE HYPOTHALAMUS

1. Where is the hypothalamus located within the brain?

The structure of the hypothalamus is highly organized, reflecting a diversity of functional components (Fig. 1). It is located at the base of the diencephalon, where it surrounds the third ventricle; it is delimited anteriorly by the optic chiasm and lamina terminalis and posteriorly at the level of the mammillary nuclei. Superiorly, the hypothalamus is contiguous with the thalamus. The inferior portion of the hypothalamus includes the infundibulum, a stalk by which it is attached to the pituitary gland, forming an intimate neuronal as well as vascular relationship by which control of the endocrine system is exerted.

2. How is the hypothalamus divided anatomically?

On a gross level, the hypothalamus can be subdivided longitudinally into periventricular, medial, and lateral zones (Fig. 2). The **periventricular zone** borders the third ventricle and is a thin layer of cells comprised of many of the small (parvocellular) neurosecretory neurons involved in the control of anterior pituitary function. The ventral-most portion of the zone is more voluminous, and it is referred to as the *arcuate nucleus*.

The **medial zone** includes some of the most well-delineated nuclei of the hypothalamus, such as the preoptic and suprachiasmatic nuclei rostrally; the paraventricular, dorsomedial, and ventromedial nuclei in the mid-region; and the posterior and mammillary nuclei caudally. The *fornix* forms a border between the medial zone and the lateral zone.

The **lateral zone** is comprised of a network of loosely scattered cells that typically cannot be divided into specific nuclei, with the exception of the lateral tuberal nuclei located along the floor of the caudal lateral hypothalamus. The lateral zone is traversed by many longitudinally oriented projection systems, most notably the medial forebrain bundle, which connects widespread regions including the cerebral cortex and basal ganglia with the brain stem and spinal cord. This bundle also is composed of numerous ascending aminergic fiber systems originating in the brainstem. In addition, the lateral zone includes neurons having widespread projections to the cerebral cortex and to the spinal cord, as well as numerous multisynaptic short-fiber projections.

3. Do the hypothalamic nuclei partition by function?

It can be said that most, if not all, hypothalamic nuclei serve a variety of specific functions. This is perhaps most clearly evident in the paraventricular nucleus, which contains distinct neuronal populations that project: (1) to the posterior pituitary, thereby controlling fluid/electrolyte balance and maternal responses, (2) to the median eminence, thereby influencing release of anterior pituitary hormones and thus an array of effects including growth, metabolic, reproductive, socio-behavioral, and emotional responses, and (3) to brainstem and spinal cord centers concerned with control of the autonomic nervous system.

Another example is the arcuate nucleus, in which two separate populations of neurons influence the secretory activity of the anterior pituitary.

4. What important fiber systems are found within the hypothalamus?

In addition to the aforementioned medial forebrain bundle, a number of distinct fiber tracts are clearly recognizable in the hypothalamus. The **fornix** and **stria terminalis** interconnect the hypothalamus with medial temporal lobe structures (i.e., hippocampal formation and amygdala, respectively). The mammillary nuclei project to the anterior thalamus and brainstem tegmentum by way of

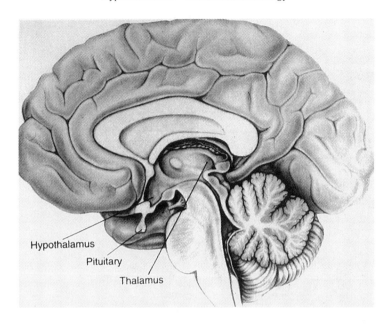

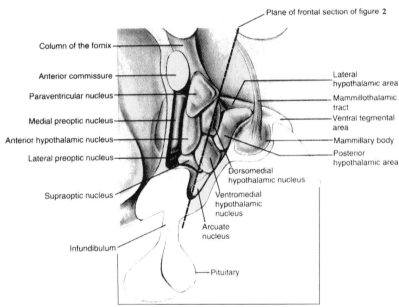

Column of the fornix

Anterior commissure

Paraventricular nucleus

Medial preoptic nucleus

Anterior hypothalamic nucleus

Lateral preoptic nucleus

Supraoptic nucleus

Infundibulum

Plane of frontal section of figure 2

Lateral hypothalamic area

Mammillothalamic tract

Ventral tegmental area

Mammillary body

Posterior hypothalamic area

Dorsomedial hypothalamic nucleus

Ventromedial hypothalamic nucleus

Arcuate nucleus

Pituitary

Figure 1. Location and structure of the hypothalamus. (From Kandel ER, Schwartz JH, Jessel TM (eds): Principles of Neural Science, 3rd ed. New York, Elsevier, 1991; with permission.)

the **mammillothalamic** and **mammillotegmental** tracts, respectively. The **dorsal longitudinal fasciculus** connects caudal hypothalamic areas to brainstem regions. The **hypothalamohypophyseal tract**, which contains the descending axons of neurons from the paraventricular and supraoptic nuclei, projects to the median eminence and posterior pituitary.

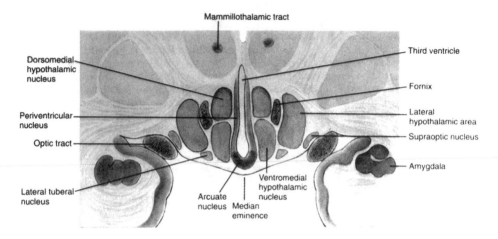

Figure 2.   Three anatomic zones of the hypothalamus. (From Kandel ER, Schwartz JH, Jessel TM (eds): Principles of Neural Science, 3rd ed. New York, Elsevier, 1991; with permission.)

HYPOTHALAMIC-LIMBIC INTERACTIONS

5. How does the hypothalamus interact with the limbic system?

The hypothalamus is intimately associated with the limbic system in large part by its connections via the fornix and stria terminalis and by its interconnections with various subcortical targets of limbic cortical regions, including the nucleus accumbens, septum, amygdala, and bed nucleus of the stria terminalis (BST).

The concept of a limbic system was originally put forward in 1937 by James Papez, who emphasized a critical role for the hypothalamus in mediating responses to stimuli of an emotional nature. The **Papez circuit** described an anatomic substrate for this function (Fig. 3). Papez proposed that higher cortical centers influence the hypothalamus through connections to the cingulate gyrus and then to the hippocampal formation (via the cingulum bundle). The hippocampal formation relays the information to the mammillary bodies of the hypothalamus via the fornix. The hypothalamus, in turn, provides a return of processed information to the cingulate cortex through a relay in the anterior nucleus of the thalamus. This circuit, though not confirmed experimentally, helped provide a framework within which to begin to understand emotional behavior.

Based on anatomic data, the concept of a limbic system has been expanded considerably to include additional subcortical areas that are extensively interconnected. The septum, for example, which is reciprocally connected with the hippocampus, also is heavily interconnected with the hypothalamus and BST. The BST has been confirmed to receive a prominent innervation from the hippocampal formation, and is reciprocally connected with the hypothalamus and amygdala. The amygdala also possesses reciprocal connections with the hypothalamus. Further, a number of additional cortical regions have been included by some authors (e.g., medial prefrontal cortical regions).

6. What are the most prominent limbic-hypothalamic neural interactions?

While there exists no consensus on limbic system components and their specific functional roles, a few generalizations may be made regarding the contributions of some prominently featured components with respect to hypothalamic function.

- The hypothalamus integrates motor or output signals concerning maintenance of physiologic equilibrium and reproductive function.
- The hippocampus, noted primarily for its role as a learning and memory center, assigns salience for a given set of stimuli and relays this information to appropriate hypothalamic output structures.

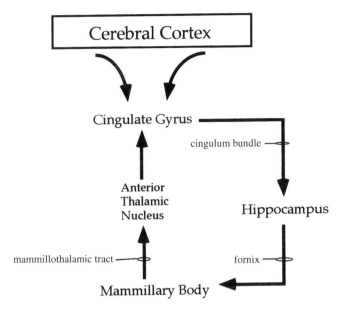

Figure 3.   The Papez circuit.

• The amygdala, which performs a critical role in emotional responses, accesses hypothalamic output structures either relatively directly (through its projections in the stria terminalis and ventral amygdalofugal pathways) or via additional forebrain structures in a position to serve as hypothalamic relays (e.g., BST).

7. How do circumventricular organs influence hypothalamic activity?

Circumventricular organs provide an important source of nonsynaptic sensory information to the hypothalamus. These specialized brain regions are associated with the cerebral ventricles and have fenestrated capillaries, allowing relatively large molecules normally excluded by the blood-brain barrier to affect neurons.

The principal circumventricular organs providing neurohumoral signaling from the periphery to hypothalamic cells are the **organum vasculosum of the lamina terminalis** and the **median eminence**, both of which are located within the hypothalamus, and the **subfornical organ** and **area postrema**, which have extensive projections to hypothalamic nuclei involved in neuroendocrine and autonomic function. Circumventricular organs are critical structures at the interface between humoral factors and limbic/hypothalamic integration because they allow the hypothalamus to provide feedback regulation in response to blood-borne chemosensory signals (e.g., sodium, cytokines).

HYPOTHALAMIC-PITUITARY INTERFACE

8. What are the two main types of pathway through which the hypothalamus controls pituitary function?

Direct pathway: Neuropeptides (e.g., arginine vasopressin or oxytocin) are synthesized in magnocellular neuron cell bodies located in the supraoptic nuclei and lateral paraventricular nuclei of the hypothalamus (Fig. 4). These peptides are transported down long axons that traverse the internal zone of the median eminence and the infundibulum and terminate on capillaries located in the posterior pituitary. When input into these magnocellular neurons increases, action potentials originating in the cell bodies travel down the axons and cause release of the peptides into the blood capillaries in the posterior pituitary. From there, the peptides drain into the cavernous sinuses and the systemic circulation, where they exert biological effects. Therefore, the posterior pituitary hormones are synthesized in the brain.

Indirect pathway: Neuropeptides or catecholamines are synthesized in parvocellular neuron cell bodies located in the more medial hypothalamic nuclei (e.g., arcuate). These releasing factors/hormones or inhibiting factors/hormones are transported down short axons that terminate on a capillary plexus in the external zone of the median eminence. When input to the parvocellular neurons induces an action potential, releasing or inhibiting factors are released into the capillary plexus, which drains into long portal blood vessels that carry the hypothalamic factors to capillaries in the anterior pituitary. These factors either stimulate or inhibit the release of anterior pituitary hormones. This system has been called the hypothalamic-hypophophyseal portal system (see Question 14).

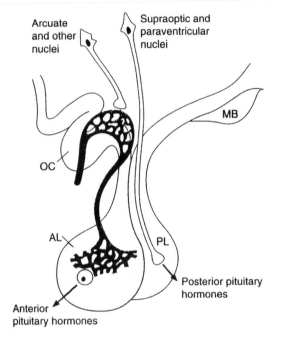

Figure 4. Hypothalamic control of pituitary function. AL = anterior lobe of the pituitary, MB = mamillary bodies, OC = optic chiasm, PL = posterior lobe of the pituitary. (From Ganong WF: Review of Medical Physiology. Appleton & Lange, Stamford, CT, 1997; with permission.)

9. Why is arginine vasopressin also called antidiuretic hormone?

Arginine vasopressin (AVP) also is called antidiuretic hormone because of its effect of decreasing free water excretion from the kidney.

10. How is the release of arginine vasopressin from the posterior pituitary controlled?

There are two main controllers of AVP secretion:

Osmotic control: An increase in plasma osmolality (primarily plasma sodium) stimulates osmoreceptors located in the anterior hypothalamus. Input into the magnocellular AVP neurons from osmoreceptors in the anterior hypothalamus and (possibly) the inherent osmosensitivity of the magnocellular neurons result in an increase in AVP secretion into the systemic circulation. AVP increases the passive reabsorption of water in the kidney, which helps to return plasma osmolality to normal. Osmoreceptor stimulation also increases thirst, such that water intake is optimized to return plasma osmolality to normal. If osmolality is too low (hyponatremia), AVP release is inhibited, renal free water excretion is increased, and osmolality is returned toward normal.

Nonosmotic control: There are many nonosmotic stimuli to AVP release, including nausea, pain, hypoxia, and hypotension. Probably the most important and best studied are the cardiovascular inputs to vasopressin. If blood volume decreases (normotensive hypovolemia), stretch receptors within the heart decrease their input to the central nervous system (CNS) which results in an increase in AVP. By decreasing free water excretion, blood volume is normalized. If the hypovolemia is severe enough to lead to arterial hypotension, high-pressure baroreceptors located in the carotid bifurcations also can stimulate AVP release and increase vasoconstriction to return arterial pressure to normal.

11. What are the major disorders of arginine vasopressin control?

Real or apparent underproduction: **Diabetes insipidus** is either of central/pituitary origin (neurogenic diabetes insipidus), in which vasopressin release is subnormal, or of renal origin (nephrogenic diabetes insipidus), in which the renal collecting ducts do not respond normally to AVP. In either case, free water loss from the kidney is excessive; hence the name diabetes (siphon—excess urine) insipidus (tasteless—hypotonic). This loss leads to plasma hyperosmolality (hypernatremia) and a stimulation of thirst. The end result is polydipsia (excessive water intake) and polyuria (excessive urine volume).

Overproduction: The **syndrome of inappropriate antidiuretic hormone** (SIADH) can be due to a variety of causes, including ectopic AVP production, intracranial disorders, and granulomatous diseases. In any case, AVP secretion is excessive, which leads to increased water retention and hypotonicity (hyponatremia). AVP excess persists despite hypotonicity.

Importantly, there are many causes of hyponatremia not directly related to abnormal AVP secretion.

12. What are some of the intracranial disorders that can lead to SIADH?

They include meningitis, head injury, abscess, inflammation, subarachnoid hemorrhage, and psychosis.

13. How is the secretion of oxytocin controlled?

Uterine contraction: In a full-term, pregnant woman, the head of the fetus pushes on the cervix, which has spinal afferents with input to the hypothalamus via the median forebrain bundle. Cervical stretch results in a stimulation of oxytocin release, which increases uterine contraction. This positive feedback results in increasing oxytocin release and uterine contractility, leading to parturition.

Milk ejection: In the postpartum woman, milk production is stimulated by prolactin. When the baby nurses, receptors in the nipple are stimulated, with impulses carried by spinal afferents to the hypothalamus via the median forebrain bundle. This input to magnocellular neurons increases oxytocin release into the systemic circulation, which results in contraction of myoepithelial cells in the mammary glands, leading to milk ejection (milk let-down).

Higher centers: Cortical influences to oxytocin release can be stimulatory (e.g., the sound of a baby crying can induce milk let-down) or inhibitory (anxiety-induced decrease in milk ejection).

14. List the established hypothalamic releasing/inhibiting factors, their nuclei of origin, and the anterior pituitary hormones they control.

Hypothalamic Hormones	Hypothalamic Nucleus	Controlled Pituitary Hormone
RELEASING		
Thyrotropin-releasing hormone (TRH)	Paraventricular	Thyrotropin (TSH), prolactin
Corticotropin-releasing hormone	Paraventricular	Adrenocorticotropin
Gonadotropin-releasing hormone (GnRH)	Preoptic area	Luteinizing hormone (LH), follicle-stimulating hormone (FSH)
Growth-hormone-releasing hormone	Arcuate	Growth hormone
INHIBITING		
Dopamine	Arcuate	Prolactin
Somatostatin	Periventricular region	Growth hormone

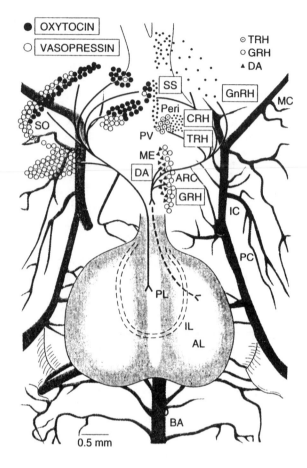

Figure 5. Hypophysiotropic nuclei. Ventral view of the rat hypothalamus and pituitary. Magnocellular cell bodies are shown on left; parvocellular on right. AL = anterior lobe, ARC = arcuate nucelus, BA = basilar artery, DA = dopamine, GH = growth hormone, GHRH = growth hormone releasing hormone, IC = internal carotid artery, IL = intermediate lobe, MC = middle cerebral artery, ME = median eminence, PC = posterior cerebral artery, Peri = periventricular nucleus, PL = posterior lobe, PV = paraventricular nucleus, SO = supraoptic nucleus, SS = somatostatin. (From Ganong WF: Review of Medical Physiology. Appleton & Lange, Stamford, CT, 1997; with permission.)

15. What is the overall hypothalamic-hypophyseal feedforward/feedback control system?

The classic system is the hypothalamic-pituitary-adrenocortical (HPA) axis (Fig. 6).

Feedforward control: The neurons from which corticotropin-releasing hormone (CRH) originates are located within the paraventricular nucleus of the hypothalamus. They receive input from a variety of sources, including circadian rhythm (suprachiasmatic nuclei), afferent stress pathways (e.g., pain-nociception, hypoxia-chemoreceptors, hemorrhage-hypotension-baroreceptors), hypoglycemia (hypothalamic glucostat), and emotional/psychological disturbances (cerebral cortex, limbic forebrain). This input leads to increased CRH release into the long portal vein, which leads to increased secretion of adrenocorticotropin (ACTH) from the anterior pituitary. ACTH stimulates the release of cortisol from the adrenal gland, which exerts a variety of biological effects.

Feedback control: Cortisol can limit its own release via negative feedback exerted on at least three anatomic sites. Cortisol directly inhibits ACTH secretion from the pituitary and CRH release from the hypothalamus, and indirectly inhibits CRH release via an action likely mediated by input from limbic central regions (e.g., hippocampus). Also, cortisol may attenuate afferent input to the hypothalamus.

16. What are the other hypothalamic-hypophyseal control loops?

In the following list, main differences from the HPA axis are italicized.

• **GHRH/somatostatin—GH—insulin-like growth factor 1:** GHRH stimulates GH, *while somatostatin inhibits* GH. GH exerts direct metabolic effects (e.g., increases hepatic glucose production)

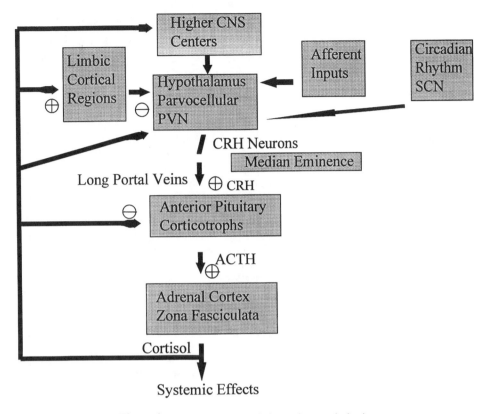

Figure 6.   The hypothalamic-pituitary-adrenocortical axis.

and indirectly increases linear growth velocity in children by increasing insulin-like growth factor 1 (somatomedin C) released from the liver.

• **GnRH—FSH/LH—testosterone/inhibin (male):** GnRH stimulates *both* of the gonadotropins, LH and FSH. LH primarily stimulates testosterone secretion, while FSH primarily stimulates inhibin release. Testosterone primarily inhibits LH, while inhibin primarily decreases FSH secretion. Therefore, this system represents *dual, parallel feedback control loops.*

• **GnRH—FSH/LH—estrogen/inhibin (female):** Similar to male except that during the middle of the menstrual cycle, *estrogen can stimulate LH and FSH release (positive feedback).*

• **TRH—TSH—thyroid hormone:** TRH stimulates TSH, which stimulates thyroid hormone release. *Most of the negative feedback of thyroid hormone is exerted at the anterior pituitary.*

• **Dopamine—prolactin:** *Primary controller of prolactin release appears to be inhibition by dopamine from the hypothalamus.* Dopamine is a *catecholamine*, rather than a peptide/protein like the other hypophysiotropic factors. Various prolactin-releasing factors have been proposed (e.g., TRH, vasoactive intestinal peptide), but none are firmly established as the one.

17. Name examples of syndromes characterized by anterior pituitary hormone over- or underproduction.

Hormone	Overproduction	Underproduction
ACTH	Cushing's disease	Secondary adrenal insufficiency
GH	Acromegaly/gigantism	Short stature in children

Table continued on facing page

Hormone	Overproduction	Underproduction
FSH/LH	Pituitary adenomas (rare)	Hypogonadotropic hypogonadism
TSH	Secondary hyperthyroidism (rare)	Secondary hypothyroidism
Prolactin	Hyperprolactinemia (adenoma or stalk compression)	?
All	—	Panhypopituitarism

18. Do hypothalamic neuropeptides have extrahypothalamic effects?

Yes. CRH neurons are located in or project to limbic structures (e.g., amygdala, bed nucleus of the stria terminalis) and nuclei related to autonomic control. Parvocellular nuclei can synthesize AVP and oxytocin with projections to the locus coeruleus, the solitary nucleus, the dorsal vagal complex, and the intermediolateral cell column of the spinal cord.

19. Do peripheral hormones under pituitary control influence the CNS?

Yes. Receptors for cortisol (glucocorticoid receptors) and aldosterone (mineralocorticoid receptors) are located throughout the brain. Cortisol is known to have a variety of behavioral and psychiatric effects.

Receptors for thyroid hormone also are located throughout the brain. Thyroid hormone is necessary for normal fetal and neonatal brain development.

20. Do any of the pituitary hormones have effects within the CNS?

There are several pituitary hormones that appear to have effects within the CNS. Note, however, that large peptides and glycoproteins must penetrate the blood brain barrier to exert an effect. It has been hypothesized that arginine vasopressin derived either from neuronal pathways or from the systemic circulation alters memory. It also has been hypothesized that prolactin can alter reproductive behavior, at least in lower animals. It probably accesses the brain via the choroid plexus and the cerebrospinal fluid.

21. What are the endogenous opioids?

Endorphin (endogenous morphine-like) is the generic name for a class of substances that bind to the different types of morphine receptors in the CNS. Among these are the pentapeptides met-enkephalin and leu-enkephalin as well as beta-, alpha-, and gamma-endorphin. The endorphins are synthesized by posttranslational processing of pro-opiomelanocortin, which also is a precursor for ACTH, and from two proenkephalins.

22. Where are the endogenous opioids located, and what do they do in these locations?

Location	Function
ENKEPHALINS	
Spinal cord	Associated with the dorsal gray matter corresponding to nerve endings of primary sensory neurons; may modulate pain perception
Vagal nucleus	Emetic and antitussive effects
Locus coeruleus	Euphoria
Amygdala	Euphoria
β-ENDORPHIN	
Pituitary; primarily in the intermediate lobe	Not firmly established

TEMPERATURE REGULATION

23. How is temperature regulated by the hypothalamus?

Regulation of body temperature requires the integration of autonomic, endocrine, and skeletomotor responses. Thermosensitive neurons have been located centrally within the preoptic and anterior areas of the hypothalamus, where temperature reception is likely to occur based on local blood temperature levels. Peripheral temperature receptors are located primarily in the skin and viscera. Posterior hypothalamic areas, while not directly involved in sensing temperature levels, do play an important role in thermoregulatory responses.

Based on studies in which the hypothalamus was electrically stimulated in unanesthetized animals, anterior hypothalamic areas appear to regulate heat dissipation, producing dilation of blood vessels in the skin, suppression of shivering, and production of panting. Conversely, posterior hypothalamic stimulation produces an opposite set of responses resulting in heat conservation. These studies find additional support from numerous ablation studies in a variety of species.

The hypothalamus controls endocrine responses to altered temperature. For example, long-term exposure to cold is known to increase thyroxine and glucocorticoid levels, via TRH-TSH and CRH-ACTH, respectively. In addition, the preoptic region plays a role in fever production, likely by receiving inputs from the organum vasculosum of the lamina terminalis (OVLT), which transduces signals from circulating cytokines into neural activity directed at appropriate hypothalamic neuronal populations. Finally, the hypothalamus controls the circadian rhythmicity of body temperature by integrating inputs from the suprachiasmatic nucleus and other hypothalamic nuclei, thereby affecting appropriate body responses via autonomic outputs. In each of these cases the precise neuronal pathways involved remain to be firmly established.

TEMPORAL RHYTHMS

24. What is the main daily rhythm in humans? Which hypothalamic nucleus is responsible?

The primary rhythm in the daily life is a diurnal rhythm that is characterized by a peak of activity upon awakening and a nadir at bedtime. Perhaps the best characterized is the circadian rhythm of the HPA axis, with ACTH driving an 0800 hour peak and midnight nadir in cortisol. The suprachiasmatic nucleus (SCN) appears to be the dominant pacemaker ("zeitgeber") for most mammalian circadian rhythms. In addition to the HPA axis, the SCN appears to drive diurnal rhythms in melatonin from the pineal gland, as well as sleep-wake cycles, changes in body temperature, and locomotor activity.

25. Are there extrahypothalamic influences on daily rhythms?

Although the SCN does have an endogenous rhythm slightly longer than 24 hours, it is entrained to 24 hours by light cues. Input to the SCN from the eyes via the retinohypothalamic fibers as well as the lateral geniculate nuclei entrain (synchronize) daily rhythms to the 24-hour cycle.

26. Are there types of neuroendocrine temporal rhythms other than circadian?

The best described is pulsatile GnRH release from the arcuate nucleus. GnRH is released in pulses with a frequency of about 90 minutes. This pulsatility is required for normal secretion of LH and FSH from gonadotrophs in the anterior pituitary.

HYPOTHALAMIC CONTROL OF FEEDING

27. What is the general role of the hypothalamus in feeding?

The hypothalamus is one of a number of brain regions involved in the regulation of food intake, playing a vital role in the integration of neural and hormonal signals and exerting influence over feeding primarily via autonomic outflow to the viscera. Following food consumption, sensory pathways innervating visceral structures (e.g., via vagal afferents) are stimulated, and satiety signals are relayed to the hypothalamus via the nucleus tractus solitarius (NTS) in the medulla. In addition, hormones released from the viscera following food consumption influence hypothalamic neuronal activity via the area postrema. These hypothalamic neurons also are under direct hormonal feedback control from visceral structures.

28. How does the paraventricular nucleus regulate feeding?

The paraventricular nucleus (PVN) plays a pivotal role in the control of feeding through its descending outputs to brain stem autonomic centers and to the spinal cord. For example, parvocellular PVN neurons that release oxytocin are known to project to the dorsal vagal complex (a region that includes the NTS), as well as to sympathetic preganglionic neurons, and have been implicated in reducing food intake. PVN cells also are influenced by afferents from the arcuate nucleus, which releases neuropeptide Y (NPY). Infusion of NPY to the PVN stimulates food intake; NPY-containing neurons in the arcuate nucleus are inhibited by the adipose cells–secreting hormone leptin, which exerts a more long-term inhibitory signal. Arcuate NPY-containing neurons also are sensitive to local insulin levels, with low insulin levels promoting food intake, and high insulin levels having the opposite effect.

29. What additional hypothalamic systems alter feeding?

A number of chemically specific afferent neurotransmitter systems modulate hypothalamic areas involved in feeding control. These include ascending brainstem projections that release both norepinephrine and galanin, and serotoninergic projections of brainstem origin. Stress also is known to decrease food intake, and various stressors activate the HPA axis. Corticotropin-releasing factor, a key mediator of these effects, is produced in the PVN and decreases food intake when delivered to cerebral ventricles. Also, leptin interacts with numerous additional hypothalamic sites to inhibit food intake (Fig. 7).

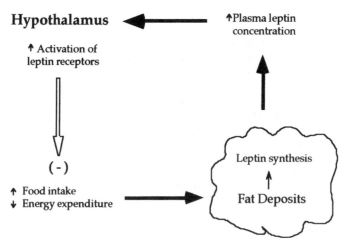

Figure 7. Leptin inhibition of food intake.

30. Summarize current general concepts on the overall control of feeding.

There remain considerable differences of opinion on the control of food intake, despite a long history of research. One view holds that eating is the result of the depletion of energy stores in adipose tissue, reduced use of metabolic fuels (glucose or lipid), or both. Food intake therefore reduces a signal to eat by satisfying levels of energy reserve or utilization of energy fuels. A second view considers animals primed to eat unless inhibited by certain signals (humoral and neural) provided by meals. The hypothalamic neural circuitry regulating the control of feeding in either scenario undoubtedly is highly complex.

31. Are there hypothalamic "centers" that control feeding?

Earlier notions of a "satiety center" and a "feeding center" located within the ventromedial hypothalamic nucleus (VMH) and lateral hypothalamus (LH), respectively, are oversimplified, although these regions do appear to at least participate in such formerly ascribed functions. For example, VMH lesions profoundly reduce sympathetic outflow while increasing parasympathetic tone and vagal reflexes, and also appear to increase food intake by resultant increases in levels of insulin. LH lesions, in contrast, reduce parasympathetic tone, decreasing feeding by lowering insulin levels and inhibiting gastric emptying.

REGULATION OF THIRST, FLUID INTAKE, SODIUM BALANCE, AND VASCULAR VOLUME

32. What are the two main factors involved in the control of drinking?

Tissue osmolality: The concentration of effective osmolytes (primarily sodium) in the extracellular fluid is the primary controller of thirst. An increase in osmolality (e.g., hypernatremia) is sensed by osmoreceptors. There is some dispute about the location of the osmoreceptors, but they probably are located in the anterior hypothalamus. Regardless, an increase in extracellular osmolality surrounding the osmoreceptive neurons results in a loss of intracellular water, leading to shrinking-induced activation of these neurons and stimulation of thirst. Conversely, hypo-osmolality (e.g., hyponatremia) leads to an influx of water into the osmoreceptive cells, such that swelling decreases their activity, leading to a decrease in thirst.

Vascular volume: An isotonic decrease in blood volume also appears to increase thirst, probably by increasing activity of the renin-angiotensin system. The resultant increase in angiotensin II appears to stimulate drinking by an action at the subfornical organ (SFO) and, possibly, at the OVLT. The SFO and OVLT are circumventricular organs located outside the blood-brain barrier, where they are accessible to circulating hormones. The resultant increase in fluid intake helps to restore blood volume. Baroreceptor activation also may participate in this process via ascending inputs from the medulla to the hypothalamus.

33. What prevents drinking too much after a prolonged dehydration?

It is quite amazing that animals (including humans) subjected to dehydration will drink almost exactly the amount of their water deficit, such that when the fluid is absorbed from the gastrointestinal tract, plasma hypotonicity does not ensue. This is thought to be regulated by a combination of afferents from oropharyngeal, gastrointestinal, and hepatic portal receptors (via the vagus nerve).

34. Is there a disorder of fluid intake?

Primary polydypsia is a fascinating psychiatric disorder in which fluid intake is dramatically increased. Usually, the hypotonicity and subsequent decrease in AVP allow the excess water to be excreted by the kidney. However, in some psychiatric patients, the failure to adequately increase free water clearance results in hyponatremia and hypotonicity. A supervised water restriction often allows the diagnosis to be made.

35. What is the renin-angiotensin-aldosterone system?

Renin is a proteolytic enzyme released by the kidney into the systemic circulation. It starts a cascade of events, beginning with renin-mediated cleavage of the peptide angiotensin I from a large hepatic globulin called angiotensinogen (also known as renin substrate). Angiotensin I is essentially devoid of biological activity, but is the substrate for the production of the biologically active angiotensin II. This reaction is catalyzed by angiotensin converting enzyme, which is located in virtually all vascular endothelia.

Angiotensin II has a wide variety of biological effects, including stimulation of aldosterone release from the adrenal cortex, vasoconstriction, stimulation of thirst (see Question 32), and direct inhibition of renin release (negative feedback). Aldosterone also inhibits renin release indirectly by increasing extracellular fluid volume (Fig. 8).

It has been demonstrated that there are tissue renin-angiotensin systems that exert local effects. Many, if not all, of the components of the brain renin-angiotensin system, for example, are expressed within the CNS.

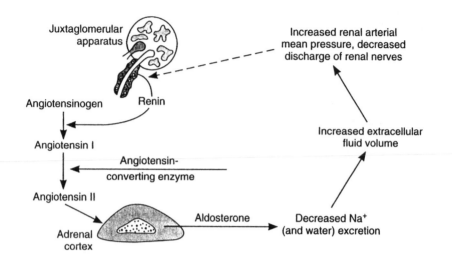

Figure 8. The renin-angiotensin-aldosterone system. Dashed arrow indicates inhibition. (From Ganong WF: Review of Medical Physiology. Appleton & Lange, Stamford, CT, 1997; with permission.)

36. What are the major effects of the renal renin-angiotensin-aldosterone system?

The main functions of this system are to decrease sodium and water excretion, which leads to an increase in extracellular fluid volume (see Fig. 8), and increase total peripheral resistance. These effects are accomplished via angiotensin II, which is a vasoconstrictor that also directly increases renal proximal tubule reabsorption. Angiotensin II acts indirectly by increasing adrenocortical production of the mineralococorticoid aldosterone, which stimulates sodium reabsorption and potassium secretion in the distal portions of the nephron.

37. How is the secretion of renin from the kidney controlled?

• Activation of the renal sympathetic nerves directly increases renin release.
• A reduction of sodium chloride delivery to the macula densa stimulates renin release from juxtaglomerular cells.
• Reduction in renal perfusion is sensed by intrarenal baroreceptors, leading to an increase in renin release.
• Angiotensin II inhibits renin release (negative feedback).

38. Give two examples of physiologic conditions in which renin is important.

• Low sodium diet: renin release is increased, maximizing renal sodium reabsorption (directly and indirectly through aldosterone).
• High sodium diet: renin release is decreased, allowing sodium to be excreted.

39. Are there primary disorders of renin release?

Yes. If renal perfusion is compromised in renovascular disease, renin release can be increased, leading to hypertension (due to vasoconstriction and increased sodium reabsorption).

Although rare, there are tumors of the kidney from which renin is secreted.

A failure of the kidney to produce renin is called hyporeninemia.

BIBLIOGRAPHY

1. Aron DC, Findling JW, Tyrrell JB: Hypothalamus and pituitary. In Greenspan FS, Strewler GJ (eds): Basic and Clinical Endocrinology. Stamford, CT, Appleton & Lange, 1997, pp 95–156.

2. Ganong WF: Central regulation of visceral function. In Ganong WF (ed): Review of Medical Physiology. Stamford, CT, Appleton & Lange, 1997, pp 217–239.

3. Heimer L: The Human Brain and Spinal Cord, 2nd ed. New York, Springer-Verlag, 1995.

3a. Herman JP, Cullinan WE: Neurocircuitry of stress: central control of hypothalamo-pituitary-adrenocortical axis. Trends Neurosci 20:78–84, 1997.

4. Kupfermann I: Hypothalamus and limbic system: Peptidergic neurons, homeostasis, and emotional behavior. In Kandel ER, Schwartz JH, Jessel TM (eds): Principles of Neural Science, 3rd ed. New York, Elsevier, 1991, pp 736–749.

5. Kupfermann I: Hypothalamus and limbic system: Motivation. In Kandel ER, Schwartz JH, Jessel TM (eds): Principles of Neural Science, 3rd ed. New York, Elsevier, 1991, pp 750–760.

6. Raff H: Endocrine physiology. In Raff H (ed): Physiology Secrets. Philadelphia, Hanley & Belfus, 1998, pp 175–219.

7. Reichlin S: Neuroendocrinology. In Wilson JD, Foster DW (eds): Williams Textbook of Endocrinology. Philadelphia, WB Saunders Co, 1992, pp 135–219.

8. Saper CB: Hypothalamus. In Paxinos G (ed): The Human Nervous System. San Diego, Academic Press, 1990.

9. Woods SC, Stricker EM: Food intake and metabolism. In Zigmond MJ, et al (eds): Fundamental Neuroscience. San Diego, Academic Press, 1999.

17. THE THALAMUS

Henry J. Ralston III, M.D.

The thalamus (from the Greek word thalamos, *a room or antechamber) is intimately linked with the cerebral cortex, and neither can function properly without the proper functioning of the other. The developmental origin of the thalamus is the dorsal diencephalon, the second major component of the forebrain along with the telencephalon, from which the cerebral cortex arises. The thalamus receives afferent input from sensory, motor, and limbic systems, modifies these inputs, and then transmits them to specific regions of the cerebral cortex. The cortex, in turn, can modify the activities of thalamic neurons, thus influencing the messages sent from the thalamus to the cortex.*

1. How is the thalamus related to other structures of the forebrain?

Like most structures in the central nervous system (CNS), the thalamus is bilaterally symmetrical, measuring about 30 mm long (anteroposterior) and 15 mm wide at its widest point. It consists of an egg-shaped aggregation of neurons that lie medial to the internal capsule and form the lateral walls of the third ventricle (Figs. 1 and 2). A thin sheet of neurons, the **thalamic reticular nucleus**, surrounds the thalamus on all but its medial aspect, like an eggshell encasing an egg (Fig. 3). The thalamus is composed of groups of anatomically and functionally distinct nuclei, each with its own set of afferent and efferent connections.

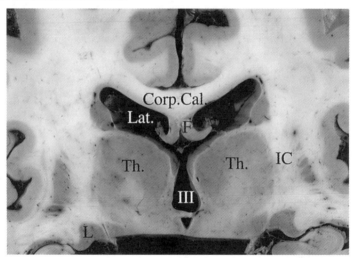

Figure 1. Coronal (transverse) specimen of the human thalamus. The thalamus (Th.) is a bilaterally symmetrical structure that forms the lateral walls of the lateral ventricle (III), which in turn is bounded laterally by the internal capsule (IC). Lat. = lateral ventricle; F= fornix; Corp. Cal. = corpus callosum.

2. How are the neuronal circuits of the thalamus organized?

There are two types of neurons: the **thalamocortical projection (TCP) cells**, which represent about 75% of the total neuronal population, and the **local circuit interneurons (LCN)**, which constitute about 25%. As its name implies, the TCP neuron sends its axon to the cerebral cortex, where it releases an excitatory neurotransmitter (most likely glutamate) to activate cortical neurons. The LCN releases γ-aminobutyric acid (GABA) on TCP cells to inhibit them.

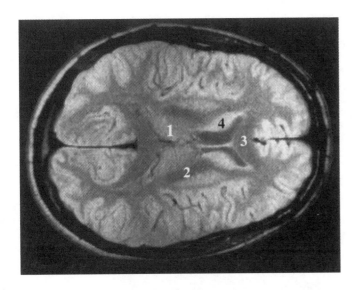

Figure 2. A magnetic resonance image in the axial (horizontal) plane. The frontal lobes are to the right, the occipital lobes to the left. 1 = thalamus; 2 = internal capsule; 3 = corpus callosum; 4 = head of the caudate nucleus.

Both TCP and LCN cells receive afferent projections from a principal afferent source, such as the retina, spinal cord, or cerebellum. Although some of the thalamic motor nuclei receive inhibitory afferents from the basal ganglia, in most cases this input is excitatory (depolarizing). Depolarization causes the TCP to send a signal to the cortex. The TCP neurons are then promptly inhibited (hyperpolarized) by the GABAergic LCN.

In addition, the TCP send a collateral branch to neurons of the thalamic reticular nucleus (TRN), which also contain the inhibitory neurotransmitter GABA. TRN cells send axonal branches to the TCP and LCN cells so that both are inhibited. The cerebral cortex, which has received excitatory afferent projections from the thalamic TCP cells, sends excitatory axons back to all thalamic cell types, so that the TCP neurons as well as the inhibitory LCN and TRN neurons are activated by cortical inputs. Finally, neurons of the rostral brainstem project to thalamic neurons.

Different groups of brainstem neurons release different neurotransmitters, particularly norepinephrine, acetylcholine, and serotonin. These different transmitters may activate or inhibit thalamic neurons.

3. What is the role of the thalamus in this circuitry?

The transmission of information by the thalamus to the central cortex is *highly modified*. The thalamus is not merely a simple relay of information between afferent centers and the cortex, but is responsible for processing this information and thus influencing cortical function.

4. Give a specific example of thalamic circuitry.

A nucleus of the somatosensory thalamus (the **ventroposterolateral nucleus**) receives information from the spinal cord and dorsal column nuclei. The afferent somatosensory axons of the medial lemniscus release an excitatory neurotransmitter (glutamate) on TCP and LCN dendrites. The LCN dendrites are specialized in that they contain synaptic vesicles with the neurotransmitter GABA; thus, excitation (depolarization) of LCN by the medial lemniscal afferents leads to release of GABA onto the dendrites of TCP neurons. The medial lemniscal input first *excites* TCP neurons and then *inhibits* them via the interposed neurons. The spinothalamic tract (STT) afferents usually have simple synapses on TCP dendrites, with little modulation of the input by LCN GABA-containing dendrites. Thus, the signaling properties of TCP cells vary depending on the nature of the medial lemniscal, compared to spinothalamic, input.

A similar differential organization has been shown for different types of retinal inputs to the thalamic nucleus for visual processing, the **lateral geniculate nucleus**.

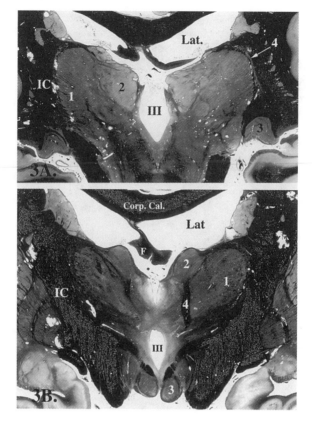

Figure 3. Two sections stained by the Weigert method cut through the thalamus in the coronal plane. **A**, Caudal level. 1 = ventrobasal nucleus (ventroposterolateral and -medial nuclei); 2 = mediodorsal nucleus; 3 = lateral geniculate nucleus; 4 = thin thalamic reticular nucleus; III = third ventricle; Lat. = lateral ventricle; IC = internal capsule. **B**, Rostral level. 1 = ventrolateral and ventroanterior nuclei; 2 = anterior nucleus; 3 = mammillary nucleus of the hypothalamus; 4 = mammillothalamic tract; F = fornix; Corp. Cal. = corpus callosum.

5. How does the thalamus function in sleep-wake mechanisms?

Thalamic neurons that project to the cerebral cortex have two intrinsic patterns of activity: a **depolarized mode**, in which they respond faithfully to afferent sensory input (waking), and a **hyperpolarized oscillatory burst mode**, in which they are relatively uninfluenced by sensory input (sleep). Thalamic neurons are depolarized by the neurotransmitters acetylcholine, norepinephrine, and serotonin produced by various brainstem nuclei. The activities of depolarized thalamic neurons are transmitted to the cerebral cortex to produce the desynchronized electroencephalogram characteristic of the waking state.

About 20 seconds before the onset of sleep, the brainstem cholinergic and monoaminergic neurons reduce their firing rate; the effects of GABA produced by intrinsic thalamic interneurons become predominant; and the thalamic projection neurons become hyperpolarized and enter the burst/oscillatory mode. Thus, the cortex is led to the progressively synchronized activity seen in the deeper stages of sleep (slow wave sleep). After a passage of hours, the activities of the brainstem neurons increase, setting thalamic neurons into the depolarized firing mode and waking up the cerebral cortex. Without these thalamic activities, there is absence of normal function of the cerebral cortex.

6. How does the thalamus participate in coma?

Coma is defined as *unarousable unresponsiveness* to the most intense sensory stimuli. About 50% of cases are due to diffuse brain dysfunction as a result of endogenous or exogenous toxins, or as a result of profound ischemic insult such as that seen following cardiac arrest. The entire cerebral cortex is damaged or malfunctioning in such instances. Focal lesions of the brain, such as those caused by hemorrhage or infarct, may induce coma if they cause **bilateral damage** to much of the thalamus, or damage the midbrain and/or rostral pons bilaterally. It is believed that such lesions destroy the fiber systems between the monoamine and cholinergic systems of the brainstem and thalamus—systems that are necessary to induce arousal of the forebrain.

Lesions in more caudal areas of the brainstem generally do not result in coma.

7. How are nuclei of the thalamus linked to other regions of the central nervous system?

The thalamus is composed of groups of anatomically and functionally distinct nuclei, each with its own set of afferent and efferent connections. The thalamus may be divided into five functional regions:

Connections of Major Thalamic Nuclei

NUCLEI	AFFERENT INPUT	CORTICAL PROJECTIONS	FUNCTION
Ventral/Posterior			
Ventrobasal complex (VPL/VPM)	Spinothalamic tract Medial lemniscus Trigemino-thalamic tract	Somatosensory cortex VPL—limbs and torso VPM—face	Touch; joint position; pain (contralateral limbs, torso, face)
Lateral geniculate nucleus	Retina	Visual cortex	Vision (contralateral visual field)
Medial geniculate nucleus	Inferior colliculus	Auditory cortex	Hearing (bilaterally)
Ventral/Anterior			
Ventrolateral	Deep cerebellar nuclei	Motor cortex	Coordination of movement
Ventroanterior	Basal ganglia	Motor cortex	Initiation of movement
Dorsal/Posterior			
Pulvinar Lateral	Parietal/occipital and temporal cortices	Parietal/occipital and temporal cortices	Processing of multimodal information*
Anterior			
Anterior	Mammillary nuclei	Cingulate cortex	Emotional behavior (limbic system)
Medial			
Mediodorsal nucleus	Amygdala; olfactory cortex	Frontal cortex	Memory, cognition, emotional behavior**

VPL/VPM = ventroposterolateral and -medial nuclei.
* Integration of visual, tactile, and auditory inputs—e.g., the knowledge that a face is that of someone you love.
** In humans, the major medial nucleus is the mediodorsal nucleus that is interconnected with the frontal lobes of the cortex, a region responsible for many of our complex cognitive processes.
Note: The connections and functions of thalamic nuclei are presented as general statements; details have been omitted. For instance, the connections of the thalamic motor nuclei are considerably more complex than indicated by the table.

8. What is the "thalamic pain syndrome"?

Lesions of the somatosensory afferent pathways within the CNS, including their terminations in the thalamus, may result in a *central pain syndrome*, characterized by **hemianesthesia** (loss of sensation of the limbs and torso on one side), with spontaneous, often excruciating, burning pain in the regions that are anesthetic. For example, a patient may exhibit reduced sensory perceptions, such as those of light touch, pinprick, and proprioception, in the right arm and hand, but complain of severe burning pain in the same limb. Pain resulting from injuries to the CNS, whether peripheral or central, is referred to as **neuropathic pain** and is often difficult to treat.

Neuropathic pain may be due to localized infarcts of a somatosensory thalamic nucleus, particularly the ventroposterolateral nucleus (VPL), which receives both spinothalamic tract and medial lemniscal afferents carrying information from the contralateral limbs and torso. A lesion of VPL interrupts the transfer of ascending somatosensory information to the cerebral cortex.

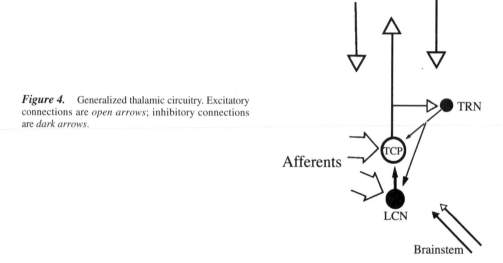

Figure 4. Generalized thalamic circuitry. Excitatory connections are *open arrows*; inhibitory connections are *dark arrows*.

The reason for the loss of sensation is readily understood; the reason for the pain in the anesthetic region is not. Experimental evidence in animals indicates that changes in the somatosensory circuitry are responsible for the abnormal pain syndrome. Whether such changes occur in humans with thalamic injury is not yet known.

9. Are most cases of central pain due to thalamic injury?

No. Studies of several hundred patients with pain following CNS injury have determined that most patients have lesions of the spinothalamic tract in the spinal cord. A substantial majority of patients with spinal cord injury have transient pain, and some have permanent pain symptoms. These patients have diminished perceptions of pinprick and temperature, but innocuous stimuli lead to severe, burning pain in the affected region.

Evidence in animals and humans indicates that there is a loss of normal inhibitory functions that modify the activities of thalamic neurons, leading to abnormal firing of thalamic neurons that transmit to the cerebral cortex.

Case Studies of Thalamic Functions

Patient 1. A 47-year-old, right-handed woman with a history of hypertension suddenly loses consciousness. She is brought to the emergency department, where she gradually awakens. The examining physician finds diminished tactile, proprioceptive, and pain and temperature sensation of the left limbs and torso. She also has a left homonymous hemianopia; visual field testing confirms the hemianopia and demonstrates a zone of preserved vision along the horizontal meridian.

10. What region of the nervous system is damaged in Patient 1?

Injury to many different regions of the brainstem or forebrain might explain the somatosensory findings. But, when combined with the visual deficits, it is very likely that her lesion is in the **right caudal ventrolateral thalamus**, and involves both the VPL and the nearby lateral geniculate nucleus (LGN; see Fig. 3). The zone of preserved visual field along the horizontal meridian is a localizing finding for injury of the LGN, rather than the optic tract or visual cortex. The arterial supply to this region of the thalamus is the anterior choroidal artery, a branch of the middle cerebral artery;

branches of the posterior cerebral artery also supply much of the caudal thalamus. A lesion of this region of the thalamus on the right results in **contralateral deficits** of the visual field and somatosensory system.

Patient 2.   An 88-year-old woman underwent a neurosurgical procedure in 1953, when she was 42, to treat her "hysteria." Prior to surgery, she was said to be combative and "difficult to get along with." Her family stated that she exhibited compulsive behaviors, characterized by repeated hand-washings to "rid herself of evil thoughts." The surgical procedure involved bilateral lesions of the connections between her thalamus and her frontal lobes. For the rest of her life, she was "easier to manage," but showed little interest in her surroundings. She was able to care for herself, but had difficulty remembering past or recent events. She willed her brain to her local medical school for study following her death.

11. What region of the thalamus was damaged in Patient 2?

This women underwent a procedure known as **prefrontal lobotomy**, the intent being to change her behavior. Prefrontal lobotomy is a misnomer, as the frontal lobes are not removed, but many of their connections with the thalamus and other regions of the brain are severed. This procedure was performed on several thousand patients during the 1940s and 1950s, when it was supplanted by the development of drugs that could be used to treat many psychological disorders. Examination of this patient's brain revealed profound degeneration of the projection neurons of the **mediodorsal nucleus** (MD; see Fig. 3), which is the principal source of thalamic projections to the frontal lobes. Thalamic projection neurons undergo retrograde degeneration following injury to their axonal arbors, in this case the axons from MD projection cells to the frontal lobes. Bilateral damage to the frontal lobes, whether by trauma, disease, or surgical procedure, results in substantial changes in cognition, behavior, memory, and language skills.

BIBLIOGRAPHY

THALAMIC ORGANIZATION
1. Blomqvist A, Ericson AC, Craig AD, Broman J: Evidence for glutamate as a neurotransmitter in spinothalamic tract terminals in the posterior region of owl monkeys. Exp Brain Res 108:33–44, 1996.
2. Kim U, Sanchez-Vives mV, McCormick DA: Functional dynamics of GABAergic inhibition in the thalamus. Science 278:130–134, 1997.
3. Ralston HJ III: The fine structure of the ventrobasal thalamus of the monkey and cat. Brain Res 356:228–241, 1984.
4. Ralston HJ III, Ralston DD: Medial lemniscal and spinal projections to the Macaque thalamus: An electron microscopic study of differing GABAergic circuitry serving thalamic somatosensory mechanisms. J Neurosci 14:2485–1502, 1994.
5. Ralston HJ III, Ohara PT, Meng XW, et al: Transneuronal changes of the inhibitory circuitry in the macaque somatosensory thalamus following lesions of the dorsal column nuclei. J Comp Neurol 371:325–335, 1996.
CLINICAL STUDIES/PAIN
1. Boivie J, Leijon GD, Johansson I: Central post-stroke pain: A study of the mechanisms through analyses of the sensory abnormalities. Pain 37:173–185, 1989.
2. Bradley WG, Daroff RB, Fenichel GM, Marsden CD: Neurology in Clinical Practice. Boston, Butterworth-Heinemann Medical, 1999.
3. Canavero S, Bonicalzi V: The neurochemistry of central pain: Evidence from clinical studies, hypothesis, and therapeutic implications. Pain 74:109–114, 1998.
4. Dougherty PM, Li YJ, Lenz FA, et al: Evidence that excitatory amino acids mediate afferent input to the primate somatosensory thalamus. Brain Res 728:267–273, 1996.
5. Lenz FA, Kwan HC, Martin R, et al: Characteristics of somatotopic organization and spontaneous neuronal activity in the region of the thalamic principal sensory nucleus in patients with spinal cord transection. J Neurophysiol 72:1570–1587, 1994.
6. Lenz FA, Garonzik IM, Zirh TA, Dougherty PM: Neuronal activity in the region of the thalamic principal sensory nucleus (ventralis caudalis) in patients with pain following amputations. Neuroscience 86:1065–1082, 1998.
7. Lenz FA, Gracely RH, Baker FH, et al: Reorganization of sensory modalities evoked by microstimulation in region of the thalamic principal sensory nucleus in patients with pain due to nervous system injury. J Comp Neurol 399:125–138, 1998.

18. CEREBRAL CORTEX

Margaret T. T. Wong-Riley, Ph.D.

The cerebral cortex covers a surface area of approximately 2.5 sq ft, but it is extremely convoluted so that two-thirds of it are buried in the depths of sulci or fissures. The cortex varies in thickness from 4.5 mm in the motor cortex to 1.5 mm in the visual cortex. At birth, the human brain weighs about 400 gm. By the end of the third year, the weight is tripled, and by the 18th year, the adult weight of ~ 1400 gm (~3 lbs) is reached. The cortex can be considered our prize possession. It helps us perceive our external and internal environment through our various senses; masterminds our actions and reactions, both simple and complex; and enables us to perform intricate mental functions, experience a variety of emotions, and integrate past memories with present events. Much has been uncovered in the past century about the cortex, but much remains to be explored. Recent functional MRI studies have revealed that the living cerebral cortex responds dynamically to varying conditions and stimuli.

1. What is the embryonic derivation of the cerebral cortex?

The cerebral cortex develops from the **telencephalon**, which is at the rostral end of the neural tube. Two lateral cerebral vesicles are formed rostral and dorsal to the optic vesicles during the seventh week of gestation, and they constitute the primordia of the cerebral hemispheres. The cerebral vesicles expand dorsally, rostrally, and caudally to eventually overshadow the underlying diencephalon, mesencephalon, and cerebellum. Each vesicle has a cavity that forms the lateral ventricle, which connects to the third ventricle of the diencephalon via the interventricular foramen of Monro. Cortical neurons arise from the pseudostratified epithelium lining the ventricular wall. (See Chapter 3, Development of the Nervous System).

2. What phylogenetic terms have been used to describe the cortex?

Most of the human cerebral cortex is made up of six-layered *isocortex* (or *neocortex*). The deeply-lying hippocampus and the dentate gyrus (at one time known as the *archicortex*) are only three-layered. The olfactory cortex (or *paleocortex*) includes the *uncus, parahippocampal gyrus, prepyriform cortex, anterior perforated substance,* and some small, adjacent areas of cortex. The phylogenetic terms archi-, paleo-, and neo-cortex have been rejected by recent investigators on the basis that all vertebrates exhibit at least three pallial subdivisions in the roof of their cerebral hemispheres: medial (hippocampal), lateral (olfactory), and dorsal cortical formations. There is no clear justification to distinguish between old (archi-) and new (neo-) portions of cortex based on phylogeny.

Northcutt RG, Kaas JH: The emergence and evolution of mammalian neocortex. Trends Neurosci 18:373–379, 1995.

3. What are the major anatomical subdivisions of the cortex?

The cerebral cortex is subdivided into three poles (frontal, occipital, and temporal) and six lobes. Each lobe is subdivided into individual gyri or lobules (Fig. 1).

- **Frontal lobe:** precentral, superior frontal, middle frontal, inferior frontal (orbital, triangular, and opercular), orbital, and straight (rectus) gyri, plus anterior portion of paracentral lobule
- **Parietal lobe:** postcentral gyrus, superior parietal lobule, inferior parietal lobule (supramarginal and angular gyri), precuneus, and posterior part of paracentral lobule
- **Temporal lobe:** superior temporal (includes transverse gyri of Heschl beneath the lateral fissure), middle temporal, inferior temporal, and medial occipitotemporal (fusiform) gyri
- **Occipital lobe:** lateral occipital, cuneus, and ligual gyri
- **Insular lobe** (Island of Reil): short and long gyri
- **Limbic lobe:** subcallosal, cingulate, parahippocampal gyri, plus uncus, hippocampus, and dentate gyrus

A

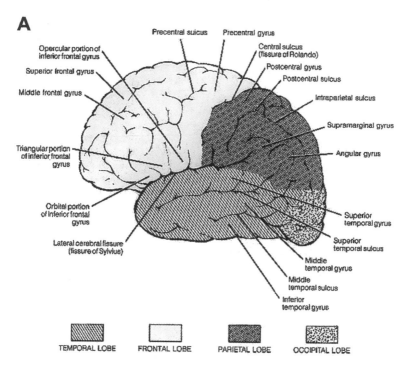

Precentral sulcus
Precentral gyrus
Opercular portion of inferior frontal gyrus
Central sulcus (fissure of Rolando)
Superior frontal gyrus
Postcentral gyrus
Middle frontal gyrus
Postcentral sulcus
Intraparietal sulcus
Supramarginal gyrus
Triangular portion of inferior frontal gyrus
Angular gyrus
Orbital portion of inferior frontal gyrus
Superior temporal gyrus
Lateral cerebral fissure (fissure of Sylvius)
Superior temporal sulcus
Middle temporal gyrus
Middle temporal sulcus
Inferior temporal gyrus

TEMPORAL LOBE   FRONTAL LOBE   PARIETAL LOBE   OCCIPITAL LOBE

B

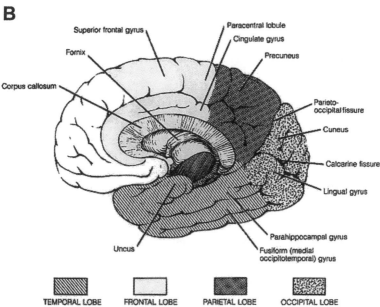

Superior frontal gyrus
Paracentral lobule
Cingulate gyrus
Fornix
Precuneus
Corpus callosum
Parieto-occipital fissure
Cuneus
Calcarine fissure
Lingual gyrus
Parahippocampal gyrus
Uncus
Fusiform (medial occipitotemporal) gyrus

TEMPORAL LOBE   FRONTAL LOBE   PARIETAL LOBE   OCCIPITAL LOBE

Figure 1. Lateral (**A**) and medial (**B**) views of the cerebral cortex showing the frontal, parietal, temporal, and occipital lobes. The insular lobe is deep within the lateral fissure and is not visible. The limbic lobe includes the cingulate, parahippocampal, and subcallosal gyri, as well as the hippocampus and the dentate gyrus deep to the parahippocampal gyrus. (From deGroot J, Chusid JG: Correlative Neuroanatomy, 12th ed. San Mateo, Appleton & Lange, 1988; with permission.)

4. What major arteries supply the cerebral cortex?

The cortex is supplied by two pairs of arteries: the internal carotid arteries and the vertebral arteries. Each internal carotid gives rise to a small **anterior cerebral artery** (ACA) and a large **middle cerebral artery** (MCA). The two vertebral arteries join at the base of the brainstem to form the basilar artery, which in turn bifurcates to form the two **posterior cerebral arteries** (PCA).

The ACA supplies the medial and anterior portions of the cortex (Fig. 2A); the MCA distributes branches to much of the frontal, parietal, occipital, and temporal cortical areas (Fig. 2B); and the PCA supplies most of the posterior portion of the cortex.

The **Circle of Willis** is formed by the three major pairs of arteries (anterior, middle, and posterior cerebral arteries) and two pairs of communicating arteries (the short **anterior communicating artery** between the two anterior cerebral arteries and the longer **posterior communicating arteries**, which join the middle and the posterior cerebral arteries) (Fig. 3). This system of anastomosis ensures collateral circulation if one of the branches is occluded. However, such compensatory circulation may not always be functionally adequate, especially in elderly individuals.

5. What constitutes the major venous drainage of the cortex?

The cerebral veins do not run with the arteries, and their pattern of distribution is distinct from that of the arteries. The fine branches arising from the brain parenchyma form a plexus in the pia mater. From there they form larger cerebral veins, which run in the pia and eventually through the subarachnoid space to empty into the cerebral venous sinuses (Fig. 4). The cerebral veins and the venous sinuses do not have valves, and the thin walls of the veins have no muscular tissue. The sinuses are located between the meningeal and periosteal layers of the dura mater. The **superior sagittal sinus** lies along the superior border of the falx cerebri, while the **inferior sagittal sinus** is along the inferior border. At its posterior end, the inferior sagittal sinus is joined by the **great cerebral vein of Galen** (which drains the deep structures of the brain), and they both empty into the **straight sinus** (rectus sinus). The straight sinus joins the superior sagittal sinus to form the two **transverse sinuses**, one for each side. These curve laterally and downward as the **sigmoid sinuses**, which eventually drain into the internal jugular veins.

The confluent sinus (confluens sinuum) is the site where the superior sagittal, straight, and transverse sinuses come together. It also is joined by a small occipital sinus that ascends within the falx cerebelli.

6. What are the six cellular layers of the cerebral cortex?

   I: The **molecular layer** is fiber-rich but cell-sparse (Fig. 5). Apical dendrites of pyramidal cells from deeper layers ramify amidst the plexus of axons.

   II: The **external granular layer** contains densely packed granule or stellate cells as well as some small pyramidal cells.

   III: The **external pyramidal layer** contains medium-sized pyramidal cells that project either to other cortical areas in the same hemisphere (via association fibers) or the opposite hemisphere (via commissural fibers).

   IV: The **internal granule layer** is rich in small granule or stellate neurons. It is well-developed in primary sensory cortical areas and is greatly expanded in the primary visual cortex (into multiple sublayers). It is the principal recipient site for thalamic afferents.

   V: The **internal pyramidal layer** contains the largest-sized pyramidal cells. It is particularly prominent in the primary motor cortex (home of the Betz cells) and other motor areas of the cortex. Pyramidal cells of this layer are known to project to the basal ganglia, the brainstem, or the spinal cord.

   VI: The **multiform layer** contains many cells with spindle-shaped cell bodies. The pyramidal cells in layer VI project to the thalamus.

7. What major types of neurons are found in the cerebral cortex?

The human cerebral cortex has 10 to 20 billion neurons. They are subdivided into two major cell types: pyramidal and nonpyramidal. *(Answer continues on page 262.)*

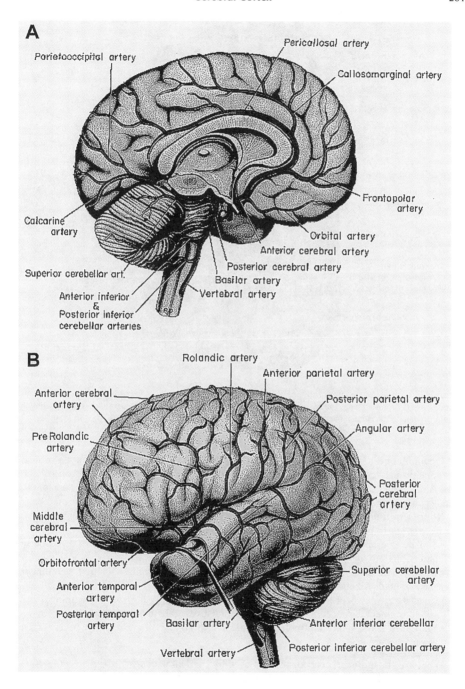

Figure 2. **A,** The major arteries on the medial surface of the brain include the anterior cerebral artery and its branches, the posterior cerebral artery, and arteries that supply the brainstem and cerebellum. **B,** The major arteries of the lateral surface of the brain include the prominent middle cerebral artery and its branches. (From Carpenter MB: Human Neuoranatomy, 7th ed. Baltimore, Williams & Wilkins, 1976; with permission.)

Note: see color panel.

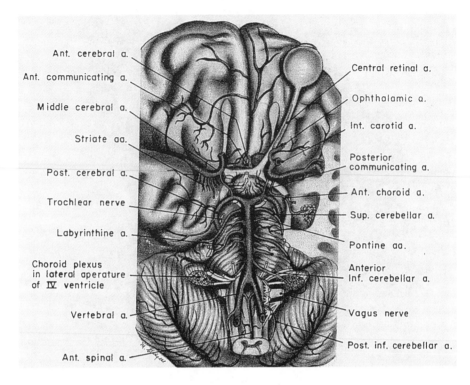

Figure 3. Arteries on the inferior surface of the brain. The Circle of Willis is formed by pairs of anterior, middle, and posterior cerebral arteries; the two posterior communicating arteries; and the anterior communicating artery. (From Carpenter MB: Human Neuroanatomy, 7th ed. Baltimore, Williams & Wilkins, 1976; with permission.)
Note: see color panel.

Pyramidal cells have spine-decorated apical and basal dendrites that ramify in the vertical and horizontal planes, respectively. The axon leaves the cortex for other cortical and subcortical destinations. A recurrent collateral often arises from the main axon and branches in the immediate vicinity to end primarily on stellate neurons. Pyramidal cells are the projection neurons of the cortex.

Nonpyramidal cells, best visualized by the Golgi silver stain, are a diverse group of interneurons whose axons do not leave the cortex:

- Stellate or granule cells: subdivided according to the presence or absence of dendritic spines (spiny, smooth, or sparsely-spined stellates)
- Bipolar, horizontal, fusiform, chandelier, and double-bouquet cells: classified according to the shapes and distribution of their dendrites and/or axons
- Cajal-Retzius cells or horizontal cells of Cajal: axons ramify horizontally within layer I; are very prominent during early development but relatively rare in the adult cortex
- Martinotti cells: small multipolar cells present in almost all cortical layers; axons ascend toward the surface

8. What are the major neurotransmitters used by cortical neurons?

Most, if not all, of the pyramidal relay neurons use **glutamate** (and/or aspartate) as their major excitatory neurotransmitter. The spiny stellate neurons have been reported to be glutamatergic, as well. The majority of the other nonpyramidal neurons, particularly the aspinous or sparsely spinous stellates and the chandelier cells, are inhibitory and use gamma-aminobutyric acid (**GABA**) as their predominant neurotransmitter. Some of the cortical neurons also contain nitric oxide synthase, an enzyme that synthesizes **nitric oxide**, a gaseous neurotransmitter.

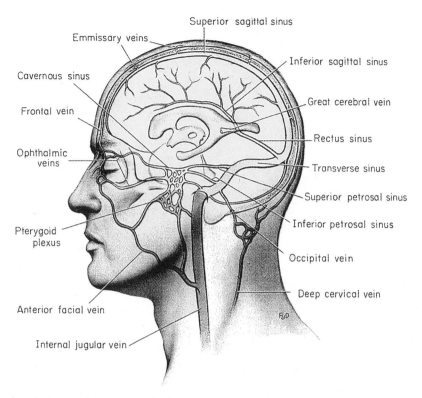

Figure 4.   The intracranial venous sinuses and extracranial veins drain primarily into the internal jugular veins. (From Carpenter MB: Human Neuroanatomy, 7th ed. Baltimore, Williams & Wilkins, 1976; with permission.)   ***Note: see color panel.***

In addition to neurotransmitters, cortical neurons express one or several neuropeptides as modulators of synaptic transmission. These neuropeptides include cholecystokinin, somatostatin, substance P, neuropeptide Y, and vasoactive intestinal polypeptides. Calcium-binding proteins, such as calbindin and parvalbumin, also are expressed by some cortical neurons.

9. Does the cortex receive monoaminergic input?

Yes, there are three monoaminergic pathways projecting to wide areas of the cortex. They are: (1) the **serotonergic pathway** from the midline raphe nuclei of the brainstem, (2) the **noradrenergic (norepinephrine) pathway** from the locus coeruleus, and (3) the **dopaminergic pathway** from the ventral tegmental area of the midbrain (mesolimbic and mesocortical projections). These pathways act through the second messenger system (e.g., cAMP) and affect ion channel activity. They are involved in attention, arousal, mood, motivation, and other complex cognitive functions. Monoamines are implicated in mental and neurologic disorders, such as depression, schizophrenia, drug addiction, and Parkinson's disease. The actions of each neurochemical vary depending on the subtype of receptors expressed as well as on other neurotransmitters or neuromodulators in the synaptic circuit.

10. What is phrenology?

During the late 18th and early 19th century, Franz Josef Gall, an anatomist in Vienna and Paris, proposed that bumps and depressions were correlated with localized brain functions. A bump represented a well-developed gyrus and, therefore, a greater faculty for a particular behavior. A depression represented an underdeveloped gyrus and reduced capacity. Originally, Gall's system had 27

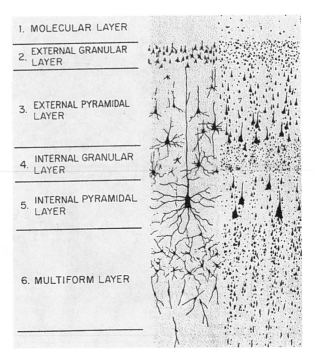

1. MOLECULAR LAYER

2. EXTERNAL GRANULAR LAYER

3. EXTERNAL PYRAMIDAL LAYER

4. INTERNAL GRANULAR LAYER

5. INTERNAL PYRAMIDAL LAYER

6. MULTIFORM LAYER

Figure 5. The six cellular layers of the cerebral cortex are revealed by the Golgi stain *(left column)* and the thionine stain *(right column)*. (Modified from Brodal P: The Central Nervous System. New York, Oxford University Press, 1992.)

faculties, including constructiveness, destructiveness, secretiveness, benevolence, and hope. This practice is known as phrenology or the study of the mind and character based on the shape of the skull. As phrenology expanded there were increasing numbers of faculties. Today, we know that such inference has no sound physiologic basis.

11. How did Brodmann study the cerebral cortex?

Korbinian Brodmann (1868–1918) was a German neurologist who, in 1909, classified the human cerebral cortex into 52 areas according to their cytoarchitecture (cellular organization) and suggested that each area was functionally distinct. He started with area 1 in the postcentral gyrus and ended with area 52 in the anterior transverse temporal gyrus (anterior to area 41) (Fig. 6). His numbering system has been widely implemented because different areas were found to have different functions and connections. However, this system is useful only in a general sense and is less precisely associated with specific functions. The boundaries of Brodmann's areas are not always coincidental with those of functional areas. Area 19, for example, has been found to consist of multiple functional areas in the occipital cortex.

Today, the number of functional cortical areas far exceeds that envisioned by Brodmann.

12. What did Wilder Penfield find when he studied the living cerebral cortex?

Wilder Graves Penfield was a Canadian neurosurgeon who worked at the Montreal Neurological Institute in the mid 1900s. He studied the cortex of conscious patients during therapeutic brain surgery for epilepsy. To ensure that the surgery would not compromise the patient's communication skills, Penfield stimulated different parts of the cortex to determine if he could elicit disorders of speech. He confirmed Wernicke's findings that electrical stimulation of Broca's area (areas 44 and 45) and Wernicke's area (area 22) arrested speech in conscious patients. Penfield also found that stimulation elicited voluntary movements of different parts of the body, indicating a topographical representation of somatic muscles of the contralateral body in the precentral gyrus. This was the basis of the **motor homunculus**. Stimulation of the postcentral gyrus produced tactile sensations such as paresthesias (numbness, tingling) and pressure in the contralateral body surface. This was the basis for the **sensory homunculus**. *(Answer continues on page 266.)*

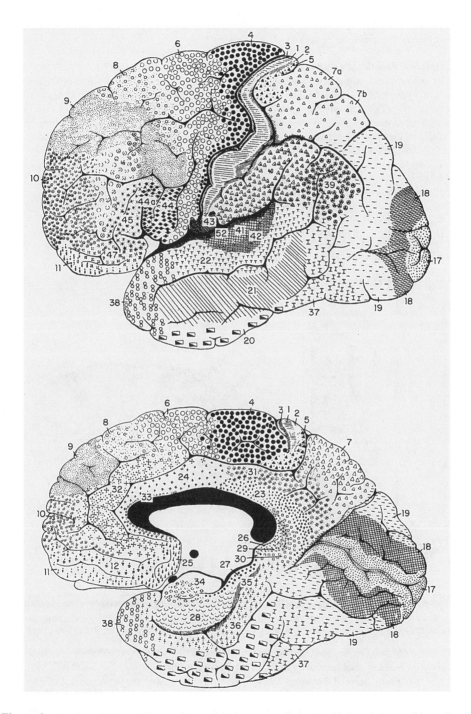

Figure 6. Brodmann's cytoarchitectural map of the human cerebral cortex designates areas with numbers and symbols. (From Brodal P: The Central Nervous System, 2nd ed. New York, Oxford University Press, 1998; with permission.)

Penfield's work followed those of many others, notably Gustav Fritsch and Eduard Hitzig, who described in 1870 how electrical stimulation of discrete areas of the precentral gyrus elicited movement of the contralateral limbs in dogs.

13. How was functional columnar organization discovered in the cortex?

In 1956, Vernon Mountcastle (at Johns Hopkins University) discovered that cells in the somatosensory cortex are organized into functional columns that extend vertically through the six cellular layers (Fig. 7). As he advanced his microelectrodes perpendicularly to the surface of the cortex, he encountered neural units that responded to the same sensory submodality (such as light touch), but when his electrodes were advanced obliquely or tangentially to the surface, he detected a series of units with different submodalities.

The concept of a vertical column as a basic functional unit has widespread applicability, as evidenced by the discovery of ocular dominance and orientation columns in the visual cortex by David Hubel and Torsten Wiesel (see Chapter 5, The Visual System). Even cortico-cortical connections have a columnar organization: cells within a cortical column are connected to cells within another cortical column in either the same hemisphere or opposite hemisphere.

Hubel DH, Wiesel TN: Shape and arrangement of columns in cat's striate cortex. J Physiol 165:559–568, 1963.

Mountcastle VB: Modality and topographic properties of single neurons of cat's somatic sensory cortex. J Neurophysiol 20:408–434, 1957.

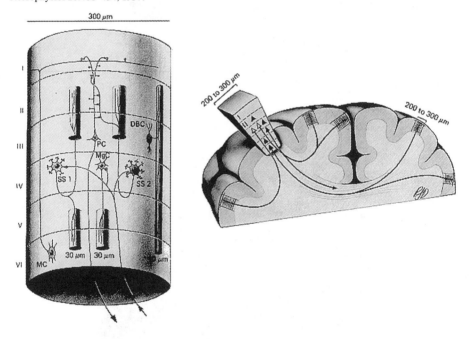

Figure 7.   A cortical column *(left)* and intercortical columnar connections *(right)*. DBC = double bouquet cell; MC = Martinotti cell; MgC = microgliaform cell; PC = pyramidal cell; SS =spiny stellate cell. (Modified from Noback CR, Demarest RJ: The Human Nervous System, 3rd ed. New York, McGraw-Hill, 1981; with permission).

14. How do cortical cells interact within a functional column?

It is thought that layer IV neurons receive excitatory input from the thalamus and transmit the information to layers II and III. Neurons from these supragranular layers project to the infragranular layers V and VI, which provide efferent fibers to subcortical centers. Layer VI sometimes projects back to layer IV. In some cortical areas, such as the visual cortex, layers I, II/III, and VI also receive direct thalamic input.

Such vertical interconnections enable cells within the same column to share similar receptive field properties. Cells within the same ocular dominance column, for example, are driven either exclusively by one eye (layer IV) or predominantly by one eye (supra- and infragranular layers).

15. What are modules in the cortex?

Modules are organized groupings of neurons that are structurally and/or physiologically distinct from surrounding regions within a given area of cortex or a previously defined cortical field. Modules often are sites of high metabolic activity and can be conveniently demonstrated with a metabolic marker, a mitochondrial enzyme cytochrome oxidase. Examples of modules are:

- In the primary visual cortex of primates, including humans, a module has the neural machinery to process visual signals from a specific locus in the visual field (see Chapter 5, The Visual System). These visual signals include eye preference, orientation, color, and spatial frequency. In the macaque monkey, a module contains a minimal representation of different types of functional columns and has a surface area of ~1–2 mm^2. Modules are arranged in a retinotopic fashion throughout the primary visual cortex.
- In the somatosensory cortex of rodents, the modular organization is in the form of layer IV barrels, each representing a single, contralateral mystacial vibrissa. A barrel has a cell-dense wall and a cell-sparse center, the latter of which receives excitatory thalamic input and has a high level of metabolic activity associated with vibrissal sensory whisking.
- In addition to sensory cortex, modules or module-like organization has been described for association cortex such as the retrospinal, perirhinal, and entorhinal cortex. The precise functions of these modules are not known, but entorhinal cortex is intimately associated with the hippocampus and is involved in memory consolidation.

Hevner RF: Cytochrome oxidase and neuroanatomical patterns. In Gonzalez-Lima F (ed): Cytochrome Oxidase in Neuronal Metabolism and Alzheimer's Disease. New York, Plenum Press, 1998.

Purves D, Riddle D, LaMantia AS: Iterated patterns of brain circuitry (or how the cortex gets its spots). Trends Neurosci 15:362–368, 1992.

16. How has the cortex been broadly divided into functional areas?

Classically, the cerebral cortex has been divided into a number of functional areas. Motor cortex, for example, is anterior to the central sulcus (primarily in the precentral sulcus). Somatosensory cortex is posterior to the central sulcus (mainly in the postcentral gyrus, visual cortex is along the two banks of the calcarine fissure (cuneus and lingual gyri), and auditory cortex is ventral to the lateral sulcus in the superior temporal gyrus (Fig. 8). A large expanse of cortex in the parietal, occipital, and temporal lobes is devoted to integrating input from one or more modalities and is known as association cortex. The prefrontal cortex is involved in higher cortical functions such as abstract thinking, mathematical calculations, and other executive functions. The cingulate gyrus and the parahippocampal gyrus are intimately associated with the limbic system.

These classic subdivisions have been useful in parceling general functions to large regions of the cortex. However, they provide only a first step in our understanding of cortical functioning.

17. Is there only a single map for each modality in the cortex?

Contrary to the classic view of the cortex, microelectrode recordings and tract tracings in the last few decades have revealed that each modality, such as somatic sensation, vision, and audition, is represented many times in the cortex. There actually are **multiple maps** in the cortex for each modality. However, although each map represents the same or similar receptive surface, it processes a slightly different aspect of the modality. For example, areas 3a, 3b, 1, and 2 do not form a single somatosensory map of the contralateral body surface, but rather four separate maps, each emphasizing cutaneous, joint, or muscle sensation (see Chapter 4, The Somatosensory System). The somatosensory/motor system includes at least 13 cortical areas. The processing of vision involves as many as 25 visual cortical areas and seven visual-association areas. The processing of audition involves 15 or more areas.

Felleman DJ, Van Essen DC: Distributed hierarchical processing in the primate cerebral cortex. Cereb Cortex 1:1–47, 1991.

Kaas JH, Hackett TA: Subdivisions of auditory cortex and levels of processing in primates. Audiol Neurootol 3:73–85, 1998.

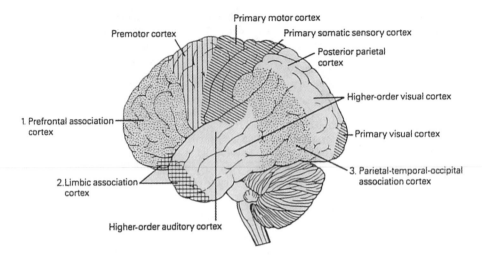

Figure 8. Major functional areas on the lateral surface of the cerebral cortex. (From Kandel ER, Schwartz JH, Jessell TM: Principles of Neural Science, 3rd ed. New York, Elsevier, 1991; with permission.)

18. How is the cortex related to the thalamus?

The cortex is intimately associated with the thalamus (see Chapter 17, The Thalamus). The primary sensory cortices (auditory, somatosensory, and visual) and the primary motor cortex are reciprocally connected with the specific thalamic nuclear groups from which they receive their primary input. If a specific thalamic nuclear group is destroyed, especially during development, the size and organization of the primary cortex will be altered (as shown in rodent and monkey studies). Alternatively, cortical lesions cause severe retrograde degeneration of thalamic neurons that normally project to those areas. Chronic and acute suppression of neuronal activity in primary somatosensory cortex, for example, induces an enlargement of receptive fields in the ventroposterior nucleus of the thalamus.

19. What are the thalamic connections and functions of the major cortical areas?

Cortical Area	Location/ Brodmann's Area	Thalamic Input	General Functions
Primary somato-sensory	Postcentral gyrus Areas 3a, 3b, 1, 2 (S1)	VPL, VPM	3b & 1: cutaneous sensations 3a & 2: muscle receptor sensations Somatotopic representation of contralateral body and face
Primary motor	Precentral gyrus Area 4 (M1)	VL	Voluntary movements of contralateral body and face
Premotor	Area 6 (lateral)	VA	Control of visually guided movements; initiation of action
Supplementary motor area	Area 6 (medial)	VL	Organize & plan complex movements; mediate appropriate motor response to sensory stimuli
Visual	Calcarine Area 17 (V1)	LGN	Contralateral visual field representation; visuotopic organization
Auditory	Superior temporal gyrus Areas 41, 42 (A1)	MGN	Tonotopic representation of sound

Table continued on following page

Cortical Area	Location/ Brodmann's Area	Thalamic Input	General Functions
Association	Posterior parietal Areas 5 and 7	LDN, LP, pulvinar	Somatosensory and visual integration for goal-directed voluntary movements and manipulation of objects; visual guidance of movements
	Parietal, temporal, & occipital Areas 39, 40; portions of 19, 21, 22, 37		Polysensory integration (somatosensory, visual, and auditory) for perception and language
Limbic	Cingulate gyrus, orbitofrontal, parahippocampal	Anterior thalamic nucleus; MD	Motivation, attention; emotions that affect motor planning
Prefrontal	Areas 9–12	MD	Higher mental functions; cognitive behavior; motor strategies & motor planning; emotion

A1 = primary auditory cortex, LDN = lateral dorsal nucleus, LGN = lateral geniculate nucleus, LPN = lateral posterior nucleus, MD = medial dorsal nucleus, MGN = medial geniculate nucleus, M1 = primary motor cortex, S1 = primary sensory cortex, VA = ventral anterior nucleus, V1 = primary visual cortex, VL = ventral lateral nucleus, VPL = ventroposterolateral nucleus, VPM = ventroposteromedial nucleus.

20. Is topographical organization an over-riding theme in the cortex?

Electrical recordings since the early 20th century have revealed precise topographical organization in many major areas of the cortex. The primary motor (M1) and primary sensory (S1) areas each has a somatotopic map of the contralateral half of the body and face. The visual cortex (V1) has a visuotopic map of the contralateral visual field, and the auditory cortex (A1) has a tonotopic map of sound frequencies. These maps are not precisely topographical, however, but rather are skewed toward high-sensitivity areas, such as the face and hand for M1 and S1, and foveal representation for V1. Thus, more cortical areas are devoted to the processing of these key areas than of other body parts or visual space.

In recent years, researchers have found that beyond the "primary" areas of cortex, many association cortical areas have topographical organization as well. Their individual maps, whether somatosensory, somatomotor, visual, or auditory, may be complete or incomplete. In short, the cortex is a well-designed structure, with many organized infrastructures.

21. How is topographical organization illustrated by the Jacksonian epilepsy?

This is a form of an epileptic fit (seizure) that is characterized by unilateral clonic movements that start in one part of the body (or one group of muscles) and spread systematically to adjacent parts. The focal site of the seizure is the contralateral M1, and so the seizure follows a somatotopic map of the contralateral half of the body and face (e.g., tongue, mouth, face, hand, shoulder, trunk, thigh, leg, and toes).

22. Do different cortical areas talk to each other?

Indeed they do, in a panoply of interconnections. There are many association fibers that interconnect functionally related areas in the same and different cortical lobes. S1, for example, is connected to M1 in the frontal lobe and area 5 in the parietal lobe. M1 is connected to the premotor cortex and the supplementary motor cortex in the frontal lobe, as well as to S1, S2, and area 5 in the parietal lobe. Together, the somatosensory/motor system in the macaque has no less than 62 known interconnections. Area 7 in the parietal lobe projects to a polysensory area in the temporal lobe, area 46 in the prefrontal lobe, as well as limbic areas medially (the cingulate gyrus and the parahippocampal gyrus). The visual cortex is extensively interconnected with association areas in the parietal, temporal, and occipital lobes. In fact, there are more than 300 connections among the 32 areas of visual representation found in the macaque, a primate that is closely related to humans. The visual hierarchy includes 10 levels of cortical processing.

Many cortico-cortical connections are reciprocal. These short and long interconnections presumably promote both convergent and divergent processing of information representing the same modality or related modalities, as well as the integration of sensory and motor functions.

23. Are cortical areas of the two hemispheres interconnected?

Yes. Parts of M1 representing the trunk and proximal extremities of the two hemispheres are linked by commissural fibers. Visual cortices representing the vertical meridian in the two hemispheres have reciprocal connections across the corpus callosum. These connections ensure continuity of representation along the midline. Callosal connections also exist for many cortical areas, but they are distinctly absent in most of V1 and in S1 and M1 areas that represent distal extremities (hands and feet).

24. How do neurons in M1 and S1 differ in their response to voluntary movements?

Cells in M1 increase their firing rate immediately *before* the commencement of a voluntary movement. Cells in S1 become active *after* the onset of movement. This indicates that S1 neurons respond to sensory signals from the moving parts, but they do not initiate the movements.

25. Is M1 necessary for learning new motor skills?

M1 is necessary for producing skilled voluntary movements. Recent studies in animals indicate that it may also participate in learning new motor skills. Several lines of evidence lend credence to this concept: (1) Adult M1 representations have been found to be modifiable. (2) The morphology of M1 pyramid cell dendrites can be changed by experience. (3) The efficacy of connections among M1 neurons can change in an activity-dependent, long-term manner. (4) The strength of horizontal intracortical connections in layers II/III of M1 is increased with motor skill learning.

Thus, the capacity for change in adult neurons indicates that both structural and functional reorganization occur in M1 with new learning.

Rioult-Pedotti M-S, Friedman D, Hess G, Donoghue JP: Strengthening of horizontal cortical connections following skill learning. Nature Neurosci 1:230–234, 1998.

26. Are all movements controlled by M1?

No. While M1 is critical for initiating and executing the movement, other cortical areas also exert a strong influence on control of the motor act. For example, the somatosensory cortex contributes sensory information necessary for gauging the motor response, and the premotor and supplementary motor areas are vital in programming and planning the motor response (see Chapter 11, The Motor Cortex).

27. What is the premotor area?

The premotor area (PMA) is located in front of the primary motor cortex, on the *lateral* side of the frontal lobe in Brodmann's area 6. Penfield stimulated this area in humans and evoked complex movements of either side of the body. PMA has a somatotopic motor map concerned with higher-order, skilled, voluntary movements, such as precise hand movements in performing rhythmic sequences (playing the piano) or coordinating visually guided, unilateral or bilateral movements (grasping an object, swinging a golf club). PMA neurons fire after the appearance of a sensory signal for a certain movement, but *before* the onset of the movement.

Damage to the PMA does not cause paralysis, but rather a difficulty in coordinating skilled movements. There also is a tendency to repeat the same movement over and over again, even though the movement may be incorrect and does not accomplish the intended goal. This tendency is known as **perseveration**, and is common among patients with prefrontal lobe lesions.

PMA receives input from the prefrontal lobe and projects to M1 and to reticulospinal neurons that control proximal motor units. It also is connected with the red nucleus, the basal ganglia, and, indirectly, with the cerebellum. Moreover, visually guided behavior requires a strong connection with extrastriate cortical areas.

28. What does the supplementary motor area do?

The supplementary motor area (SMA) is located on the *medial* side of the frontal lobe, in front of the primary motor cortex, again in Brodmann's area 6. Like PMA, it is somatotopically organized, but unlike PMA—which indirectly controls proximal motor units—SMA directly innervates distal motor units. It is concerned with programming and performing *complex* movements, either real or imagined, that are appropriate to specific sensory stimuli. Cells in SMA respond to sensory cues (visual, somatosensory) that signal certain voluntary movement, and SMA neurons respond earlier than those in M1. Damage to SMA results in an inability to perform a previously facile task, such as both hands cooperating in a complex motor act.

SMA receives input from the ventrolateral nucleus of the thalamus as well as from the prefrontal cortex. It projects to M1, the reticular formation, and the spinal cord. Thus, the SMA contributes directly and indirectly to the corticospinal pathway.

29. Are there other motor areas in the medial wall of the frontal cortex?

Besides SMA, researchers have uncovered at least three motor areas buried within the cingulate sulcus and a pre-SMA in front of the SMA proper in the monkey frontal cortex. Most of these areas probably have their counterparts in the human, as suggested by positron emission tomographic studies.

While the cingulate gyrus is part of the limbic system, the cingulate motor areas in the depth of the cingulate sulcus are related to the motor system. These areas are involved in the initial ("higher-order") stages of movement generation as well as in various simple and complex tasks, such as in speech production and targeted eye movements.

The pre-SMA appears to be involved in the selection and preparation of movement, especially during the initial stages of skill acquisition, while the SMA is more concerned with the execution of complex motor acts. For example, the pre-SMA is activated when an individual is playing an unfamiliar piece of music that has cognitive/motor demands, and the SMA is activated when the individual is playing a well-rehearsed set of scales. SMA and pre-SMA are reciprocally involved during motor learning. Both areas also participate in targeted eye movements and in speech.

Picard N, Strick PL: Motor areas of the medial wall: A review of their location and functional activation. Cereb Cortex 6:342–353, 1996.

30. What are the functions and connections of areas 5 and 7 in the posterior parietal cortex?

Areas 5 and 7 of the parietal association cortex mediate somatosensory and visual integration for purposeful motor actions. They receive input from somatosensory, visual, and auditory cortical areas, and they project to motor and premotor areas. Area 5 is essential for linking somatosensory information to goal-directed voluntary movements and to object manipulations. Area 7 integrates visual and somatosensory information for coordinated eye and hand movements. Through their connections with the prefrontal cortex and the cingulate gyrus, the posterior parietal cortex influences attention, emotions, and motivation associated with behavior elicited by various sensory modalities (Fig. 9).

Mountcastle first described neurons in the posterior parietal cortex as units that increased their firing before the animal moved its arm toward an object of interest. For example, a monkey sees a banana and reaches out to get it. Mountcastle suggested that **command neurons** might direct the animal's motivated action toward a perceived sensory target.

31. What happens when there is a lesion in the posterior parietal cortex?

Bilateral lesions of the posterior parietal cortex often lead to difficulty in knowing or understanding the meaning of a previously familiar sensory stimuli in the absence of sensory loss. This **agnosia** (inability to recognize) can be manifested as visual agnosia, tactile agnosia, or asterognosis (inability to recognize objects by their three-dimensional form). Agnosia often leads to an inability to perform a visually guided movement because the patient has difficulty gauging the size and distance of objects or the spatial relationship of objects. The patient also cannot seem to attend to more than one detail at a time. The inability to carry out purposeful movements in the absence of paralysis or other motor or sensory impairment is known as **apraxia**. Constructional apraxia is an inability to place objects in their proper two-dimensional or three-dimensional framework.

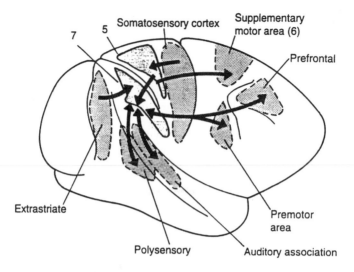

Figure 9. Cortico-cortical connections of the posterior parietal cortex (areas 5 and 7, also called parietal association cortex) in a monkey brain, which closely resembles the human brain. Connections with the limbic cortical areas are not shown. (From Brodal P: The Central Nervous System, 2nd ed. New York, Oxford University Press, 1998; with permission.)

32. Can agnosia and apraxia occur with lesions outside of the posterior parietal cortex?

Yes. Patients with lesions in the prefrontal cortex, the thalamus, or the basal ganglia can have similar symptoms. These areas all have connections to the parietal cortex.

33. What is the functional significance of the parietal-temporal-occipital association cortex?

As the name implies, these are association areas in the parietal, temporal, and occipital lobes, including Brodmann's areas 39, 40, and portions of 19, 21, 22, and 37 (see Fig. 6). They receive input from primary sensory areas (somatosensory, visual, and auditory) and project to premotor, limbic, and prefrontal areas of the cortex. These areas mediate polymodal sensory integration for purposeful actions, and they are involved in the control of multisensory perception, movement, and motivation. They also are intimately concerned with language processing.

The superior temporal gyrus (area 22) is intimately associated with the auditory cortex, while the inferior temporal cortex (IT; parts of areas 37 and 19) is dominated by processed visual information from the extrastriate cortex. Neurons in IT often respond to familiar faces or objects. Lesions in IT lead to **visual agnosia** (psychic blindness) that is manifested by an inability to distinguish complex visual patterns and difficulty in recognizing previously familiar objects and persons. Stimulation of the temporal association cortex may elicit recalled memories of past events or imagined events, while bilateral lesions of the temporal association cortex result in profound amnesia.

34. What is Gerstmann's syndrome?

Josef Gerstmann (born in 1887) was a Vienna neurologist who described a host of symptoms resulting from lesions in the **angular gyrus** (Brodmann's area 39) of the *dominant* hemisphere (usually the left). These symptoms include finger agnosia (inability to recognize one's own or another's fingers), right-left disorientation, agraphia (inability to put thoughts into writing), acalculia (inability to do simple mathematical calculations), and, often, constructional apraxia (inability to copy simple drawings or to reproduce models with building blocks). In some cases, alexia (inability to read and comprehend previously known words) also is present.

Gerstmann J: Syndrome of finger agnosia, disorientation for right and left, agraphia and acalculia. Arch Neurol Psychiat (Chic) 44:398, 1940.

35. What happens with a lesion in the angular gyrus on the nondominant side?

Unilateral lesion of the nondominant (usually right) angular gyrus can result in **contralateral neglect**. This is a unilateral spatial deficit in which the patient ignores the existence of objects, features, and even his or her own body parts contralateral to the side of the lesion. Thus, the patient draws the face of a clock with all the numbers on the right side and nothing on the left, or dresses only the right side of the body. The patient's own left extremities are viewed as foreign objects. Parietal lesions also affect initial stages of motor planning as well as perception. These symptoms indicate that the inferior parietal cortex may be critically involved in visual awareness (see Chapter 20, Higher Cortical Functions).

Driver J, Mattingley JB: Partial neglect and visual awareness. Nature Neurosci 1:17–22, 1998.

36. Where is Wernicke's area?

This cortical area is named after Karl Wernicke, a German neurologist (1848–1905), who, in 1876, described a type of aphasia that involved a disturbance in the comprehension rather than the execution of speech. Wernicke proposed that Broca's area controlled the motor program of speech, while the sensory perception of speech was in the temporal lobe area. Thus, Wernicke's area originally was a speech center in the posterior portion of the superior temporal gyrus. In time, the area has included the supramarginal and angular gyri of the inferior parietal lobule, as well. These parietal association cortical areas are where spoken or written words are converted to an auditory code used in both speech and writing.

Lesions in this area result in **sensory (receptive) aphasia**. Patients can speak, but have difficulty comprehending previously familiar spoken and written language. However, studies in recent years indicate that language processing is more complex than the "one area: one deficit" concept.

37. Where is Broca's area?

Pierre Paul Broca (1824–1880) was a French anatomist, anthropologist, and surgeon who, in 1861, described a patient who could understand language but could neither speak grammatically nor in full sentences. In 1863, he documented eight cases in which language was affected by damage to the left frontal lobe, and in the following year he proposed that language expression was controlled mainly in the left cortex. Broca's area is located in parts of the triangular and opercular portions of the inferior frontal gyrus (parts of Brodmann's areas 45 and 44, respectively) and is dominant in most individuals in the left hemisphere.

Lesions in this area result in **motor (expressive) aphasia**. Patients understand, but cannot express themselves in spoken or written language. Milder forms may involve incorrect word choices or grammatical constructions in a patient who previously knew the correct form. As mentioned above, language processing probably is more complex than the "one area: one deficit" concept.

38. What is the arcuate fasciculus?

This is the arching fibrous tract that connects Wernicke's area with Broca's area (Fig. 10). Its function is thought to be the transformation of sensory (auditory) aspects of speech to motor execution of spoken and written language.

Lesions of the arcuate fasciculus lead to **conduction aphasia**. Patients understand spoken and written words, but cannot repeat simple phrases. They can speak fluently, but use incorrect words and pronunciations.

39. What is the Wada procedure?

The procedure was developed by John Wada of the Montreal Neurological Institute to test for the cerebral dominance of language. An injection of a barbiturate, usually sodium amytal, is made into the internal carotid artery to anesthetize the ipsilateral hemisphere for about 10 minutes. If the anesthetized hemisphere is dominant for speech, the patient will be transiently aphasic. However, if the anesthetized hemisphere is not dominant, then the patient's language function will not be interrupted.

Wada's procedure revealed dominance of the left hemisphere for speech in 96% of right-handed individuals and 76% of left-handed people. Interestingly, bilateral representations of speech are present only among left-handed people.

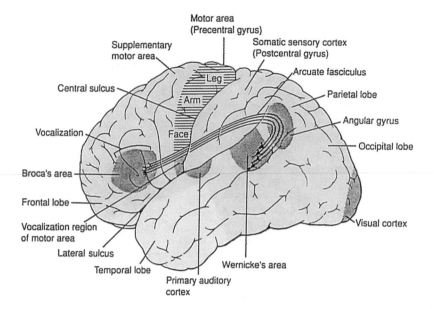

Figure 10. The major cortical areas involved in language (including Wernicke's area, Broca's area, and angular gyrus). The arcuate fasciculus is the major fiber tract linking these areas. (From Kandel ER, Schwartz JH, Jessell TM: Principles of Neural Science, 3rd ed. New York, Elsevier, 1991; with permission.)

40. How functionally significant is the prefrontal association cortex?

The prefrontal association cortex (areas in front of the premotor area [PMA] and the supplementary motor area [SMA]) has great functional significance. It is a "general-purpose central executive" involved in attention, affect, emotion, memory, and motor aspects of behavior. It participates in higher mental processing, such as mathematical calculations, analysis, judgment, foresight, and motivation. It confers the ability to form and retain concepts of objects in time and space when the objects are no longer visible, and contributes to "working" memory (rather than associative memory) when the individual performs a visuo-spatial delayed-response task. It also is important in the planning and execution of complex voluntary movements and in organizing goal-oriented behavior.

41. What are the connections of the prefrontal association cortex?

Prefrontal association cortex receives input from the parietal, occipital, and temporal association cortex and the cingulate gyrus (Fig. 11). The major subcortical inputs arise from the medial dorsal nucleus (MD) of the thalamus and the basolateral amygdala. The prefrontal cortex projects to the PMA, SMA, and parietal and temporal association cortex, as well as to the caudate nucleus, hypothalamus, and back to the MD and amygdala. It is in a position to integrate and organize input from various sensory modalities with the emotional and motivational state of the individual in the execution of goal-directed complex movements and mental tasks.

42. True or false: Prefrontal cortex comprises one processing domain.

False. Recent findings indicate that the prefrontal cortex contains separate processing mechanisms for remembering the "what" and "where"of an object, similar to the "what" and "where" processing streams of the visual system. This implies that input from the two visual streams is somewhat segregated in the prefrontal cortex for encoding working memory of spatial location and object identity. For example, an area in the inferior convexity of the prefrontal cortex contains neurons that respond to pictures of faces or specific objects. This area receives direct projections from an area in the inferior temporal complex (known as TE in the monkey), where neurons also respond to complex stimuli such as faces. Imaging studies in humans support the spatial segregation of processing domains: a **spatial processing domain** located in the middle frontal gyrus (including area 46), an **object processing domain** located more inferiorly, and a **linguistic processing domain** still more inferiorly.

Damage to the prefrontal cortex results in a dysfunction of the central executive, such as disorganization, perseveration, and distractability.

Goldman-Rakic PS: The prefrontal landscape: Implications of functional architecture for understanding human mentation and the central executive. Phil Trans R Soc Lond B 351:1445–1453, 1996.

Scalaidhe SPO, Wilson FAW, Goldman-Rakic PS: Areal segregation of face-processing neurons in prefrontal cortex. Science 278:1135–1138, 1997.

Wilson FAW, Scalaidhe SPO, Goldman-Rakic PS: Dissociation of object and spatial processing domains in primate prefrontal cortex. Science 260:1955–1958, 1993.

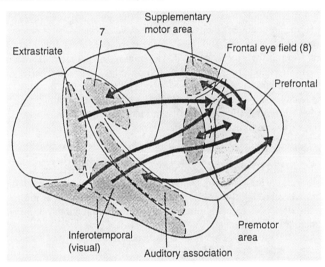

Figure 11. Extensive cortico-cortical connections in the prefrontal cortex of a monkey. Connections with the limbic cortical areas are not shown. (From Brodal P: The Central Nervous System, 2nd ed. New York, Oxford University Press, 1998; with permission.)

43. What are the consequences of prefrontal lobe lesions?

Lesions of the prefrontal lobe result in few or no sensory or motor deficits, but there is usually a dramatic change in mood and personality. Formerly sociable, garrulous, and well-adjusted individuals often become apathetic, indifferent, depressed, withdrawn, and quiet, or irreverent, indulgent, profane, immature, and lacking in social graces. The individual typically is unable to change a response when the stimulus changes (perseveration) and, at the same time, is easily distracted and unable to remain attentive or perform continuous activities.

44. Who was Phineas Gage?

Phineas Gage was a young foreman at a railroad construction in Vermont when an accidental dynamite explosion sent an iron rod through his head, from under his left eye through his left frontal lobe. The rod was 3 ft 7 in long, with a diameter of 1.25 in at its widest point. Phineas survived the incident, but underwent a marked personality change. From a well-balanced, smart, and capable individual, he became fitful, impatient, obstinate, and profane. This famous case was documented by Dr. John Harlow in 1848 (the year of the accident) and as a follow-up in 1868. It demonstrates the importance of the frontal lobe in emotional expressions, behavior, and personality traits.

Blumer D, Benson DF: Personality changes with frontal and temporal lobe lesions. In Benson DF, Blumer D (eds): Psychiatric Aspects of Neurologic Disease. New York, Grune and Stratton, 1975.

45. Where is the limbic association cortex?

It is parceled among portions of the parietal, frontal, and temporal lobes. It is concerned with emotional and motivational aspects of behavior and with memory. Deep within the temporal lobe is the hippocampus, which also is critical for memory (see Chapter 19, The Limbic System).

46. How is memory stored in the cortex?

Although memory generally is thought of as being stored in many regions of the cerebral cortex, different types of memory are stored in different portions of the brain.

A famous case involved a young patient (H.M.) who underwent bilateral removal of the medial portion of the temporal lobe as a therapeutic treatment against uncontrollable seizures. He suffered a profound loss of the ability to transfer most types of learning from short-term memory (lasting seconds and minutes) to long-term memory (lasting days or longer). However, H.M. retained his memory of events that preceded his surgery, and he had intact short-term memory. He also could learn new motor skills normally. These facts suggested that there are different types of memory.

Lesions of the medial temporal lobe disrupt long-term storage of *new* memory. The hippocampus stores new memory temporarily and transfers the learned information to other cortical areas for more permanent storage. Memory comes in two major forms: explicit and implicit. **Explicit memory** deals with facts and the *what* aspect of knowledge. **Implicit memory** involves learning *how* to do things. The **medial temporal lobe** is concerned with explicit learning and memory, and it includes the hippocampus, the entorhinal cortex (which projects to the hippocampus), the subiculum (which receives input from the hippocampus), and the parahippocampal cortices. Implicit learning and memory of perceptual and motor skills often has an automatic or reflexive quality, and memory of a specific task involves the **specific sensory or motor system** that learns such tasks and stores the learned information.

Recent functional MRI studies showed that the dorsolateral prefrontal cortex and the parahippocampal cortex are active during the encoding of memories. Specifically, the left prefrontal and the left parahippocampal cortex jointly promote memory formation for verbalizable experiences (word memory), while the right posterior prefrontal cortex and bilateral parahippocampal cortex are activated by visual memory (picture memory).

Brewer JB, Zhao Z., Desmond JE, et al: Making memories: Brain activity that predicts how well visual experience will be remembered. Science 218:1185–1187, 1998.

Kandel ER, Schwartz JH, Jessell TM (eds): Essentials of Neural Science and Behavior. Norwalk, Appleton and Lange, 1995.

Wagner AD, Schacter DL, Rotte M, et al: Building memories: Remembering and forgetting of verbal experiences as predicted by brain activity. Science 281:1188–1191, 1998.

47. Does sensory deprivation during early stages of postnatal development cause lasting changes in the cortex?

Studies conducted over the last three decades on macaque monkeys have shown that sensory deprivation, such as eyelid suture, during the first 6–12 months of life can impart persistent changes in the structural and physiological properties of cortical neurons. Behaviorally, the animal no longer responds appropriately to visual cues, even when vision is restored to both eyes.

Absence or deprivation of a primary sensory input during early development can result in the expansion of other sensory modalities into parts of the cortex not normally devoted to such modalities (see Chapter 25, Neural Plasticity).

48. Can cortical maps reorganize in the adult?

This is an interesting question. The adult brain has been perceived as a relatively static entity with little, if any, ability for plastic change. Major changes in the adult brain have been attributed to trauma, aging, dementia, and other types of pathology, with resultant loss of function.

Studies in the last few decades, however, have clearly pointed to a much more dynamic brain capable of plastic changes even in the normal adult. Cortical areas deprived of usual sensory input undergo physiological and structural (e.g., synaptic) reorganization and respond to neighboring receptive surfaces. Some of the reorganizations are disorderly and transient. However, other changes appear to be the basis for learning, memory, functional adaptation to changing environment, and functional recovery after injury.

Noninvasive human studies using focal transcranial electric and magnetic stimulation have shown reorganization of cortical representation in (1) motor maps after amputation, spinal cord injury, and hemispherectomy, and (2) sensorimotor maps of finger representation induced by learning in blind, Braille-reading individuals. In addition, animal studies have demonstrated the reorganizing capacity within the adult visual, auditory, somatosensory, and motor cortical areas. Plasticity can be induced in cortical output as well as in cortical receptive areas.

In short, the adult cortex can no longer be viewed as a static entity with hard-wired circuits.

Kaas JH: Plasticity of sensory and motor maps in adult mammals. Annu Rev Neurosci 14:137–167, 1991.

Pascual-Leone A, Cohen LG, Hallett M: Cortical map plasticity in humans. Trends Neurosci 15:13–14, 1992.

Wong-Riley MTT: Primate visual cortex: Dynamic metabolic organization and plasticity revealed by cytochrome oxidase. In Peters A, Rockland K (eds): Cerebral Cortex, Vol. 10—Primary Visual Cortex in Primates. New York, Plenum Press, 1994, pp 141–200.

BRAIN IMAGING STUDIES

49. In what ways can the living cortex be studied?

In addition to the study of clinical signs and symptoms and postmortem analysis, the cortex can be studied invasively and noninvasively. When the skullcap is removed during therapeutic surgery, the living cortex can be stimulated directly (see Question 12). Both extracellular and intracellular recordings are used in animal studies. The living brain is imaged less invasively by ultrasound, computed tomography, positron emission tomography (PET), single photon emission computed tomography (SPECT), magnetoencephelography (MEG), magnetic resonance imaging (MRI), magnetic resonance spectroscopy (MRS), and functional MRI. Functional MRI, in particular, is based on changes in blood flow, blood volume, and oxygenation when specific regions of the brain are activated. These noninvasive techniques have delineated various functional regions of the living brain and detected abnormalities previously postulated or demonstrable only postmortem. (See Chapter 22, Neuroimaging.)

50. What is the Talairach coordinate space?

The Talairach coordinate space is the prevailing standard used in functional neuroimaging studies for reporting the location of brain foci being activated. The stereotaxic atlas is based on a series of sparsely sampled sections through a postmortem brain.

Talairach J, Tournoux P: Coplanar stereotaxic atlas of the human brain. New York, Thieme, 1988.

51. What is the "Visible Man"?

The "Visible Male" is a computerized digital atlas of the human body published by Spitzer, et al. in 1996. Van Essen's group has extended this atlas and generated surface reconstructions and cortical flat maps based on the geometry, geography, and functional organization of the human cerebral cortex. They also used cardinal coordinate axes based on the Talairach stereotaxic atlas (1988), but the Visible Man's brain is slightly smaller than the Talairach brain. The advantage of the Visible Man atlas is its high resolution in both volume and surface reconstructions.

Spitzer V, Ackerman MJ, Scherzinger AL, Whitlock DJ: The Visible Male: A technical report. J Am Med Informat Assoc 3:118–130, 1996.

Van Essen DC, Drury HA: Structural and functional analyses of human cerebral cortex using a surface-based atlas. J Neurosci 17:7079–7102, 1997.

52. Which cortical area is involved in the analysis of the temporal aspect of sound?

Recent brain imaging studies, such as PET, have revealed that the processing of short-term (pitch computation) temporal information resides bilaterally in the superior temporal gyrus (STG) near the primary auditory cortex of Heschl. The processing of longer-term (melodic pattern) temporal information occurs bilaterally in the STG posterior to the Heschl's gyrus and bilaterally in the superior temporal sulcus/middle temporal gyrus.

Griffiths TD, Rees G, Rees A, et al: Right parietal cortex is involved in the perception of sound movement in humans. Nature Neurosci 1:74–79, 1998.

53. What does functional MRI reveal about cortical areas for fine and complex movements?

Functional MRI showed that simple finger movements activate the contralateral primary motor cortex, as expected. However, it also revealed that complex hand movements activate additional areas, including the supplementary motor area (SMA), bilateral premotor area, and contralateral somatosensory cortex. During imagined complex movements, the SMA and, to a lesser degree, the premotor cortex are activated. The SMA also is found to be involved in the explicit timing of movements. Furthermore, there is a hemispheric asymmetry whereby the right primary motor cortex is activated by contralateral finger movements, and the left motor cortex is activated by both contralateral and ipsilateral movements. This effect is more pronounced in right-handed individuals.

Kim S, Ashe J, Hendrich K, et al: Functional magnetic resonance imaging of motor cortex: Hemispheric asymmetry and handedness. Science 261:615–617, 1993.

Rao SM, Binder JR, Bandettini PA, et al: Functional magnetic resonance imaging of complex human movements. Neurol 43:2311–2318, 1993.

54. What cortical areas are activated by language processing in functional MRI studies?

Functional MRI has revealed that many more areas are activated by language functions than previously recognized. The left prefrontal cortex beyond the classical Broca's area, for example, is activated across a variety of language tasks and is involved in language comprehension. In addition, the left middle temporal gyrus, inferior temporal gyrus, and angular gyrus cortex surrounding Wernicke's area (posterior superior temporal gyrus [STG]) play a more important role in comprehension at a linguistic-semantic level than the classical posterior cortical areas known to be involved in language. The STG (including Wernicke's area and the planum temporale) is reported to be critical for complex sound analysis but not for language per se. This assertion is based on the finding that STG is not modulated by the semantic content (meaningfulness) of language or by the type of cognitive task involved in language. Rather than a transcortical concept center for language, new functional MRI data suggest that there is a left-hemisphere-dominant language network with a distributed system of knowledge regarding semantic relationships and linguistic symbols representing these relationships.

Binder JR: Neuroanatomy of language processing studied with functional MRI. Clin Neurosci 4:87–94, 1997.

BIBLIOGRAPHY

1. Bear MF, Connors BW, Paradiso MA: Neuroscience: Exploring the Brain. Baltimore, Williams and Wilkins, 1996.
2. Brodal P: The Central Nervous System. New York, Oxford University Press, 1992.
3. Buonomano DV, Merzenich MM: Cortical plasticity: From synapses to maps. Annu Rev Neurosci 21:149–186, 1998.
4. Kandel ER, Schwartz JH, Jessell TM (eds): Principles of Neural Science. 3rd ed. New York, Elsevier Publishing Co., Inc., 1991.
5. Kandel ER, Schwartz JH, Jessell TM (eds): Essentials of Neural Science and Behavior. Norwalk, Appleton and Lange, 1995.
6. Ross MH, Romrell LJ, Kaye GI: Histology: A Text and Atlas. 3rd ed. Baltimore, Williams and Wilkins, 1995.
7. Swanson G (ed): Special Issue: Evolution and Development of the Cerebral Cortex. Trends Neurosci, Vol 18, 1995.
8. Talairach J, Tournoux P: Co-Planar Stereotaxic Atlas of the Human Brain. New York, Thieme Medical Publishers, 1988.

19. THE LIMBIC SYSTEM

Sara J. Swanson, Ph.D., and Elliot A. Stein, Ph.D.

INTRODUCTION AND HISTORY

1. What is the limbic system?

A functional anatomic system of interconnected cortical and subcortical structures including the hippocampal formation, parahippocampal gyrus, amygdala, fornix, septal area, cingulate gyrus, mammillary bodies, and anterior thalamus. It is an area of intimate interaction between hypothalamic activity and cortical information processing. The limbic system plays a role in emotions, learning, and autonomic regulation. Its structures are considered a unified system because of their rich reciprocal anatomic interconnections and common behavioral, physiologic, and neurochemical properties.

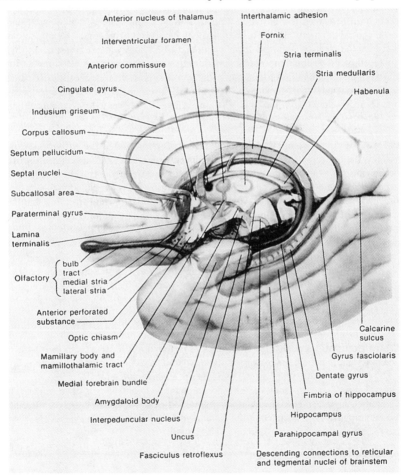

Figure 1. The limbic system. (From Netter FH: The Ciba Collection of Medical Illustrations. Volume 1, The Nervous System. Part I, Anatomy and Physiology. Brass A, Dingle RV (eds): CIBA, 1986; with permission.)

Note: see color panel.

2. What is the origin of the term limbic?

The 1878, Paul Broca coined the term "le grande lobe limbique," which means border or hem, to designate a group of anatomically related structures that were in close proximity to the olfactory system and formed a border between the hypothalamus and cerebral cortex. Because of the anatomic interconnections between the olfactory system and limbic structures, the limbic system was originally thought to have developed to process olfactory information. Together, the olfactory and limbic structures were called the rhinencephalon (smell-brain).

3. What was the original Papez's circuit?

Papez, a neurologist, proposed in 1937 that the limbic structures formed a circuit:

cingulate → hippocampus → fornix → mammillary bodies → anterior thalamus → cingulate

Papez's ideas were considered revolutionary at the time since he was proposing an anatomic substrate for emotion. He believed that input from cortical areas entered the circuit, was elaborated as emotion, and then ultimately influenced the hypothalamus to release appropriate hormones. These structures and their interconnections "constitute a harmonious mechanism which may elaborate the functions of central emotions as well as participate in emotional expression." Emotional awareness was achieved in the cingulate, which added "emotional color" to psychic processes.

More recently, the mammillary nuclei, anterior nucleus of the thalamus, and hippocampus have been shown to be more important for memory function than emotion (see questions 10, 23, and 40). Limbic areas that did not figure prominently in the original Papez circuit, such as the septal area, nucleus accumbens (NAcc), ventral tegmental area (VTA), and amygdala, appear to have emotional functions.

Papez JW: A proposed mechanism of emotion. Arch Neurol Psychiatry 38:725–744, 1937.

4. What was MacLean's contribution to current understanding of the limbic system?

He coined the term limbic system and reintroduced Papez's theory that limbic structures might be the neuroanatomic substrate for emotion. MacLean's work and theories were based on experimental data suggesting that cortical and hypothalamic information is integrated in the limbic system. He diminished the role of olfaction, laying to rest the "smell brain" and stressing that the limbic system is a target of multisensory input. He added structures more vital for emotional regulation, including the amygdala, septal area, and orbital frontal cortex. MacLean described two main functional subdivisions within the limbic system: (1) the septal pathway (septal region, cingulate, and hippocampus), important for species preservation, including social and sexual behavior, and (2) the amygdala pathway (amygdala and frontotemporal regions), with a presumptive role in self-preservation behaviors such as fighting, feeding, and fleeing, as well as visceral functions.

NEUROANATOMY OF LIMBIC STRUCTURES

5. List the primary fiber pathways of the limbic system and the structures they interconnect.

- Medial forebrain bundle: interconnects hypothalamic nuclei and forebrain (septum, amygdala, and hippocampus with midbrain VTA and interpeduncular nuclei.
- Fornix: connects the septum with the hippocampus and hypothalamus (mammillary nucleus).
- Mammillothalamic tract: connects mammillary bodies and anterior nucleus of the thalamus.
- Ventral amygdalofugal path: connects the amygdala with the hypothalamus, dorsal medial nucleus (DMN) of the thalamus, and rostral cingulate.
- Perforant path: connects neurons in layer II of the entorhinal cortex (EC) with dentate gyrus and CA_3 region of the hippocampus.
- Stria terminalis: connects the posterior aspect of the amygdala with the bed nucleus of the stria terminalis, NAcc, septum, and anterior hypothalamus (Figs. 2 and 3).

6. In what direction is information carried along the fiber pathways between limbic structures?

Almost all limbic fiber tracts are bidirectional.

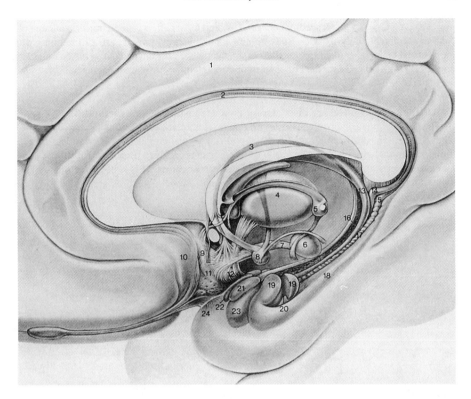

Figure 2.   Structures of the human limbic system, midsagittal perspective. 1 Gyrus cingulus, 2 Indusium griseum, 3 Stria terminalis, 4 Nucleus medialis thalami, 5 Nuclei habenulae, 6 Nucleus ruber, 7 Fasciculus telencephalicus medialis, 8 Corpus mamillare, 9 Septum verum, 10 Area subcallosa, 11 Gyrus diagonalis, 12
Fibrae amygdalofugales ventrales, 13 Crus fornicus, 14 Gyrus fasciolaris, 15 Fasciola cinerea, 16 Fissura
choroidea, 17 Gyrus dentatus, 18 Subiculum, 19 Cornu ammonis, 20 Site of limbus Giacomini, 21 Nucleus
corticalis amygdalae, 22 Nucleus anterior amygdalae, 23 Nuclei basalis + lateralis amygdalae, 24 Cortex
prepiriformis. (From Nieuwenhuys R, Voogd J, van Huijzen Chr: The Human Central Nervous System: A
Synopsis and Atlas, 3rd ed. Berlin, Springer-Verlag, 1988; with permission.)

7. Describe the anatomic connection between the hippocampus and the mammillary body.

White matter fibers called the **alveus** originate in the hippocampus and converge in a bundle
called the **fimbria**. The fimbria exits the posterior aspect of the hippocampus as the crus of the fornix.
The two crura are in close proximity to the undersurface of the corpus callosum and converge into the
body of the **fornix**. The fornix is an arched bundle of over one million fibers. The body of the fornix
splits anteriorly into the columns of the fornix, which connect with the mammillary bodies (Fig. 4).

8. Describe the gross anatomy of the hippocampal formation.

The hippocampal formation consists of the hippocampus ("sea horse"), which extends through
the floor of the temporal horn of the lateral ventricle, parahippocampal gyrus, and dentate ("tooth")
gyrus. The hippocampus proper (Ammon's horn) forms an interlocking "C" with the dentate gyrus,
so named because of its notched appearance. The parahippocampal gyrus consists of the subiculum,
presubiculum, parasubiculum, and EC (Fig. 5).

9. How is the hippocampal formation internally organized?

The hippocampus proper is divided into four subfields designated by the letters CA for cornu
Ammonis or Ammon's horn. The superior part of the hippocampus is called CA_1, and the inferior

portion is CA_3. CA_2 is a small section between CA_1 and CA_3. CA_4 is a small transitional area of hippocampus and dentate gyrus. This basic organization is identical in all parts of the hippocampus. The principal cell type of the hippocampus is the pyramidal cell; the dentate gyrus contains mainly granule cells. Basket cells are the principal inhibitory interneurons in both the dentate gyrus and the hippocampus proper (Fig. 6; also see Fig. 5).

10. Which thalamic nuclei are most closely associated with limbic structures?

The anterior nuclear group (AN) of the thalamus receives projections from the mammillary bodies and is reciprocally connected to the hypothalamus and cingulate. It is considered the "most limbic" of the thalamic nuclei. The DMN of the thalamus received projections from the temporal lobe and amygdala and projects to the entire prefrontal cortex. It is critical for memory and is thought to integrate sensory information with emotions. The AN and DMN are functionally significant for emotional tone and recent memory.

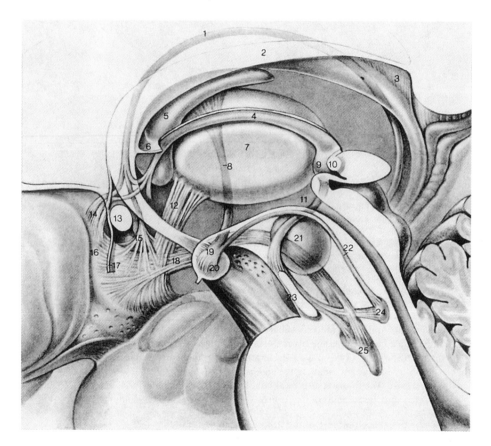

Figure 3. The central parts of the human limbic system, illustrating tracts and nuclei. 1 Stria terminalis, 2 Fornix, 3 Commissura fornicis, 4 Stria medullaris thalami, 5 Nucleus anterior thalami, 6 Tela choroidea ventriculi tertii, 7 Nucleus medialis thalami, 8 Tractus mamillothalamicus, 9 Nuclei habenulae, 10 Commissura habenulae, 11 Tractus habenulointerpeduncularis, 12 Pedunculus thalami inferior, 13 Commissura anterior, 14 Precommissural components (stria terminalis, stria medullaris thalami, fornix), 15 Stria terminalis postcommissuralis, 16 Septum verum, 17 Lamina terminalis, 18 Fasciculus telencephalicus medialis, 19 Fasciculus mamillaris princeps, 20 Corpus mamillare, 21 Nucleus ruber, 22 Tractus mamillotegmentalis, 23 Nucleus interpeduncularis, 24 Nucleus tegmentalis dorsalis, 25 Nucleus centralis superior. (From Nieuwenhuys R, Voogd J, van Huijzen Chr: The Human Central Nervous System: A Synopsis and Atlas, 3rd ed. Berlin, Springer-Verlag, 1988; with permission.)

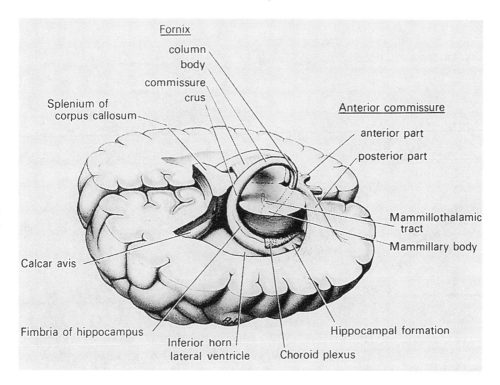

Figure 4. Horizontal section showing the fimbria, fornix (crus, body, and columns), hippocampal formation, and mammillary body. (From Parent A: Carpenter's Human Neuroanatomy, 9th ed. Baltimore, Williams & Wilkins, 1996, with permission.)

11. Describe the entorhinal cortex.

The EC is located in the anterior part of the parahippocampal gyrus, Brodmann's area 28. It is located on the medial surface of the temporal lobe, and its cytoarchitecture suggests that it is a transitional zone between hippocampus and temporal neocortex. EC receives afferent fibers from many neocortical regions, while the efferent fibers from the EC project primarily to hippocampus, but also to anterior cingulate, dentate gyrus, and amygdala. For this reason, the EC is considered a relay station, transferring sensory, motor, and cognitive information from the neocortex to the hippocampus and thus the entire limbic system.

12. Describe the anatomic location, afferents, and efferents of the cingulate gyrus.

Cingulate cortex is a large limbic structure located primarily dorsal to the corpus callosum. It is the main target for the AN of the thalamus and is one of the key efferent targets of the hippocampal formation. Projections from the subicular complex and EC convey information processed in the hippocampus. The cingulate receives input from more thalamic nuclei than any other cortical area. Pyramidal neurons in the cingulate cortex project to motor areas and the striatum (caudate, NAcc, and putamen), accounting for the role of the anterior cingulate in motor, premotor, and executive functions. Thalamic connections to cingulate likely account for its role in behavioral responses to nociceptive stimuli. A portion of caudal anterior cingulate is considered nociceptive cortex (see Fig. 10). Other anterior cingulate projection sites appear to regulate visceromotor, autonomic, and endocrine functions, and emotional vocalizations.

Devinsky O, Morrell MJ, Vogt BA: Contributions of anterior cingulate cortex to behaviour. Brain 118:279–306, 1995.

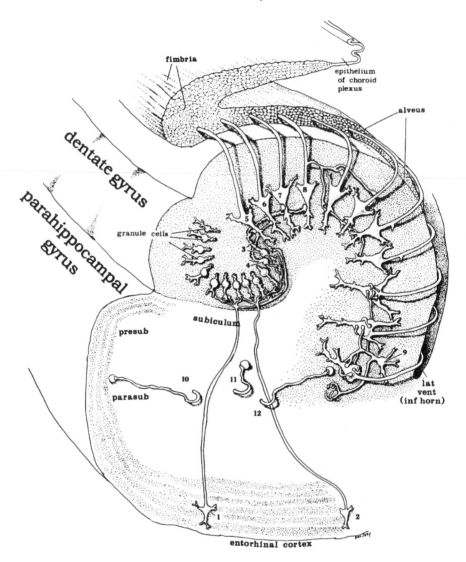

Figure 5. Hippocampal formation including the dentate gyrus and parahippocampal gyrus (subiculum, presubiculum, and parasubiculum). Neurons 1 and 2 project from medial and lateral entorhinal cortex to the dentate gyrus, where they synapse with granule cells. Granule cells 3 and 4 of the dentate gyrus synapse with hippocampal pyramidal cells 5, 6, 7, and 8. These pyramidal cells extend toward the lateral ventricle where they form the alveus. Also shown is a basket cell (9), which makes synaptic baskets around several pyramidal neurons in Ammon's horn. (From Poritsky R: Neuroanatomy: A Functional Atlas of Parts and Pathways. Philadelphia, Hanley & Belfus, Inc., 1992; with permission.)

13. What are the main divisions of the amygdala?

The amygdala is an almond-shaped group of nuclei in the dorsomedial portion of the temporal lobe, continuous with the uncus of the parahippocampal gyrus. The major divisions include the mediocentral nuclei, the cortical portions, and the basolateral complex (basal, lateral, and accessory basal nuclei).

The major connections to the amygdala can be separated into subcortical and cortical origins.

14. Describe the *subcortical* connections to the amygdala.

Olfactory tract: projects mainly to corticomedial nuclei and indirectly from piriform cortex to basolateral nuclei; reciprocal connections back to olfactory bulb

Basal forebrain: reciprocal link includes nucleus basalis of Meynert

Striatum: perhaps one of most substantial efferents of amygdala, with prominent outputs to NAcc, putamen, and caudate

Hippocampus: projections to EC, hippocampus, and subiculum; only meager projections back to amygdala

Thalamus: to DMN, which then projects to same region of orbitofrontal cortex that receives direct amygdala projections; no reciprocal projections from DMN back to amygdala; also reciprocal projections to nucleus reuniens and centralis midline nuclei

Hypothalamus: from corticomedial to anterior hyopthalamic, supraoptic, paraventricular, and ventromedial nuclei (few reciprocal hypothalamic connections back to amygdala)

Brainstem: to autonomic nervous system (ANS) regulatory structures including periaqueductal gray, parabrachial nuclei, dorsal motor nucleus of vagus, and reticular formation; prominent projections from substantia nigra pars compacta and VTA, providing potent dopamine connections; locus coeruleus provides norepinephrine input and the dorsal raphe nucleus provides serotonergic input.

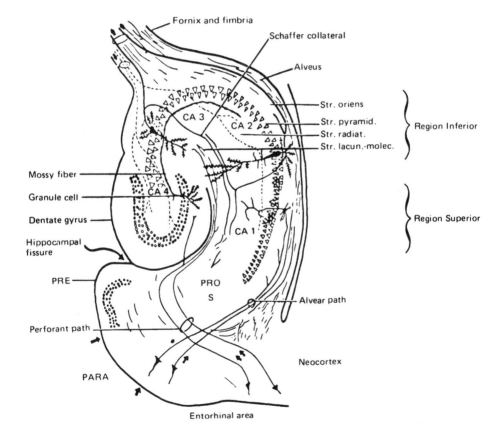

Figure 6. Internal organization of the hippocampal formation showing the cornu Ammonis subfields. Str. oriens = stratum oriens; Str. pyramid = stratum pyramidale; Str. radiat. = stratum radiatum; Str. lacun.-molec = stratum lacunosum-moleculare; PRE = presubiculum; PARA = parasubiculum; PRO = prosubiculum; S = subiculum. (From Isaacson RL: The Limbic System, 2nd ed. New York, Plenum Press, 1982; with permission. Adapted from Brodal A: Neurological Anatomy. New York, Oxford University Press, 1969.)

15. Describe the *cortical* connections to the amygdala.

Most sensory-related cortical regions: prominent reciprocal connections;inputs from visual, auditory, and somatosensory cortex (are from upstream processing regions, not primary sensory cortex)

Cingulate temporal areas, insula, and perirhinal and frontal cortex: amygdala likely receives enormous amounts of convergent sensory information; via its outputs, can influence and activate emotions and modulate sensory processing based on affective states (Fig. 7).

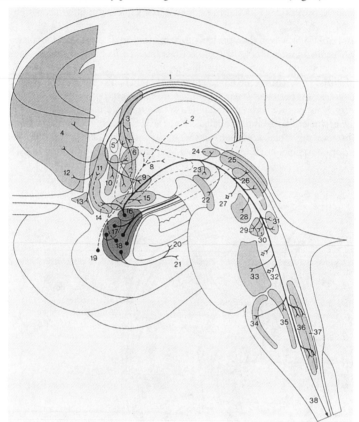

Figure 7. Amygdala efferent projections to the hippocampus and subcortical structures. 1 Stria terminalis; 2 Nucleus medialis thalami, pars medialis; 3 Nucleus interstitialis striae terminalis; 4 Nucleus caudatus + putamen; 5 Commissura anterior; 6 Nucleus paraventricularis; 7 Nucleus anterior hypothalami; 8 Area lateralis hypothalami; 9 Nucleus ventromedialis; 10 Nucleus preopticus; 11 Nuclei septi + nucleus gyri diagonalis, pars dorsalia; 12 Nucleus accumbens; 13 Tuberculum olfactorium; 14 Nucleus gyri diagonalis, pars ventralis; 15 Substantia innominata; 16 Nucleus centralis amygdalae; 17 Nuclei corticalis + medialis amygdalae; 18 Nuclei basalis + lateralis amygdalae; 19 Cortex periamygdaloideus; 20 Subiculum; 21 Cortex entorhinalis; 22 Substantia nigra, pars compacta; 23 Area tegmentalis ventralis; 24 Nucleus peripeduncularis; 25 Griseum centrale mesencephali; 26 Nucleus raphes dorsalis; 27 Nucleus cuneiformis; 28 Nucleus centralis superior; 29 Nucleus coeruleus; 31 Nuclei parabrachiales; 32 Formatio reticularis rhombencephali; 33 Nucleus raphes magnus; 34 Nucleus raphes pallidus; 35 Nucleus raphes obscurus; 36 Nucleus dorsalis nervi vagi; 37 Nucleus solitarius; 38 Fibrae amygdalospinales. (From Nieuwenhuys R, Voogd J, van Huijzen Chr: The Human Central Nervous System: A Synopsis and Atlas, 3rd ed. Berlin, Springer-Verlag, 1988; with permission.)

16. Discuss the internal organization and principal projections of the septum.

The septal gray matter generally is divided into medial and lateral septal nuclei. The medial group is composed of the medial septal nucleus and the nucleus of the diagonal band of Broca. Cells in this area primarily contain the neurotransmitters acetylcholine and GABA and project principally to the hippocampus, EC, and presubiculum, mostly via the fornix.

The lateral nuclei comprise multiple subdivisions, including the septofimbral nucleus, with nerve cells strung along the fornix and fimbria.

The principal descending outputs of the septum enter either the medial forebrain bundle, descending through the hypothalamus (including lateral hypothalamus, preoptic area, and mammillary nuclei) and terminating in the midbrain tegmentum, or the stria medularis, which connects the septum to the habenula. Afferents into the septum include fibers from the hippocampus and amygdala. Most inputs, however, enter via the medial forebrain bundle, carrying information from the hypothalamus, VTA (dopaminergic), raphe (serotonergic), and locus coeruleus (adrenergic) (Fig. 8).

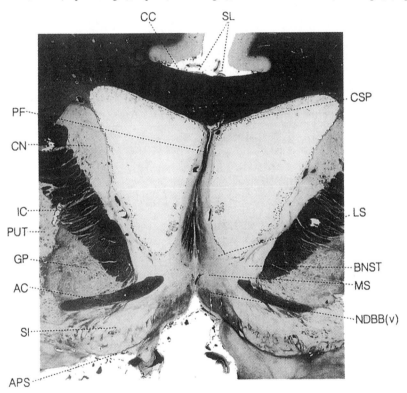

Figure 8. Coronal section of the human brain through the level of the lateral ventrical and septum. AC = anterior commissure, APS = anterior perforated substance (tuberculum olfactorium), BNST = bed nucleus of the stria terminalis, CC = corpus callosum, CN = caudate nucleus (head), CSP = cavum septi, GP = globus pallidus, IC = internal capsule, LS = lateral septal nucleus, MS = medial septal nucleus, NDBB(v) = nucleus of the diagonal band of Broca, PF = precommissural fornix, PUT = putamen, SI = substantia innominata, SL = striae Lancisii mediales of indusium griseum. (From Gloor P: The Temporal Lobe and Limbic System. New York, Oxford University Press, 1997; with permission.)

17. What is the main olfactory pathway?

Olfactory receptors at the top of the nasal cavities are bundled to form the olfactory nerve (cranial nerve I), which penetrates the cribriform plate and synapses in the olfactory bulb, a multi-layered analog of the retina. The olfactory tract is a band of white matter that serves as the output of the olfactory bulb. The olfactory tract runs beneath the orbital frontal area to the anterior perforated substance, where it separates into the medial and lateral olfactory stria. The medial stria cross the anterior commissure and extend to the opposite olfactory bulb. The lateral stria project to the **ipsilateral periamygdaloid and prepiriform areas**, considered the primary olfactory cortex.

From primary olfactory cortex, fibers project to EC, DMN of the thalamus, amygdala, hypothalamus, and septal area. The anatomic association between olfactory afferents and limbic structures likely accounts for the role of olfaction in eating, social and sexual behavior, and memory (Fig. 9).

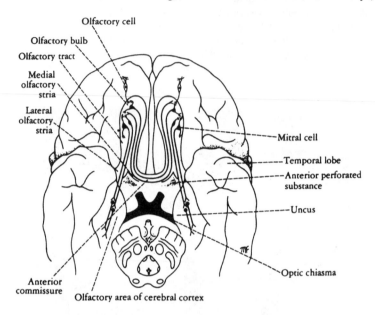

Figure 9.   The olfactory pathway. Cranial nerve I synapses in the olfactory bulb and extends as the olfactory tract, which separates into the medial and lateral olfactory stria. (From Snell RS: Clinical Neuroanatomy for Medical Students, 4th ed. Philadelphia, Lippincott-Raven, 1997; with permission.)

18. What differentiates the olfactory system from other sensory systems?

First, together with gustation, olfaction is the only sensory information that is processed primarily in limbic and paralimbic structures. Second, olfactory tracts connect primarily with ipsilateral pyriform cortex, whereas other sensory systems are crossed. Third, the olfactory system is the only sensory system in which afferent fibers do not synapse in the thalamus prior to reaching cortex.

FUNCTIONAL NEUROANATOMY

19. What are the broad functional divisions of the limbic system?

The **rostral** limbic system—amygdala, septum, orbitofrontal cortex, anterior insula, and anterior cingulate—is important for emotion. The **caudal** limbic system—hippocampus, posterior parahippocampal cortex, and posterior cingulate gyrus—is important for memory and visual spatial functions.

20. What are the principal functional roles ascribed to the amygdala?

The amygdala is critical for assigning affective significance to stimuli by forming stimulus-reinforcement associations. More specifically, the amygdala is thought to be involved in:

- **Preservation of self behaviors:** feeding, fighting, self-protection, and autonomic and emotional responses
- **Learning:** coordination of information from different sensory modalities and association of stimuli with emotional responses (as shown by amygdala's importance in the acquisition of classically conditioned emotional responses)

• **Emotional processing:** amygdaloid lesions in humans produce deficits in recognition of facial emotions. Positron emission tomography (PET) studies show activation in the amygdala when humans process fearful faces. Primates with amygdaloid lesions no longer show emotional responses to threatening stimuli. Intracranial recording studies demonstrate that amygdaloid activity increases with increasing emotional significance and social ambiguity in monkeys. Amygdalectomized wild monkeys become social isolates, because they are no longer able to interact socially; they eventually wander off to die.

Morris JS, Friston KJ, Büchel C, et al: A neuromodulatory role for the human amygdala in processing emotional facial expressions. Brain 121:47–57, 1998.

21. What are the functional consequences of a septal lesion in humans?

Lesions of the septum, often as a consequence of a ruptured anterior communicating artery, can cause amnesia. The amnesia usually is anterograde and limited to memory dependent on hippocampal function, and can be both verbal and nonverbal, but does not include procedural memory or priming. Cell loss in the septum has been strongly correlated with Alzheimer's disease, although it is uncertain how much of the pathology is due to loss of acetylcholine or GABA influence on the hippocampus. There are reports of septal lesions occurring during intraventriculoperitoneal shunt placement, resulting in hypersexuality in humans.

22. Is the cingulate gyrus considered functionally and anatomically homogenous?

No. The cingulate (Brodmann's areas 24, 25, 32) is divided into the **anterior executive region**, which is considered important for integrating affective and motor behavior, and the **posterior cingulate**, which is important for visual spatial and memory functions. The anterior cingulate has important visceromotor regulatory functions: electrical stimulation of this area can modulate virtually all ANS and most endocrine functions. The anterior and posterior cingulate regions differ in cytoarchitecture, connections, and functions (Fig. 10).

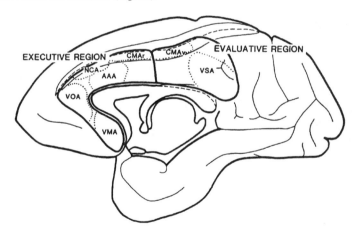

Figure 10. Functional divisions of the cingulate gyrus in a rhesus monkey brain, medial view. The major divisions are the executive and evaluative regions *(thick outlines)*. The executive region is further divided into the visceromotor (VMA), vocalization (VOA), nociceptive (NCA), attention to action (AAA), and rostral cingulate motor (CMAr) areas. The evaluative region is divided into the ventral cingulate motor (CMAv) and the visuospatial (VSA) areas. (From vogt BA, Finch DM, Olson CR: Functional homogeneity in cingulate cortex: The anterior executive and posterior evaluative regions. Cereb Cortex 2:435–443, 1992; with permission.)

23. What is thought to be the principal function of the hippocampus?

Both animal and human research has clearly demonstrated that the hippocampus is critical for establishing new memories (called recent, long-term, episodic, or declarative memory). Bilateral lesions to the hippocampus result in amnesia, which is the inability to acquire new information such as facts and events (declarative memory). However, skill-based or procedural memory and immediate memory (span memory) are preserved. The hippocampus also is involved in spatial recognition and learning in lower animals.

24. Is there a distinct emotional learning circuit in the brain?

Pioneering work by the laboratory of Dr. Joseph LeDoux and others has revealed a central role for the amygdala, notably the basolateral region, in emotional memory formation and expression. Using a rat fear-conditioning model, the amygdala has been shown to integrate sensory and emotional stimuli arriving from primary sensory, association, and polymodal cortices (including an EC-hippocampus-subiculum link) and the thalamus. The amygdala then outputs information for emotional expression via the bed nucleus of the stria terminalis (BNST) and anterior pituitary to regulate stress hormone release; via the parabrachial and dorsal motor nucleus of the vagus to regulate parasympathetic function; via the peri-aqueductal gray for emotional and behavioral expression; via the lateral hypothalamus and medulla for sympathetic regulation; and via the nucleus borsalis of Meynert to modulate attention and arousal.

LeDoux JE: Emotion: Clues from the brain. Annu Rev Physiol 46:209–235, 1995.

25. How can the spectrum of behavioral changes associated with the anterior cingulate be accounted for?

The anterior cingulate (AC) is considered an area where thought, motivation, emotion, and movement are integrated. The AC amplifies and filters affective states and is important for making the transition from early premotor to behavioral states. Thus, excessive amplification of emotions and motor responses may lead to anxiety, tics, impulsivity, and obsessive compulsive disorder. Excessive filtering may lead to apathy and akinesias such as akinetic mutism seen with bilateral cingulate lesions.

26. What are the roles of the entorhinal cortex and hippocampus in epilepsy?

Nissl-stained tissue from patients with temporal lobe seizures show pronounced cell loss in layer III of rostral medial EC. The preferential neuronal death in this area is thought to be due to oversecretion of excitatory amino acids (e.g., glutamate) during seizures and may have a functional impact on target neurons in the hippocampus.

Ammon's horn or hippocampal sclerosis is a common histologic finding in patients with idiopathic complex partial seizures. Hippocampal cell loss is considered both a cause and a consequence of repeated seizures. Early brain injury or febrile convulsions may lead to cell loss in the dentate gyrus—neurons that have an inhibitory effect on hippocampal neurons—resulting in a hyperexcitable state. Repeated seizures lead to additional cell loss and eventually the full syndrome of hippocampal sclerosis. Removal of the sclerotic hippocampus often results in seizure freedom.

Du F, Schwarcz R, Tamminga CA: Entorhinal cortex in temporal lobe epilepsy. Am J Psychiatry 152:826, 1995.
Sloviter RS, Tamminga CA: The hippocampus in epilepsy. Am J Psychiatry 152:659, 1995.

27. Describe the cytoarchitecture arrangement of limbic cortex.

In contrast to the six-layered neocortex, the hippocampus is three-layered allocortex. The cingulate gyrus or outer ring of the limbic system represents a transitional area between neocortex and allocortex, and is referred to as mesocortex.

28. Stimulation of which limbic structures is most likely to result in emotional and experiential phenomena?

Pierre Gloor's work showed that electrical stimulation of the temporal lobe limbic structures with intracerebrally implanted electrodes in epilepsy patients resulted in experiential phenomena. The most common psychic and experiential phenomena included fear, déjà vu (an inappropriate sense of familiarity), jamais vu (a feeling that a familiar place is unfamiliar), elementary and complex visual and auditory hallucinations, illusions, memories, forced thinking, and emotional distress. Of all the limbic system structures, stimulation of amygdala, hippocampus, or both together were most likely to result in the experience of these psychic or emotional phenomena.

Gloor P, Olivier A, Quesney LF, et al: The role of the limbic system in experiential phenomena of temporal lobe epilepsy. Ann Neurol 12:129–144, 1982.

29. What are the behavioral effects of lesions and stimulation to the structures of the limbic system?

Structure	Lesion	Stimulation	_patient[?]_ [handwritten]	Bilateral Lesions
Hippocampus	R ↓ nonverbal memory L ↓ nonverbal memory	Emotions, illusions, memories, fears	↘	Anterograde amnesia
Amygdala	↓ Emotion, placidity ↓ Social reactivity ↓ Affective response to stimuli Indiscriminant hypersexuality ↓ Facial learning ↓ Discrimination of facial emotions ↓ Affective vocalizations	Rage or fear Complex experiential, emotional, and perceptual experiences in humans Autonomic and behavioral defense responses Changes in gut activity		Klüver-Bucy syndrome
Septal region	Hypersexuality Rage Hyperemotionality ↓ Memory	Sexual arousal, orgasm, pleasure, euphoria		
Mammillary bodies				Korsakoff's syndrome*
Anterior cingulate	↓ Anxiety ↓ Social awareness R lesion—contralateral motor neglect Apathy, depression Disinhibition Pain relief Abolition of conditioned emotional vocalizations Reduction of obsessive compulsive behaviors Impaired motor initiation	Heightened arousal Affective vocalizations Aggression Penile erection Autonomic and endocrine changes Visceromotor changes Rituals		Akinetic mutism Docile behavior

* Usually in combinations with lesions in medial thymus and hypothalamus
R = right, L = left

30. Discuss the anatomy of the mesocorticolimbic system and its role in reinforcement.

The mesocorticolimbic (MCL) system is one of three dopamine-containing tracts in the central nervous system (CNS) (Fig. 11). The others are the nigrostriatal system, between the substantia nigra, pars compacta, and the caudate putamen, and the tuberoinfundibular path from the arcuate nucleus of the hypothalamus to the pituitary. MCL system cell bodies originate within the mesencephalic ventral tegmental area (VTA), and axons project rostrally to terminate in such limbic regions as the amygdala, nucleus accumbens (NAcc; mesolimbic division), and neocortical frontal lobe including the orbitofrontal, medial frontal, and anterior cingulate cortex (mesocortical division).

The MCL system has been implicated in positive reinforcement behaviors including feeding, drinking, sexual activity, and drug abuse (cocaine, opiates, ethanol, and marijuana). In humans, disregulation within this system has been implicated in the positive and negative symptoms of schizophrenia.

31. Why is the nucleus accumbens thought to play a prominent role in reinforced behavior?

The NAcc, a component of the ventral striatum, is said to lie at the limbic-motor interface, whereby emotions are translated into actions (Fig. 12). It receives prominent inputs from the hippocampus, frontal lobes, VTA, EC, amygdala, and several thalamic nuclei. After integration, the outputs of the NAcc are motor and ANS regulatory centers, including the ventral pallidum, globus pallidus, entopeduncular nucleus, BNST, pedunculopontine nucleus, and various hypothalamic nuclei involved in emotional expression.

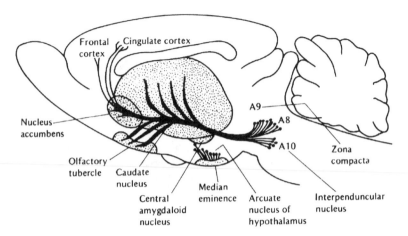

Figure 11. Central dopamine pathways, with major nerve terminal regions *(dots)*. (From Cooper JR, Bloom FE, Roth RH: The Biochemical Basis of Neuropharmacology, 4th ed. New York, Oxford University Press, 1982; with permission. Modified from Ungerstedt U: Acta Physiol Scand Suppl 367, 1971.)

32. What is LAMP?

LAMP or limbic system–associated membrane protein was described by Levitt and colleagues and is considered a marker for the limbic system. It is a neuron-specific glycoprotein that was isolated from rat hippocampus. LAMP is expressed extracellularly on the cell membranes of limbic structure neurons (especially cingulate cortex and anterior thalamic nuclei) and on structures connected with the limbic system. LAMP immunoreactivity is observed early in fetal development. The protein is considered a genetically-controlled cell-recognition molecule, which may be crucial for establishing connections between limbic system structures.

Levitt P, Eagleson KL, Chan AV, et al: Signaling pathways that regulate specifications of neurons in developing cerebral cortex. Dev Neurosci 19:6–8, 1997.

33. What is kindling?

Kindling, an animal model of epileptogenesis, is a process by which repeated subthreshold electrical stimulation to a brain region eventually leads to spontaneous convulsions. The hippocampus and amygdala are the areas most susceptible to kindling. It is thought that the electrical stimulation, similar to the interictal EEG abnormalities observed in epilepsy patients, results in strengthening of synaptic connections. Kindling may account for the progressive nature of seizure disorders and possibly for the interictal personality changes that occur in some individuals with intractable epilepsy.

MEMORY

34. Who is H. M.?

H. M. is a famous patient who developed a dense anterograde amnesia after undergoing bilateral medial temporal lobe resection in 1953 for the treatment of intractable epilepsy. Examination of H. M. revealed the role of mesial temporal structures in memory. Postoperatively, H. M.'s intelligence was high average and well preserved. Language functions, visual spatial abilities, and personality were unchanged, but he was amnestic for all information and events since the time of the surgery. H. M. was unable to enter new information into long-term memory or establish any permanent memories following the surgery. He stated: "Every day is alone in itself, whatever enjoyment I've had and whatever sorrow I've had." (Milner, et al., 1968)

Scoville WB, Milner B: Loss of recent memory after bilateral hippocampal lesions. J Neurol Neurosurg Psychiatry 20:11–21, 1957.

Milner B, Corkin S, Teuber HL: Further analysis of the hippocampal amnesic syndrome: 14-year follow-up study of H. M. Neuropsychologia 6:215–234, 1968.

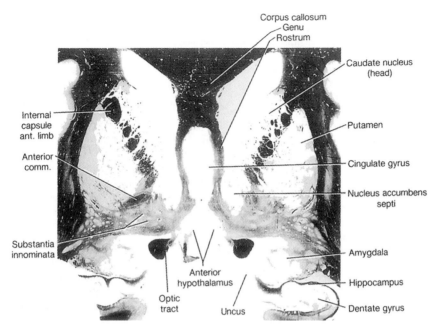

Figure 12. Coronal section through the genu of the corpus callosum revealing NAcc ventromedial to the caudate. The NAcc is in close proximity to both limbic and motor structures, likely accounting for its role in translating emotions into actions. The substantia innominata contains the large hyperchromic neurons known as the basal nucleus of Meynert, a major source of cholinergic innervation for the brain. (From Parent A: Carpenter's Human Neuroanatomy, 9th ed. Baltimore, Williams & Wilkins, 1996; with permission.)

35. What are the differences between immediate, recent, and remote memory?

Immediate memory, also known as short-term, working, primary, or span memory, refers to the focus of current attention, workspace, or memory buffer in which information is maintained while it is being processed. For example, immediate memory is used to hold a telephone number in mind long enough to dial the telephone.

Recent memory, also known as long-term, delayed, declarative, or episodic (memory for current life events), refers to memory for newly learned information or the ability to recall recent events.

Remote memory, also known as autobiographical, tertiary, or semantic memory, refers to past memories and acquired knowledge. It includes knowledge of the world, facts, concepts, and vocabulary.

Squire LR, Zola SM: Episodic memory, semantic memory, and amnesia. Hippocampus 8:205–211, 1998.
Squire LR: Memory and Brain. New York, Oxford University Press, 1987.
Baddeley A: Working Memory. Oxford, Carendon Press, 1986.

36. Differentiate the major neurobehavioral syndromes based on their effects in immediate, recent, and remote memory.

	Memory Function		
	IMMEDIATE	RECENT	REMOTE
Confusional states (delirium)	−	−	+
Dementia	+	−	−
Dementia with confusion	−	−	−
Primary amnesia	+	−	+
Attentional disorder (aprosexia)	−	+	+

Data from Hamsher K deS: Specialized neuropsychological assessment methods. In Goldstein G, Hersen M (eds): Handbook of Psychological Assessment, 2nd ed. New York, Plenum Press, 1990.

37. What neurologic disorders are associated with amnesia?

Degenerative dementias, limbic encephalitis associated with a paraneoplastic syndrome, Wernicke-Korsakoff syndrome, transient global amnesia, anoxic encephalopathy, herpes simplex encephalitis, post-traumatic amnesia following closed cranial trauma, and cerebrovascular disease including strokes involving the posterior cerebral artery or thalamic penetrating arteries and aneurysms to the anterior communicating artery.

38. Which arteries perfuse the hippocampus?

The anterior third of the hippocampus is perfused by the anterior choroidal artery, a branch of the internal carotid artery. The posterior two-thirds of the hippocampus are perfused by the hippocampal artery that arises form segment P2 of the posterior cerebral artery.

39. Which neurotransmitter system is important for memory?

Acetylcholine. The nucleus basalis of Meynert within the substantia innominata (see Fig. 12) and the septal nuclei provide the cholinergic input for the brain, which appears necessary for intact memory.

40. What are the clinical and neuroanatomic correlates of Wernicke-Korsakoff syndrome?

This syndrome occurs in patients with chronic alcoholism and nutritional deficiencies (thiamine). It occasionally occurs in nonalcoholic patients with vitamin deficiencies secondary to malabsorption disorders. The acute stage of the illness, Wernicke's encephalopathy, is characterized by ataxia, ophthalmoplegia, confusion, and disorientation. When the confusional state clears, the patient may be left with a permanent, severe anterograde amnesia and a temporally graded retrograde amnesia. Confabulation, apathy, impaired awareness, and meager conversational content are common.

Korsakoff's amnesia previously was attributed to lesions in the mammillary bodies. However, more recent autopsy data indicate that patients with lesions to the mammillary bodies alone developed Wernicke's encephalopathy, but not Korsakoff's amnesia. Lesions in the amnestic patients typically were found in *both* the mammillary bodies and dorsomedial nucleus of the thalamus.

DRUGS, PAIN, AND PLEASURE

41. What did early searches for a pleasure center in the brain reveal about the anatomic correlates of self-stimulation?

In 1953, Olds and Milner reported that rats would cross electrified grids and forfeit food, water, and sex to obtain electrical stimulation to septal and hypothalamic regions. Exhausted rats dragged themselves to a lever pressing at a rate of more than 2000 times per hour for 24 hours. Subsequently, Olds and others demonstrated that rewarding effects also could be produced by stimulating a number of limbic system sites, including the lateral hypothalamus, medial forebrain bundle, septal region, portions of amygdala and hippocampus, VTA, and anterior cingulate.

Olds J, Milner P: Positive reinforcement produced by electrical stimulation of septal area and other regions of rat brain. J Comp Physiol Psychol 47:419–427, 1954.

42. What are some of the behavioral characteristics of electrical intracranial self-stimulation (ICS)?

- Heavy work loads for extended periods of time, i.e., relatively insatiable
- Rapid extinction after current is turned off
- Acceptance of pain to obtain ICS
- Choice of ICS over food, water, sleep, and sex
- No known drive state, although ICS performance increases with hunger, thirst, and drug abuse (e.g., heroin, cocaine), speaking to the generalization of this putative common reward mechanism
- Seizures with ICS in limbic structures (e.g., hippocampus)

43. What neurotransmitter(s) and neuroanatomic structure(s) has been implicated in positive reinforcing brain mechanisms?

The mesocorticolimbic (MCL) system.

Kiyatkin EA: Functional significance of mesolimbic dopamine. Neurosci Biobehav Rev 19:573–598, 1995.

44. What evidence exists to support a role for the MCL system in positive reinforcement?

Evidence from extensive animal experimental data includes the following: firing rates in the VTA increase in the presence of several reinforcers; dopamine release increases in the NAcc in the presence of food, drugs of abuse, and sexual behavior; lesions of the NAcc or neuroleptics (dopamine antagonists) in the NAcc decrease or block reinforced behavior; MCL supports ICS; ICS behavior is enhanced in the presence of food deprivation and acute administration of abused drugs.

45. Discuss the interactions of the endogenous opioid peptide system, the MCL system, and reinforced behavior.

Three principal types of opiate receptors (called mu, delta, and kappa) have been identified, cloned, and their distributions mapped in the CNS. Three families of opioid peptides also have been identified and sequenced (beta-endorphin, the enkephalins, and dynorphins). Numerous links between the opioid and MCL systems exist, including extensive receptors and peptide terminals in the NAcc and VTA. Opioid peptides (and such opiate drugs as morphine and heroin) modulate VTA dopamine-output neurons, mostly by inhibiting GABAergic inhibitory interneurons.

Behavioral evidence suggesting a functional interaction includes: (1) increase in food and water consumption occurs with direct exogenous opioid peptide administration into various hypothalamic and MCL sites, (2) the opiate receptor antagonist, naloxone, decreases food and water intake in deprived animals, (3) sweet foods increase β-endorphin release in the hypothalamus, and (4) opiate self-administration is blocked by dopamine antagonists and MCL lesions.

Goldstein A (ed): Molecular and Cellular Aspects of Drug Addictions. Springer-Verlag, New York, 1989.

46. What is the physiologic mechanism for the reinforcing properties of cocaine?

Cocaine inhibits reuptake of all three monoamines (serotonin, dopamine, and norepinephrine). However, it is the potentiation of dopaminergic neurotransmission in the MCL system that is considered the critical reward substrate.

Kuhar MJ, Ritz MC, Boja JW: The dopamine hypothesis of the reinforcing properties of cocaine. Trends Neurosci 14:299–302, 1991.

47. Is the limbic system involved in pain perception?

Yes. (1) Nociceptive information is carried to the thalamus (intraluminar nuclei, ventroposterolateral and -medial nuclei, lateral posterior nucleus) and relayed to the limbic system via a number of pathways, including a direct spinoamygdalar pathway. (2) Limbic and forebrain structures contain a high density of opioid receptors that probably are involved in the affective component of pain. (3) The periaqueductal gray (PAG)—that region of the midbrain surrounding the cerebral aqueduct—is involved in at least five major functions, including pain processing and modulation, autonomic regulation (cardiovascular [CV]), fear and anxiety, sexual motor/postural behaviors, and vocalization. All of these functions interact to some extent. Emotional events such as fear, anxiety, anger, and pain can significantly alter blood pressure and heart rate, indicating the involvement of higher centers in CV regulation via inputs from the amygdala, prefrontal and insular cortex, and hypothalamus. In fact, the largest number of afferents into the PAG is from the hypothalamus, most from the lateral and medial preoptic anterior areas.

Willis WD, Westlund KN: Neuroanatomy of the pain system and of the pathways that modulate pain. J Clin Neurophysiol 14:2–31, 1997.

EMOTION AND PSYCHIATRIC STATES

48. What is the Klüver-Bucy syndrome?

A seminal series of experiments, performed by Klüver and Bucy between 1937 and 1940, described the effects of large bilateral temporal lobe lesions in rhesus monkeys. The lesions included the uncus, amygdala, and parts of the hippocampus. Prior to surgery, the animals were aggressive, assaulting anyone who tried to handle them. Following surgery, the animals were placid and tame, making no motor or vocal responses to stimuli that normally elicited fear and anger. The monkeys experienced psychic blindness in that they no longer recognized or knew the meaning of objects presented visually (visual agnosia), despite intact visual discrimination. In addition, strong oral exploratory tendencies, hypersexuality, and hypermetamorphosis (excessive tendency to take notice of and react to visual stimuli) were observed. These symptoms persisted unchanged during several years of experimental observations.

Klüver H, Bucy PC: Preliminary analysis of functions of the temporal lobes in monkeys. Arch Neurol Psychiatry 42:979–1000, 1939.

49. Does the Klüver-Bucy syndrome occur in humans?

Yes. Less than 200 human cases have been reported in the literature. Frequently humans do not show the full syndrome, and more complex behavioral changes are characteristic, including aphasia, amnesia, and dementia. The etiology of human Klüver-Bucy syndrome includes post-traumatic encephalopathy, herpes encephalitis, anoxia, Alzheimer's and Pick's diseases, subarachnoid hemorrhage, bitemporal infarction, and focal status epilepticus. Neuroanatomically, all autopsied cases have extensive lesions, involving bilateral anterior, medial, and inferior temporal lobes and amygdala.

50. Describe the interictal personality syndrome that is reported to occur in patients with complex partial seizures arising from the temporal lobes.

A unique syndrome of personality and behavioral changes, frequently referred to as the **Geschwind syndrome**, has been reported in individuals with temporal lobe seizures. This syndrome is characterized by increased concern with philosophical, cosmic, or religious issues; hypergraphia; altered sexual behavior (frequently hyposexuality); viscosity or a tendency toward interpersonal "stickiness"; and irritability.

Geschwind N: Behavioral changes in temporal lobe epilepsy. Psychol Med 9:217–219, 1979.

Bear DM, Fedio P: Quantitative analysis of interictal behavior in temporal lobe epilepsy. Arch Neurol 34: 454–457, 1977.

51. What is the relationship between interictal personality and Klüver-Bucy syndrome?

In many ways, the behavioral changes and pathogenesis of the Klüver-Bucy and Geschwind syndromes are polar opposites. Klüver-Bucy syndrome is considered a *disconnection* syndrome, wherein the primary sensory and sensory associations areas are disconnected from limbic structures that provide the affective significance and meaning to perception and thought. This might account for the increase in exploratory behavior and the visual agnosia. In contrast, the basis of interictal personality changes is thought to be sensory limbic *hyperconnection* due to kindling associated with repeated seizures. There is a heightened tendency to attach emotional significance to neutral environmental stimuli, leading to a hyperconditionable state.

Studies of these syndromes have contributed to the field of neuropsychiatry and our understanding of how perturbations in the limbic system account for the remarkable spectrum of psychiatric disorders.

52. What features of partial seizures support the notion of the limbic system as a circuit involved in the experience of emotion?

Partial (simple partial and complex partial) seizures are differentiated from generalized seizures based on whether there is clinical or electrographic activation of neurons limited to part of one cerebral hemisphere. Simple and complex partial seizures typically arise from the temporal lobe or limbic structures. Such seizures are often preceded by an olfactory, gustatory, epigastric, or autonomic aura, and can be accompanied by psychic phenomena such as fear, intense joy or depression, laughter (gelastic epilepsy), illusions, and hallucinations. These emotions, together with the observation that temporal lobe seizures spread rapidly within limbic structures rather than to the neocortex, lend credence to the notion of a limbic circuit.

Dreifuss FE, Henriksen O: Classification of epileptic seizures and the epilepsies. Acta Neurol 140(Suppl): 8–17, 1992.

Nayel M, Awad LA, Larkins M, Lüders H: Experimental limbic epilepsy: Models, pathophysiologic concepts, and clinical relevance. Cleve Clin J Med 58:521–530, 1991.

53. What is the evidence supporting the role of the anterior cingulate in Gilles de la Tourette syndrome?
- The relationship between the anterior cingulate (AC) and affective vocalizations is well documented. For example, AC lesions in animals can abolish conditioned emotional vocalizations. Thus, aberrations in this area may lead to an inability to inhibit vocalizations.
- Dopaminergic hyperactivity is postulated as the principal neurochemical abnormality in Tourette syndrome. There is a dopaminergic pathway from the VTA to the AC cortex.
- Electrical stimulation to the AC in humans results in movements that are similar to tics.
- Tourette syndrome patients have decreased cerebral glucose utilization in the AC.
- AC lesions can reduce obsessive-compulsive behaviors, and obsessive-compulsive disorder is an associated feature of Tourette syndrome.
- Disconnection of the AC and the thalamus results in a reduction in Tourette symptoms.

54. Are there hemispheric asymmetries in emotions?
Yes. Left hemisphere lesions are more likely to give rise to negative affective states such as depression and "catastrophic reactions." Right hemisphere lesions are more likely to result in euphoria, anosagnosia, and hemispatial neglect. Patients with right hemisphere lesions are more likely to be unconcerned or unaware of their deficits and show disorders of abnormal awareness. Similarly, electrophysiologic studies of normal patients reveal that greater right activation is associated with depression, and great left activation is associated with happiness. It is thought that left lesions release the right (sad or negative) hemisphere from inhibition and that right lesions release the left (positive) hemisphere from inhibition.

Different emotional changes are observed with left and right hemianesthesia during Wada or intracarotid sodium amytal testing. The Wada test involves producing a temporary hemianesthesia by injecting sodium amytal into the internal carotid artery (ICA). Right ICA injections are more likely to lead to euphoria or disinhibition, while left ICA injections are more likely to result in sadness or tearfulness. The hemispheres are thought to have different pharmacologic systems as well, with the left hemisphere being primarily cholinergic and dopaminergic and the right hemisphere being primarily noradrenergic.

55. What are the two main functional subdivisions within the frontal lobe that are associated with distinct behavioral syndromes?
The **orbital frontal** and the **dorsolateral**. Lesions or damage to the orbital frontal/anterior temporal region lead to disinhibition, tactlessness, impulsivity, and reduced concern for social conventions. Individuals with orbital frontal lesions may show deficient self-awareness, perseveration, lack of concern for hygiene, and an inability to profit from experience.

In contrast, individuals with dorsolateral lesions are apathetic, bradyphrenic, lacking in drive and initiative, and show a lack of concern for the past or future. They have difficulty engaging in goal-directed behaviors.

NEUROSURGERY

56. What is psychosurgery?
Psychosurgery is the neurosurgical treatment of mental disease. After learning that monkeys could be made docile through bilateral frontal lobotomy, Antônio Egas Moniz, a Portuguese neurologist, proposed that psychiatric disorders were a result of frontal lobe pathology, which might be treated surgically. The first attempt at psychosurgery was conducted in 1935, when Moniz and his neurosurgeon, Almeida Lima, injected alcohol into the frontal lobes of a patient to perform a frontal leucotomy. More than 5000 lobotomies were performed between 1942 and 1952 in the United States, and in 1949 Moniz was awarded the Nobel prize for his discovery of the benefits of frontal lobotomy.

57. What led to the diminished role of psychosurgery in modern medicine?
Psychosurgery proceeded without adequate experimental testing, and follow-up assessment of treatment effects and morbidity was poor. It later became evident that the benefits of frontal lobotomy

were limited and that some patients suffered serious, negative side effects. Ironically, Moniz was shot in the back by one of his lobotomized patients. Psychosurgery fell out of favor in the 1960s with the advent of psychotropic medication.

58. Which disorders benefit from psychosurgical approaches?

Currently, psychosurgery is used rarely, primarily for severe and refractory cases of obsessive-compulsive disorder (OCD). Cingulotomy, anterior capsulotomy, limbic leucotomy, and subcaudate tractomy, all of which interrupt connections between the frontal lobes and thalamus/basal ganglia, have resulted in significant improvement in severe OCD patients. Stereotactic cingulotomy is the surgical treatment of choice for OCD because of the lower complication rates.

Stimulation or the production of a stereotactic lesion is used in the treatment of severe tremor (thalamic stimulator implantation), Parkinson's disease (pallidotomy), pain (cingulotomy and, rarely, stereotactic lesioning of the nucleus ventralis posterolateralis), and epilepsy (temporal lobectomy). Interestingly, patients who have undergone cingulotomy for chronic pain report no diminution in their pain sensation, but rather that they are no longer bothered by their pain (i.e., the affective component has been separated form the sensory properties).

Marino R Jr, Cosgrove GR: Neurosurgical treatment of neuropsychiatric illness. Psychiatr Clin North Am 20:933–943, 1997.

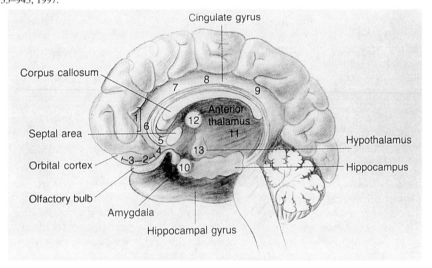

Figure 13. Targets of psychosurgical procedures: 1–bimedial leukotomy; 2–yttrium lesions to subcortical white matter; 3–orbital undercutting; 4–bifrontal stereotaxic subcaudate tractotomy; 5–anterior capsulotomy; 6–mesoloviotomy; 7, 8, and 9–anterior, middle, and posterior cingulotomies; 10–amygdalectomy; 11–thalamotomy (dorsomedial, contromedian, or parafascicular nuclei); 12–anterior thalamotomy; 13–hypothalamotomy. (From Kolb B, Whishaw IQ: Fundamentals of Human Neurophysiology, 3rd ed. New York, W.H. Freeman and Company, 1990; with permission. Adapted from Valenstein ES (ed): The Psychosurgery Update. San Francisco, WH Freeman, 1980.)

59. What is the mesial temporal lobe epilepsy syndrome?

Because this is considered a surgically remedial epilepsy syndrome, greater emphasis has been placed on identifying its core features. The defining feature of the mesial temporal lobe syndrome is hippocampal sclerosis. Early age at onset of recurrent seizures is typical, usually in the first decade of life. Often there is a history of febrile convulsions. Hippocampal volume asymmetries, memory asymmetries on Wada testing, and better seizure outcome following temporal lobectomy also are common.

Seidenberg M, Hermann B, Wyler AR, et al: Neuropsychological outcome following anterior temporal lobectomy in patients with and without the syndrome of mesial temporal lobe epilepsy. Neuropsychology 12: 303–316, 1998.

FUNCTIONAL NEUROIMAGING

60. What have functional MRI and PET studies revealed about human memory?

The hippocampus and medial temporal lobe structures are critical for the formation of new declarative and episodic memories. Medial temporal lobe activation occurs automatically when events are experienced, making it difficult for researchers to select control or contrast tasks when studying memory encoding. The strength of activation in these structures increases with how well or how deeply the material is encoded (e.g., making a decision about the meaning of a word rather than performing a feature detection task on a word), novelty, and the forming of semantic associations. Greater activation is observed in right hemisphere structures when tasks involve novelty detection and in left hemisphere structures when tasks involve semantic (deep) processing. In addition, encoding of episodic memories has been associated with greater left prefrontal and cingulate activation, while retrieval of episodic memories was associated with right prefrontal cortex and bilateral precuneus.

Fletcher PC, Frith CD, Grasby PM, et al: Brain systems for encoding and retrieval of auditory-verbal memory: An *in vivo* study in humans. Brain 118:401–416, 1995.

Henke K, Weber B, Kneifel S, et al: Human hippocampus associates information in memory. Proc Natl Acad Sci 96:5884–5889, 1999.

Martin A: Automatic activation of the medial temporal lobe during encoding: Lateralized influences of meaning and novelty. Hippocampus 9:62–70, 1999.

61. What cognitive process results in consistent activation of the cingulate and dorsolateral prefrontal cortex in PET and functional MRI experiments?

The anterior cingulate and dorsolateral prefrontal cortex are consistently activated by tasks that involve working memory. The working memory system is divided into two parts: (1) short-term storage, which is necessary for active maintenance of information over a period of seconds while the information is manipulated, and (2) executive process operations (such as selective attention and task management) performed on the contents of short-term storage.

Smith EE, Jonides J: Storage and executive processes in the frontal lobes. Science 278:1657–1661, 1999.

62. How have functional brain imaging studies implicated the amygdala and cingulate in psychiatric disease?

PET studies show increased blood flow in the amygdala in patients with post-traumatic stress disorder who are undergoing symptom provocation, and before and after pharmacologic treatment in patients with familial depression. Hyperactivity in orbitofrontal and anterior cingulate areas has been demonstrated with functional MRI and PET in patients with OCD. This brain activation is accentuated in limbic regions during symptom provocation (e.g., exposing patients with hand-washing compulsions to a stimulus that they are led to believe is contaminated).

Breiter HC, Rauch SL, Kwong KK, et al: Functional MRI of symptom provocation in obsessive-compulsive disorder. Arch Gen Psychiatry 53:595–606, 1996.

63. What is the role of the amygdala in human emotion?

A number of functional imaging studies are beginning to elucidate the role of the amygdala in emotional processing. For example, rapid presentation of happy and fearful faces, interspersed with slower presentation of neutral faces, causes subjects to report seeing only the neutral faces. Nevertheless, the amount of activity in the amygdala increases when the "masked" (i.e., presented too quickly to be consciously seen) fearful face is presented and decreases to the masked happy face, suggesting that the amygdala activity differentially reflects emotional valence of external stimuli.

These data are supported by the finding that selective bilateral amygdala damage impairs the recognition of fear and of multiple emotions in a face, but does not alter facial discrimination and recognition of familiar faces.

Whalen PJ, Rauch SL, Etcoff NL, et al: Masked presentations of emotional facial expressions modulate amygdala activity without explicit knowledge. J Neurosci 18:411–418.

Adolphs R, Tranel D, Damasio H, Damasio A: Impaired recognition of emotion in facial expression following bilateral damage to the human amygdala. Nature 372:669–672, 1994.

64. What brain structures mediate the perception of pain? Can this perception be distinguished from anticipation?

Functional MRI and PET imaging experiments have revealed a network of cortical and subcortical brain regions activated following painful peripheral stimulation (generally produced experimentally by noxious heat). These regions include the anterior cingulate; insular, prefrontal, and primary and secondary somatosensory cortices; and thalamus. The frontal lobe, insula, and cerebellum appear to be able to distinguish between pain perception and anticipation, with distinct regions of each structure involved in each aspect of pain.

Ploghaus A, Tracey I, Gati JS, et al: Dissociating pain from its anticipation in the human brain. Science 284:1979–1981, 1999.

65. What role does the limbic system play in drug craving?

Cues that are able to induce a craving state in experienced cocaine addicts have a distributed system of cortical structures, including medial temporal limbic regions involved in conditioned emotional responses (amygdala), working memory circuits in dorsolateral prefrontal and orbitofrontal cortex, and posterior parietal and cingulate regions in attention/arousal system. This emerging picture of widespread neuronal involvement may reflect the participation of a number of cognitive and emotional processes working to concert to produce the subjective craving experience.

Childress AR, Mozley PD, McElgin W, et al: Limbic activation during cue-induced cocaine craving. Am J Psychiatry 156:11–18, 1999.

Grant S, London ED, Newlin DB, et al: Activation of memory circuits during cue-elicited cocaine craving. Proc Natl Acad Sci USA 93:12040–12045, 1996.

BIBLIOGRAPHY

1. Aggleton JP: The Amygdala: Neurobiological Aspects of Emotion, Memory, and Mental Dysfunction. New York, Wiley-Liss, 1992.
2. Bear DM, Fedio P: Quantitative analysis of interictal behavior in temporal lobe epilepsy. Arch Neurol 34:454–467, 1977.
3. Braak H, Braak E, Yilmazer D, Bohl J: Functional anatomy of human hippocampal formation and related structures. J Child Neurol 11:265–275, 1996.
4. Cabeza R, Nyberg L: Imaging cognition: An empirical review of PET studies with normal subjects. J Cog Neurosci 9:1–26, 1997.
5. Davidson RJ: Cerebral asymmetry, emotion, and affective style. In Davidson RJ, Hugdahl K (eds): Brain Asymmetry. Cambridge, The MIT Press, 1995.
6. Devinsky O, Morrell MJ, Vogt BA: Contributions of the anterior cingulate cortex to behaviour. Brain 118:279–306, 1995.
7. Devinsky O, Theodore WH (eds): Epilepsy and Behavior. Frontiers of Clinical Neuroscience 12. New York, Wiley-Liss, 1991.
8. Gloor P: The Temporal Lobe and Limbic System. New York, Oxford University Press, 1997.
9. Heilman KM, Satz P: Neuropsychology of Human Emotion. New York, The Guilford Press, 1983.
10. Isaacson RL: The Limbic System, 2nd ed. New York, Plenum Press, 1982.
11. Kalivas PW, Barnes CD: Limbic Motor Circuits and Neuropsychiatry. Boca Raton, CRC Press, 1993.
12. MacLean PD: Some psychiatric implications of physiological studies on frontotemporal portion of limbic system (visceral brain). EEG Clin Neurophysiol 4:407–418, 1952.
13. Squire LR: Memory and Brain. New York, Oxford University Press, 1987.
14. Vogt BA, Gabriel M: Neurobiology of Cingulate Cortex and Limbic Thalamus. Boston, Birkhäuser, 1993.

20. HIGHER CORTICAL FUNCTIONS: LANGUAGE, COGNITION, LEARNING AND MEMORY

Henry J. Ralston III, M.D.

CENTRAL LANGUAGE AREA

The most distinct and definable aspects of higher cortical function are those having to do with the production and comprehension of language. Language is defined as the ability to communicate through the use of common symbols. Speech, writing, and American sign language are all examples of language. These functions rely upon, but are distinct and separable from, the neural mechanisms underlying primary auditory, visual, and motor functions of the brain. For example, a parrot can mimic the sounds of human speech, but cannot communicate abstract concepts with these sounds. Human beings can listen to, read, or even faithfully copy a foreign language with no more understanding than a tape recorder has of the words it is recording. In short, language implies comprehension and communication of abstract ideas.

1. How does language develop?

Most humans first learn language in the auditory (speech) mode, the principal exception being those babies who are deaf or who are raised by nonspeaking parents (e.g., deaf-mute parents). For all infants, **early exposure** to language, whether verbal or by signing (American sign language), is crucial for normal language development in any mode (speech, writing, signing). Thus, it is important to determine whether an infant has normal hearing, and if not, to provide appropriate exposure to other, nonverbal language modes early in development.

2. Where are the language areas in the cortex?

The central language area consists of a receptive, symbol-decoding region (**Wernicke's area**, which comprises portions of Brodmann's areas 22, 39, 40) immediately adjacent to the primary auditory cortex on the left. The sounds of verbal language (speech) reach the auditory cortex on both sides of the brain. From the auditory cortex on the left side of the brain the sound is transferred to Wernicke's area, where the auditory language content is decoded. Wernicke's area is connected via a subcortical bundle of white matter to a motor language-programming, word-sequencing region located on the left posterior-inferior frontal cortex (**Broca's area**, which comprises Brodmann's areas 44, 45). The neurons of Broca's area activate the appropriate zone of the adjacent motor cortex for language production, i.e., face, mouth, tongue, larynx, and diaphragmatic centers for speech; arm, wrist, and hand for writing or signing.

In addition to the cortical regions involved in speech, a region of the left parieto-occipital cortex, located caudal to the central speech area, is concerned with the visual-symbolic information involved in reading.

3. Do language dominance and handedness always go hand-in-hand?

About 90% of humans are *right handed*, and their dominant cerebral hemisphere for handedness and for language is the *left hemisphere*. About 50% of left-handed people also have language dominance in the left hemisphere, or the language functions are shared between the two hemispheres. The remaining left-handed individuals have their language function primarily in the right hemisphere, on the same side as that dominant for their handedness. (See figure on following page.)

4. Is there any structural asymmetry to some of the language-associated areas?

There is a structural asymmetry of the two hemispheres in most right-handed people (less obvious for those who are left handed). The region of the auditory association cortex on the superior

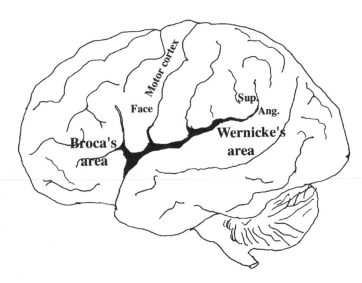

Language zones of the left hemisphere. Wernicke's area and the adjacent angular (Ang.) and supramarginal (Sup.) gyri constitute the symbol-decoding area for language. They are interconnected with Broca's area via a subcortical white pathway, the arcuate fasciculus. Other cortical speech areas are in the immediately adjacent frontal, parietal, and posterior temporal cortices. Note that the face area of the primary motor cortex is immediately caudal to Broca's area, and shares much of the same blood supply.

aspect of the left temporal gyrus—the planum temporale—is about one-third larger on the left than on the right. This asymmetry is present in newborns, suggesting that it is genetically predetermined.

5. How important are cortico-cortical connections to language functions?

For reproduction of sounds, the development of expressive language ability requires cortico-cortical connections between auditory regions associated with Wernicke's area (superior temporal gyrus, angular gyrus, supramarginal gyrus) and Broca's area in the inferior frontal lobe. The connections involve subcortical white matter pathways through the parieto-frontal operculum known as the **arcuate fasciculus**. It should be stressed that each site within the central language area functions by virtue of its connections to other language-related cortical (and subcortical) areas.

6. What new insight have we gained about the classic language areas?

What the neurons in each site contribute to language function is a current object of study. For example, positron emission tomography (PET) and functional magnetic resonance imaging (MRI) have shown that Broca's area, traditionally considered to be associated with the *expression* of language (e.g., talking, writing), has increased activity during a language *discrimination* task. Furthermore, patients with lesions in Broca's area have subtle but significant difficulties understanding material with even slightly complex semantics. Thus, one cannot assign a purely language-receptive function to Wernicke's area, or a purely language expressive function to Broca's area.

Normally, reading and writing are learned several years after a person has extensive auditory-vocal language exposure. The graphic-symbolic systems of reading and writing are added onto pre-existing speech functions and must occur primarily between visual association areas of the occipital lobe and the parieto-frontal intermodal language areas. One would expect a more posterior (parieto-occipital) concentration of neurons concerned with reading than with auditory language skills. In fact, certain parieto-occipital lesions can destroy writing and/or reading ability while leaving auditory language skills intact. In contrast, lesions of auditory-intermodal association areas destroy both reading and auditory comprehension, since the auditory associations are primary in language development.

7. Briefly map the brain's involvement in language.

The central language area consists of a symbol-decoding region (Wernicke's area) connected via the arcuate fasciculus to a motor language-programming, word-sequencing region (Broca's area) that then activates the appropriate zone of motor cortex for language production. Adjacent to this central language area are groups of cells more concerned with auditory-intermodal, visual-symbolic, and other, less well defined symbolic manipulation. Recent studies using PET and functional MRI have shown many regions of the brain in both the dominant and nondominant hemispheres to have heightened activity during language tasks. Thus, although the central language area is crucial for normal language function, regions active in language are widely distributed in the forebrain and cerebellum.

Case Study A

The family of a 72-year-old right-handed woman states that she has had a sudden change in her speech. You find that her speech consists of a series of disconnected words that are understandable, but do not form comprehensible sentences. She does not respond appropriately to verbal or written commands. She has normal movements of her face and of all extremities.

8. What is your diagnosis?

The patient exhibits **aphasia**, which is defined as an acquired disorder of language (including, but not limited to, speech) secondary to injury of one or more regions of the brain. Conversely, mutism and dysarthria (slurred speech) are motor disturbances, which do not necessarily imply a language disturbance. Similarly, deafness does not imply lack of language comprehension.

9. Which region of the brain is damaged in this patient?

The patient does not appear to comprehend spoken or written language, although she can produce a series of words that have little meaning to others. Her lesion is in the posterior region of the central language area (left superior temporal lobe, angular gyrus, supramarginal gyrus, Wernicke's area). The rapid onset of the aphasia in this patient indicates that the lesion is probably due to impairment of the blood supply provided by posterior branches of the middle cerebral artery, such as the temporo-occipital artery.

Case Study B

A 57-year-old right-handed man collapses in a restaurant. He is conscious when admitted to the emergency department, but he can only say simple, one- or two-syllable words. He responds appropriately to written and verbal commands, such as "Raise your left arm." The right lower two-thirds of his face is weak. He has normal movements of all four extremities.

10. What is your diagnosis?

This patient also exhibits aphasia (see Case Study A). In contrast to the previous patient, he appears to comprehend spoken and written language, although he can say very little. His disorder is more than that of improper articulation of speech (**dysarthria**), as he is unable to say series of words in a coherent fashion, and would have the same difficulty if asked to write sentences.

11. Which region of the brain is damaged in this patient?

His lesion is in the anterior region of the central language area and involves not only the posterio-inferior left frontal lobe (Broca's area) but also the adjacent region of the facial motor cortex, leading to a right facial weakness (dysfunction of the central or upper motor facial neurons). The sudden onset of the aphasia indicates that the lesion is probably due to impairment of the blood supply provided by anterior branches of the middle cerebral artery, such as the precentral artery.

12. Weakness of the right lower two-thirds of the face is more common in patients with an expressive (Broca's) aphasia than in patients with receptive (Wernicke's) aphasia. Explain this finding.

This type of weakness is more common in patients with a Broca's aphasia because the posterio-inferior left frontal lobe is immediately adjacent to the primary motor cortex of the precentral gyrus.

Case Study C

During surgery for a brain tumor, the surgeon uses an electrical stimulus to explore the cortex of a conscious, right-handed patient. The patient is asked to count from 1 to 10; stimulation of a particular cortical region causes an arrest in the counting, which the patient resumes when the stimulus is removed.

13. What region of the brain is being electrically stimulated in this patient?

The surgeon has electrically stimulated Broca's area, causing an arrest of the production of speech. Such stimulation is done commonly during neurosurgical procedures in the language-dominant hemisphere, so that language-associated areas may be spared, if at all possible.

LANGUAGE DISTURBANCES ASSOCIATED WITH CEREBRAL LESIONS

14. What are the major types of aphasia?

Clinically, aphasia syndromes fall into two major categories: those of the central language area (Wernicke's area, Broca's area, and the cortex that overlies the arcuate fasciculus; see Figure on page 302) and those of adjacent associated cortex (frontal, parietal, and posterior temporal).

The two most distinctive syndromes of the central language area are Broca's (motor, expressive, verbal) aphasia and Wernicke's (sensory, receptive) aphasia. These syndromes have in common a deficit in repetition. Patients are unable to repeat a short sentence without error.

Common Aphasia Syndromes

SYNDROME	SPONTANEOUS SPEECH	COMPREHENSION	REPETITION
Broca's	Nonfluent	Preserved	Lost
Wernicke's	Fluent	Lost	Lost
Global	Nonfluent	Lost	Lost
Conduction	Fluent	Preserved	Lost
Anomic	Fluent	Preserved	Preserved

15. What are the characteristics of Broca's aphasia?

Patients with Broca's aphasia have sparse, labored, dysarthric speech. Small grammatical words are omitted. Pronunciation of single words improves with repetition, but combinations of more than three words are extremely difficult. Comprehension is relatively normal. The patient often exhibits weakness of the right lower two-thirds of the face and the right arm, because a lesion of Broca's area may extend to involve the adjacent primary motor cortex. Patient's with Broca's aphasia frequently are depressed, because they know that others cannot understand their speech.

16. How is Wernicke's aphasia different from Broca's aphasia?

The patient with a lesion of Wernicke's area is unconcerned, often euphoric, and has fluent, paraphasic speech. (In paraphasia, a substitute word is used for the obviously correct one, e.g., cutter for knife.) Comprehension is impaired. It is difficult to say whether repetition is impaired since the patient doesn't know what is being requested. Hemiplegia usually is not present, and this type of patient may be given a mistaken diagnosis of a psychiatric disorder.

17. What is global aphasia?

Global aphasia occurs with large lesions of the left hemisphere, usually in the territory of the middle cerebral artery. Patients have extensive damage to both the posterior and anterior regions of the central language area, so that all forms of understanding and production of language are impaired.

18. What causes conduction aphasia?

Conduction aphasia arises as a result of damage to the interconnections between the posterior (Wernicke's) and anterior (Broca's) regions. Patients exhibit a major deficit in being able to repeat spoken or written words, although their spontaneous speech may be reasonably fluent. However, they often are hesitant and use incorrect words. The lesion involves some component of the arcuate fasciculus, typically in the left superior temporal or inferior parietal region.

19. How is anomic aphasia manifested?

Of the aphasias resulting from lesions outside the central language area, anomic aphasia is the most common. These patients have fairly normal comprehension, but have great difficulty finding the correct name. They might call a wristwatch a "wand" (paraphasia) or "the thing you tell time with" (a circumlocution). Anomic aphasia often is due to a discrete vascular lesion of the parietal lobe, near the angular gyrus or above it. It also has been reported in association with lesions of the left pulvinar nucleus of the thalamus. This type of aphasia may be seen in diffuse dementias, metabolic encephalopathy, and brain tumors in any location. Anomic aphasia may occur in the absence of any other neurologic defects.

20. Can aphasia be treated?

Unfortunately, in spite of years of careful study and the use of different therapeutic approaches, there is little that can be said with confidence about the treatment of aphasia. In general, patients with preserved comprehension and motivation to improve have the best prognosis. Patients with conduction aphasia and Broca's aphasia benefit from speech therapy. Improvement can continue for up to 3 years after the initial insult, but if there has been no improvement by 3 months, the prognosis is poor.

HEMISPHERE DOMINANCE

21. What do we know about cerebral dominance for language?

A source of confusion in the clinical analysis of language deficits is the fact that the degree of left hemisphere dominance for motor dexterity (i.e., handedness) varies from great (most right-handed persons) to nil (ambidextrous) to negative (left-handed). Furthermore, motor dominance and speech dominance are not always linked. For example, following the intracarotid injection of the short-acting barbiturate, amytal (which should selectively put one hemisphere to sleep), dysphasia may be produced by inactivation of the nondominant hemisphere in 1% of right-handed people and in about 15% of left handers. This indicates that both hemispheres participate in language function in many left-handed people. It follows that since cerebrovascular lesions are equally likely in either hemisphere, left-handed people are more likely to become aphasic with stroke. On the other hand, statistically speaking, they may improve more rapidly and completely.

Case Study D

A 32-year-old woman fails to put her left arm in her sleeve while dressing. Her family reports that she insists that the left arm is not her own. Her visual fields are normal.

Case Study E

A 58-year-old man ran the left side of his car into a light pole because he failed to see the pole. His visual fields are normal. You note that the left side of his face is poorly shaved compared to the right.

22. What region of the brain is the likely site of a lesion in case studies D and E?

Lesions in the **right parietal lobe**, specifically the angular and supra-marginal gyri, give rise to striking deficits in manipulation of spatial concepts. Patients may not recognize the left half of their own bodies and, therefore, do not clean or shave the left side of their face, or do not put clothing on their left extremities. Such patients often cannot recognize the existence of objects or people in the left visual hemifield (**spatial neglect**), even though their visual fields may be intact. When asked to draw or copy a figure, such as a clock, they may crowd all 12 numbers onto the right half of the clock face, or simply omit the numbers 7–12 that normally occupy the left half of the figure.

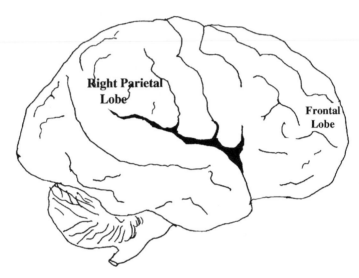

The right parietal lobe is served by posterior branches of the middle cerebral artery. Impairment of the blood supply to this region, or other types of lesions, can result in "neglect" syndromes in the contralateral visual field, even though the patient may have normal visual fields.

COGNITION

Case Study F

A 41-year-old man was thrown into the windshield during an automobile accident. Several months later, his family states that he has become argumentative and abusive, and that he lost his job because of poor work performance. His cognitive functions, such as orientation for time and place, appear normal.

23. What may be the cause of the above symptoms?

Bilateral lesions of the frontal lobes frequently are associated with changes in personality. The patient also may have altered attention spans, reduced mathematical skills, and/or impaired language comprehension.

Case Study G

A 47-year-old man is brought to you by his wife because he did not appear to recognize her the day before. In fact, he is unable to recognize his wife *and* his children. When he looks into a mirror, he does not recognize his own face. He has normal visual fields, and he can read, write, and identify objects. However, he states that the color is "drained out" of objects, and he is unable to perceive colors in any part of his visual fields.

24. What is the basis of this patient's deficits?

There is a remarkable deficit, **prosopagnosia**, associated with lesions of the inferior aspect of one or both temporal lobes. Prosopagnosia is characterized by an inability to recognize previously known human faces—even one's own face viewed in the mirror. This deficit occurs even though the affected individual can describe the face (e.g., blue eyes, dark hair, prominent cheekbones). The lesion frequently is caused by ischemic events arising from decreased blood supply in the territories of the posterior cerebral arteries. These patients often exhibit **achromatopsia**, an impairment of the perception of color. The inferior temporal lobes process higher-order aspects of visual perception, in which visual information is integrated. Such complex deficits illustrate injuries to cortical regions responsible for higher-order integration and processing of sensory-motor information characteristic of multimodal association cortex.

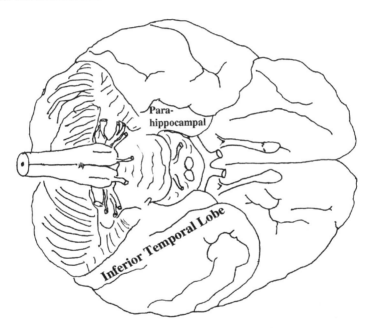

The inferior temporal lobes are supplied by branches of the posterior cerebral arteries. Impairment of the blood supply to this region, or other types of lesions, can result in visual agnosias or other deficits in higher-order visual processing. The parahippocampal gyrus is shown on the inferior aspect of the right temporal lobe.

LEARNING AND MEMORY

25. What constitutes learning and memory?

The terms "learning" and "memory" imply an acquisition of knowledge of facts, experiences, and skills. During learning and memory, knowledge, understanding, and skills are gained by study, instruction, or experience. This information is stored (encoded) in the brain, and can be recalled (retrieved), either consciously or unconsciously. The information may be unimodal (e.g., lists of words, a telephone number), but often is multifaceted, with verbal, visual, auditory, and emotional components (e.g., the memory of a loved one who has died).

Current evidence about memory systems is based on clinical examination of individuals with focal brain lesions that impair one or another form of memory, imaging of brain areas that are activated during memory tasks (PET, functional MRI) in normal humans or in patients with brain injury, and numerous experimental studies of animals during learning and memory tasks. We now believe that memory is not a unitary phenomenon, but involves multiple, interrelated systems that can be distinguished from one another. **Amnesia** is an impairment of one or more components of memory (see Case Study H).

Case Study H

A 27-year-old man had a history of intractable seizures. He underwent bilateral surgical resections of both medial temporal lobes, and his seizures improved. However, he developed a striking memory deficit in which he was unable to remember short series of words or numbers for more than a few minutes. He would meet with others or read the daily newspaper and be able to discuss the meeting or the news for a few minutes afterward, but then would have no recollection of the meeting or of the newspaper. He had no long-term memories of events that occurred after the time of his surgery, although he could remember most of the major events of his life prior to his surgery. Interestingly, when he practiced a new motor skill he improved from week to week, even though he had no recollection of ever having performed the task before.

Scoville WB, Milner B: Loss of recent memory after bilateral hippocampal lesions. J Neurol Neurosurg Psych 20:11–21, 1957.

26. What forms of memory are impaired and preserved in this subject?

Case Study H is a summary report of one of the most famous clinical studies in cognitive neuropsychology. It demonstrates that there are multiple forms of memory, and that each must involve different regions of the brain. This patient, known to history as H.M., was operated on at the Montreal Neurological Institute in September, 1953. For him, life's clock stopped at that time, and he remained 27 years old. This and many subsequent studies have shown that bilateral damage to the ventromedial aspects of the temporal lobes, structures that include the hippocampus, adjacent parahippocampal gyrus, and amygdala, seriously impair the ability to acquire new **declarative** (also known as **explicit**) **memories**, with little effect on other forms of memory.

27. What is declarative memory?

Declarative (explicit) memory is defined as the conscious recollection of factual information and past experiences. It often is subdivided into **episodic memory**, which deals with the recollection of events in one's personal past (What did you do on your vacation last summer? Which high school did you attend?), and **semantic memory**, a general knowledge of facts and concepts (What city is the capitol of England? Where is the primary visual cortex?). The acquisition of *new* declarative memories (both episodic and semantic) depends on the integrity of structures in the medial temporal lobes. Imaging studies have shown that the *retrieval* (recall) of earlier (stored) memories involves the activation of both medial temporal and frontal lobe structures. H.M. had a severe deficit in his declarative memory function for events occurring after the surgical removal of his medial temporal lobes (**anterograde amnesia**), but he was able to recall episodic and semantic memories of information and events that occurred prior to his surgery.

28. Is an amnesic patient able to learn new motor skills?

H.M. was able to learn new motor skills (called **procedural** or **motor skill memory**) by practicing the motor tasks each week, even though he could not remember the practice sessions themselves. Others with similar injuries to medial temporal lobe structures exhibit the same dissociation between failing to remember the practice sessions and the ability to acquire new motor skills. Clinical studies of patients with basal ganglia and/or cerebellar diseases, as well as imaging studies of normal people during motor task acquisition, have shown that learning of new motor skills depends on the integrity of the motor cortical, basal ganglia, and cerebellar circuitry. H.M.'s preserved procedural memory indicates that such motor learning can continue even in the absence of the medial temporal lobes.

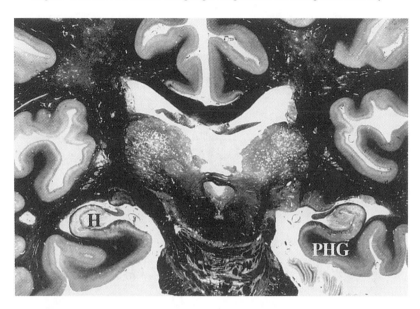

A coronal section of the human brain stained for myelin (black-Weigert stain) to show the hippocampus (H). PHG = parahippocampal gyrus.

29. Imaging studies are carried out on normal volunteers who are asked to remember a string of eight numbers and then recite them within 30 seconds. What region(s) of the brain are activated during the study?

The short-lived memory involved with a task is called **working memory**. A common form of working memory is looking up a telephone number, remembering it long enough to make a phone call, and then forgetting the number. Another example is meeting someone new at a party, introducing that person to someone else shortly thereafter, and then forgetting the name. Human and animal studies have shown neuronal populations of the **prefrontal cortex** to be activated during such memory tasks.

Working memory is distinct from semantic memory. H.M. and others with medial temporal lobe lesions have relatively preserved working memory, but patients with lesions of the frontal lobes (or sometimes the parietal lobes) have working memory deficits with preserved declarative memory.

Three Forms of Memory

MEMORY TYPE	FUNCTION	NEURAL SYSTEM
Declarative memory	Conscious memories of facts and events	Medial temporal lobe
Procedural (motor) memory	Acquisition of new motor skills	Motor cortex, basal ganglia, cerebellum
Working memory	"On-line," short-term, problem-solving memory	Prefrontal cortex, parietal cortex

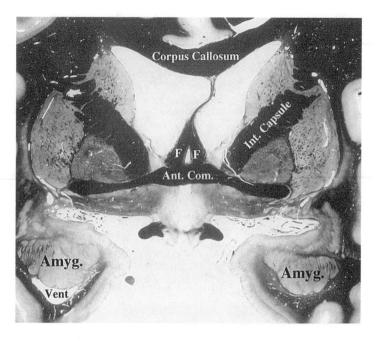

A coronal section of the human brain at a more rostral level than the previous figure, to show the large amygdaloid nuclei (Amyg.). The medial structures of the temporal lobe are essential for declarative memory functions. Procedural memory depends upon the integrity of the basal ganglia. Ant. Com. = anterior commissure; F = fornix; Vent. = ventricle (inferior horn).

BIBLIOGRAPHY

Language
 1. Binder JR, Frost JA, Hammeke TA, et al: Human brain language areas identified by functional magnetic resonance imaging. J Neurosci 17:353–362, 1997.
 2. Damasio AR: Aphasia. New Engl J Med 326:531–539, 1992.
 3. Fitch RH, Miller S, Tallal P: Neurobiology of speech perception. Annu Rev Neurosci 20:331–353, 1997.
 4. Frackowiak RSJ: Functional mapping of verbal memory and language. Trends Neurosci 17:109–115, 1994.
 5. Nobre AC, Plunkett K: The neural system of language: Structure and development. Curr Opin Neurobiol 7:262–268, 1997.
 6. Petersen SE, Fiez JA: The processing of single words studied with positron emission tomography. Annu Rev Neurosci 16:509–530, 1993.

Learning and Memory
 7. Cabeza R, Mangels J, Nyberg L, et al: Brain regions differentially involved in remembering what and when: A PET study. Neuron 19:863–870, 1997.
 8. Eichenbaum H: To cortex: Thanks for the memories. Neuron 19:481–484, 1997.
 9. Eichenbaum H, Cahill LF, Gluck MA, et al: Learning and memory: Systems analysis. In Zigmond MJ, Bloom FE, Landis SC, et al (eds): Fundamental Neuroscience. San Diego, Academic Press, 1999, pp 1455–1486.
10. Fletcher PC, Frith CD, Rugg MD: The functional neuroanatomy of episodic memory. Trends Neurosci 20:213–218, 1997.
11. Goldman-Rakic PS: Cellular basis of working memory. Neuron 14:477–485, 1995.
12. Willingham DB: Systems of memory in the human brain. Neuron 18:5–8, 1997.

21. REGULATION OF THE CEREBRAL CIRCULATION

Christopher G. Sobey, Ph.D., and Frank M. Faraci, Ph.D.

ANATOMICAL ASPECTS OF BLOOD SUPPLY TO THE BRAIN

1. What are the blood supply requirements of the brain?

Although the brain is only about 2% of total body weight, it receives almost 15% of total resting cardiac output. If blood supply to the brain is stopped for just a few seconds, consciousness is lost, and irreversible pathological changes occur within just a few minutes of ischemia. Therefore, mechanisms that regulate cerebral blood flow are required to maintain adequate brain perfusion over a broad range of conditions. In contrast to most other organs, the rate of total cerebral blood flow is held within a relatively narrow range, and in humans it is approximately 55 ml/min per 100 g of brain.

2. Which arteries supply blood to the brain?

The brain is supplied by four major arteries: the right and left internal carotid arteries, and the right and left vertebral arteries. In primates, the carotid and vertebral systems provide similar contributions to total cerebral blood flow. The vertebral arteries, arising from the subclavian arteries, join to form the basilar artery. The two common carotid arteries arise from the aortic arch and undergo bifurcation, and the internal carotid arteries unite with the basilar artery to form a complete anastomotic ring around the base of the brain known as the circle of Willis.

Heistad DD, Kontos HA: Cerebral circulation. In Shepherd JT, Abboud FM (eds): Handbook of Physiology—The Cardiovascular System. Baltimore, Williams and Wilkins Co., 1983, pp 137–182.

Purves MJ: The Physiology of the Cerebral Circulation. New York NY, Cambridge University Press, 1972.

Sokoloff L: Anatomy of cerebral circulation. In Welch KMA, Caplan LR, Reis DJ, et al (eds): Primer on Cerebrovascular Diseases. San Diego, Academic Press, 1997, pp 3–5.

3. What is the function of the circle of Willis?

The circle of Willis is thought to normally function as an anterior-posterior shunt rather than a side-to-side shunt, because arterial blood pressure usually is similar on both sides of the brain. The circle of Willis gives rise to three pairs of arteries: the anterior, middle, and posterior cerebral arteries. These arteries cover the external surface of the corresponding areas of cerebral cortex, and divide into smaller arteries that penetrate the brain tissue and supply blood to specific regions. The cerebellum and brainstem are supplied by branches of the vertebral and basilar arteries.

4. What influence does the cranium have on the cerebral circulation?

A unique feature of the cerebral circulation is that it lies within a rigid structure, the cranium. Since intracranial contents are incompressible, any increase in arterial inflow, as with arteriolar dilation, must be associated with a comparable increase in venous outflow. In brain, unlike in most tissues, the volume of blood and extracellular fluid is relatively constant, and changes in either of these fluid volumes must be accompanied by a reciprocal change in the other.

Sokoloff L: Anatomy of cerebral circulation. In Welch KMA, Caplan LR, Reis DJ, et al (eds): Primer on Cerebrovascular Diseases. San Diego, Academic Press, 1997, pp 3–5.

5. How is blood drained from the brain?

The brain is drained by a complex venous system that generally consists of three main groups of valveless veins. These are: (1) the superficial cortical veins, which drain the cortex and are located in the pia mater on the cortical surface, (2) the deep or central veins that drain the brain's interior, and (3) the venous sinuses within the dura, where most of the cerebral venous blood eventually drains (e.g., the superior sagittal, inferior sagittal, cavernous, and straight sinuses). Continuations of the superior sagittal sinus (on the right side of the cortex) and of the straight sinus (on the left side of the cortex) extend downward into the internal jugular veins. The internal jugular veins thus provide the exit for most of the cerebral venous blood return.

Sokoloff L: Anatomy of cerebral circulation. In Welch KMA, Caplan LR, Reis DJ, et al (eds): Primer on Cerebrovascular Diseases. San Diego, Academic Press, 1997, pp 3–5.

CHARACTERISTICS OF CEREBRAL BLOOD VESSELS

6. What are some distinctive features of the cerebral circulation?

Several features distinguish cerebral blood vessels from much of the peripheral vasculature, including the blood-brain barrier, the level and functional significance of innervation, the coupling of flow to metabolism, the effects of hypercapnia and hypoxia, the importance of autoregulation, and the role of large arteries in regulating brain vascular resistance.

7. What is the blood-brain barrier?

The endothelial layer forms a tight blood-brain barrier that limits access of many humoral stimuli to smooth muscle of cerebral vessels. This endothelial barrier is structurally much tighter than in most other vascular beds, with a filtration coefficient 70 times less than in skeletal muscle vessels, and 800 times less than in mesentery. There is also an enzymatic aspect to the blood-brain barrier, with a prevalence of monoamine oxidase (which degrades norepinephrine and serotonin), cholinesterases, and other enzymes to prevent passage of humoral neurotransmitters from entering the central nervous system.

Bradbury MWB: The blood-brain barrier. Exp Physiol 78:453–472, 1993.

8. Do nerves play a role in regulation of cerebral blood flow?

Cerebral blood vessels have relatively abundant innervation—from autonomic and sensory fibers—but, in general, the functional significance of this innervation is poorly defined. The innervation is by sympathetic nerves (mainly from the superior cervical ganglion), parasympathetic fibers (mainly from the sphenopalatine, otic, and internal carotid ganglia), and the trigeminal nerve (from the trigeminal ganglion).

9. What do autonomic nerves do in the cerebral circulation?

In contrast to other vascular beds, sympathetic stimulation has little effect on cerebral blood flow under normal conditions. This may be because in response to sympathetic stimulation large arteries constrict, but small vessels downstream dilate as an autoregulatory response to the decrease in perfusion pressure. Despite this modest effect of sympathetic stimuli under normal conditions, there is a profound and important effect of sympathetic activation during acute hypertension. Under this condition, activation of sympathetic nerves attenuates increases in cerebral blood flow and protects the blood-brain barrier. The functional significance of parasympathetic fibers is less clear.

Heistad DD, Kontos AA: Cerebral Circulation. In Shepherd JT, Abboud FM (eds): Handbook of Physiology—The Cardiovascular System. Baltimore, Williams and Wilkins Co., 1983, pp 137–182.

10. Do sensory nerves affect cerebral blood flow?

Sensory fibers can modulate constriction of cerebral blood vessels, and appear to contribute to increases in cerebral blood flow that occur during meningitis, cortical spreading depression, seizures, and reactive hyperemia.

11. Is cerebral blood flow coupled to brain metabolism?

Changes in cerebral blood flow are closely coupled to changes in brain metabolism. For example, increases in neuronal activity, probably by multiple mechanisms, produce increases in local blood flow. These mechanisms may involve coupling of local blood flow to local metabolism by substances such as glutamate, nitric oxide, adenosine, potassium ion, or dopamine.

12. How does the cerebral circulation respond to hypercapnia and hypoxia?

Hypercapnia and hypoxia are potent vasodilators. Vasodilatation in response to hypercapnia appears to be dependent upon formation of nitric oxide, or at least sufficient basal levels of nitric oxide or cyclic GMP need to be present. Some evidence suggests that activation of potassium channels also plays a role in the response to hypercapnia. Adenosine and activation of potassium channels appear to be important mechanisms of cerebral vasodilatation in response to hypoxia.

13. Is cerebral blood flow autoregulated?

Autoregulation is particularly effective in the brain, whereby changes in perfusion pressure produce marked changes in cerebrovascular resistance so that blood flow is maintained relatively constant over a large range of perfusion pressures (~60 to 140 mmHg). Myogenic mechanisms, metabolic factors, neural mechanisms, and activation of potassium channels are thought to be important in the autoregulation of cerebral blood flow.

14. Do the large cerebral arteries play a role in regulation of cerebral blood flow?

Large arteries play a key role in regulation of brain vascular resistance, whereas large vessels are only moderately involved in coronary vascular resistance, and play little role in mesenteric and skeletal muscle vasculature. In the brain, the ~50% of the total resistance to blood flow is contributed by arteries > 200 μm, whereas arteries of this size probably contribute ~10% to vascular resistance in the heart, mesentery, and skeletal muscle. Thus, constriction and dilatation of large cerebral arteries make a critical contribution to regulation of cerebral blood flow.

Faraci FM, Heistad DD: Regulation of large cerebral arteries and cerebral microvascular pressure. Circ Res 66:8–17, 1990.

IMPORTANCE OF ENDOTHELIUM

15. What important vasoactive factors are released from cerebral endothelium?

The cerebral endothelium exerts an important influence on vascular tone through the production and release of a diverse group of vasoactive factors (Fig. 1). Relaxing factors produced by endothelium include nitric oxide, a hyperpolarizing factor, and prostacyclin. Endothelium-derived contracting factors include cyclo-oxygenase products of arachidonic acid and endothelin.

Faraci FM, Heistad DD: Regulation of the cerebral circulation: Role of endothelium and potassium channels. Physiol Rev 78:53–97, 1998.

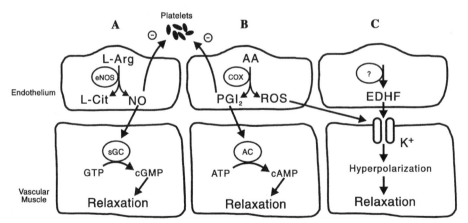

Figure 1. Cerebral endothelial cells synthesize several vasoactive factors. **A,** Nitric oxide (NO) is produced by the conversion of L-arginine (L-Arg) to L-citrulline (L-Cit) by eNOS-type III nitric oxide synthase. NO diffuses into the underlying vascular muscle cells and activates soluble guanylate cyclase (sGC). sGC generates the second messenger molecule, cyclic guanosine monophosphate (cGMP),which causes vascular muscle relaxation and vasodilatation. **B,** Arachidonic acid (AA) is a substrate for cyclo-oxygenase (COX) in cerebral endothelium, resulting in production of prostacyclin (PGI₂) and reactive oxygen species (ROS). PGI₂ stimulates adenylate cyclase in vascular muscle to generate cyclic adenosine monophosphate (cAMP), which causes relaxation. Both NO and PGI₂ also inhibit intraluminal platelet aggregation. **C,** Endothelium-derived hyperpolarizing factor (EDHF), like ROS, activates potassium channels in vascular muscle, causing hyperpolarization and relaxation. Some data indicate that EDHF may be a metabolite of AA.

16. What is nitric oxide?

Nitric oxide (NO) is a gaseous molecule produced in many cell types by a family of isoenzymes known as NO synthases. In general, NO synthases include: type I—constitutively present in neurons (nNOS); type II—induced by proinflammatory stimuli often in immunological cells (iNOS); and type III—constitutively present in endothelium (eNOS). These enzymes convert molecular oxygen and L-arginine to NO and L-citrulline. NO is a potent vasodilator. The finding that inhibitors of NO synthase produce marked constriction of cerebral arteries suggests that NO is released in significant amounts under basal conditions by cerebral endothelium.

17. What cellular second messenger system does nitric oxide stimulate?

NO stimulates soluble guanylate cyclase in vascular smooth muscle cells, which results in intracellular accumulation of cyclic GMP and muscle relaxation. Nitrovasodilator drugs such as nitroglycerin and sodium nitroprusside produce vasodilatation by acting as NO donors. NO also can potentially relax vascular smooth muscle independently of cyclic GMP production, although the physiologic importance of this mechanism may be limited for the relatively low concentrations of NO that are produced endogenously under normal conditions.

Moncada S, Palmer RMJ, Higgs EA: Nitric oxide: Physiology, pathophysiology, and pharmacology. Pharmacol Rev 43:109–142, 1991.

Sobey CG, Faraci FM: Effects of a novel inhibitor of guanylyl cyclase on dilator responses of mouse cerebral arterioles. Stroke 28:837–843, 1997.

18. What is the role of endothelium-derived nitric oxide in regulation of cerebral blood flow?

In addition to tonic release in the cerebral circulation by endothelial cells under basal conditions, NO is released as the major mediator responding to endothelium-dependent vasodilators, such as acetylcholine, substance P, bradykinin, arginine vasopressin, oxytocin, and trypsin. Moreover, increases in shear stress (which occur in the presence of intraluminal blood flow) produce endothelium-dependent NO-mediated vasodilatation, which undoubtedly is an important stimulus for basal NO release. NO released from endothelium is also an important inhibitor of platelet and leukocyte aggregation.

19. Is nitric oxide a physiologic mediator in the cerebral circulation?

NO is the major endothelium-derived relaxing factor released in response to stimuli such as acetylcholine and shear stress, and it appears to play an important role in modulating cerebral vascular tone in response to other stimuli. NO may be released from neurons following activation, and this process elicits dilatation of nearby blood vessels. In this way, neuronally-derived NO is thought to be important in the mechanism of coupling local cerebral blood flow to the level of neuronal metabolic activity.

Iadecola C: Regulation of the cerebral microcirculation during neuronal activity: Is nitric oxide the missing link? Trends Neurosci 16:206–214, 1993.

20. Is nitric oxide a pathologic mediator in the cerebral circulation?

NO also may act as an inflammatory mediator in the circulation when it is produced by the immunologic isoform of NO synthase (type II, iNOS). Type II NO synthase is not expressed constitutively, but is synthesized in response to inflammatory stimuli such as bacterial lipopolysaccharide (endotoxin) and some cytokines (such as tumor necrosis factor α, interleukin β, and interferon γ). The activity of this enzyme (unlike isoforms I and III) is not dependent on increased intracellular levels of calcium ions, and thus can generate large quantities of NO under basal conditions, especially by astrocytes and glia.

iNOS is expressed in brain following ischemia, and also can be detected in the presence of meningitis, multiple sclerosis, encephalitis, and Alzheimer's disease. When produced in excessive amounts, NO may be cytotoxic, and effects in the brain can include neuronal damage, excessive vasodilatation, and increased permeability of the blood-brain barrier.

Huang Z, Huang PL, Panahian N, et al: Effects of cerebral ischemia in mice deficient in neuronal nitric oxide synthase. Science 265:1883–1885, 1994.

Iadecola C: Bright and dark sides of nitric oxide in ischemic brain injury. Trends Neurosci 20:132–139, 1997.

21. What is the role of endothelium-derived arachidonic acid metabolites?

Prostacyclin, a cyclo-oxygenase metabolite of arachidonic acid, is released by endothelial cells. Like NO, prostacyclin produces cerebral vascular relaxation and is a powerful inhibitor of platelet aggregation (see Fig. 1). Prostacyclin generally relaxes cerebral arteries by activation of adenylate cyclase and accumulation of cyclic AMP in vascular muscle. In some instances, endothelium-derived prostacyclin may be a significant mediator of the cerebral vasodilator responses to bradykinin and thrombin.

In addition to prostacyclin, an endothelium-derived hyperpolarizing factor (EDHF) could be another metabolite of arachidonic acid (see Question 17). There is considerable uncertainty over the identity of this factor at present.

22. Is there an endothelium-derived hyperpolarizing factor in cerebral arteries?

In addition to production and release of NO and prostacyclin, endothelium may produce relaxation of underlying vascular muscle by release of an EDHF. Although difficult to bioassay and not yet conclusively identified, there is some evidence that EDHF is a diffusible factor released from endothelium which hyperpolarizes vascular muscle via activation of potassium channels. Possible candidate molecules for the identity of EDHF include: cytochrome P450 metabolites of arachidonic acid (e.g., epoxyeicosatrienoic acids), anandamide (an endogenous cannabinoid), and potassium ion.

EDHF may be less important in the cerebral circulation under normal conditions than, for example, coronary or mesenteric vessels because, in most species studied, endothelium-dependent cerebral vasorelaxation can be greatly attenuated by inhibitors of NO synthase, suggesting that NO release accounts for the majority of the response. Current evidence suggests that in some blood vessels EDHF is simply potassium ion released by endothelium. Whether such a mechanism is important in the cerebral circulation is not known.

Faraci FM, Sobey CG: Role of potassium channels in regulation of cerebral vascular tone. J Cereb Blood Flow Metab 18:1047–1063, 1998.

23. What is the role of endothelin in the cerebral circulation?

In addition to relaxing factors, cerebral endothelium can release contractile substances, the most notable of which is endothelin. Endothelin is generated from big-endothelin by endothelin-converting enzyme (Fig. 2). Endothelin can contract *or* relax cerebral vessels, depending on the location of the receptor being stimulated. Stimulation of either of the two endothelin receptor types (endothelin-A and endothelin-B) on vascular muscle cells results in vasoconstriction, whereas stimulation of endothelial cell receptors (commonly just endothelin-B receptors) results in vasodilatation.

The contractile effect of endothelin on cerebral arteries is potent and long-lasting, and is dependent on extracellular calcium and, in part, activation of protein kinase C. Most evidence suggests that endothelin does not play a physiologic role in the regulation of cerebral blood flow, but may become a significant factor contributing to the delayed and persistent cerebral vasospasm that occurs after subarachnoid hemorrhage (see Question 31). Local production of endothelin also may contribute to the pathophysiology of cerebral ischemia.

Salom JB, Torregrosa G, Alborch E: Endothelins and the cerebral circulation. Cerebrovasc Brain Metab Rev 7:131–152, 1995.

24. Are reactive oxygen species physiologic mediators in the brain?

Reactive oxygen species, such as superoxide anion, hydrogen peroxide, and hydroxyl radical, may be produced in brain and are vasodilators of cerebral vessels. In cerebral arterioles, the mechanism of vasodilatation in response to bradykinin and arachidonic acid appears to involve the formation of reactive oxygen species, indicating that these mediators probably play a physiologic role in the regulation of cerebral microvascular tone.

Faraci FM, Sobey CG: Role of potassium channels in regulation of cerebral vascular tone. J Cereb Blood Flow Metab 18:1047–1063, 1998.

Kontos HA: Oxygen radicals in cerebral vascular injury. Circ Res 57:508–516, 1985.

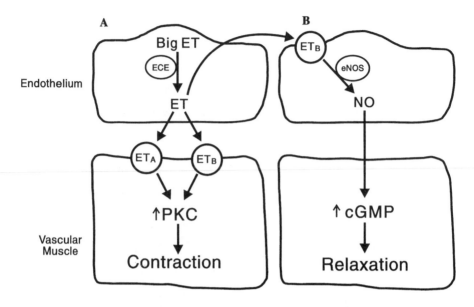

Figure 2. **A**, Endothelin (ET) is synthesized in cerebral endothelial cells by conversion from big-endothelin (Big ET) by endothelin converting enzyme (ECE). ET activates ET-A and ET-B receptors on vascular muscle to cause vasoconstriction, in part via activation of protein kinase C (PKC). **B**, ET also may induce vasodilatation by stimulating ET-B receptors on endothelium, causing NO production by eNOS and cGMP-mediated vascular relaxation.

ELECTROPHYSIOLOGY OF CEREBRAL ARTERIES

25. What is the membrane potential of cerebral arteries?

In vascular muscle, membrane potential is a major determinant of cytosolic free calcium and, thus, vascular tone. The membrane potential of cerebral arteries has not been measured *in vivo* but, based on *in vitro* data, it is probably –40 mV (Fig. 3). A wide variety of vasoactive stimuli elicit their changes in cerebral artery diameter by altering membrane potential. Stimuli that depolarize the vascular muscle membrane (i.e., cause membrane potential to move towards zero) produce vasoconstriction; examples are histamine, serotonin, endothelin, neuropeptide Y, alkalosis, and increased intravascular pressure. On the other hand, hyperpolarizing stimuli (which move membrane potential further away from zero) produce vasodilatation; examples include ADP, ATP, acetylcholine, substance P, adenosine, NO, and acidosis.

Faraci FM, Sobey CG: Role of potassium channels in regulation of cerebral vascular tone. J Cereb Blood Flow Metab 18:1047–1063, 1998.

26. Are potassium channels important in cerebral arteries?

Yes, potassium channels are a major determinant of membrane potential in arterial smooth muscle. When a potassium channel in the vascular muscle cell membrane opens, potassium ions flux out of the cell down their electrochemical gradient, causing the membrane potential to approach the equilibrium potential for potassium, typically about –85mV (i.e., hyperpolarization from a resting potential of approximately –40mV). Membrane hyperpolarization causes closure of voltage-operated calcium channels, leading to a decreased intracellular calcium concentration and, consequently, vascular muscle relaxation (Fig. 4). It now is established that opening (or activation) of potassium channels is a major mechanism of vasodilatation in cerebral arteries. Stimuli that activate potassium channels include: NO/cyclic GMP, cyclic AMP, arachidonic acid, hypoxia, hypercapnia, and synthetic openers such as cromakalim. Closure (or inhibition) of potassium channels decreases the outward flux of potassium ions, causing membrane depolarization and vasoconstriction.

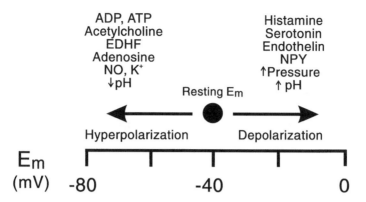

Figure 3. Several vasoactive stimuli affect membrane potential (E_m) in cerebral vascular muscle. Hyperpolarization occurs when E_m is moved to a more negative value, and vasodilator stimuli such as adenosine diphosphate (ADP), adenosine triphosphate (ATP), acetylcholine, EDHF, adenosine, NO, potassium ions (K⁺), and acidosis (decreased pH) will do this. Vasoconstrictor stimuli, such as histamine, serotonin, endothelin, neuropeptide Y, increased blood pressure, and alkalosis (increased pH), cause cerebral vascular depolarization.

27. What types of potassium channels are functional in cerebral arteries?

There are at least four types of potassium channels present in cerebral arteries: calcium-activated (K_{Ca}); ATP-sensitive (K_{ATP}); voltage-dependent (K_V); and inwardly rectifying (K_{IR}) (Fig. 5). To date, the best-studied of these are the K_{Ca} and K_{ATP} channels.

Nelson MT, Quayle JM: Physiological roles and properties of potassium channels in arterial smooth muscle. Am J Physiol 268:C799–C822, 1995.

28. What is known about K_{Ca} channel function in cerebral arteries?

K_{Ca} channels are the most abundant potassium channels in vascular smooth muscle, and are activated under physiologic conditions by increasing intracellular levels of calcium, cyclic AMP, or

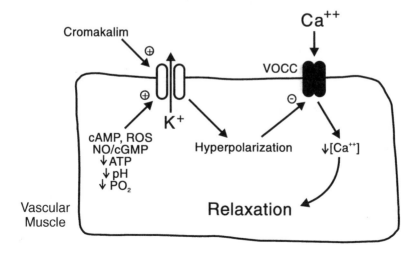

Figure 4. Activation of a potassium channel (left) causes K⁺ to flux from the cell, leading to hyperpolarization. Hyperpolarization causes closure of voltage-operated calcium channels (VOCC), resulting in decreased intracellular calcium concentration ([Ca⁺⁺]) and vascular relaxation.

K⁺ Channels in Cerebral Arteries

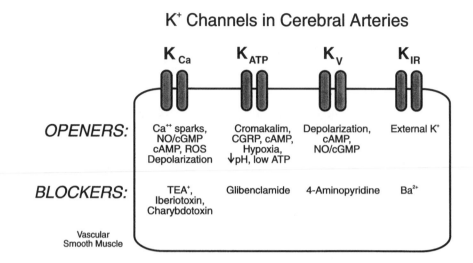

Figure 5.   There are at least four types of potassium channels in cerebral arteries: calcium-activated (K_{Ca}), ATP-sensitive (K_{ATP}), voltage-dependent (K_V), and inward rectifier (K_{IR}). TEA⁺ = tetraethylammonium ion; CGRP = calcium gene-related peptide; Ba²⁺ = barium ion.

cyclic GMP. The cyclic nucleotides, cyclic AMP and cyclic GMP, are thought to stimulate localized "sparks" of calcium to be released from the sarcoplasmic reticulum in close proximity to the K_{Ca} channels, thus causing channel activation. K_{Ca} channels may be especially important in buffering contractions of cerebral arteries (associated with increases in intracellular calcium levels), such as myogenic contractions that occur in response to increases in cerebral intra-arterial pressure. Inhibitors of K_{Ca} channels, such as tetraethylammonium ion, charybdotoxin, and iberiotoxin, cause constriction of larger cerebral arteries, suggesting that K_{Ca} activity exists in these vessels under normal conditions.

Nelson MT, Cheng H, Rubart M, et al: Relaxation of arterial smooth muscle by calcium sparks. Science 270:633–637, 1995.

29. What is known about K_{ATP} channel function in cerebral arteries?

The activity of K_{ATP} channels may reflect the metabolic state of the vascular muscle cell, as intracellular ATP inhibits the channel activity. Thus, reduced levels of ATP, as well as metabolically related stimuli such as hypoxia and acidosis (and synthetic openers like cromakalim), cause K_{ATP} channel opening and cerebral vasodilatation. Since inhibitors of K_{ATP} channels such as glibenclamide have little or no effect on resting diameter of cerebral arteries, there appears to be minimal basal activity of cerebral K_{ATP} channels in cerebral arteries.

Quayle JM, Nelson MT, Standen NB: ATP-sensitive and inwardly rectifying potassium channels in smooth muscle. Physiol Rev 77:1165–1232, 1997.

PATHOPHYSIOLOGY OF CEREBRAL ARTERIES

30. How does chronic hypertension affect cerebral artery function?

Chronic hypertension causes both structural and functional changes in the cerebral circulation (Fig. 6). Structurally, there is remodeling of the arterial wall, with a decreased luminal area and an increased wall thickness. Endothelial function appears to be particularly affected by chronic hypertension. In large cerebral arteries and cerebral arterioles, vasodilator responses to endothelium-dependent agonists such as acetylcholine, ADP, and bradykinin are impaired during chronic hypertension, whereas responses to endothelium-independent agonists (which act directly on vascular muscle) such as NO, nitroglycerin, and adenosine are preserved. The mechanism of these changes appears to differ according to the vessel size. It appears that in large arteries the abnormality is due to reduced production or activity of endothelium-derived nitric oxide, whilst in cerebral arterioles there may be an increased production of an endothelium-derived contractile factor that counteracts the effects of NO.

Faraci FM, Heistad DD: Regulation of the cerebral circulation: Role of endothelium and potassium channels. Physiol Rev 78:53–97, 1998.

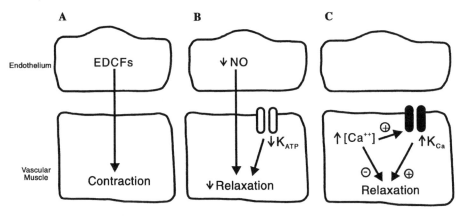

Figure 6. Abnormalities in cerebral artery function in chronic hypertension. **A,** In cerebral arterioles, unidentified endothelium-derived contractile factors (EDCFs) inhibit responses to endothelium-dependent vasodilators. **B,** Decreased production or activity of NO may occur, and activity of K_{ATP} channels also may be decreased. **C,** Activity of K_{Ca} channels appears to be increased during chronic hypertension, perhaps in response to increased levels of intracellular calcium ($[Ca^{++}]$).

31. Is potassium channel function altered by chronic hypertension?

Data so far indicate that the function of potassium channels in cerebral vessels is differentially altered by hypertension. For example, basal activity of K_{Ca} channels is increased during hypertension, perhaps as a compensatory response to the increased myogenic contractility. In contrast, cerebral vasodilator responses to openers of K_{ATP} channels appear to be markedly impaired in hypertension.

32. How do hypercholesterolemia and atherosclerosis affect cerebral artery function?

Although it is well established that atherosclerosis causes impairment of release or activity of endothelium-derived NO in *extra*cranial vessels, the effect of atherosclerosis on the function of *intra*cranial vessels is less clear. These vessels appear to develop atherosclerotic lesions more slowly than extracranial vessels, and endothelium-dependent vasodilatation can still be normal in intracranial vessels when a similar response is markedly impaired in the peripheral circulation.

Vasoactive effects of platelets and platelet products appear to be altered by atherosclerosis. In the presence of atherosclerosis in the carotid and other large arteries supplying the brain, constrictor responses to serotonin and thromboxane A_2 are enhanced. Intracarotid injection of collagen, which activates platelets, normally increases carotid blood flow due to the release of ADP and subsequent endothelium-dependent vasodilatation. In contrast, collagen decreases carotid blood flow in the presence of atherosclerosis.

Faraci FM, Heistad DD: Regulation of the cerebral circulation: Role of endothelium and potassium channels. Physiol Rev 78:53–97, 1998.

33. Is dietary treatment of hypercholesterolemia effective in improving cerebral artery function?

Reduction in dietary cholesterol produces regression of atherosclerotic lesions and restores toward normal the impaired endothelium-dependent relaxation and augmented constrictor responses to serotonin of extracranial arteries. Importantly, significant functional improvement appears to precede structural regression of cerebral and noncerebral atherosclerotic lesions, and occurs within a few months of dietary treatment. Thus, the benefits of cholesterol therapy may be relatively fast.

Sobey CG, Faraci FM, Piegors DJ, Heistad DD: Effect of short-term regression of atherosclerosis on reactivity of carotid and retinal arteries. Stroke 27:927–933, 1996.

34. How does diabetes mellitus affect cerebral artery function?

Endothelial dysfunction can occur in diabetes mellitus. Mechanisms of these abnormalities appear to be similar to those in hypertension. The increased release of an endothelium-derived contractile factor that activates a prostaglandin H_2/thromboxane A_2 receptor appears to cause reduced endothelium-dependent dilatation of cerebral arterioles, but not in large cerebral arteries. Moreover, hyperglycemia per se appears to impair endothelium-dependent dilatation of cerebral arterioles. Activity of K_{ATP} channels and responses to β-adrenergic agonists also are impaired in cerebral arteries in diabetes mellitus. However, responses to endothelium-independent vasodilators (such as NO donors) are not impaired, indicating that not all vasodilator mechanisms are nonspecifically attenuated.

35. What is known regarding the mechanisms of impaired cerebral vasodilatation in diabetes mellitus?

Recent evidence suggests that treatment with dimethylthiourea, an inhibitor of hydroxyl radical, restores to normal the impaired dilator responses of the basilar artery to acetylcholine in diabetic rats. Therefore, the impairment of cerebral endothelial function in diabetes mellitus, now recognized as a disease state involving increased oxidant stress, may be related to excessive production and/or release of reactive oxygen species.

Mayhan WG, Patel KP: Treatment with dimethylthiourea prevents impaired dilatation of the basilar artery during diabetes mellitus. Am J Physiol 274:H1895–H1901, 1998.

36. How does subarachnoid hemorrhage affect cerebral artery function?

Subarachnoid hemorrhage (SAH) commonly is due to cerebral aneurysm or trauma, and often results in abnormalities of cerebral artery function that involve impaired vasodilator responsiveness and increased vasoconstriction. The most critical cerebrovascular complication of SAH is delayed cerebral vasospasm—a sustained constriction of cerebral arteries exposed to the blood clot. This vasospasm does not usually begin to develop in patients until 3 days after SAH, and typically reaches a maximum on days 6–8.

The mechanism of cerebral vasospasm is poorly understood, and there are still no adequate pharmacologic treatments, although recent evidence suggests that increased endothelin-induced vasoconstriction may play an important role. Endothelin levels in the CSF are increased after SAH, and treatment with endothelin-A antagonists may reduce vasospasm. Hemoglobin and thrombin, also present in the CSF after SAH, can enhance endothelin production and release (Fig. 7).

Sobey CG, Faraci FM: Subarachnoid hemorrhage: What happens to the cerebral arteries? Clin Exp Pharmacol Physiol 25:867–876, 1998.

37. What happens to the nitric oxide-cyclic GMP vasodilator pathway in cerebral arteries after SAH?

Vasodilatation via the NO-cyclic GMP pathway appears to be especially attenuated following SAH. This may be partly due to damaged endothelial cells as well as oxyhemoglobin contained in erythrocytes, causing impaired production or activity of endothelium-derived NO, respectively. However, cerebral vasodilator responses to NO donor drugs (e.g., nitroglycerin and sodium nitroprusside) often also are impaired after SAH, indicating that responsiveness of vascular muscle to NO is diminished. This may be due to decreased activity of soluble guanylate cyclase and/or reduced levels of cyclic GMP in vascular muscle.

38. Is potassium channel function altered in cerebral arteries after SAH?

Changes in activity of potassium channels may contribute to spasm of cerebral arteries after SAH. Partial depolarization of cerebral vascular muscle after SAH appears to be due to decreased

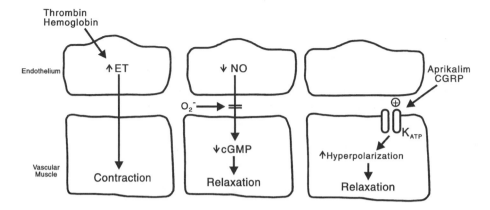

Figure 7. Abnormalities in cerebral vessels following SAH. **A,** Thrombin and hemoglobin stimulate production of endothelin (ET), a potent vasoconstrictor. **B,** Superoxide anion ($O2^-$) may be formed from hemoglobin in the CSF and may inactivate NO, thus impairing vasorelaxation. **C,** Vasodilation in response to activation of K_{ATP} channels (e.g., by aprikalim or calcitonin gene-related peptide [CGRP]) appears to be augmented following SAH, which may represent a direction for therapy against cerebral vasospasm after SAH.

membrane conductance to potassium ions. Since CGRP, nicorandil, aprikalim, and cromakalim (all K_{ATP} channel openers) are reported to be effective cerebral vasodilators after experimental SAH, treatment with activators of potassium channels may have beneficial effects during vasospasm following SAH (Fig. 7).

39. How does ischemia affect cerebral artery function?

Formation of reactive oxygen species, which is known to occur during post-ischemic reperfusion, seems to cause significant impairment of endothelium-dependent cerebral vasodilatation. Compelling evidence for this conclusion is that impaired vasodilatation can be restored to normal experimentally by treatment with superoxide dismutase and catalase (which destroy superoxide anion and hydrogen peroxide, respectively). Sources of reactive oxygen species in the cerebral circulation after ischemia may include the cyclo-oxygenase pathway, the nitric oxide synthase pathway (in the absence of adequate substrate L-arginine), and the NADH oxidase pathway in leukocytes. Activation of leukocytes and adherence of these cells to endothelium may therefore be an important factor in causing brain injury during post-ischemic reperfusion.

40. Is nitric oxide beneficial or harmful in cerebral ischemia?

NO produced by cerebral endothelium (type III, eNOS) appears to be protective for the brain during and after ischemia, whereas it is not clear whether NO produced by the immunologic form of the enzyme (type II, iNOS) is harmful or beneficial under these conditions.

Iadecola C: Bright and dark sides of nitric oxide in ischemic brain injury. Trends Neurosci 20:132–139, 1997.

41. How does hyperhomocysteinemia affect cerebral artery function?

Moderate elevation of plasma homocysteine appears to be an independent risk factor for stroke and, like hypercholesterolemia, is caused by both genetic and dietary factors and may contribute to vascular disease in a large number of patients. Dietary supplementation with folic acid can decrease moderate hyperhomocysteinemia, suggesting that this is a treatable risk factor. Mechanisms causing vascular disease may involve hydrogen peroxide or other reactive oxygen species, and include impairment of endothelium-dependent NO-mediated vasodilatation, increased platelet-mediated vasoconstriction, and decreased thrombomodulin-dependent activation of the anticoagulant protein C.

BIBLIOGRAPHY

1. Bevan RD, Bevan JA (eds): The Human Brain Circulation: Functional Changes in Disease. Totowa, New Jersey, Humana Press Inc., 1994.
2. Bradbury MWB: The blood-brain barrier. Exp Physiol 78:453–472, 1993.
3. Faraci FM, Heistad DD: Regulation of the cerebral circulation: Role of endothelium and potassium channels. Physiol Rev 78:53–97, 1998.
4. Heistad DD, Kontos HA: Cerebral circulation. In Shepherd JT, Abboud FM (eds): Handbook of Physiology: The Cardiovascular System. Baltimore, Williams and Wilkins Co., 1983, pp 137–182.
5. Purves MJ: The Physiology of the Cerebral Circulation. New York NY, Cambridge University Press, 1972.

22. NEUROIMAGING: TECHNOLOGY AND CLINICAL APPLICATIONS

Kathleen M. Donahue, Ph.D., and John L. Ulmer, M.D.

The dramatic influx of technologies into the field of neuroradiology over the last two decades has resulted in some of the most significant developments to date in the diagnosis and management of neurological diseases. It is now possible to evaluate brain morphology, tissue structure, metabolite concentrations, molecular movements, and neuronal function using noninvasive imaging techniques. These techniques are in a constant state of evolution and refinement. The following chapter outlines some of the more commonly used imaging methods for evaluating the brain, as well as newly developed techniques that are increasing our understanding of neurological function and disease every day. Selected clinical applications of these techniques are provided to illustrate their widespread clinical utility.

IMAGING TECHNOLOGY

1. Which modalities are used most often for clinical brain imaging?

Computed tomography (CT), magnetic resonance imaging (MRI), and x-ray angiography. Of these, CT and MRI now create the majority of clinical brain images generated throughout the world.

Computed Tomography

2. What is computed tomography?

CT is similar to conventional radiographs (i.e., x-rays) in that the images are produced by the differential absorption of x-rays, but it is much more sensitive. The CT scan is an image of a single plane or section of tissue; hence, the term tomography. A section of a tomogram is a true two-dimensional representation of a two-dimensional object (the thin plane), in contrast to a conventional x-ray, which represents a three-dimensional object in two dimensions.

3. How does computed tomography work?

Like conventional planar x-rays, x-radiation is transmitted across a patient and detected with a radiation detector on the opposite side. With CT, x-ray transmission data is obtained by scanning an area from many different directions. This data then is digitally reconstructed to provide two-dimensional anatomical information.

4. How is image contrast achieved with computed tomography?

In CT, the attenuation of x-ray beams passing through a given tissue region is measured directly. Dark areas correspond to regions of high x-ray transmittance, and light areas correspond to areas of low x-ray transmittance. In this way, the signal differences between tissues (i.e., the image contrast) is based on differences in the absorbency of radiation.

5. Describe the nature of CT image contrast in brain tissue.

The skull and calcium-accumulating tissues appear bright due to their high absorption of x-radiation. Conversely, air absorbs very little radiation and appears dark. Also, due to computer-analyzed x-ray transmission profiles, resolution of gray and white matter, blood, and cerebrospinal fluid is possible despite very small differences in radiodensity (less than 2%).

6. Can CT image contrast be further enhanced?

Intravenous injection of iodinated radiopaque material further enhances the contrast between tissue constituents in regions that have either increased vasculature or impaired blood-brain barrier functions. By this means, blood vessels, tumors, and abscesses can be visualized effectively.

Magnetic Resonance Imaging

7. What is magnetic resonance imaging?

Magnetic resonance imaging is a medical technology that uses a strong magnetic field and radiofrequency waves to create an image of tissue water.

8. How does MRI work?

First, a patient is placed in a strong magnetic field, typically 100,000 times the strength of the earth's magnetic field. Then, a pulse of radio frequency (rf) energy is transmitted into the patient under controlled and prescribed conditions. Finally, the patient responds to this stimulation by emitting a radio frequency signal that is computer processed to produce an image.

9. What does the magnet do?

Water protons, which comprise 80–90% of our body tissues, have a certain property allowing them to be magnetized. This property is analogous to that of a compass needle, which points north in response to the earth's magnetic field. Consequently, when a patient is placed within a large magnetic field, the water protons become oriented along the direction of the main field. More specifically, they rotate or precess around an axis that is aligned with the main field, much like a rotating top, spinning around the earth's gravitational field (Fig. 1). The frequency of precession (ω_0, given in radians per second) is termed **Larmor frequency**, and is equal to the product of the nuclei's gyromagnetic ratio (γ, which is unique to each nuclear species) and the strength of the main magnetic field (B_0). This is the Larmor equation:

$$\omega_0 = \gamma B_0$$

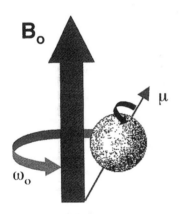

Figure 1. A water proton (represented by the sphere) in the presence of an external magnetic field, B_0. When a patient is placed within a large magnetic field, the water protons become oriented along the direction of B_0. More precisely, they rotate around their own axis (generating a magnetic movement, μ) while precessing around B_0, with a precession or Larmor frequency, ω_0.

10. Why do we image primarily water protons and not another nuclear species that also can be magnetized?

The strength of a nuclei's magnetization is a property of the type of nucleus and determines its detection sensitivity. Of the nuclei that can be magnetized, ^1H nuclei (protons) possess the strongest magnetization when in a magnetic field, which, together with the high biological abundance of hydrogen, makes it the nucleus of choice for MRI.

11. What does "resonance" have to do with magnetic resonance imaging?

In order to measure the tissue water magnetization and its properties (which are influenced by the chemical environment of the tissue water), the equilibrium magnetization state must be perturbed. Energy is effectively transmitted into the system only when it is of the same frequency as the precessing water protons. This same-frequency condition is called resonance. And it turns out that the range of resonance frequencies required for MRI are the same as those used for an FM radio, thus explaining the use of radio frequency (rf) energy.

12. How do we detect the signal emitted by the patient?

The rf pulse "flips" some or all of the tissue water magnetization, which originally was aligned with the main field (i.e., by convention in the z-direction when using a Cartesian coordinate system), into the xy or transverse plane (Fig. 2). After the rf pulse is turned off, the magnetization in the xy plane begins to decay back toward equilibrium in a time-dependent manner. This time-varying magnetic field induces a current in a receiver coil, enabling detection of the rf signal emitted from the patient.

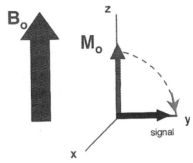

Figure 2.   The radiofrequency energy transmitted into an equilibrium system of aligned water protons (M_O) results in some or all of the tissue water magnetization being "flipped" into the transverse or xy plane. It is the transverse component of the MRI signal that is detected and measured.

13. How is the MRI signal mapped to a given location? In other words, how are images created?

By superimposing linear gradients of magnetic field on the main field, unique spatial information can be derived from the received signal. The term "gradient" designates that the magnetic field is altered as a function of position along a selected direction (Fig. 3).

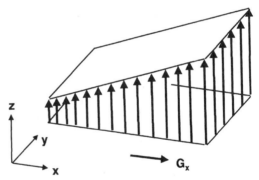

Figure 3.   A magnetic field gradient in the x direction, G_x. By superimposing a gradient of magnetic field on the main magnetic field, the frequency of water protons varies as a function of position, as described by the Larmor equation (see Question 9). Application of gradients in three perpendicular directions (G_x, G_y, G_z) enables the unique spatial localization of the MRI signal and the formation of an image.

14. How do these magnetic field gradients provide the necessary spatial information?

According to the Larmor equation (see Question 9), if the magnetic field is varied linearly along a certain direction, then the Larmor or resonance frequency of the water protons also varies with location. Therefore, by determining the frequency content of the received signal we know where the signal is coming from and how much signal is in a given location. Specifically, a mathematical process called the Fourier transform converts the time-dependent MRI signal, which is what we measure, to a frequency distribution of the signal, giving the amount of signal present at each frequency (location).

15. How are these gradients used to provide unique information in each image location (voxel)?

Gradients of magnetic field are applied in three orthogonal directions (e.g., x, y, and z). Application of these gradients in each of the directions is termed slice selection, phase encoding, and frequency encoding, respectively.

16. What gives magnetic resonance images their excellent soft tissue contrast?

MRI soft tissue contrast results from a combination of intrinsic tissue parameters and user-controlled manipulation of the image sequence timing parameters. In addition, exogenous contrast agents frequently are used to improve contrast, especially between normal and pathologic tissues.

17. What are the intrinsic tissue parameters that influence MRI contrast?

After turning off the rf transmission pulse, which produces some net magnetization in the transverse plane, the time-varying magnetization begins to both relax back toward equilibrium, i.e., grow in the z-direction, and decay in the transverse or xy plane. The time constants describing these growth and decay processes are termed **T1** and **T2**. These time constants, together with the density of water protons, compose the intrinsic tissue parameters that provide the basis for the image contrast.

18. What are some typical values for T1 and T2 in brain tissue?

At a magnetic field strength of 1.5 Tesla, the T1s of cerebrospinal fluid (CSF), gray matter, and white matter are 2650 milliseconds (ms), 760 ms, and 510 ms, respectively (Fig. 4A). For these same tissues, the T2 values are approximately 280 ms, 77 ms, and 67 ms (Fig. 4B). Except in pure water, T2 is always less than T1.

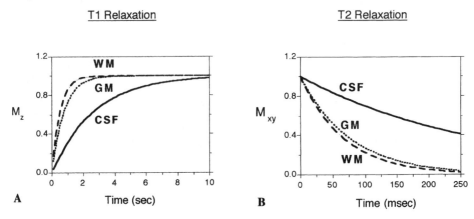

Figure 4. Relaxation of time constants in white matter (WM), gray matter (GM), and cerebrospinal fluid (CSF). **A**, T1 relaxation describes the growth of the magnetization in the z-direction (M_z) as a function of time. **B**, T2 relaxation describes the decay of the magnetization in the transverse or xy plane (M_{xy}).

19. How can we control the image contrast?

T1, T2, and proton density are intrinsic tissue parameters over which the user has no control. However, the operator can alter tissue contrast and signal-to-noise by the choice of the imaging sequence parameters. Specifically, images can be obtained in which tissue contrast is determined primarily by (i.e., weighted toward) T1, T2, or proton density characteristics. This weighting is achieved in a variety of ways. For example, various image contrast weightings can be obtained by varying: the time between the rf excitation and the measurement of the signal (the echo time, TE); the time between successive rf excitations (the repetition time, TR); or the strength of the rf pulse.

20. What is the appearance of a strongly T1-weighted brain image?

Since the T1 of CSF is longer than that of the gray and white matter (the CSF z-axis signal requires more time to return to its equilibrium state of magnetization), its T1-weighted signal is lower. Thus, the CSF appears dark on a strongly T1-weighted MRI.

21. What is the appearance of a strongly T2-weighted brain image?

Since the T2 of CSF is longer than that of the gray and white matter (the CSF transverse magnetization takes more time to decay to zero), its T2-weighted singal is higher. Thus, the CSF appears bright on a strongly T2-weighted MRI.

22. What are MRI contrast agents?

MRI contrast agents are exogenously administered media that alter the T1 and T2 relaxation times in the tissues in which they distribute.

23. Are MRI contrast agents different from x-ray and nuclear medicine contrast agents?

MRI contrast agents are different from those used in x-ray and radionuclide imaging techniques in two important ways. First, they are nonionizing. Second, unlike nuclear medicine and x-ray studies in which the signal attenuation is a direct measure of contrast concentration, the MRI signal is indirectly related to contrast media concentration. Specifically, with MRI it is the *effect* of the contrast agent on the tissue water magnetization that is directly measured.

24. Can MRI be used to evaluate tissue physiology and function?

Yes. Several of the more common applications include MRI evaluation of blood flow, perfusion (blood delivery to tissues), blood volume, and diffusion (the molecular movement of tissue water within tissue). There are two general approaches for measuring perfusion: one uses endogenous (natural) contrast, and the other uses exogenous (injectable) contrast.

25. Briefly describe the perfusion techniques that use injectable contrast agents.

With high-speed imaging techniques, the first pass of a contrast agent through tissue vasculature can be observed. Using standard tracer kinetic theory, blood flow, perfusion, and blood volume can be calculated from this dynamic information.

26. Briefly describe the MRI perfusion methods that are based on endogenous contrast.

Currently there are two general approaches under investigation. The first is based on the radiofrequency labeling of blood water. These **arterial spin labeling (ASL)** techniques, as they are called, are relatively new and not yet widely used. The second approach is based on **blood oxygenation level–dependent (BOLD) contrast** and is currently the method of choice to monitor brain activity. Specifically, with high-speed echo planar imaging (EPI) techniques it is possible to observe changes in the blood oxygenation level in the brain, which occur with increases in brain activity. EPI commonly is termed functional MRI (Fig. 5). Though functional MRI currently is used primarily as a research tool, clinical applications are growing steadily.

27. How are MRI images made sensitive to diffusion?

The application of extra, very large, magnetic field gradients to the standard imaging techniques makes the MRI images highly sensitive to the molecular motion of water. The resulting images are therefore said to be **diffusion-weighted**, in that areas of slower diffusion appear bright (e.g., ischemic tissue), and tissues with faster diffusion (e.g., a cyst) appear dark. By acquiring images at several different gradient levels, the diffusion constant can be determined absolutely in units of mm^2/sec. Diffusion imaging is becoming important in the evaluation of acute stroke (see Question 78).

28. What is the time resolution of MRI?

Depending on the chosen imaging sequence, images take between tens of milliseconds to many minutes to acquire. The standard or conventional imaging sequences, which also provide very high spatial resolution, take several minutes. Fast imaging sequences, such as fast gradient echo sequences, can be acquired in seconds. Finally, high-speed imaging sequences such as EPI can be acquired in less than 100 ms. In general, as the time resolution increases the spatial resolution decreases.

X-ray Angiography

29. What is angiography?

Angiography provides images of blood vessels and lymphatics. Presently, x-ray angiography is the most common method used for this purpose.

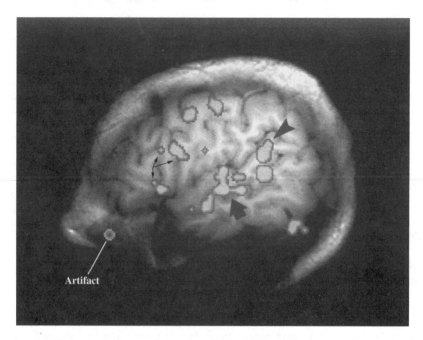

Figure 5.   Functional MRI of auditory and language cortical activation in the dominant left hemisphere, in response to a text-listening task. There is cortical activation in primary and auditory association cortex *(thick
arrow)* and in the posterior language area *(arrowhead)*. Additional cortical activation is evident in the left inferior
frontal lobe, corresponding to anterior language-relevant cortex *(triple arrow).*   ***Note: see color panel.***

30. How does x-ray angiography work?

In x-ray angiography, the patient receives an intravascular injection of a radio-opaque material (contrast medium). Following this injection, serial x-rays are taken in rapid sequence.
This results in the precise delineation of blood vessels that contain the circulating radio-opaque
material.

31. What are the primary advantages and drawbacks of x-ray angiography?

X-ray angiography provides a wealth of information on the anatomy of the cerebral vasculature
and the speed of blood circulation in the brain in normal and diseased regions. In particular, it can
identify aneurysms, vascular malformations, occlusive strokes, and vascular tumors, and is the optimal procedure for diagnosing lesions of the intracranial vascular system. Primary drawbacks are that
it is invasive, and it involves intravascular injection of radio-opaque material, which can cause neurological complications.

32. Can angiograms be acquired with MRI-based methods?

Yes. In particular, recent advances in MRI allow intracranial vessels to be imaged through a
noninvasive technique termed magnetic resonance angiography (MRA). Although MRA has poor
resolution compared to conventional angiography, with technical advances it may supplant invasive
angiography.

33. Is the information derived from an MRA different from an x-ray angiogram?

It can be. Specifically, while x-ray angiography provides purely anatomical information about
vessels, MRA techniques delineate vessels by sensitivity to flow. In fact, MRA methods are based
on the same principles as flow quantitation techniques.

Diagnostic Methods Sensitive To Tissue Chemistry and Metabolism

34. Are there diagnostic methods available to evaluate brain tissue chemistry and metabolism?

Positron emission tomography (PET), single photon emission computed tomography (SPECT), and magnetic resonance spectroscopy (MRS) are used in the evaluation of tissue chemistry and metabolism.

35. What is positron emission tomography?

PET is a diagnostic modality in which the distribution of positron-emitting radioisotopes in tissue is imaged.

36. What is a radioisotope?

Atoms of a given element that differ in number of neutrons and consequently in mass are called *isotopes* (e.g., carbon-12 and carbon-14). Isotopes that are unstable undergo radioactive decay and are known as *radio*isotopes.

37. What is a positron-emitting radioisotope?

A small number of radioisotopes are unstable because their nuclei contain an excess number of protons with respect to a more stable configuration of neutrons and protons. These radioisotopes get rid of their excessive energy by emitting a *positron*, a particle that has the same mass as an electron but the opposite charge.

38. Gives examples of positron-emitting isotopes.

Carbon, oxygen, nitrogen, and hydrogen each have at least one isotope that decays through positron emission. This is a very fortunate feature for PET, since these elements constitute most of living matter. The importance of being able to follow *in vivo* the fate of such compounds and their metabolites is obvious.

39. Describe the essential steps in the performance of a PET study.

Early each day, the radionuclide(s) to be used in that day's PET studies are generated in an on-site cyclotron (except for a few generator-produced radionuclides). Some compounds are available for use at the end of the cyclotron production cycle or shortly thereafter. Others require synthetic procedures leading to a variety of labeled, organic compounds, which are then used in metabolic and other measurements of biochemistry and function. Prior to radioisotope administration, a transmission scan is performed to determine the attenuation of gamma rays along each image scan line. Following transmission scanning, the positron-emitting tracer is injected intravenously, and static or sequential images are acquired.

40. How is the distribution of the radioisotopes detected?

The radioisotope emits a positron that eventually collides with one of the many electrons in the tissue, at which time a spontaneous annihilation occurs (Fig. 6). In this annihilation event, the masses of the positron and electron are converted into electromagnetic radiation in the form of two high-energy protons, or gamma rays. These two gamma rays travel in opposite directions, and each gamma ray is detected by the PET machine's scintillation detectors. The near-simultaneous detection of two oppositely-directed photons enables the tissue localization of the radioisotope.

41. What are the primary advantages and disadvantages of PET imaging?

PET is a powerful and comprehensive tool for studying tissue metabolism noninvasively. It often is used as a gold standard to which other noninvasive imaging results and measures of metabolism are compared. However, the need for an on-site cyclotron, the use of radioactive tracers, and poor image resolution ($\approx$ 8 mm in-plane resolution in the most advanced PET scanners) has precluded the widespread use and availability of PET imaging.

42. What is single photon emission computed tomography?

As the name suggests, SPECT techniques entail imaging the distribution of radionuclides that emit single photons.

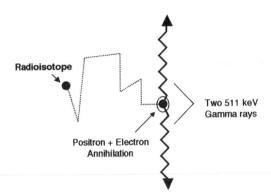

Figure 6.   A positron emitted from a radioisotope. Due to collisions, the positron travels in a zig-zag path through the tissue. As its loses its velocity it binds to an electron, with which it annihilates, creating two 511-kiloelectron volt (keV), oppositely-directed gamma rays, or photons.

43. How are SPECT images obtained?

Multiple angular projections are accumulated as a gamma camera rotates around the subject's head. Computerized techniques are applied, resulting in three-dimensional, tomographic data sets.

44. What are some of the more common radionuclides used in SPECT imaging?

Some of the more common radionuclides imaged with SPECT include ^{133}Xe gas and ^{99m}Tc-hexamethylpropyleneamineoxime. Both are used for the measurement of regional cerebral blood flow.

45. What is the spatial resolution of SPECT images?

Typical SPECT scanners provide a spatial resolution of 10–16 mm. However, advanced scanners dedicated to brain imaging can achieve spatial resolutions as good as 8 mm.

46. What is magnetic resonance spectroscopy?

MRS, like MRI, is a technology based on the phenomenon of nuclear magnetic resonance. However, MRS does not provide the same high-resolution spatial information available with MRI. Instead, MRS provides more specific information about tissue chemistry, obtaining a plot of intensity versus frequency (a spectrum) of nuclei in different local magnetic field environments for a given tissue sample (Fig. 7).

47. What is the source of the intrinsic magnetic field environments?

These local magnetic field environments result from differences in the chemical structure of the molecule in which the nuclei reside. Recall that each nucleus is surrounded by a cloud of electrons—moving, charged particles that generate their own magnetic fields. These magnetic fields either add to or subtract from the main (external) magnetic field. According to the Larmor equation (Question 9), slightly different magnetic fields result in slightly different resonance frequencies.

48. What information does MRS provide?

Study of a variety of nuclei, other than protons, that are visible by nuclear magnetic resonance has allowed evaluation of different aspects of metabolism, such as energetics and compartmentalization. Consequently, MRS techniques are able to identify detailed molecular structures and conformations, local pH and temperature, biochemical pathways, and metabolite kinetics.

49. How is MRS information obtained?

The process of acquiring MRS data is essentially the same as that described for MRI, with the important exception that the MRS signal is collected in the absence of magnetic field gradients (i.e., no frequency encoding of position).

50. Why must the MRS signal be acquired in the absence of magnetic field gradients?

The acquired signal frequency distribution (spectrum) must represent local magnetic field differences due to the tissue's chemical environment, and not differences imposed by an external gradient.

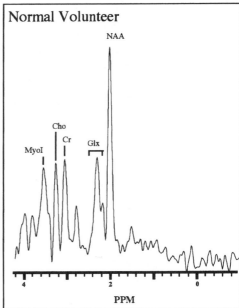

Figure 7. A proton MRS spectrum from a normal volunteer. Spectral peaks corresponding to myo-inositol (MyoI), choline (Cho), creatine (Cr), glutamate and glutamine (G1x) and n-acetyl aspartate (NAA) are apparent.

51. Can MRS information be acquired for each tissue location?

Yes. The technique that accomplishes this is termed chemical shift imaging, which is an MRI technique that provides spectral resolution and some degree of spatial localization. However, obtaining spectroscopic information from many voxels, instead of one, results in less signal-to-noise per voxel (given that the total imaging time is the same in both cases).

CLINICAL APPLICATIONS

Intracranial Hemorrhage

52. What is the imaging method of choice for evaluating acute subarachnoid hemorrhage?

Computed tomography (CT) is usually the initial imaging method of choice to confirm and localize clinically suspected subarachnoid hemorrhage (bleeding in the subarachnoid space) in patients with suspected cerebral aneurysm rupture. Subarachnoid hemorrhage results in increased attenuation of the cerebrospinal fluid (CSF)-filled basal cisterns relative to adjacent brain (Fig. 8). However, the continual production and resorption of CSF and the mixing of CSF with hemorrhage can make subarachnoid blood undetectable by CT within 1–2 days, depending upon the original amount of blood present. MRI is at least as sensitive as CT in detecting subarachnoid hemorrhage, but the cost-effectiveness, practicality, and speed with which a CT can be obtained renders it the first choice at most institutions.

53. When is lumbar puncture and CSF analysis indicated despite a negative CT scan of the head?

Clinical symptoms of subarachnoid hemorrhage occurring more than 2 days prior to presentation is an indication for a lumbar puncture (spinal tap) and CSF analysis, despite the absence of subarachnoid hemorrhage identified on a CT scan. While CT is sensitive for the presence of acute subarachnoid hemorrhage, tiny hemorrhages mixed with CSF may not be apparent even in the acute phases. Lumbar puncture may be clinically indicated for this scenario, as well.

54. What is the imaging method of choice for evaluating cerebral hemorrhage?

At most institutions, CT is the initial imaging method of choice for evaluating acute cerebral or brainstem hemorrhage because of its sensitivity, cost-effectiveness, and availability. However, MRI

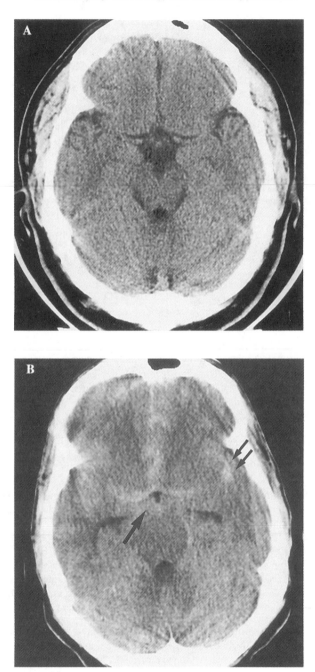

Figure 8. **A,** Normal CT scan of the base of the brain and CSF-filled basal cisterns. Note that brain parenchyma has greater x-ray attenuation (i.e., appears denser) compared with low-density CSF within the basal cisterns and sylvian fissures. **B,** CT scan of a young female with subarachnoid hemorrhage, secondary to rupture of a cerebral aneurysm. Note the increased x-ray attenuation in the basal cisterns *(large arrow)* and in the sylvian fissures *(small arrows)* due to mixing of hemorrhage with CSF.

is more sensitive in detecting intraparenchymal hemorrhage, particularly in brainstem areas that are difficult to visualize with CT imaging (due to beam-hardening artifacts). Once hemorrhage has been established with CT, MRI—with its superior soft tissue contrast—often is used to diagnose the source of the bleeding. This two-step process has application in hemorrhagic stroke, hemorrhagic neoplasm, hypertensive hemorrhage, amyloid angiopathy, drug-induced hemorrhage, and hemorrhage from a vascular malformation.

55. Describe the evolution of intracranial blood products on CT.

Parenchymal or contained extra-axial (e.g., subdural or epidural) hemorrhagic blood products initially are hyperattenuating relative to normal brain on CT (Fig. 9A). Within 1–6 weeks, the attenuation of hemorrhage decreases to approach that of brain as the blood products are liquified and resorbed (Fig. 9B). Hemorrhage may be difficult to distinguish from normal brain during this phase of evolution. At 4–6 weeks, the attenuation of hemorrhage begins to decrease below that of surrounding brain tissue.

56. What causes the increased x-ray attenuation of intracranial hemorrhage?

Increased attenuation of x-rays seen in intracranial hemorrhage is due to coagulation, molecular cross-linking, and retraction of the globin molecule within the blood clot. Contrary to popular misconceptions, the heme molecule contributes little to the clot density observed with CT. Thus, physiologic factors such as hematocrit, hydration states, and coagulation status can impact the density and evolution of hemorrhage on CT scanning. In the setting of a low hematocrit or coagulation disorder, hemorrhage can be isodense to brain acutely.

57. Describe the evolution of intracerebral blood products on MRI.

MRI is more differentiating than CT in identifying the various stages of evolution of intracranial hemorrhage. On MRI, hyperacute (minutes to hours old) hemorrhage containing oxyhemoglobin produces signal that is isointense on T1-weighted images and hyperintense on T2-weighted images relative to brain, due to increased free water content. Acute hemorrhage (several hours old) is characterized by isointense signal on T1-weighted images (Fig. 10A) and hypointense signal on T2-weighted images, secondary to the desaturation of oxyhemoglobin to deoxyhemoglobin. After several days, oxidative denaturation increases methemoglobin concentrations in subacute hemorrhages, causing increased signal on T1-weighted images (Fig. 10B) and hypo- to hyperintense signal on T2-weighted images. These signals parallel the relative intracellular and extracellular methemoglobin concentrations, respectively. Methemoglobin may persist for days to months.

Hemosiderin and ferritin within old hemorrhage sites produce decreased signal on T2-weighted images that may persist for years or indefinitely. T2-weighted gradient-echo sequences are the most sensitive imaging method to detect magnetic susceptibility effects associated with deoxyhemoglobin (Fig. 11) and hemosiderin/ferritin.

Cerebrovascular Diseases

58. Which imaging modalities are best suited to evaluate carotid and vertebral artery stenosis?

Contrast-enhanced CT angiography (CTA) and MR angiography (MRA) are precise techniques that can quantify the extent of stenosis in the cervical carotid and vertebral vasculature. Occlusions causing stroke can be identified by both of these imaging modalities. Conventional (x-ray) angiography can be used to document carotid or vertebral disease when MRA and CTA results are equivocal or limited by technical artifacts.

59. What are the criteria for diagnosing a "significant" stenosis of the internal carotid artery in asymptomatic patients?

The North American Symptomatic Carotid Endarterectomy Trial and the European Carotid Surgery Trial have shown a clinical benefit from carotid endarterectomy when a stenosis of 70–99% is present in the internal carotid. Thus, a precise estimate of stenosis identified on x-ray, CT, or MR angiography is paramount. Stenosis can be calculated by the diameter ratio of stenotic

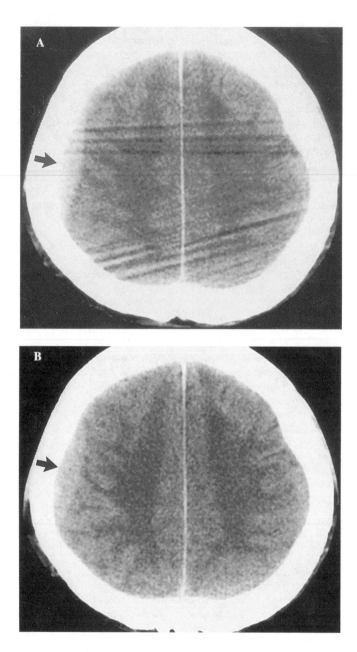

Figure 9.   **A**, Post-traumatic CT scan of a right-sided subdural hematoma *(arrow)*, obtained at 10 days. The diagonal lines running through the image are a result of the metal head restraint worn by the patient. This restraint, common in trauma situations, attenuates the x-ray beam and creates a beam-hardening artifact. **B**, CT scan at 18 days after the trauma. Notice that the hyperattenuating subdural hematoma has become less dense with time, as blood products are degraded and resorbed. It is nearly equivalent in density to adjacent, normal cortical gray matter.

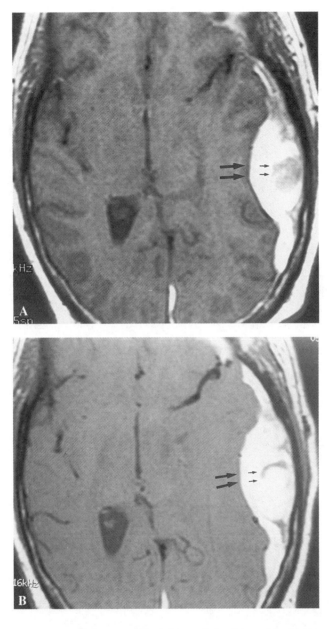

Figure 10. **A,** Post-traumatic MRI (same patient as Figure 9) showing a subdural hematoma *(large arrows)* on T1-weighted images, at 4 days. Note that the subdural blood is largely hyperintense due to methemoglobin within the hematoma. The central portion of the hematoma *(small arrows)* demonstrates relatively low signal compared to the surrounding portions of the hematoma, due to the presence of a deoxyhemoglobin. **B,** T1-weighted images 6 days after the trauma. As the subdural blood aged, the central portion of the hematoma *(small arrows)* became as hyperintense as the rest of the subdural blood, due to the conversion of deoxyhemoglobin to methemoglobin. Note that CSF within the right lateral ventricular atrium and cerebral fissures/sulci has low signal relative to adjacent brain, due to its long T1 relaxation time. Brain tissue has a T1 relaxation time and signal that is intermediate between CSF (low signal, long T1) and subdural methemoglobin (high signal, short T1).

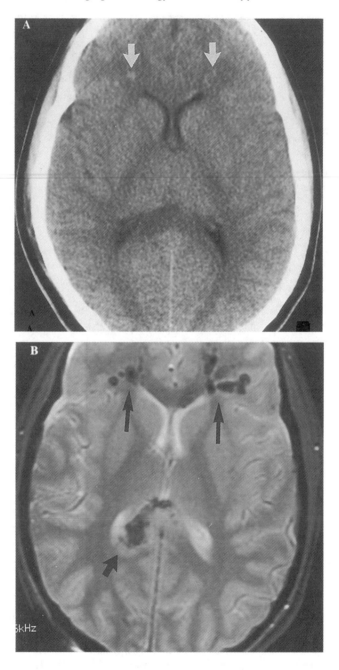

Figure 11.   **A**, Post-traumatic CT scan of a young man with diffuse axonal injury. A few scattered areas of hyperattenuating focal blood are present within the frontal lobe white matter *(white arrows)* and the anterior aspect
of the corpus callosum, indicating the presence of axonal shearing injury to the brain. **B**, T2-weighted gradient-
echo MRI obtained several hours after the CT scan reveals improved visualization of frontal lobe *(top arrows)* and
anterior corpus callosum blood products, due to magnetic susceptibility effects produced by deoxyhemoglobin.
Additionally, blood products are seen involving the posterior aspect of the corpus callosum *(bottom arrow)* that
were not detectable on the CT scan, demonstrating the superior sensitivity of MRI.

to distal uninvolved internal carotid vessel lumen, multiplied by 100. Occasionally, a second, tandem stenosis is seen by angiography, most commonly in the carotid siphon (intracranial portion).

60. What imaging techniques are used to diagnose cerebral aneurysms?

CTA and MRA are sensitive techniques in detecting most cerebral aneurysms, but x-ray arteriography still is required to exclude the smallest aneurysms (Fig. 12). With continued developments, conventional x-ray angiography as a method of diagnosing cerebral aneurysms likely will be replaced in the near future by these noninvasive techniques. However, it always will be required for endovascular treatments of aneurysms and other cerebrovascular diseases.

61. What are the clinical limitations of CTA and MRA in evaluating cerebrovascular disease?

CTA and MRA are not yet adequate to evaluate diseases of the most peripheral cerebral vessels, because of limited spatial resolution. In the proper clinical setting, multiple infarcts demonstrated on CT or MRI may suggest vasculitis or other vasculopathies of the smaller cerebral vessels. However, such diagnoses only can be confirmed with conventional x-ray angiography. CTA and MRA can effectively reveal focal stenoses of the larger intracranial arteries. Due to the large size of the draining venous structures, MR or CT venography are preferred methods for documenting and determining the extent of dural sinus and deep cerebral vein thrombosis.

62. What are common locations of cerebral aneurysms?

Saccular cerebral aneurysms occur at the branch points of large intracranial arteries, particularly about the circle of Willis. Common locations detected by angiography include the anterior communicating artery (30%), the posterior communicating artery (30%), the middle cerebral artery bifurcation (20%) (see Fig. 12A and B), the basilar tip (5%) (see Fig. 12C and D), and other sites in the intracranial vertebra-basilar circulation. There is a 1–2% risk per year of saccular aneurysm rupture and a 20–50% risk of nonoperated aneurysm re-bleeding. Mycotic aneurysms result from septic emboli causing inflammation and destruction of the arterial wall, and occur in the more distal cerebral arteries.

63. Which imaging method is commonly used to support the diagnosis of brain death?

Technetium-99m cerebral perfusion agents and SPECT imaging techniques commonly are used to evaluate cerebrovascular blood flow. These agents can be employed to evaluate hypoperfusion in neurodegenerative and other disorders, as well as focal regions of hypoperfusion in patients with stroke. However, they are most widely used to support the diagnosis of brain death, confirming a lack of arterial flow to the brain and brainstem.

Stroke

64. What are the early signs of stroke on CT imaging?

The earliest indication of a stroke on CT imaging is the **dense middle cerebral artery (MCA) sign**, identified by a hyperattenuating, clot-filled MCA on the side of the stroke, relative to the unaffected side (Fig. 13). However, this sign is seen in only a minority of cases. Generally, there are no diagnostic findings of stroke identified on CT within the first 12 hours after onset.

At 12–24 hours, subtle effacement of the cortical sulci and loss of the gray-white matter differentiation may be identified as an early indication of stroke. At 24–72 hours, cytotoxic edema results in hypoattenuation of the infarcted area, relative to normal brain, and may cause considerable associated mass effect on adjacent brain structures (Fig. 14A).

Small strokes and brainstem strokes may not be evident on CT at any stage; MRI may be indicated to confirm such events. CT usually is obtained immediately after the onset of an acute stroke, to exclude the presence of associated intracranial hemorrhage. Hemorrhagic transformation can occur 1–3 days after the stroke onset, however.

65. What are the early findings indicating a stroke on conventional MRI?

Within the first several hours, conventional MRI may show no findings of cerebral or brainstem infarction. Contrast-enhanced T1-weighted images may show vascular engorgement in the distribution

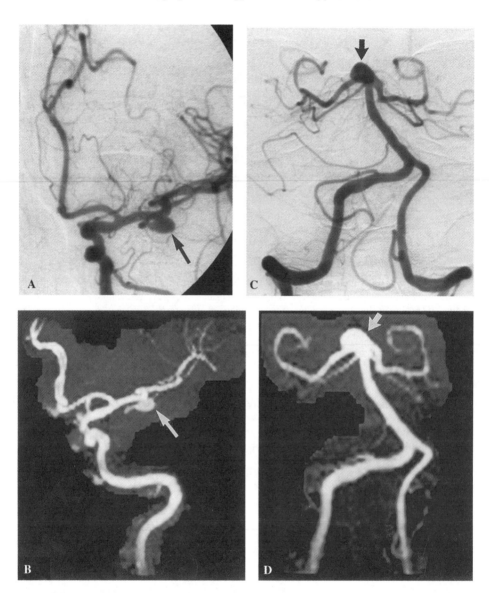

Figure 12. Conventional x-ray angiograms *(top images)* and 3D time-of-flight MR angiograms *(bottom images)* in a young man. **A and B**, Cerebral aneurysms are visible in the middle cerebral artery bifurcation *(arrows).* **C and D**, They also are evident at the basilar artery tip *(arrows).* While MRA is adequate to identify relatively large aneurysms, it does not yet adequately visualize the smallest aneurysms. Because individuals commonly have more than one cerebral aneurysm, conventional angiography still is required to fully evaluate the cerebrovasculature prior to aneurysm surgery.

of the stroke, due to loss of cerebrovascular auto-regulation. When large vessel occlusion is the cause of the cerebrovascular accident (stroke), a lack of intravascular flow–related signal void on MRI or a lack of signal enhancement on MRA can be demonstrated immediately. T1-weighted images reveal morphologic changes of subtle mass effect and altered gray-white matter contrast.

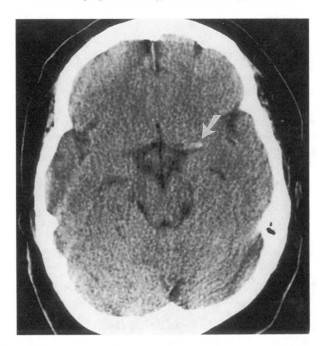

Figure 13. CT scan of a 46-year-old woman with symptoms of left hemispheric stroke. Note the hyperattenuating (hyperdense) left middle cerebral artery (MCA; M1 segment), relative to the other side. The M1 segment of the MCA is a relatively common place for an embolus to lodge; therefore, the dense MCA sign is one of the earliest indications of stroke on a CT scan.

Within 12 to 24 hours, hyperintense signal becomes apparent in infarcted regions on long TR (repetition time) sequences (e.g., proton density–weighted and T2-weighted sequences). Over the next several days, regions of infarction are delineated by very hyperintense signal on long TR images (Fig. 14B) and may show gadolinium enhancement on T1-weighted images. (Presently, the most common MRI contrast agents used clinically are gadolinium-chelated contrast agents.) Hemorrhage associated with infarction undergoes evolutionary stages described in Question 57.

66. How is diffusion MRI used to evaluate acute strokes?

Diffusion imaging can detect acute stroke instantaneously, by virtue of its sensitivity to the restricted molecular motion of water in intracellular compartments. Ischemia results in reduced capacity of the sodium-potassium ATPase to maintain ionic gradients across the cell membrane. This loss of membrane integrity allows the influx of water into the intracellular compartment, where the water diffusion is more restricted, leading to an overall decrease in the molecular diffusion of tissue water and increased signal on a diffusion-weighted image (DWI) (Fig. 15). This effect may last for up to 14 days, after which diffusion begins to increase in infarcted tissue above that of normal brain.

The diffusion abnormality associated with a stroke usually indicates irreversibility and cell death. Because old stroke is characterized by increased diffusion, DWI can be used to distinguish old from acute regions of infarction.

67. How is perfusion MRI used to evaluate acute strokes?

Perfusion imaging relies on intravascular gadolinium contrast agents administered during high-speed MRI to document areas of reduced perfusion within the brain. The perfusion abnormality may be larger than the diffusion abnormality—the area of mismatch indicates regions of brain that are at

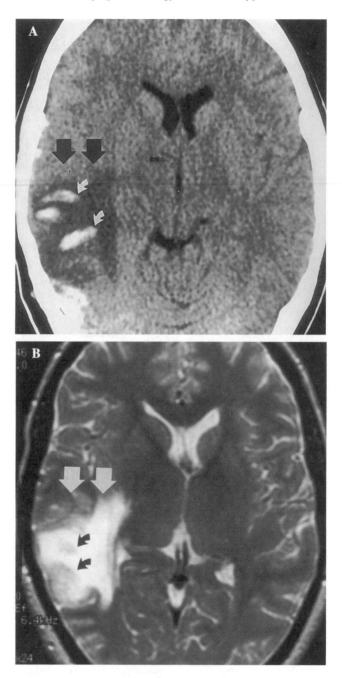

Figure 14. A right posterior temporal stroke *(large arrows)* 4 days after the event. **A**, CT scan reveals hemorrhagic transformation of the infarct by hyperdense blood *(small white arrows)* surrounded by hypodense cytotoxic edema. **B**, T2-weighted MRI reveals hyperintense signal related to the long T2 relaxation time of edema. Blood products *(small black arrows)* are mildly hyperintense to brain and hypointense to edema, secondary to methemoglobin within the hemorrhage. Because of the hemorrhagic transformation within the infarct, this patient's thrombolytic therapy was halted to prevent progressive intracranial hemorrhage.

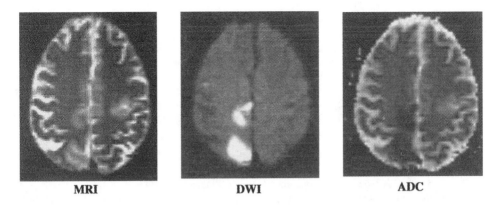

| MRI | DWI | ADC |

Figure 15. T2-weighted MRI, diffusion-weighted image (DWI), and corresponding apparent diffusion coefficient (ADC) map from a patient with both chronic and subacute strokes. In the subacute stroke, present in the patient's right hemisphere (left side of each image), the signal is somewhat increased on the MRI, bright on the DWI, and decreased on the ADC map. These results are consistent with the decreased diffusion associated with a stroke of a couple of days. Note that in the case of very early ischemia (minutes to hours), signal increases on the T2-weighted MRI would not have occurred yet, but the DWI and ADC results would be similar. The chronic stroke visible in the patient's left hemisphere (right side of each image), demonstrates high signal on the T2-weighted image, no signal change on the DWI, and increased signal on the ADC map. These observations are consistent with the increased diffusion associated with chronic stroke.

risk and potentially salvageable with thrombolytic agents and other treatments. Therapies are effective only in the earliest stages of a stroke, making the advent of new MRI techniques capable of characterizing acute strokes potentially very important. When intra-arterial thrombolytic therapy is indicated, conventional diagnostic x-ray angiography is performed to identify the site of thrombus within the intracerebral vasculature before therapy.

Craniocerebral Trauma

68. What is the imaging modality of choice for evaluating brain contusions?

CT is the initial imaging method of choice to document cranial and facial trauma and to document the presence of brain injury. Cortical contusions are characterized by edema, with or without hemorrhage, located within the peripheral brain tissue that has been thrown against bony structures of the skull base during trauma. Hemorrhagic contusions cause focal high (blood) and low (edema) attenuation regions on CT. The amount of hemorrhage, edema, and associated mass effect can increase dramatically over several days following a trauma. MRI is more sensitive than CT in detecting cerebral contusions, but usually is reserved for cases that are equivocal on CT or for patients with a confusing clinical picture.

69. What are the etiologies of epidural and subdural hematomas?

Epidural hematomas result from skull fractures (85–95%) traversing and tearing the middle meningeal artery or dural venous sinuses. On CT and MRI, these are seen as extra-axial, bioconvex blood collections that may cross dural attachments, but not sutures. The displaced dural lining may be visible on MRI.

Subdural hematomas (see Figs. 9 and 10) result from tearing of bridging cortical veins due to sudden changes in head velocity. They are crescentic-shaped collections located between dura and arachnoid, and are limited by dural attachments, but not sutures. Subdural hematomas account for high mortality and can occur in the setting of minor trauma, particularly in older individuals.

MRI is more sensitive than CT for visualizing subdural and epidural hematomas, due to the lack of cranial artifact with MRI.

70. What are the findings indicative of traumatic vascular injury on CT?

Cervical carotid and vertebral arteries are most susceptible to injury during trauma by virtue of their location within the neck, containment within bony structures (i.e., vertebral arteries), and transition from extra- to intracranial course. Traditional head CT imaging usually cannot detect vascular injury directly, but associated findings of arterial infarction, large amounts of subarachnoid hemorrhage, skull fractures extending through vascular channels (e.g., carotid canal) or clinical indications of a stroke may stimulate further imaging workup to evaluate vessel integrity. When this is the case, conventional angiography, CTA, or MRA may be necessary to exclude the possibility of vertebral or carotid artery dissections or lacerations.

71. What are the findings indicating diffuse axonal injury on CT and MRI?

Diffuse axonal injury (DAI) is caused by sudden rotational or acceleration/deceleration injuries of the cranium and is generally not apparent on initial CT scans obtained immediately after a trauma, despite profound neurological impairment. DAI often occurs in association with cerebral contusions and is a major cause of head trauma deaths. Within 24–48 hours after DAI, focal hemorrhages and edema (see Fig. 11) generally become apparent at gray-white matter interfaces of the cerebral hemispheres, brainstem, corpus callosum, and basal ganglia regions. MRI also can document these foci by detecting blood and edema, but is generally reserved to diagnose DAI in patients with a negative head CT scan. Chronically, DAI often results in brain atrophy.

72. What is the significance of subarachnoid hemorrhage in the setting of trauma?

It is not unusual to identify subarachnoid hemorrhage in association with intracranial injury, but large amounts of subarachnoid blood raise the possibility that a hemorrhagic event actually caused the head trauma. When this is the case, x-ray angiography may be indicated to exclude the presence of a ruptured cerebral aneurysm, or the rare case of intracranial vascular injury.

Intracranial Neoplasms

73. What is the imaging method of choice for evaluating intracranial tumors?

Due to superior soft tissue contrast, MRI is vastly superior to any other imaging method in identifying the location and extent of intracranial neoplasms. In many instances, MRI is specific in identifying the type of tumor present within the cranium or brain. MRI is the most sensitive method for detecting metastases. Brain tumors generally are characterized by iso- and hypointense signal on T1-weighted images (Fig. 16A) and hyperintense signal on long TR (proton density–weighted) images. Most, but not all, brain tumors enhanced with gadolinium administration are characterized by dramatically increased signal on T1-weighted images (Fig. 16B).

74. What are the common intracranial tumors?

Approximately two thirds of brain tumors are primary neoplasms, and one third are metastatic lesions arising from extracranial primaries. Of the primary neoplasms, gliomas make up the majority (50%), followed by meningiomas, primitive neuroectodermal tumors, nerve sheath tumors, pituitary tumors, and others. The most common metastatic tumors include lung cancer, breast cancer (Fig. 17), melanoma, and gastrointestinal/genitourinary neoplasms. Metastatic intracranial tumors can arise from virtually any primary cell type and can involve the skull, dura, leptomeninges, subarachnoid space, brain parenchyma, and ventricular system.

75. What is the significance of gadolinium contrast enhancement in brain tumors?

Intravenous administration of gadolinium results in increased signal on T1-weighted images in regions of neoplasm where there has been breakdown of the blood-brain barrier. Despite popular misconceptions, gadolinium enhancement does not correlate with hypervascularity, and occasionally conventional cerebral angiography is required to identify hypervascular regions of a cerebral neoplasm prior to biopsy or resection. Fast imaging sequences acquired during injection of intravenous contrast can be used to calculate blood volume maps (Fig. 18) within cerebral neoplasm, prior to surgical intervention and during therapy with agents that inhibit angiogenesis (growth of new blood vessels).

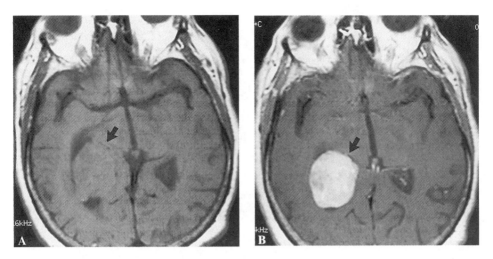

Figure 16. T1-weighted MRI scans of an intraventricular meningioma. **A**, Prior to intravenous administration of gadolinium contrast, note that the meningioma *(arrow)* is nearly isointense to brain. **B**, After administration of gadolinium, the image reveals dramatically shortened T1 relaxation time and increased signal. Enhancement is related to leakage of intravascular gadolinium into the interstitial space.

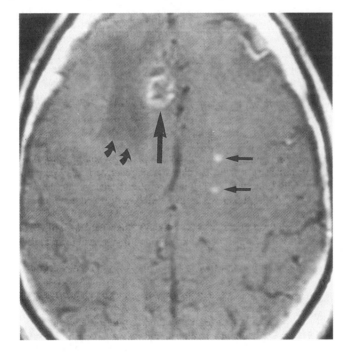

Figure 17. T1-weighted MRI scan of breast cancer metastases to the brain of a 46-year-old woman, after the administration of intravenous gadolinium contrast. A rim of enhancement surrounds necrotic portions of a metastasis in the right frontal lobe *(large arrow)*. Regions of low signal surround the right frontal lobe metastasis *(left arrows)*, due to vasogenic edema that has a long T1 relaxation time. Small left frontal metastatic lesions *(right arrows)* were not apparent on CT, demonstrating the superior sensitivity of MRI in identifying enhancing lesions of the brain. In brain tissue, gadolinium enhancement is a reflection of a breakdown of the blood-brain barrier, which normally prevents larger molecules from entering the interstitial space.

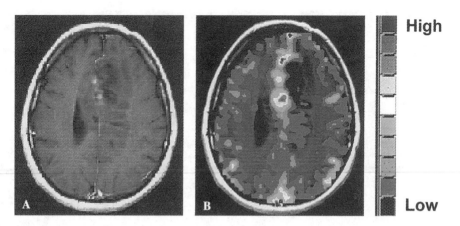

Figure 18. Demonstration of the utility of blood volume maps in the evaluation of brain neoplasms. This patient has a grade III astrocytoma. **A**, The post-contrast T1-weighted image demonstrates negligible enhancement. **B**, The blood volume map, shown in color and superimposed on the T1-weighted image, shows a significant signal increase in the lesion area. This result is consistent with the highly vascular and therefore aggressive nature of this tumor. ***Note: see color panel.***

76. What is the clinical indication for functional MRI in patients with brain tumors?
Functional MRI is a new technique capable of mapping eloquent cortex and its proximity to cerebral neoplasms preoperatively. When a patient performs a task, increased oxyhemoglobin concentrations and decreased deoxyhemoglobin concentrations in the microvascular network of activated cortex results in increased signal on T2*-weighted fast imaging sequences, such as echoplanar imaging. Functional MRI exploits this blood oxygen level–dependent (BOLD) contrast, assessing the risk of surgery (Fig. 19). FMRI also can be used to determine language dominance in seizure patients prior to temporal lobe surgery (see Fig. 5). With future developments, functional MRI is expected to contribute to the workup of a variety of neurological and psychiatric conditions in clinical practice.

77. What is the indication for magnetic resonance spectroscopy in patients with brain tumors?
Magnetic resonance spectroscopy (MRS) can differentiate between neoplastic and similar appearing non-neoplastic lesions of the brain by detecting elevated choline metabolites in tumors associated with cellular turnover (Fig. 20). N-acetyl-aspartate is a neuronal marker and is decreased in brain neoplasms. Markedly elevated choline and absent N-acetyl-aspartate is characteristic of meningiomas and other intracranial tumors located outside of the brain. Spectroscopic analysis of intracranial masses can be utilized to differentiate between neoplasms and other etiologies such as stroke, radiation necrosis, and infection.

78. How can diffusion-weighted imaging contribute to the evaluation of brain tumors?
Molecular diffusion is decreased in most cerebral neoplasms, while diffusion is increased in vasogenic brain edema often associated with neoplasms. Thus, DWI can be used to differentiate tumor margin from surrounding vasogenic edema, yielding a more precise estimate of tumor extent. Necrotic tumors and pyogenic abscesses usually are not distinguishable on CT and traditional MRI. Because diffusion is restricted in pyogenic abscesses and increased in tumor necrosis, DWI can be used to differentiate between these lesions.

Neurodegenerative Diseases

79. What is the role of imaging in dementias?
Dementias generally are diagnosed by clinical criteria, but imaging studies may be supportive of a difficult diagnosis. Regional atrophy can support the diagnosis of particular types of dementias

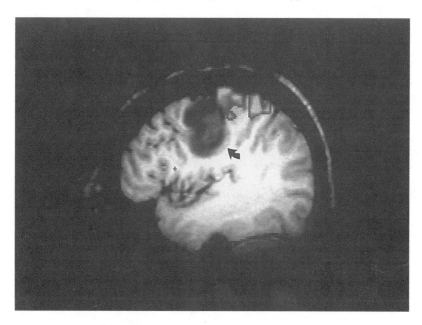

Figure 19.   Functional MRI of the left hemisphere in a 22-year-old woman with a primary brain tumor *(arrow)*. Right finger tapping task results in sensory and motor cortical activation and demonstrates eloquent cortex to be located immediately posterior and adjacent to the edge of the grade III astrocytoma. This information aided the neurosurgeon in planning an approach to resect the brain tumor, while avoiding a postoperative motor deficit.   ***Note: see color panel.***

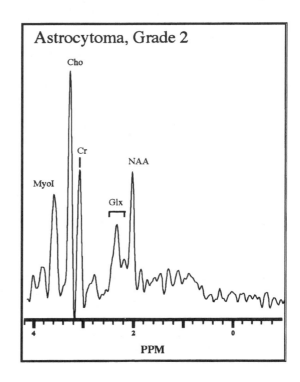

Figure 20.   MRS results from a patient with a grade II astrocytoma. Note the markedly increased choline (Cho) and decreased n-acetyl-aspartate (NAA) in this spectrum relative to the normal spectrum shown in Figure 7.

such as Alzheimer's (temporal lobe atrophy) or Pick's disease (temporal and frontal lobe atrophy), but morphologic brain imaging patterns are not sensitive or specific for these types of dementias. MRI can, however, distinguish vascular from nonvascular dementias. Hydrocephalus on MRI or CT in the setting of dementia may indicate normal pressure hydrocephalus, a diagnosis that can be supported with nuclear medicine studies of CSF dynamics. Modalities such as PET and SPECT demonstrate characteristic features in certain dementias, by virtue of reduced cerebral metabolism or blood flow: Alzheimer's disease shows reduced activity in the temporo-parietal regions, and Pick's disease and non-Alzheimer's type FLD (frontal lobe dementia) show reduced activity in the frontal lobes, in particular.

Because of its capacity to assess brain function, functional MRI may increase the role of imaging in the diagnosis and management of patients with dementia. Evaluation of brain metabolites with MR spectroscopy has promise in evaluating dementias, as well.

80. What is the role of imaging in psychiatric diseases?

Generally, imaging is not an integral part of the diagnosis and management of psychiatric diseases at most institutions. However, imaging may be required to exclude other diseases of the brain that may mimic psychiatric diseases, including diffuse axonal injury and brain tumors. Occasionally, radionuclide studies can be used to support the diagnosis of a particular illness. Some psychiatric diseases show hypometabolic regions with PET imaging. For example, schizophrenia is characterized by hypometabolism in the frontal regions, particularly in the prefrontal cortex. Many believe that with further research and development, functional MRI will significantly impact our understanding of psychiatric diseases, as PET has done.

81. Which neurodegenerative diseases are best evaluated with MRI?

MRI is exquisitely sensitive to degenerative diseases of myelinated white matter. Since myelin contains hydrophilic binding sites, it restricts the motion of free water and considerably alters the behavior of water molecules in the presence of a magnetic field. As a consequence, the contrast of white matter on MRI is dramatically altered by the destruction of myelin. Thus, MRI is a mainstay in the work up of white matter diseases. For example, MRI is a sensitive indicator of multiple sclerosis, showing focal, high-signal white matter lesions on proton density–weighted and T2-weighted images with a periventricular dominance (Fig. 21). Viral and post-viral inflammatory conditions, such as acute disseminated encephalomyelitis and toxic lesions of white matter, are readily detected by MRI, as well.

82. What is the normal developmental pattern of white matter myelination?

Because MRI is sensitive to brain myelin, the stages of white matter myelination occurring after birth are well demonstrated on long TR sequences. At birth, the medulla, dorsal midbrain, inferior/superior cerebellar peduncles, posterior internal capsule, and ventrolateral thalamus white matter are myelinated. At 1 month of age, cerebellar, corticospinal tract, pre/post central gyrus, and optic nerve/tract white matter become myelinated. At 3 months of age, middle cerebellar peduncle, ventral midbrain, optic radiation, anterior internal capsule, occipital subcortical U fiber, and corpus callosum splenium white matter structures become myelinated. By 8 months, most of the frontal cerebral white matter, most of the subcortical U fibers, and the anterior corpus callosum are myelinated. At 18 months, myelinated white matter takes on the appearance of the adult brain.

Inborn diseases that interfere with white matter myelination, such as leukodystrophies (Fig. 22), show confluent, hyperintense signal in the cerebral white matter on proton density–weighted and T2-weighted images.

83. How can MR spectroscopy contribute to the diagnosis of inborn errors of metabolism?

MR spectroscopy can show altered brain metabolites that reflect inborn errors of metabolism. For example, spectroscopy generally demonstrates elevated lactate concentrations in the gray matter of patients with mitochondrial encephalopathy. Elevated lactate concentrations in these patients may even be seen in the absence of signal abnormality on traditional MRI. Spectroscopy may add certainty to the diagnosis of amino acidopathies, as well, by demonstrating elevated corresponding amino acid metabolites.

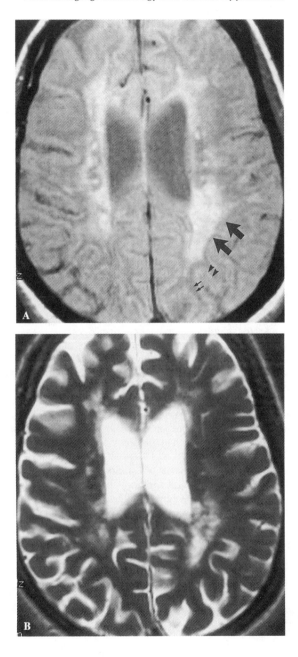

Figure 21. MRI scans of a 36-year-old woman with multiple sclerosis. **A,** In the proton density–weighted scan, signal differences between a large area of demyelination *(large arrows)*, normal white matter *(small arrows)*, and normal gray matter *(arrow heads)* are evident. The hydrophilic nature of myelin binding sites and their interactions with tissue water result in relatively low signal on proton density–weighted and T2-weighted images of the normal brain. However, destruction of myelin causes a reduction of tissue-water interactions and increased T2 relaxation time, resulting in hyperintense signal in the white matter of patients with multiple sclerosis. CSF is relatively low-signal here. **B,** In the T2-weighted scan, CSF is hyperintense. Note the differences in tissue and lesion contrast between the two images.

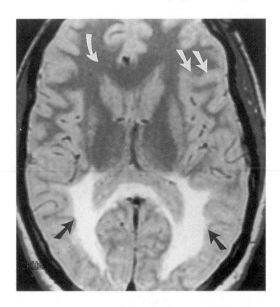

Figure 22. Proton density–weighted MRI of a 44-year-old man with adult-onset adrenoleukodystrophy, demonstrating confluent, abnormal hyperintensity in the posterior cerebral white matter *(black arrows)*. The difference in signal intensity between the posterior white matter lesion, normal white matter *(left white arrow)*, and normal gray matter *(double white arrows)* is shown.

84. How does MRI impact the diagnosis of movement disorders?

In general, traditional MRI plays little role in the diagnosis of movement disorders. MRI findings such as increased iron and decreased signal in the basal ganglia and midbrain may be seen on T2-weighted images in Parkinson's disease and Parkinson's-like syndromes, but they are not required to make the diagnosis, and they are not specific. However, imaging is used at many institutions to localize globus pallidus or thalamic structures for stereotactic ablation or stimulator placement as a treatment for Parkinson's disease symptoms. Wallerian degeneration (increased T2 signal) along the corticospinal tracts indicates amyotrophic lateral sclerosis, but is an insensitive finding. Caudate nucleus atrophy seen with Huntington's disease contributes infrequently to the management of such patients. Functional MRI may increase the role of imaging in the management of patients with movement disorders because of its capacity to assess brain function and interconnections. Future developments in glutamate spectroscopy may provide an assessment of glutamate excitotoxicity in these and other neurodegenerative disorders.

BIBLIOGRAPHY

1. Mettler F, Guiberteau MJ (eds): Essentials of Nuclear Medicine Imaging. Grune and Stratton, 1986.
2. Mitchell DG (ed): MRI Principles. Philadelphia, W.B. Saunders, 1999.
3. Stark DD, Bradley Jr WG (eds): Magnetic Resonance Imaging. St. Louis, Missouri, Mosby Year Book, 1992.
4. Sutton D (ed): A Textbook of Radiology and Imaging. Churchill Livingstone, 1993.

23. MOLECULAR BASIS OF NEUROLOGICAL DISEASES

BethAnn McLaughlin, Ph.D., and Pat Levitt, Ph.D.

1. What is a neurological disease?

Neurological diseases affect the central and peripheral nervous systems, including the brain, spinal cord, and nerves plus the muscles they innervate. Neurological dysfunction can occur as a result of a genetic defect; exposure to toxins, contagions, or direct trauma; or other factors. For the purposes of this chapter, neurological diseases are defined as those not directly associated with an acute traumatic event (such as spinal cord injury and stroke) and not congenital (present at birth). Even using this narrow definition, there are dozens of diseases that affect the nervous system.

2. How are neurological diseases contracted?

Neurological diseases can be divided broadly into three groups based on their mode of transmission: (1) diseases that are inherited, (2) diseases that are the result of an infectious process, and (3) diseases for which the mode of transmission is unclear (idiopathic). The molecular mechanisms that cause neurological disease are best understood in the inherited neurodegenerative disorders. In this group of diseases, genetic mutations from either or both parents are passed on to the affected individual. These mutations may cause grave neurological consequences, which are apparent in the first few years of life, or subtle changes in the CNS that can go undetected for decades.

3. What are the greatest risk factors for contracting neurological diseases?

The two greatest risk factors for contracting neurological disease are positive family history and age. While not all neurological disorders are inherited, diseases such as Alzheimer's disease (AD), Parkinson's disease (PD), and amyotrophic lateral sclerosis (ALS) can be inherited, and genetic screening is available for many at-risk individuals. The prevalence of neurodegenerative disorders such as AD and PD increases dramatically with age. In fact, AD is the most common progressive neurodegenerative disease, affecting approximately 5–10% of people over the age of 65, while PD affects approximately 1% of people over 60.

4. How are neurological diseases inherited?

The three modes of inheritance are autosomal dominant, autosomal recessive, and X linked. In **autosomal dominant** mutations, only one copy of the disease gene from only one parent is required for offspring to show symptoms of the disorder. In order to contract an **autosomal recessive** disease, offspring must inherit mutated copies of the disease gene from both parents. **X-linked** diseases affect the male offspring of a mother with genetic mutations on the X chromosome.

5. Why is it so difficult to identify genes associated with neurological disorders?

There are a number of obstacles in determining the genetic components of neurological diseases: (1) inappropriate clinical categorization of patients, (2) the fact that a single genetic mutation can cause very different clinical manifestations, and (3) the finding that not all diseases are caused by mutations in one gene, but can result from alterations in multiple genes (multigenic).

Clinical diagnosis can be too narrow and exclude conditions that are actually quite similar. For example, when the genetic defects associated with members of the spinal cerebellar ataxia family were mapped to their chromosomal loci, it was determined that mutations in the same gene had been diagnosed as several different clinical conditions. Clinical diagnosis also can be broad, leading to the grouping of heterogeneous disorders into one larger diagnosis. For instance, patients diagnosed with schizophrenia may have symptoms ranging from withdrawal and avoidance to delusions and mania.

These so-called negative and positive symptoms may be the result of divergent genetic mutations under one diagnosis.

Incomplete penetrance also makes genetic localization of disease genes difficult. Penetrance refers to the ability of the gene to be expressed fully. For example, myotonic muscular dystrophy is an autosomal dominantly inherited disorder with variable penetrance, which results in a range of severity from asymptomatic carriers to severely affected infants with gross motor and intellectual deficits.

In the context of penetrance, it is also possible that **multiple genes** or environmental factors, or a combination of both, may be required for clinical manifestations of a given disease. For instance, there are three variants of the cholesterol transport protein, apolipoprotein. Patients with late-onset AD who are homozygous for the ApoE4 allele have increased numbers of neuronal plaques. However, simply being homozygous for ApoE4 does not alter the risk of contracting AD on its own. The ApoE genotype is probably the first in a series of susceptibility factors to be identified that can increase the onset or progress of neurological diseases.

In spite of these difficult issues, more than 200 genes that cause or contribute to neurologic disease have been identified.

6. How are genes linked to certain diseases?

Genetic mapping in human pedigrees (families) is the typical manner in which genes are identified as being linked to or causal of diseases. Gene mapping is very tedious, but has been enhanced by the development of methods that allow more rapid screening for gene mutations in the population. Linkage to a disease requires analysis of a large number of pedigrees with affected individuals, so that investigators can follow the segregation of a genetic characteristic with the expression of the disease.

7. What methods are used to map genetic characteristics?

New methods, developed just prior to and in the context of the Human Genome Project, have greatly aided in the analysis of genetic diseases. One method focuses on variability in DNA sequence and uses restriction endonucleases to cut DNA and identify **restriction fragment length polymorphisms** (see Figure). Differences in the length of DNA fragments arise after enzymatic treatment because certain restriction sites, which are created by specific base sequences that are cleaved by the endonucleases, are absent, or novel sites are present. These base changes, due to point mutations, deletions, insertions, or variable number of tandem repeats of bases (see Questions 9 and 10) may be present in noncoding regions of genes that have nothing to do with function or disease. Alternatively, they may be present in regions of the gene that alter gene expression or protein function, and thus can be linked to a particular disease through pedigree analysis of affected and unaffected individuals.

Even more rapid methods for performing pedigree analysis and linkage rely on new information from the Human Genome Project. Unique **sequence-tagged sites** (STSs), present once per haploid gene, mark domains in the human genome that can be specifically amplified from libraries of genetic material and used to build a physical map of genes on chromosomes. STSs may be in areas of the genome that are outside of coding regions. **Expressed sequence tags** (ESTs) are derived from complementary DNA, which is produced from the expressed RNA in specific tissues or cells. ESTs are popular because they provide information on location of expressed genes.

Methods for isolating, cloning, and rapid sequencing of large DNA fragments, using bacterial and yeast artificial chromosomes, also has helped in the analysis of human disease.

8. Are all neurological diseases progressive?

The vast majority of neurodegenerative diseases are relentless in their progression. The symptoms, however, often fluctuate over time, especially early in the disease process. For example, of the approximately 1 in 100 people who seek treatment for **schizophrenia**, very few experience only a single episode and remain symptom-free afterward. More commonly, symptoms of the disease reappear over several decades, with each recurrence leading to increased impairment. The factors that determine which patients will suffer chronic disability and which will be impaired only temporarily are unknown. Neurological diseases of affect or mood (e.g., depression)—which are not typified by appreciable neuron death—can, in some instances, resolve themselves.

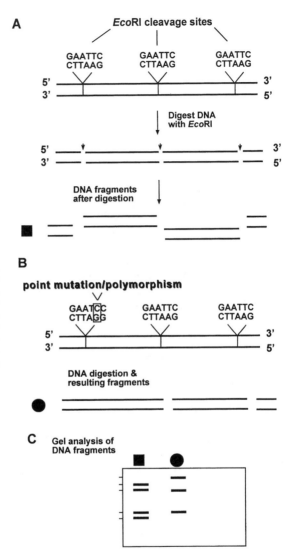

Steps in analysis of DNA polymorphisms between individuals. Polymorphisms may result from large-scale differences in base sequences or from point mutations. **A**, Here, three sites have a base sequence specific for digestion by the enzyme EcoRI. Digestion results in four DNA fragments of distinct size. This represents a pattern of digestion from one individual *(black square)*. **B**, A point mutation at one of the EcoRI restriction sites prevents cleavage of the DNA at that site. Digestion of the DNA from this individual *(black circle)* results in three fragments. **C**, These differences can be visualized by doing gel analysis, in which the DNA fragments from each individual are separated by size.

9. If the same genes are present in every cell, then why aren't all cells equally vulnerable to neurological diseases?

While most cells in the body have the same genetic makeup, the subset of proteins that are synthesized in a given cell or population of cells can vary considerably. The nervous system has a remarkable amount of temporal and spatial heterogeneity in the complement of proteins that are expressed in any given brain region. This heterogeneity is due to complex differential regulation of gene expression. It is though that the varied profile of protein expression within specific neuron types, coupled with unique, regionally specific factors, such as the extent of oxygenation, energetic demands, and neurochemical composition, contribute to the vulnerability of certain neurons to neurological disease.

10. Can different genes or infectious agents cause the same disease?

It has been recognized widely that multiple mutations can occur within a single gene and result in the same disease. ALS is one example of a disease that is caused by mutations of different genes.

ALS is a progressive disease that is characterized by loss of upper and lower motoneurons, which results in muscle weakness and degeneration. Approximately 10% of patients with ALS suffer from an inherited form of the disease, and a subset of these individuals have point mutations in the Cu^{2+}/Zn^{2+} superoxide dismutase gene. This enzyme is a critical part of the cellular defense against reactive oxygen species. There are, however, no known mutations in this gene in the vast majority of patients with ALS, suggesting that alternative, yet unidentified, genes also can cause this disorder.

It also is becoming increasingly clear that multiple genes or exposures to viruses and toxins can produce neurological conditions that are clinically and neuropathologically indistinguishable from progressive neurodegenerative diseases. This fact again demonstrates that there are multiple routes that can target the same neuronal population.

11. Are there similarities between the molecular mechanisms that cause different neurological diseases?

Yes. One of the most striking aspects of many neurodegenerative diseases is the prevalence of expanded trinucleotide repeats as the underlying genetic mutation. CAG repeats of variable lengths cause spinal cerebellar ataxia types 1, -2, -3, -6, and -7, as well as Huntington's disease, spinal and bulbar muscle atrophy, and dentatorubral-pallidoluysian atrophy. These mutations occur in the coding region (exon) of the gene, which ultimately is synthesized into a protein. It is clear that the length of the CAG repeats usually corresponds to the severity of the disease. Thus, less than 40 repeats generally are normal whereas those repeats of greater than 40 produce disease.

Fragile X syndrome, myotonic dystrophy, and Freidreich's ataxia belong to another group of neurodegenerative diseases that also have expanded trinucleotide repeats. These diseases, however, have much longer CGG, CTG, and GAA repeats in regions of the gene that are not made into proteins.

Expansion mutations of trinucleotide repeats have been implicated in several neuropsychiatric disorders, including bipolar affective disorder, schizophrenia, and autism, but the genes associated with these diseases remain largely unknown.

12. How do expanded trinucleotide repeats cause disease?

The mechanisms by which trinucleotide repeat diseases cause neurodegeneration are largely unknown. The best understood of the trinucleotide diseases is **Freidreich's ataxia**, which is caused by a mutation in the frataxin gene. The frataxin protein normally is highly expressed in the mitochondria of neurons and cardiomyocytes. Patients affected with Freidreich's ataxia lose functioning of the normal frataxin protein, which results in abnormal iron accumulation within these cells and an impaired ability to make cellular energy (ATP). The functional significance of expanded repeats in other neurodegenerative diseases remains to be determined, but it is generally thought that these repetitive sequence elements have the potential to form abnormal RNA, DNA, or protein structures that may contribute to loss of transcriptional or translational activity or abnormal protein function and interactions.

13. What is "anticipation" in inherited diseases?

Anticipation is a phenomenon observed in some inherited neurological diseases: affected individuals show earlier and and more severe symptoms in progressive generations. These events do not follow traditional genetic patterns, and have been observed in diseases such as the dominantly inherited ataxias. Anticipation is most often observed in genetic mutations that are paternally inherited, and results from lengthening of the trinucleotide repeats from parent to offspring. In the normal population, polymorphic repeats are stably inherited. The mechanisms leading to anticipation are not well understood.

14. What is the difference between a loss-of-function and a gain-of-function mutation?

Neurodegenerative disorders often are classified as loss-of-function or gain-of-function mutations. A *loss-of-function mutation* is one in which the pathological process results because a protein is no longer able to perform its normal function. One example of a loss-of-function disease is early-onset Tay-Sachs. **Tay-Sachs disease** results from the inability of a lysosomal enzyme to degrade a specific kind of lipid. Loss of function of this enzyme (hexosaminidase A) allows a fatty substance called GM2 ganglioside to accumulate in neurons. This fatal autosomal recessive disorder is characterized by progressive paralysis, blindness, and deafness.

Patients with Tay-Sachs disease and other loss-of-function mutations ultimately may be treated with enzyme replacement or gene therapy, but currently no treatment is available. It is assumed that a patient with two mutated copies of a gene (one from each parent) would be affected more severely than an individual with only one copy of the mutated gene.

Gain-of-function diseases, such as **Huntington's disease** (HD), are typified by mutated RNA, DNA, or protein. These mutations may result in a new pattern of expression or function which is deleterious to cells. In HD, there is no evidence to indicate that patients with two copies of the disease gene fare worse than those with only one copy. While the pathological processes associated with HD are unclear, it is thought that the trinucleotide expansion causes the huntingtin protein to assume an abnormal conformation that initiates an internal cell suicide program.

15. Do similar pathogenic mechanisms contribute to cell death in different diseases?

Yes. One increasingly recognized feature of several neurodegenerative disease is the presence of aberrant, **proteinaceous aggregates** in and around affected neurons. Examples include Lewy bodies of Parkinson's disease, amyloid plaques of Alzheimer's disease, prion protein aggregates of Creutzfeldt-Jakob disease, and nuclear and perinuclear aggregates observed in a number of CAG repeat diseases and some inherited forms of ALS. It remains to be determined if these aggregates are toxic entities that damage cells directly; catalysts for other neurotoxic pathways; or adaptive responses to isolate damaged proteins and reinforce cell architecture.

16. How do genetic defects result in cell death?

Both loss-of-function and gain-of-function mutations disrupt the ability of cells to maintain their homeostatic mechanisms, which maintain the chemical and molecular pathways required for normal cell function. If the cellular environment becomes sufficiently corrupted by genetic defects, numerous molecular mechanisms are in place to initiate an internal cell suicide program, called **apoptosis**. This process involves activation of enzymes that degrade protein and DNA (proteases and DNases, respectively), deconstruct the cell cytoskeleton, and package the cellular debris in such a way that the damage to surrounding cells is minimal. A second mechanism of cell damage is **necrotic cell death**, in which cells lyse. Necrosis can expose adjacent cells to potentially toxic levels of chemicals and thereby recruit damaging non-neuronal cells to the affected region. It remains to be determined to what extent apoptosis contributes to cell death in all of the neurological diseases, but extensive apoptosis and apoptosis-related enzyme activity has already been documented in AD, PD, and HD.

17. What is the role of non-neuronal cells in neurological diseases?

In addition to neurons, the nervous system contains many other cell types, including macroglia, microglia, and endothelial cells of brain capillaries. There are 10 times as many glial cells as neurons in the brain, and they are critically involved in metabolism, maintenance of ion homeostasis, reaction to infection, removal of cellular debris, development of proper neural circuitry, myelination of nerve fibers, and chemical signaling within the CNS. Neurological disorders may result when non-neuronal cells are compromised, as in demyelinating diseases like multiple sclerosis, or when these cellular elements become activated and invasive, as in HIV-induced dementia, autoimmune disorders, and most types of brain tumors.

18. Do environmental factors contribute to neurologic diseases?

Yes. Exposure to environmental toxins such as heavy metals, pollutants, herbicides, or pesticides can cause a variety of neurological conditions, ranging from subclinical behavioral changes to blindness, encephalopathy, and death. Lead poisoning is a particularly prevalent condition resulting from ingestion or inhalation of the metal. Within the brain, lead disrupts the astrocytes and microvasculature, which are important components of the blood-brain barrier, and damages the prefrontal cerebral cortex and hippocampus, which are critically involved in affect, learning, and memory.

Other compounds, such as the herbicide paraquat, have come under scrutiny as potential neurotoxins because of their structural similarities to compounds that kill dopaminergic cells in a manner similar to that observed in Parkinson's disease. Similarly, ingestion of the fungal toxin 3-nitropropionic acid results in bilateral striatal degeneration and a movement disorder than is comparable to Huntington's disease.

However, note that these compounds do not actually *cause* neurodegenerative diseases; they simply mimic the selective cell loss observed in these conditions. Environmental toxins have been used extensively by researchers to understand the factors that render groups of neurons vulnerable to cell death. The role of daily exposure to environmental factors in the pathogenesis of neurological diseases, however, remains largely unknown.

19. Are certain brain regions more vulnerable than others to neurological diseases?

Historically, neuroscientists and neurologists have based their understanding of neurological disease on the tenet that there is "selective regional vulnerability" to various disorders. That is to say, cell death in PD occurs in the substantia nigra, the striatum for HD, motoneurons for ALS, and the hippocampus and parts of the cortex for AD. This approach to disease is relevant to how these neurological disorders and cell death pathways are studied.

However, the idea that populations of cell have selective vulnerability is being replaced with the observation that those groups of neurons that may just be the first to die or are the most profoundly affected. While HD and PD do cause massive cell death in the striatum and substantia nigra, respectively, patients affected with these diseases often suffer from loss of cortical cells and dementia. Similarly, parkinsonian symptoms frequently develop in patients with AD, and individuals with ALS can develop dementia and may have altered glucose metabolism in regions such as the striatum.

20. How are idiopathic neurodegenerative diseases diagnosed?

One of the major obstacles to treating neurodegenerative diseases is that extensive cell death often occurs prior to the onset of clinical manifestations of many diseases. In **Parkinson's disease**, over 70% of the dopamine-rich, substantia nigra neurons may have degenerated before patients show any of the characteristic motor disturbances. This example serves to illustrate two important points about treating neurodegeneration. First, there is remarkable redundancy and plasticity within many regions of the CNS, which allows subpopulations of neurons to perform the tasks normally distributed among the much larger group of cells, without an appreciable loss of function. Second, the problems associated with supporting the remaining neurons and thus preventing more cell death become more difficult.

Brain imaging methods offer the immediate promise of earlier diagnosis of neurological disease. Modern scanning technology such as functional magnetic resonance imaging, positron emission tomography, and high-density arrays for analysis of evoked potentials, allow for real-time visualization of the activity and viability of regions at risk in neurodegenerative diseases. For instance, altered metabolic activity within the brain can be observed years prior to the onset of clinical manifestations of HD, AD, and PD. Early diagnosis of these conditions may prove useful in the management strategies for these and other disorders.

21. How are neurological diseases treated?

Most neurological diseases are treated with pharmacologic replacement therapy to alleviate motor or cognitive symptoms and pain and suffering. Pharmacotherapy may modulate levels of specific neurotransmitter or affect the activity of specific neurotransmitter receptors. For example, in Parkinson's disease, replacement therapy with dopamine-like drugs such as levodopa increases levels of the neurotransmitter that is diminished by the disease. The drug passes the blood-brain barrier to enter the brain and is transported into cells that contain the synthetic enzyme necessary to convert it into dopamine. Unfortunately, the therapeutic window during which levodopa is effective is somewhat limited, and symptoms often recur. Higher doses of this compound also can lead to unwanted motor effects and hallucinations. Other drugs that will decrease dopamine metabolism and mimic dopamine's action are being developed.

Similar strategies have been employed for loss of the neurotransmiter acetylcholine in AD, enhancement of aminergic neurotransmission by receptor agonist in affective disorders such as depression, and modification of glutamate and GABA transmission in epilepsy.

22. Can cell death in neurodegenerative diseases be stopped?

Not yet. Current treatments to prevent a number of congenital neurological diseases, such as spina bifida, rely on preventing cell death before it starts. There are no treatments available that halt the underlying pathological changes for the major neurodegenerative conditions. There is some evidence that therapy, e.g., vitamin E supplementation, can slow the onset of mental status changes in AD, and that blocking dopamine metabolism delays the disability associated with PD, but the treatment options for most neurodegenerative diseases involve strategies to alleviate symptoms and discomfort rather than stall or reverse the pathology.

Gene therapy techniques, in which nonfunctioning genes are replaced with healthy ones, hold promise as a means to halt neurodegeneration, particularly in loss-of-function mutations. However, the nervous system presents unique problems for gene therapy including issues related to bypassing the blood-brain barrier, targeting genes to specific brain regions and neuronal populations, sustaining the expression of foreign genes, and re-establishing accurate connections between neurons.

23. Can neuronal cells be replaced once they are dead?

The dogma that neurons in the adult brain are postmitotic and unable to self-propagate remains, but the concept that they cannot be replaced recently has been drawn into question. Stem cells in the CNS produce new progenitor and neuronal cell populations in a few areas, such as the hippocampus and olfactory bulb. Strategies to direct the progenitors towards specific neuronal phenotypes remain in the experimental stage. **Neural transplantation**, in which damaged brain cells are replaced with new neurons or cell lines, has been explored as a strategy to allow the brain to compensate for neurodegeneration. The disorder most often discussed for this treatment strategy is Parkinson's disease. PD is typified by loss of a relatively small group of neurons within the brain (the dopaminergic neurons of the substantia nigra), thereby making the replacement of these cells more tenable than in neurodegenerative diseases with widespread cell death.

24. What are important factors to consider in determining the success of cell transplantation?

There are several factors that are critical in designing cell transplantation therapy: (1) the capacity for proliferation and differentiation of the starting population of donor cells, (2) the location in the host for placement that will best support viability and function, and (3) the ability to evaluate in vivo the viability and function of the transplanted cells.

25. What types of cells can be used successfully in grafts?

Grafts can be composed of genetically engineered cells that express certain traits; autologous (derived from the affected individual) cells from other parts of the body that can produce dopamine, such as the adrenal medulla or the paraneural cells of the carotid bodies; or cells derived from fetal donors or other mammals. Successful transplants in model systems also have used embryonic and fetal cells that include primary progenitor cells with restricted abilities to differentiate into certain cell types, **embryonic stem cells** that can form any cell in the embryo and can be derived in vitro to express certain phenotypic traits, or tissue stem cells that have the capacity to form any cell type within that tissue. Even hematopoietic stem cells recently were used in graft experiments in which they formed both neurons and glia.

26. What limits the success of transplanted cells in ameliorating neurological disease?

Synaptic contacts are critical components to successful cell signaling, and one limitation of transplants derived from non-neuronal cells is that they generally do not innervate affected regions. In effect, they serve as mini-pumps to supply depleted molecules and neurotransmitters. The only group of cells that have been shown to form synapses, release dopamine, and aide in functional recovery in Parkinson's patients are neurons that have been derived from fetal brain tissue, and the latest research suggests that enhanced motor activity is only observed in patients who are younger than 60 years of age.

The issue of where transplanted tissue should be placed is critical. The relatively selective loss of a single projection pathway in Parkinson's patients makes this a less complicated decision than in other diseases, such as ALS or AD, in which larger or multiple regions of the CNS are affected. Neural transplants for Parkinson's disease are placed into the denervated area, the neostriatum.

Recent work in animal models of demyelinating disorders indicates that cells such as oligodendrocytes, which are normally highly mobile, can be replaced using a cell transplantation strategy. However, an additional major obstacle to overcome is the enhancement of transplant viability postoperatively. The large majority of transplanted neurons die within months of replacement surgery.

It is likely that, eventually, cells will be manipulated genetically in complex ways to direct the production of certain substances that are depleted in the patient and to enhance long-term survival.

BIBLIOGRAPHY

1. Asbury AK, McKhann GM, McDonald WI: Diseases of the Nervous System: Clinical Neurobiology. Philadelphia, W.B. Saunders Press, 1992.
2. Hardy J, Gwinn-Hardy K: Genetic classification of primary neurodegenerative disease. Science 282:1075–1078, 1998.
3. Kim T-W, Tanzi RE: Neuronal intranuclear inclusions in polyglutamine diseases: Nuclear weapons or nuclear fallout? Neuron 21:657–659, 1998.
4. Olanow CW, Kordower JH, Freeman TB: Fetal nigral transplantation as a therapy for Parkinson's disease. Trends Neurosci 10:102–109, 1996.
5. Paulson HL, Fishbeck KH: Trinucleotide repeats in neurogenetic disorders. Ann Rev Neurosci 19:79–107, 1996.
6. Price DL: New order from neurological disorders. Nature 399:A3–A5, 1999.
7. Ross CA: Intranuclear neuronal inclusions: A common pathogenic mechanism for glutamine-repeat neurodegenerative diseases? Neuron 19:1147–1150, 1997.
8. Shoulson I: Experimental therapeutics of neurodegenerative disorders: Unmet needs. Science 282:1072–1074, 1998.
9. Solter D, Gearhart J: Putting stem cells to work. Science 283:1468–1470, 1999.
10. Svendsen CN, Smith AG: New prospects for human stem-cell therapy in the nervous system. Trends Neurosci 22:357–364, 1999.

24. DEGENERATION, APOPTOSIS, AND REGENERATION

Carolanne E. Milligan, Ph.D.

Development of a mature, functional nervous system includes events of mitosis, differentiation, migration, maturation, and cell death. In fact, during normal development of the central nervous system (CNS), on average 50% of the neurons originally generated die. This cell death is an active process, and similar biochemical pathways appear to be reactivated following injury to the CNS and in degenerative pathologies. This chapter addresses why and how neurons die in development and examines neuronal death following CNS injury and pathology. Finally, issues related to regeneration are addressed.

1. What is programmed cell death?

There has been an explosion of research focused on cell death. Cell death that occurs during development has been referred to as "naturally occurring cell death," "developmental death," "histogenetic cell death," and "programmed cell death" (PCD). This latter term originally was coined by Lockshin and Williams in 1965 to describe the developmentally regulated loss of specific larval muscles following the emergence of the adult moth. In purest terms, PCD is the spatially and temporally specific loss of a given population of cells during development of the organism. For example, in the developing moth the intersegmental muscles die within the first day of emergence. The same population of muscles dies at the same time in each moth of the species.

Many investigators have used the term PCD to encompass many other types of cell death, including that which occurs during normal homeostasis and following pathological insult. The word "programmed" originally was used to indicate part of the developmental program of an organism. However, it now applies to any type of cell death that involves a **genetically mediated process**.

2. What is apoptosis?

In 1972, Kerr, Currie, and Wyllie employed the word "apoptosis" to describe a type of cell death that they had encountered in tumor biology. Cells that die by apoptosis have the morphological characteristics of aggregation of nuclear chromatin into compact granular masses, subsequent condensation of cytoplasm, and a breaking up of the cell into discrete, membrane-bound fragments. Cells that die by apoptosis appear to do so by an active process of the cell: they commit suicide by activating specific intrinsic biochemical and molecular mechanisms. For this reason the term apoptosis has been used synonymously with PCD. However, apoptosis is a type of cell death, and while *some* forms of PCD occur by apoptosis, not all cells that undergo PCD involve this specific process.

3. What is necrosis?

Necrosis occurs as the result of a direct injury to the cell, such as trauma, membrane toxins, or immune mediators that include complement components. The morphological features of necrosis include increased permeability of mitochondrial and plasma membranes. Due to this increased membrane permeability, cations move across concentration gradients with accompanying extracellular fluid, causing cell swelling and eventual bursting of the cell. This type of cell death does not require the cell to activate specific biochemical and molecular mechanisms.

4. Are there just two types of cell death?

No. There is a tendency to categorize cell deaths as either apoptosis or necrosis; however, ongoing research on cell death is revealing that many cells, especially neurons, die by means involving characteristics of both types of death. This is especially true in the nervous system. It is more productive to shift focus from attempts to pigeon-hole a type of death into a specific category, to analyzing the morphological changes that may provide clues to the mechanisms involved.

5. How much cell death is there in the developing nervous system?

The earliest documentation of cell death is from 1896 when John Beard discovered and described the degeneration of the Rohon-Beard cells in the skate. Rohon-Beard cells are transient sensory cells that connect the ectoderm and neural tube in amphibian and fish embryos. In 1926, Ernst proposed that there was an overproduction of dorsal root ganglion neurons, followed by their degeneration. This concept of neuronal death and degeneration was largely ignored or dismissed primarily because investigators believed that development was purely a progressive event. The observed dying cells presumably indicated only a few aberrant cells that were not considered important for overall development of the organism.

Landmark work by Victor Hamburger and Rita Levi-Montalcini provided detailed quantitative analysis of the magnitude of cell death in the developing CNS. They demonstrated that 50% of the sympathetic neurons and lumbar spinal motoneurons produced during embryogenesis died prior to birth. Neuronal death also has been documented to occur in the optic tectum, superior colliculus, retina, basal ganglion, cerebellum, pontine nuclei and inferior olive, cranial motoneurons, ciliary ganglion, sympathetic ganglion, and dorsal root ganglion.

6. Do non-neuronal cells undergo cell death during CNS development?

Cell death in the developing nervous system is not limited to neuronal cells. The astrocytes composing the transient glial sling that underlies the developing corpus callosum die. Oligodendrocytes also undergo cell death, as do Schwann cells.

Barres BA, Hart IK, Coles HS, et al: Cell death and control of cell survival in the oligodendrocyte lineage. Cell 70:31–46, 1992.

Cuitat D, Caldero J, Oppenheim RW, Esquerda JE: Schwann cell apoptosis during normal development and after axonal degeneration induced by neurotoxins in the chick embryo. J Neurosci 16:3979–3990, 1996.

Hankin M, Schneider B, Silver J: Death of the subcallosal glial sling is correlated with the formation of the cavum septi pellucidi. J Comp Neurol 272:191–202, 1988.

7. Do neurons die by apoptosis?

The best answer is that some do. Anatomical studies of PCD in different species and in different cellular lineages within a species have revealed that not all PCDs display the same morphological features.

The best characterized pattern of cell death is apoptosis, a process that involves: cellular condensation, genomic DNA fragmentation, the deposition of electron-dense chromatin along the inner margin of the nuclear envelope, the formation of membrane "blebs" that contain portions of the nucleus and intact organelles, and, ultimately, the phagocytosis of these apoptotic bodies by neighboring cells. There are subtle differences in the type of apoptosis that a neuron undergoes. For example, while apoptotic neurons demonstrate condensed cytoplasm and nuclei, their nuclear chromatin is condensed throughout the nucleus, not only at the inner margin of the nuclear membrane as originally described (Fig. 1A). Additionally, the extent of membrane blebbing in neurons has not been determined.

A characteristic biochemical marker for many, but not all, apoptotic deaths is DNA fragmentation induced by an endogenous endonuclease. This results in the cleavage of DNA into approximately 180 base pair oligonucleotide fragments. When the DNA from cells undergoing apoptosis is size-fractionated in an agarose gel, a characteristic "ladder" can be resolved. It is now possible to detect this DNA fragmentation anatomically in individual cells by performing an in situ nick translation or terminal end-labeling (TUNEL) reaction whereby biotinylated nucleotides are incorporated into the fragmented DNA. This is a very powerful tool for investigators, since it allows detection of individual apoptotic cells within tissue sections as well as easier determination of the percentage of apoptotic cells within a given population.

8. If all neurons do not die by apoptosis, what other types of cell death are there?

While the majority of programmed cell deaths occur with the stereotypic, apoptotic morphology, many nonapoptotic cell deaths are seen in the vertebrate nervous system. Pilar and Landmesser examined the ultrastructural morphology of dying ciliary ganglion cells and observed two distinct morphologies associated with cell death: **nuclear** and **cytoplasmic**. These morphologies also were

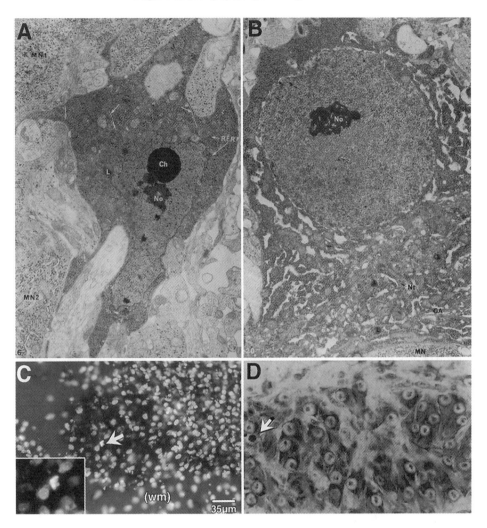

Figure 1. Dying motoneurons. **A**, Electron micrograph of an apoptotic motoneuron from an embryonic day (E) 6 spinal cord. Lumbar spinal motoneuron PCD occurs between E6 and E10. Note that the morphological characteristics of nuclear chromatin condensation, lobed nuclei, and condensed cytoplasm are prominent. MN1, MN2 = dying motoneurons, Ch = chromatin, L= lysosomes, No = nucleolus, RER = rough endoplasmic reticulum. **B**, Electron micrograph of a motoneuron from an E8 spinal cord. This cell has the morphological features of cytoplasmic type 2 cell death, in which changes within the cytoplasm are prominent and include dilation of the mitochondria. The nuclei retains its shape; chromatin condensation occurs, but to a lesser extent than in apoptosis (see *A*). Nt = neurotubules, GA = Golgi apparatus. **C**, Light micrograph of the lateral motor column of an E8 chick lumbar spinal cord. The tissue has been stained with Hoescht 33342, a DNA-binding dye, so that only the nuclei are visible. A pyknotic motoneuron is evident *(arrow)* and looks quite different from an adjacent healthy nucleus *(inset)*. wm = white matter. **D**, Nissl-stained tissue section of an E9 chick lumbar spinal cord. A pyknotic motoneuron is visible *(arrow)*.
From Chu-Wang I-W, Oppenheim RW: Cell death of motoneurons in the chick embryo spinal cord. I. A light and electron microscopic study of naturally occurring and induced cell loss during development. J Comp Neurol 177:33–58, 1978 *[images A and B]*; Barnes NY, Li L, Schwartz LM, et al: Increased production of the amyloid precursor serves as a substrate of caspase-3 in dying motoneurons. J Neurosci 18:5869–5880, 1998 *[image C]*; and Clarke PGH, Oppenheim RW: Neuron death in vertebrate development: In vivo methods. Meth Cell Biol 46:277–321, 1995 *[image D]*. All with permission.

observed subsequently in several other regions of the developing nervous system, where they were referred to as type 1 and type 2, respectively.

Although the nuclear type of cell death represents an apoptosis-type of neuronal death, the cytoplasmic type of cell death shares few structural features with apoptosis (Figs. 1A and B). While these cells undergo cytoplasmic condensation, they do not display the specific genomic DNA fragmentation that generates a "ladder," early chromatin deposition, or membrane blebbing. The initial changes associated with cytoplasmic death are found in the cytoplasm and include swelling of the mitochondria and a breakdown of ribosomes. While the cytoplasmic type of neuronal death displays certain structural features of necrosis, it involves an *active* process of the cell, and does not involve cell lysis.

There is also a third type of cell death observed in the nervous system: **autophagic neuron death**. The most prominent feature of this type is the abundant autophagic vacuoles found in the cytoplasm.

All three types of cell death are observed in normal development and in CNS injury and pathology.

9. What is a pyknotic neuron?

A degenerating neuron at the light microscopic level often is referred to as "pyknotic." The tissue is stained with a Nissl stain that identifies acidic molecules of the cell (i.e., DNA, RNA, rER) or with a DNA-binding dye. Pyknotic cells have a condensed, somewhat shrunken, darkly stained nucleus (Figs. 1C and D). Considering the morphological characteristics of apoptosis, many pyknotic cells are probably apoptotic; however, cells that die by the cytoplasmic type of cell death (see Question 8) often appear pyknotic.

10. Is there a significance to the type of cell death a neuron undergoes?

While it would be convenient to assume that these different morphologies reflect differences in species or cellular lineages, preliminary data suggest that some cells can generate *both* morphologies, depending on the signals they receive. For example, during chick embryogenesis, the majority of ciliary ganglion cells that die display a cytoplasmic pattern of death. However, when these cells are induced to die by removal of their target, essentially 100% of the dying cells display an apoptotic morphology. Therefore, it appears that the same cell can activate two different pathways for death depending on the nature of the trigger.

Alternatively, a neuron's interaction with target and afferents may be steps in its maturation, and the execution of cytoplasmic versus apoptotic cell death pathways may reflect maturation-specific choices. It is not known if these two morphologies use overlapping molecular components or are distinct.

11. What are the techniques used to detect dying cells?

Methods Used to Detect Cell Death

TECHNIQUE	COMMENTS
Electron microscopy	Most reliable technique to detect and characterize type of cell death (apoptosis vs. necrosis)
Count healthy/dying cells	Very reliable for determining extent of cell loss. Requires that criteria for healthy vs. dying cell be clearly defined
Use of DNA-binding dyes	Will identify pyknotic nuclei but not distinguish between apoptotic vs. nonapoptotic types of cell death
Gel electrophoresis to detect fragmentation of genomic DNA	Determines if a population of cells dies by apoptosis where DNA is cleaved between nucleosomes by endonucleases to produce 180 bp fragments on an agarose gel. The activation of endonucleases and the specific fragmentation is a hallmark of apoptosis. While DNA fragmentation may occur in non-apoptotic deaths, the specific fragmentation to yield 180 bp fragments is considered unique to apoptosis.

Table continued on facing page

Methods Used to Detect Cell Death (Continued)

TECHNIQUE	COMMENTS
TdT-mediated dUTP-biotin nick end labeling (TUNEL)	Reaction where TdT incorporates a biotinylated nucleotide onto the free 3′ ends of fragmented DNA. Advantageous because it allows localization of apoptotic cells in tissue sections. While theoretically only apoptotic cells should be labeled, any cell whose DNA has been nicked can be labeled.
Cell viability assays Enzymatic (MTT) or ion pump assays Cytotoxicity assays Membrane permeability assays (uptake of trypan blue) or cytoplasm leakage assays (release of LDH)	Only effective for in vitro studies of cell populations
Fluorescence-activated cell sorting	Determines percentage of apoptotic cells within an in vitro homogeneous population. For analysis cells must be suspended; therefore, this may not be the best assay for neurons that are generally attached to a surface in culture.
In situ hybridization and/or immuno-cytochemistry to detect cell death–associated messages/proteins	Most messages/proteins associated with cell death are not unique to that cellular process

LDH = low-density lipoprotein.
Note: For additional information on these techniques, see Schwartz L, Osborne BA: Cell death. Meth Cell Biol 46, 1995.

12. Why do cells die?

Considering that 50% of neurons generated undergo cell death, the question arises: Why would an organism waste the energy and resources to make so many cells, only to soon kill them? One possible reason is that PCD provides a great deal of **plasticity**. For example, an alternate strategy to insuring a specific genetic program for each individual cell would be to generate a population of cells that must successfully complete a primary developmental program to survive.

13. What is the trigger for cell death?

Given that PCD occurs within a developmental context, it is not surprising that the signals used to trigger this process are physiological, and can be used to initiate other differentiation decisions as well. The molecules that trigger PCD can act at a distance (e.g, hormones) or more intimately, via cell-cell contact. In principle, all cells in the body can be exposed to the trigger, but only a subset are programmed by lineage-specific decisions to be capable of responding to it with death. Cell death in the developing CNS appears to be influenced by several mechanisms, including target interactions such as synaptic contacts, availability of synaptic space, availability of trophic factors, axon or dendritic stability, afferent input, and, most likely, a fine balance between all of the above.

14. What is the role of trophic factor in mediating neuronal death?

While our understanding of the precise triggers for cell death is not complete, dependence on trophic (nutritional) support appears to be a critical component of survival. The first hypothesis suggesting the existence of a trophic factor was made by Levi-Montalcini and Hamburger in 1950, and was followed by a demonstration that the survival of sympathetic neurons was dependent on nerve growth factor (NGF). It is thought that the limited availability of trophic factors is one of the mechanisms by which cell populations size within the nervous system is adjusted to allow proper matching between neurons and their targets. Indeed, if the target size is surgically altered, for example by removing or transplanting an additional limb, then the number of sympathetic neurons and motoneurons changes accordingly.

15. What is the trophic factor hypothesis?

Based on studies by Hamburger and Levi-Montalcini on the role of NGF in sympathetic ganglion cell survival, the neurotrophic factor hypothesis states that during development neurons compete for limited amounts of target-derived, survival-promoting agents.

16. What is the source of trophic factor?

One source of trophic factor is target. For example, survival of the motoneuron is dependent on its interaction with muscle targets, since removal of the limb induces greater than 90% motoneuron death, and transplantation of an additional limb results in reduced cell death. Glial and supporting cells also are sources of trophic support. Afferent input provides trophic support: if afferent input from the retinal ganglion cells to the superior colliculus is removed from the visual system via enucleation at birth, then cell death in the superior colliculus is greatly enhanced.

17. Is neuronal death an active process of the cell?

Yes. The molecular mechanism mediating cell death in the nervous system is currently an area of intense research. Generally, the cell receives a signal for death (for example, the loss of trophic support), and this signal is translated by second-messenger systems into cellular responses that often include new gene expression leading to death. These cellular responses lead to activation of cytoplasmic protease, endonucleases that degrade DNA, and oxidative stress. It appears as if neuronal death can involve one or all three of these processes.

18. What are some of the genes that show increased expression in neuronal death?

New gene expression appears to be required for some neuronal deaths, as indicated by experiments in which cell death is prevented by addition of RNA and/or protein synthesis inhibitors. For example, cultured superior cervical ganglion cells deprived of NGF undergo cell death, and messages for the proto-oncogenes *c-jun*, *c-fos*, *fos B*, and *jun-B*, the transcription factor NGF-1A, the cell cycle regulator cyclin D1, and transin and collagenase are increased. The amyloid precursor protein has been shown to have increased expression in dying cells. Recently it has been reported that the increased expression of amyloid precursor protein provides a substrate for caspase 3, one of the proteases activated in dying motoneurons. While these and other genes show increased expression coincident with cell death, their causative role in the process is an area of continued research.

Barnes NY, Li L, Schwartz LM, et al: Increased production of the amyloid precursor serves as a substrate for caspase-3 in dying motoneurons. J Neurosci 18:5869–5880, 1998.

Freeman RS, Estus S, Johnson Jr EM: Analysis of cell cycle–related gene expression in postmitotic neurons: Selective induction of cyclin D1 during programmed cell death. Neuron 12:343–355, 1994.

19. What is the role of oxidative stress in neuronal death?

Oxygen free radicals have been implicated in several forms of cell death, and reactive oxygen species (ROS) interact with specific cellular components to bring about extensive damage. Since ROS are a normal component of aerobic respiration, endogenous antioxidants within the cell, such as glutathione, serve to balance the detrimental effects of ROS. ROS have been implicated in the PCD of sympathetic neurons, as well as cell death in response to ischemia and neurodegenerative diseases.

Antioxidant agents such as superoxide dismutase or N-acetylcysteine have been shown to prevent neuronal death. Interestingly, treatment of NGF-deprived sympathetic neurons with superoxide dismutase is effective only for a brief time (6–8 hours) following trophic factor deprivation, suggesting that the increase in ROS that may signal death is initial and transient. Furthermore, it has been suggested that ROS are involved in initiating new gene expression, caspase activation, and DNA damage.

20. Is there a relationship between cell cycle and cell death?

Experiments using mitotically active cells have indicated that several components of the cell cycle are involved in cell death. In fact, mistakes in regulation of the cell cycle are thought to result in cell death. Several cell cycle components have been reported to be increased in dying neurons, including cyclins, cyclin-dependent kinases, p53, and retinoblastoma tumor suppressor protein. Furthermore, cell cycle inhibitors have been shown to also inhibit cell death. This finding has led to the hypothesis that inadequate trophic support signals the cell to "de-differentiate" and attempt to re-enter the cell cycle. The neuron's failure to do this results in death. While the expression of several cell cycle molecules is increased during neuronal death, their causative role in the process has not been demonstrated conclusively.

21. What are caspases? Are they involved in neuronal death?

Caspases (cysteine aspartases) are cysteine proteases that have the unique property of cleaving their substrates specifically at a carboxyl side of aspartate (a specificity that is unusual for most mammalian proteases). The homology between mammalian interleukin-1β-converting enzyme (ICE; caspase 1) and the nematode cell death gene *ced-3* suggests an evolutionary significance for these molecules in cell death. To date, at least twelve caspase family members have been identified with sequence similarities to ICE and *ced-3*. These molecules have been assigned to one of three subfamilies according to their sequence homology. All family members appear to be capable of regulating apoptotic forms of cell death.

Caspases are synthesized as precursors that must be proteolytically processed to yield a prodomain and two subunits. The two subunits comprise the active $\alpha_2\beta_2$ tetramers. Multiple caspases that appear to act hierarchically in a proteolytic cascade are essential for initiating the final stages of the cell death pathway.

The involvement of caspases in the PCD of neurons has been demonstrated in several studies. The first evidence came from the study of CrmA, a viral serpin-like pseudosubstrate that inhibits some caspase family members. CrmA was shown to block the death of chicken dorsal root ganglion (DRG) neurons induced by trophic factor (NGF) deprivation, suggesting that ICE-like proteases play an important role in the death of DRG neurons. Another caspase, Nedd-2 (caspase 2) was found to be involved in the death of PC12 cells and sympathetic neurons after trophic factor withdrawal. Caspases 1 and 3 play a role in the cell death of motoneurons during development, while caspase 6 and 8 have little, if any, role. In addition, evidence that much of neuronal PCD fails to occur in caspase 3 knockout and caspase 9 knockout mice indicates the importance of these caspases in PCD in the mammalian brain. These observations strongly support a role for the caspases, especially caspase 3 (CCP-32), in neuronal PCD.

Kuida K, Haydar TF, Kuan C-Y, et al: Reduced apoptosis and cytochrome c-mediated caspase activation in mice lacking caspase 9. Cell 94:325–327, 1998.

Kuida K, Zheng TS, Na S, et al: Decreased apoptosis in the brain and premature lethality in CCP32-deficient mice. Nature 384:368–372, 1996.

Li L, Prevette D, Oppenheim RW, Milligan CE: Multiple caspases are involved in motoneuron cell death. Mol Cell Neurosci 12:157–167, 1998.

22. What are the molecules that serve as substrates for caspases?

Identification of caspase substrates is occurring rapidly. There are four classes of substrates for caspases. Class 1 substrates include molecules that are activated as a result of caspase cleavage. Caspases themselves belong to this class. Class 2 includes molecules that are inactivated because of cleavage. The retinoblastoma tumor suppressor protein is an example of a class 2 substrate. Class 3 substrates are structural proteins whose cleavage by caspases alters their assembly or disassembly properties. The nuclear lamins are an example of a class 3 substrate. Finally, class 4 substrates are molecules whose cleavage by caspases have no known effects on cell death. Poly-ADP-ribose polymerase, actin, fodrin, and huntingtin are examples of this class of substrates.

Villa P, Kaufmann SH, Earnshaw WC: Caspases and caspase inhibitors. Trends Biol Sci 22:388–393, 1997.

23. What are bcl-2 family members?

While caspases appear to be molecules that promote cell death, other molecules have been shown to prevent it. One such molecule is bcl-2. Bcl-2 was identified first as as consequence of a mutation that results in Burkitt's lymphoma. In this condition, a translocation brought the *bcl-2* gene under the control of the immunoglobulin enhancer, causing B cells to overproduce bcl-2 and fail to undergo cell death. The bcl-2 protein shares 22% identity with the *Caenor-habditis elegans* ced-9 protein, which prevents cell death in the nematode. As well, introduction of *bcl-2* into *ced-9* loss-of-function mutant nematodes results in the partial rescue of the phenotype, suggesting that they share functional homology.

Bcl-2 appears to be located in the outer mitochondrial membrane and perinuclear membrane, and while the specific mechanism by which bcl-2 prevents cell death is not known, it has been suggested that it acts as free radical scavenger. Recent studies have demonstrated that there is a family of bcl-2–related proteins (including bax, bcl-x$_L$, bcl-x$_S$, and bad) that appear to interact as positive and negative regulators of cell death. For example, while bcl-2 and bcl-x have protective effects, bax and bad promote death. In bax knock-out animals, there is a decrease in neuronal PCD. The role of bcl-2, bcl-x, bax, and other family members in regulating cell death is an area of ongoing research.

Adams JM, Cory S: The bcl-2 protein family: Arbitors of cell survival. Science 281:1322–1326, 1998.

Chao DT, Korsmeyer SJ: Bcl-2 family: Regulators of cell death. Ann Rev Immunol 16:395–419, 1998.

24. Are bcl-2 family members involved in neuronal death?

Yes. Bcl-2 has been shown to protect many types of neurons from death. Overexpression of bcl-2 in sympathetic neurons can prevent their death following trophic factor withdrawal; however, one report suggests that while bcl-2 has a regulatory role in the survival of sympathetic neurons during PCD, it is not involved in development of trophic factor independence. The role of bcl-2 in axonal degeneration is unclear, as it does not prevent axonal degeneration in a mouse model of motor neuron disease.

In addition to bcl-2, bcl-x and bax also play roles in mediating neuronal death. Bax appears to have a key role in this process, because its overexpression promotes sympathetic neuronal death even in the presence of NGF. Furthermore, bax knock-out mice show dramatically decreased levels of neuronal death.

Deckwerth TL, Elliott JL, Knudson CM, et al: Bax is required for neuronal death after trophic factor deprivation and during development. Neuron 17:401–411, 1996.

Garcia I, Martinou I, Tsujimoto Y, Martinou J: Prevention of programmed cell death of sympathetic neurons by the *bcl-2* proto-oncogene. Science 258:302–304, 1992.

Greenlund LJS, Korsmeyer SJ, Johnson Jr EM: Role of bcl-2 in the survival and function of developing and mature sympathetic neurons. Neuron 15:649–661, 1995.

Sagot Y, Dubois-Dauphin M, Tan SA, et al: Bcl-2 overexpression prevents motoneuron cell body loss but not axonal degeneration in a mouse model of a neurodegenerative disease. J Neurosci 15:7727–7733, 1995.

Vekrellis K, McCarthy MJ, Watson A, et al: Bax promotes neuronal cell death and is downregulated during the development of the nervous system. Development 124:1239–1249, 1997.

25. Are there other cell death inhibitory proteins?

Yes. One clinical manifestation of excessive motoneuron death during human development is the spinal muscular atrophies (SMAs). The SMAs are characterized by motoneuron depletion that is attributed to excessive or prolonged, naturally occurring motoneuron death during normal development. A mutation in the gene for neuronal apoptosis inhibitory protein (NAIP) has been found and analyzed. This deletion of the first two coding exons (found in approximately 67% of type I SMAs) is thought to result in or contribute to the pathological condition. The first two exons of the NAIP gene show homology to the baculovirus inhibitor of apoptosis protein, p35.

In addition to NAIP and p35, several other mammalian inhibitory-of-apoptosis proteins (IAPs) recently have been identified, and it has been speculated that the IAPs may interact with ICE-like proteases to prevent cell death. Another gene product, the survival motor neuron (SMN), also has been implicated in the SMAs. SMN is thought to have synergistic anti-apoptotic activity with bcl-2.

Barinaga M: Forging a path to cell death. Science 273:735–737, 1996.

Iwahashi H, Eguchi Y, Yasuhara N, et al: Synergistic anti-apoptotic activity between bcl-2 and SMN implicated in spinal muscular atrophy. Nature 390:413–417, 1997.

26. How do molecules such as bcl-2 and caspases interact to bring about cell death?

The cell death pathway, or cascade, only can be hypothesized at this point (Fig. 2). While bcl-2 is generally survival-promoting, family members bik and bax are death-promoting. Alterations in bax concentrations are thought to lead to release of cytochrome c from the mitochondria to the cytoplasm, perhaps by bax- or bik-forming pores in the mitochondrial membranes. Once in the cytoplasm, cytochrome c can activate apaf-1, a molecule that can further activate caspase 9. Activation of caspase 9 leads to subsequent activation of other caspases, including caspase 3, that can lead to cell death.

Note that the entire cascade has not been observed from beginning to end in one cell type. Additionally, there appear to be alternate, caspase-independent pathways of cell death within given populations of cells.

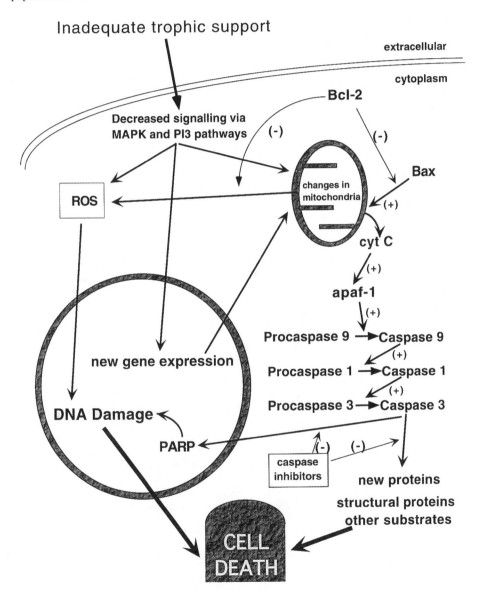

Figure 2. Neuronal cell death cascade, featuring molecules known to be involved in neuronal death (but perhaps not in every cell type) and their possible interactions. Here, the signal for death is inadequate supply of trophic support.

27. What are the responses to cell death in the CNS?

While much attention has been devoted to understanding the signals and molecular pathways that mediate PCD, less attention has been focused on how the body deals with removing the cellular debris that follows death. This is not a trivial consideration, given the number of cells that undergo PCD and the inflammatory nature of intracellular constituents; phagocytosis of the dead cell is an essential component of the cell death process. The genetics of this process are best understood in *C. elegans*, for which seven genes involved in the process of phagocytosis of the corpse have been identified. These genes appear to represent two distinct complementation groups: cell surface ligands that identify the cell as a corpse, and receptors for these signals on the phagocytosing cell. While mutations in these genes prevent corpse removal, they have no impact on the death process itself.

Although neighboring cells have been found to phagocytose dying cells, the predominant professional scavenger is the **macrophage**. In fact, almost every morphological study examining tissues displaying PCD describes the presence of macrophages. The CNS has been well characterized in this regard: macrophages/microglia remove dead cells that arise during PCD, axon retraction, and glial scaffold elimination. The phagocytosis of cells undergoing PCD is so efficient that dying cells often are found within macrophages *prior to the final death* of the cell.

28. How are cells recruited to the area of cell death/injury in the CNS?

While the pattern of macrophage recruitment during PCD is well characterized, little is known about the molecular mechanisms responsible for targeting macrophages to these regions. Since macrophages are usually not resident in the tissues where PCD occurs, chemotactic signals must recruit them to the regions where their activity is required. Given the specificity of this reaction in the CNS, some investigators have hypothesized that degenerating neuronal elements provide a chemotactic signal for macrophages. A brain-derived chemotactic factor (BDCF) has been identified in neonatal CNS injury. BDCF exhibits opioid-like activity that initiates macrophage chemotaxis via a receptor with the pharmacological characteristics of a *delta* opioid receptor. The monocyte chemotactic protein-1 and fractalkine also have been found to be increased following CNS injury.

Harrison JK, Jiang Y, Chen S, et al: Role for neuronally derived fractalkine in mediating interactions between neurons and CX3CR1-expressing microglia. PNAS 95:10896–10901, 1998.

Milligan CE, Webster L, Piros ET, et al: An opioid chemotactic factor mediates the targeting of macrophages to the site of injury-induced neuronal cell death in the developing brain. J Immunol 154:6571–6581, 1995.

Wang X, Yue T-I, Barone FC, Feuerstein GZ: Monocyte chemoattractant protein-1 messenger RNA expression in rat ischemic cortex. Stroke 26:661–666, 1995.

29. Do dying cells express specific markers that allow them to be recognized by phagocytes?

In addition to chemotaxis, some cell-cell interactions must be involved to insure that macrophages/microglia engulf dying, but not healthy, cells. The mechanisms by which macrophages identify cells to be phagocytosed appear to involve alterations in the cell surface of dying cells. These interactions appear to be mediated by a macrophage cell surface lectin that interacts with an altered vitronectin receptor on apoptotic cells. The lectin-vitronectin connection may be mediated by macrophage-secreted thrombosporin that binds to both dying cells and the integrin receptors (and other receptors) on macrophages.

Another factor that appears to mediate macrophage recognition and phagocytosis of dying cells is phosphatidylserine. While this phospholipid usually is restricted to the inner monolayer of the plasma membrane, changes in membrane hydrophobicity or charge in dying cells appears to result in the exposure of phosphatidylserine on the external surface of the membrane.

The macrophage 61D3 antigen (uncharacterized), scavenger receptors, and the mouse macrophage ABC-1 molecule (a member of the ATP-binding cassette superfamily) also have been demonstrated to mediate macrophage recognition of dying cells.

Savill J: Recognition and phagocytosis of cells undergoing apoptosis. British Med Bul 53:491–508, 1997.

30. Are phagocytes necessary for cell death?

In both nematodes and moths, cell death occurs independently of phagocytosis. The same appears to be true in mammals. For example, the initial morphological changes in neurons of the dorsal lateral geniculate nucleus associated with cell death occur prior to massive macrophage invasion into the brain. However, one report has presented evidence that macrophages may serve not just to remove debris but also to kill target cells in the developing mouse eye. In this study, the authors used transgenic mice that targeted toxin to subsets of mature macrophages, including those found in the eye cavity. In contrast to wild-type mice, the hyaloid vasculature persisted in the transgenic animals, suggesting that in the absence of hyalocytes (macrophages), death of the cells associated with hyaloid vasculature was not initiated. However, it is possible that the cell death still occurred, but in the absence of phagocytosis, gross tissue morphology was maintained. Furthermore, in some systems macrophage response following cell death may facilitate tissue remodeling during development.

31. Does cell death occur following injury to the CNS?

CNS Injuries and Pathologies Involving Neuronal Death

INJURIES	PATHOLOGY
Spinal cord injuries*	Diseases of dementia
Stroke*	Alzheimer's disease*
Head trauma*	Pick's disease
Axotomy of CNS axons*	Progressive supranuclear palsy
	Movement disorders
	Parkinson's disease*
	Huntington's chorea*
	Ataxia
	Friedreich's ataxia
	Familial cerebellar cortical atrophy
	Olivo-ponto-cerebellar atrophies
	Wilson's disease
	Hallevorden Spatz disease
	Diseases of muscle weakness
	Spinal muscular atrophies*
	Amylotrophic lateral sclerosis*

* Apoptosis is known to occur; unknown extent to which other types of cell death also occur.

32. Are mechanisms involved in neuronal PCD similar to those involved in cell death induced by injury or pathology of the CNS?

Yes. Many of the molecules that have been found to be involved in neuronal PCD during development also are involved in pathological cell death. For example, caspases, amyloid precursor protein, and bcl-2 family members have been implicated in the apoptosis associated with Alzheimer's disease, amylotrophic lateral sclerosis, and ischemia models of stroke. Additionally, the NAIP and SMA molecules were identified as defective molecules associated with the SMAs (see Question 25).

33. What happens to the axon of an injured neuron?

Let's use axotomy (cutting of the axon) as an example of injury to a neuron. The axonal part closest to the cell body is referred to as the proximal segment; the other part is the distal segment. Following axotomy, there is a spillage of axoplasm into the extracellular space; however, it is limited because the cut membranes quickly seal. The proximal and distal segments swell due to a buildup of mitochondria, vesicles, and cytoskeletal and membrane components that are transported via fast axonal transport. Keep in mind that this transport goes in both directions.

34. What are the changes in the cell body of an injured neuron?

The changes observed in the cell body following axotomy are dependent on whether the neuron can regenerate its axon. Axotomy to a peripheral axon results in characteristic changes within the cell body that are reflective of the cell's gearing up in attempt to make a new axon. The cell body swells, the nucleus moves to an eccentric position, and the rough endoplasmic reticulum (RER) dissociates and moves to the periphery of the cell body. This dissolution of the RER (visualized by the loss of Nissl staining) is called chromatolysis. Neurons whose axons are located peripherally to the CNS can regenerate the axon, and the cell body regains its normal appearance. CNS neurons cannot restore proper connections, and the cell atrophies or degenerates completely.

35. What is Wallerian degeneration?

The degeneration of the distal axonal segment following axotomy is termed Wallerian degeneration after Augustus Waller, the English physician who originally described the process. In the mature animal, this process usually occurs over 1–2 months.

36. What is terminal degeneration?

Terminal degeneration is the degeneration of synapses in the distal segment of the axon following axotomy. The maintenance of the presynaptic terminal critically depends on supply from the cell body, as indicated by the observation that almost immediately following axotomy the presynaptic terminal is lost.

37. Are neurons that are connected to the injured neuron also affected by the injury?

Yes, especially if the injured neuron degenerates. Transneuronal degeneration is the loss of cells that provide afferent input to the injured cell (retrograde transneuronal degeneration) and/or the loss of target neurons of the injured cell (anterograde transneuronal degeneration). This degeneration is thought to be the result of a loss of trophic interactions.

38. What are the non-neuronal events associated with injury to neurons?

Following axotomy, for example, there is proliferation of astrocytes (CNS) or connective tissue and Schwann cells (peripheral nervous system). These cells form a scar around the injured area. Additionally, the myelin sheath breaks down. Phagocytic cells (microglia/macrophages) invade the region and begin to phagocytize the myelin fragments and degenerating axons. In addition to the neuronal degeneration in the injured CNS, many glial cells, especially oligodendrocytes, also degenerate.

39. Can neurons regrow axons?

Peripheral nerves are capable of regeneration. In the CNS, while the developing system does show improved recovery and regeneration following injury, the mature system does not provide an environment that promotes neuronal regeneration. However, experimental manipulations of the extracellular environment of the mature CNS have demonstrated that injured neurons can recover and regrow axons, suggesting that mature neurons have an intrinsic ability for regeneration.

40. What are the events that lead to regeneration of peripheral nerves?

After scar formation, Schwann cells divide and form a bridge from the scar to the target. Neurites sprout from the proximal end of the severed or crushed peripheral axon. The Schwann cell bridge forms a pathway for the growing axons and provides a substrate for successful re-establishment of sensory and motor connections. Neurites that fail to contact the Schwann cell bridge degenerate. Microsurgical techniques that rapidly re-establish contact of severed nerves allow for a more rapid return of function. Such techniques are in part responsible for making reattachment of severed limbs a relatively routine practice.

Schwann cells appear to have a critical role in axonal regeneration. Interestingly, when Schwann cells are grafted into transected spinal cords to bridge the gap caused by the transection, axons enter and regenerate within the Schwann cell bridge. Whether brainstem or sensory axons regenerate depends on if the bridge is treated (brainstem and sensory axons) or not treated (sensory axons only) with neurotrophins, further suggesting the complexity of axonal regeneration. Unfortunately, regenerated axons do not exit the Schwann cell bridge, and therefore do not re-enter the CNS environment.

Xu MN, Chen A, Guenard V, Kleitmann N, Bunge MB: Bridging Schwann cell transplants promote axonal regeneration from both the rostral and caudal stumps of transected adult rat spinal cord. J Neurocytol 26:1–16, 1997.

Xu MN, Guenard V, Kleitman N, Bunge MB: A combination of BDNF and NT-3 promotes supraspinal axonal regeneration into Schwann cell grafts in adult rat thoracic spinal cord. Exp Neurol 134:261–272, 1959.

41. What are some differences between the developing and mature nervous system that may account for lack of regeneration in the mature CNS?

There are several factors that are thought to contribute to improved recovery and regeneration of the injured, developing CNS compared to the mature CNS (Fig. 3). All of these factors are concerned with the extracellular environment and responses of glial cells. One factor may be that there is more general production of trophic factors in the developing CNS as compared to the mature CNS. Another factor is changes in the expression of astrocyte-associated proteoglycans. The developing CNS has not completed myelination, and the presence of myelin also has been reported to inhibit axonal regrowth. Finally, the response of macrophages/microglia in the developing CNS appears to be different from the response in the mature system.

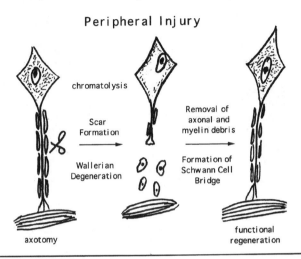

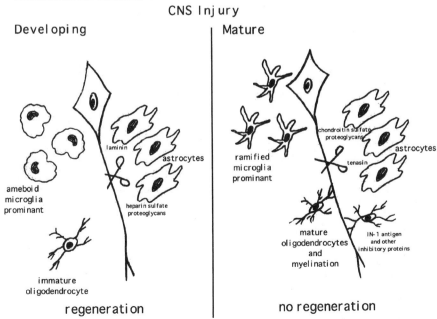

Figure 3. Differences in responses to injury in the peripheral and central nervous systems.

42. Are there regions of the CNS that do regenerate?

The neuronal population of the olfactory epithelium undergoes continuous renewal throughout the lifespan of mammals. For the olfactory system to remain functional, these peripherally derived neurons must send their axons to the CNS olfactory bulb. The continued expression of laminin and collagen IV are thought to contribute to the olfactory epithelium neuronal axonal growth/regeneration into the CNS. Additionally, olfactory ensheathing cells (olfactory astrocytes) appear to be key regulators of this process. Interestingly, when these ensheathing cells are transplanted into lesioned corticospinal tracts or transected spinal cords, regeneration of adult axons occurs. The ensheathing cells appear to provide not only a substrate for growing axons, but also appropriate factors that promote long-distance axonal growth.

Julliard AK, Hartmann DJ: Spatiotemporal patterns of expression of extracellular matrix molecules in the developing and adult rat olfactory system. Neurosci 84:1135–1150, 1998.

Li Y, Field PM, Raismann G: Regeneration of adult rat corticospinal axons induced by transplanted olfactory ensheathing cells. J Neurosci 18:10514–10524, 1998.

Ramon-Cueto A, Plant GW, Avila J, Bunge MB: Long-distance axonal regeneration in the transected adult rat spinal cord is promoted by olfactory ensheathing glia transplants. J Neurosci 18:3803–3815, 1998.

43. What is the role of astrocytes in regeneration?

Astrocytes appear to play a dual role by both promoting and inhibiting neurite outgrowth. During development, astrocytes form glial slings that aid in the formation of axonal tracts such as the corpus callosum; yet, following injury, formation of the astrocytic scar is inhibitory to axonal growth. The astrocytes themselves are similar in the developing and mature CNS, but their altered production of extracellular matrix proteins creates an environment that is permissive or inhibitory for axonal growth. During development, molecules such as laminin and heparin-sulfated proteoglycans promote neurite extension, and tenasin and chondroitin-sulfated proteoglycans are inhibitory. Regulated expression of these molecules plays a role in axonal guidance so that appropriate connections are made. While there are several factors that may contribute to the nonpermissive environment, there appears to be an up-regulation of expression of tenasin and chondroitin-sulfated proteoglycans following injury to the mature CNS. This up-regulation in part causes the glial scar to be inhibitory for axonal growth. When these sulfated proteoglycans are inhibited or blocked experimentally, axonal outgrowth is successful.

Fitch MT, Silver J: Glial cell extracellular matrix: boundaries for axon growth in development and regeneration. Cell Tissue Res 290:379–384, 1997.

44. Are oligodendrocytes involved in CNS regeneration?

One model system of CNS injury is spinal cord resections. Interestingly, when mid-thoracic transections are performed on embryonic day 10 (E10) chicks, there is regeneration and recovery of function; however, transections performed at E15 result in no regeneration or recovery of function. Therefore, within a very short time period (E10 to E15) a transition is made between an environment conducive to recovery versus one that is not. The identification of this critical period has the potential to allow for identification of cellular and molecular changes that mediate a sudden altered response to injury.

Extensive work done by Steeves and colleagues has shown that this critical period in chicks appears to be between E12 and E13, the time coincident with the onset of myelination. Additionally, when dissociated neurons are plated onto CNS frozen section, adhesion and neurite outgrowth occurs on gray but not white matter.

Hassan SJ, Nelson BH, Valenzuela JI, Steeves JD, et al: Functional repair of transected spinal cord in embryonic chick. Restor Neurol Neurosci 2:137–154, 1991.

Savio T, Schwab ME: Rat CNS white matter, but not gray matter, is nonpermissive for neuronal cell adhesion and fiber outgrowth. J Neurosci 9(4):1126–1133, 1989.

Shimizu I, Oppenheim RW, O'Brien M, Shneiderman A: Anatomical and functional recovery following spinal cord transection in the chick embryo. J Neurobiol 21:918–937, 1990.

45. What are the features of oligodendrocytes or CNS myelin that prohibit regeneration?

Growth cones that make contact with mature oligodendrocytes or CNS myelin collapse. Since peripheral nerves are capable of regeneration, and Schwann cells appear to play a role in promoting this process, there must be something unique to oligodendrocytes and/or CNS myelin that inhibits regeneration. Schwab and colleagues have identified myelin-associated inhibitors of neurite growth. Membrane proteins of CNS white matter have been isolated and found to be inhibitory to neurite outgrowth, and a monoclonal antibody, IN-1, has been raised against one of these proteins. When this antibody is applied to explants of white matter, axonal elongation is permitted. Staining patterns of IN-1 correspond to those of an antibody to myelin oligodendrocyte glycoprotein, a protein exclusively found in CNS myelin and differentiated oligodendrocytes. The inhibitory activity of the IN-1 antigen not only affects growth cone mobility, but also appears to involve a retrograde regulation of gene expression in adult CNS neurons.

Bandlow CE, Schmidt MF, Hassinger TD, Schwab ME, Kater SB: Role of intracellular calcium in NI-35-evoked collapse of neuronal growth cones. Science 259(5091):80–83, 1993.

Caroni P, Schwab ME: Antibody against myelin-associated inhibitor of neurite growth neutralizes nonpermissive substrate properties of CNS white matter. Neuron 1(1):85–96, 1988.

Rubin BP, Dusart I, Schwab ME: A monoclonal antibody (IN-1) which neutralizes neurite growth inhibitory proteins in the rat CNS recognizes antigens localized in CNS myelin. J Neurocytol 23(4):209–217, 1994.

Zagrebelsky M, Buffo A, Skerra A, et al: Retrograde regulation of growth-associated gene expression in adult rat Purkinje cells by myelin-associated neurite growth inhibitory proteins. J Neurosci 18(19):7912–7929, 1998.

46. Are trophic factors involved in axonal regeneration?

Yes. Trophic factors appear to be critical modulators of axonal regeneration. For example, following peripheral axotomy of motoneurons, production of trophic support increases in their target muscles. This increase is thought to contribute to the neurons' regeneration. In the mature CNS, addition of exogenous trophic factors has been shown to promote neuronal survival and axonal growth following injury. Furthermore, improved axonal growth following spinal cord transections is observed when tissue bridges treated with trophic factors are transplanted into the lesion site, as compared to transplants of untreated tissue bridges. Additionally, following spinal cord transection, infusion of trophic factors together with the inhibition of growth-restricting molecules such as the IN-1 antigen promotes improved recovery, as compared to either treatment alone.

Henderson CE, Huchet M, Changeux JP: Denervation increases a neurite-promoting activity in extracts of skeletal muscle. Nature 302(5909):609–611, 1983.

47. What happens to a neuron that fails to regenerate?

The first task of an injured neuron is to survive the initial insult. If survival occurs, the neuron then must regenerate its connections with afferents and/or its target to become functional. If a neuron fails to make these reconnections, it may atrophy or die. Theoretically, if sufficient trophic support can be maintained by glial cells, then a neuron may atrophy but survive. However, considering the complexity of dependence on trophic support for developing and injured neurons, it is realistic to assume that over time, without the *combination of support* from glial, afferent, and target sources, the neuron eventually will die.

The resulting damage to the CNS is far-reaching, including not only the death of the individual neuron, but the glial and extracellular response to the death (transneuronal degeneration). While this scenario presents a rather bleak picture, keep in mind that less than a decade ago there was no hope for recovery following spinal cord or brain injury. The tremendous strides made in this area of research now provide investigators with the *realistic* hope that recovery and regeneration are possible.

BIBLIOGRAPHY

1. Aubert I, Ridet J-L, Gage FH: Regeneration in the adult mammalian CNS: Guided by development. Curr Opin Neurobiol 5:625–635, 1995.
2. Clarke PGH: Apoptosis versus necrosis? How valid a dichotomy for neurons? In Koliatsos V, Rata R (eds): Cell Death in Diseases of the Nervous System. Totowa NJ, Humana Press Inc., 1997, pp 3–28.

3. Cunningham TJ: Naturally occurring death and its regulation by developing neural pathways. Intl Rev Cytol 74:163–186, 1982.
4. Fawcett JW, Geller HM: Regeneration in the CNS: Optimism mounts. Trends Neurosci 21:179–180, 1998.
5. Guth L: Regeneration in the mammalian peripheral nervous system. Physiol Rev 36:441–478, 1956.
6. Milligan CE, Schwartz LM: Programmed cell death during development in animals. In Holbrook NJ, Martin GR (eds): Cellular Aging and Cellular Death. New York, Wiley-Liss, 1996, pp 181–208.
7. Oppenheim RW: Programmed cell death. In Zigmond MJ, Bloom FE, Landis SC, et al: Fundamental Neuroscience. New York, Academic Press, 1998, pp 581–609.
8. Schwartz LM, Osborne BA: Cell death. Meth Cell Biol 46, 1995.
9. Stefanis L, Burke RE, Greene LA: Apoptosis in neurodegenerative disorders. Curr Opin Neurol 10:299–305, 1997.

25. NEURAL PLASTICITY

Jon H. Kaas, Ph.D., and Neeraj Jain, Ph.D.

1. What is neural plasticity?

Neural plasticity refers to the ability of the nervous system to change to a different structural and functional state. Circuits in the brain need not be stable. They change so that they can process information in new ways and have new functions. Plasticity during development has been studied the most. Normally, brains of the same species develop in much the same way, but under conditions of sensory deprivation or early brain injury, brains can develop in quite different ways. Other types of plastic changes occur even in mature brains. We all benefit from learning and training, and acquisition of new skills and knowledge depends on changes in the brain.

The brain also alters its functional organization during recovery from injury. Sometimes the plastic changes are helpful, and sometimes they lead to undesirable consequences.

2. Give an example of developmental plasticity.

Perhaps the most studied form of developmental plasticity is the changed development of primary visual cortex in cats and monkeys reared with one eye shut and normal vision in the other eye. Visual cortex receives input from both eyes via a relay in the thalamus, the lateral geniculate nucleus. Most neurons in visual cortex respond to a stimulus presented to either eye. If one eye is covered so that the retina receives only diffuse light from birth, almost all neurons in visual cortex of the adult cat or monkey respond only to the stimulation of the undeprived, normal eye. The brain develops differently, so that cortical neurons receive most of the connections from thalamic neurons related to the normal eye, but very few connections from thalamic neurons related to the deprived eye.

Thus, normal development depends on the two eyes receiving equal stimulation. Unbalanced stimulation leads to unbalanced growth of connections and altered function. The deprived eye becomes functionally blind.

3. Are there other types of experience that lead to altered brain growth?

Yes, one of the earliest discoveries was that rats reared in an interesting, complex environment (a special home cage) developed thicker visual cortex than rats reared in a simple environment (the normal home cage). Neurons in cortex grew more connections and became larger. The implication is that brain development can be hindered by limited sensory and motor experience, and enhanced by more experience.

4. Are other sensory systems besides the visual system plastic during development?

Yes, but the visual system has been the most studied. In rats, damage to the sensory nerves from the face or to whiskers on the snout early in development alters the structural development of somatosensory cortex (Fig. 1). In addition, if sensory inputs from a limb are damaged very early in development, the neurons normally activated by the damaged inputs in cortex become responsive to other inputs. As an example, a cut nerve regenerates to the skin with many errors, so that a mixed-up message is sent to the brain, and stimuli on the skin are mislocalized. If this mix-up occurs early in development, it can be corrected by changes in the connections of the central nervous system.

5. What is one of the most dramatic ways in which normal development of sensory cortex has been experimentally altered?

One example is in rodents and ferrets that have damaged visual and auditory systems at birth. Under some conditions when brainstem targets for projections from the retina are missing, and auditory inputs to the thalamus are eliminated, retinal afferents may grow into the auditory thalamus, so that visual information is relayed to auditory cortex. Thus, neurons in auditory cortex respond to vision. However, it is not yet known if the rodents then hear light, or see with auditory cortex.

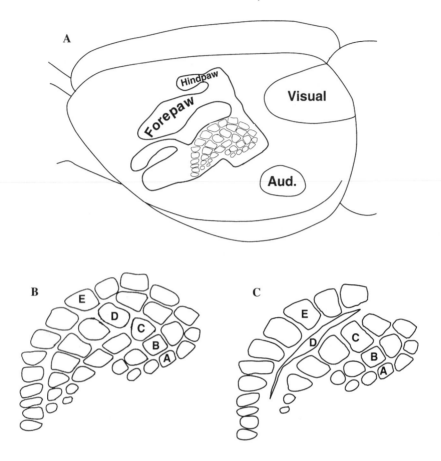

Figure 1. Developmental plasticity in the rat somatosensory cortex. **A**, The primary somatosensory cortex (S1) demonstrates a somatotopic representation of the body surface. Each whisker on the snout is represented as a discrete cluster of cells or "barrel." Primary visual and primary auditory (Aud.) regions are shown for reference. **B**, The normal representation of the whiskers in the barrel field. Each rostral to caudal row of whiskers (A to E) on the snout has a corresponding row of barrels in S1. **C**, The barrel field that results if row D of whiskers is ablated early in development. The barrels corresponding to row D shrink and fuse together, while barrels in the adjacent rows (C and E) expand and occupy larger than normal areas. A similar ablation of the whiskers in adulthood does not affect the barrel pattern, but there is reduced activity and metabolic capacity of the neurons in the deprived barrels.

6. Does this mean that any part of the cortex can develop to assume any role?

While all areas of cortex reflect a basic laminar and vertical pattern of organization, different parts have different cellular organization, and there are differences in the local circuitry between the cells. The development of the cortex is a gradual process that involves genetic specifications in the beginning. However, environment and sensory experience increasingly play a role in the final shaping of the cortical structure. It appears that if cortex is modified by the environment and experimental manipulations early enough, it can be made to assume a number of roles. However, it is unlikely that one area of cortex, such as auditory cortex, can adapt in detail to the roles of another area.

7. What are the implications for humans of the studies in developmental plasticity?

There are two main conclusions. First, providing a normal and enriched sensory environment is important. An abnormal sensory environment is detrimental. If an infant does not see properly with both eyes, then the anatomical framework for normal vision will not develop. If one eye deviates at birth, a surgical correction should be done early. Recovery to normal levels of function may be difficult or impossible after long developmental periods of sensory deprivation.

Second, compensations for brain damage and injury can be much more extensive in the developing brain than the mature brain. The developing brain has greater plasticity; thus, it is more susceptible to the damaging effects of deprivation, but also more capable of repair and compensation.

8. Why is the developing brain more plastic than the adult brain?

During development, the connections between different parts of the brain still are being formed. New growth and changes in growth patterns are feasible. Correct wiring of the brain depends on the presence of the intact target region as well as on sensory experience. If the target region is absent or damaged, the growing axons may end up in a new place, forming new connections. However, in the adult brain all the connections are already in place. Therefore, the scope of structural changes is more limited due to the limited potential for growth in the adult brain. The plastic changes are largely constrained by the anatomical framework already laid out.

9. What is the "critical period" of developmental plasticity?

The critical period is a concept that refers to the observation that some types of brain plasticity can only take place within, or are limited to, a restricted period of time during development. Imprinting—a sudden and lasting change in behavior as a result of experience—typically is confined to short periods during development and occurs by rapid and relatively permanent brain changes, although the nature of the brain changes may be unknown. Some songbirds, for example, learn their adult song patterns while still in the nest, but not afterward. For humans and other primates, the detrimental effects of visual deprivation on the visual system are greatest at early stages of development, and minor in adults. Critical periods also are called sensitive periods.

10. Is the critical period the same for all the parts of the brain?

No, the time course of normal development is different for different parts of the brain and varies for different modalities. For example, in primates the somatosensory system develops earlier than the visual system. Consequently, any changes in the sensory experience after birth have more effect on the visual system than the somatosensory system. Moreover, subcortical circuitry matures before the circuits in the cortex are formed.

11. Is brain development altered by stress?

Much evidence now indicates that early stress alters the development of the brain. High levels of stress in infants can alter the brain systems so that there are increased behavioral and endocrine responses to stress in adult life.

12. How is the course of brain development altered by experience?

Sensory experience and motor acts alter the patterns of neural activity in the brain. In many areas, neural activity is essential for the formation of a normal pattern of neural connections. Patterns of neural activity often determine the adult arrangement of neural connections.

13. How are connections in the developing brain altered by activity patterns?

It appears that "neurons that fire together wire together." Inputs that converge on the same neuron stay in place and become stronger if the two inputs are active at precisely the same time. If a weak input is active only when a strong input is inactive, the weak input may be lost. Thus, the details of how neurons interconnect are altered by stimuli that cause them to respond in different ways. In addition, the expression of many genes in neurons also is dependent on activity levels. The products of these genes can alter form and function.

14. How does closing one eye alter activity patterns?

If a cat or monkey is reared with one eye shut, ganglion cells projecting from the closed eye are poorly activated, and they fail to respond to visual objects that activate ganglion cells in the open eye. Such major differences in the activity patterns in the two eyes interfere with the preservation and strengthening of converging inputs on cortical neurons related to the two eyes, so neurons come to respond to one eye or the other, usually the eye that was open during development.

15. What is Hebbian plasticity?

The psychologist Donald Hebb attempted to account for learning and memory by postulating that learning occurs as a result of changes in synaptic efficacy that alter the properties of groups of interacting neurons. In 1949, he wrote: "Where an axon of Cell A is near enough to excite Cell B and repeatedly or persistently takes part in firing it, some growth or metabolic change takes place in one or both cells such that A's efficiency, as one of two cells firing B, is increased." This major assumption about the structural changes that make memory possible has received much experimental support. Changes in synaptic strength as a result of neural activity often are referred to as Hebbian plasticity, to recognize Hebb's theoretical contribution.

16. Where do plastic changes take place in the brain?

Probably all parts of the brain are plastic. Developmental plasticity has been studied most extensively in the visual and other sensory systems where deprivation effects are easily detected. Synaptic plasticity of the Hebbian type has been studied most in the hippocampus, which is a structure specialized for some types of learning. The cerebellum has been studied as a structure that is important in the plasticity of sensorimotor performance. Other parts of the brain, especially the neocortex, have been investigated extensively in recent years for modifications that demonstrate plasticity related to perceptual learning and motor skills. Plasticity also has been investigated in mature brains recovering from injury. Sensory systems have proven to be especially useful in these investigations, since changes in the normal order of sensory representations can be easily detected.

17. The hippocampus is considered to be a major site of neural plasticity. Why?

Two parallel lines of research have led to this view. First, many studies demonstrated that neurons could sprout and form new connections after lesions produced localized damage in the hippocampus of both developing and mature mammals. The hippocampus is a precisely organized structure where it is easy to demonstrate growth and the formation of new synapses. It now appears that such new growth can occur throughout the central nervous system.

Second, a type of functional plasticity initially was demonstrated in the hippocampus, where it has been studied most extensively. In physiological recording experiments, long-term potentiation (LTP) was demonstrated first in intact animals, then in tissue slice preparations.

18. What is long-term potentiation?

LTP is important as a leading candidate for a synaptic or cellular mechanism of rapid learning. LTP is the "long-term" (hours or longer) increase in synaptic strength between two neurons or two groups of neurons that follows brief, high-frequency electrical stimulation of the first neuron or set of neurons. After such stimulation, any subsequent stimulation produces a greater response in the second neuron or neurons, and the potentiation of the response lasts for at least hours and most typically the duration of the experiment. While electrical stimulation is used to demonstrate the plasticity, these synaptic changes are thought to be the same ones that occur in learning. LTP was first demonstrated in the hippocampus, and more recently in cortex.

19. How is long-term potentiation induced?

The powerful synaptic action that is evoked by electrical stimulation sets in motion a series of biochemical events that strengthen synapses. These biochemical events are still under study, but it is generally accepted that the induction of LTP requires the activation of postsynaptic N-methyl-D-aspartate (NMDA) glutamate receptors. Stimulation of axons releases glutamate from the terminals, which depolarizes neurons in synaptic contact with the axons. Depolarization results in the removal of a voltage-dependent block of the opening in the NMDA receptor, so that Ca^{2+} can enter the postsynaptic neurons. The increase in calcium ions is thought to trigger structural changes in the neurons, with the result that they respond more easily and strongly to subsequent stimuli.

20. What is long-term depression?

In order for LTP to work for associative learning, there must be ways of weakening synapses as well as strengthening them. A long-term depression (LTD) or weakening of synaptic strength between neurons has been demonstrated under some experimental conditions. LTD may be a reversal of LTP.

21. How does LTP work?

Cellular mechanisms of learning work at the systems level in that the properties of networks of neurons change. Theoretical studies of networks with connections of modifiable strengths show that powerful associative learning effects can emerge. LTP and LTD, as Hebbian mechanisms of use-dependent modifications in the strengths of pre-existing synaptic connections among neurons, therefore are seen as critically important in learning and memory storage.

22. Are sensory representations in cortex changed during the learning of perceptual skills?

Yes. Auditory, somatosensory, and visual inputs to cortex all relate to orderly representations of cochlear hair cells, skin receptors, or the retina. Training on a task can distort these representations slightly so that more cortical neurons are devoted to the learned tasks. For example, learning a discrimination based on tones results in more neurons in primary auditory cortex becoming responsive to the tones used during training. In monkeys trained to make difficult discriminations with their fingertips, more neurons in primary somatosensory cortex become responsive to touch on the fingertips. The changes in the primary cortical representations are small, but they may be significant in mediating the improved performance. Of course, higher-order representations also may change and contribute.

23. What happens to the central representations of the body when a nerve is damaged or a finger or a limb is lost?

This issue has been studied most in primary somatosensory cortex. One might suppose that sectors of the orderly map of the body in cortex would become silent or unresponsive to tactile stimuli after the loss of input from any part of the body. Instead, the cortical territory devoted to inputs from a missing finger or limb, or the skin subserved by a damaged nerve, becomes responsive to remaining inputs from the skin. The time course of this recovery varies from an immediate change to several months or longer, depending largely on the magnitude of the sensory loss. These different times of reactivation reflect different mechanisms for brain plasticity (Fig. 2).

24. How can a sensory representation immediately reorganize after the loss of an input?

Primary somatosensory cortex represents the skin of the digits and palm in an orderly way, with a small territory for each digit and pad of the palm (Fig. 2). With the loss of the digit or the block of sensory nerves from a digit, neurons in the cortical territory for that digit may suddenly respond to adjacent digits or the palm instead. Similar limited reorganizations of cortical maps occur after other disruptions of inputs. These immediate or extremely rapid brain changes have been referred to as **"unmasking" of latent inputs**. The premise is that the inputs necessary for the reorganization were already in place before the sensory loss, but they could not be detected because their effects were below the threshold for evoking neural activity.

25. What causes these subthreshold inputs to become above threshold?

The usual explanation is that they become **disinhibited**. The inputs that activate the normal territory of the digit, for example, also activate inhibitory neurons, and these inhibitory neurons suppress minor inputs from other digits. The removal of the activating drive of these inhibitory neurons allows subthreshold inputs from other digits to become disinhibited and rise above threshold. At a neural network level, removing an input alters the dynamic balance of the system, so that different inputs are expressed and different outputs result.

26. Are all the rapid changes in cortical maps the result of disinhibition?

No. Long-term potentiation (LTP), or Hebbian plasticity, can be extremely rapid. LTP can be demonstrated after a few seconds of electrical stimulation of brain circuits, and frequent electrical

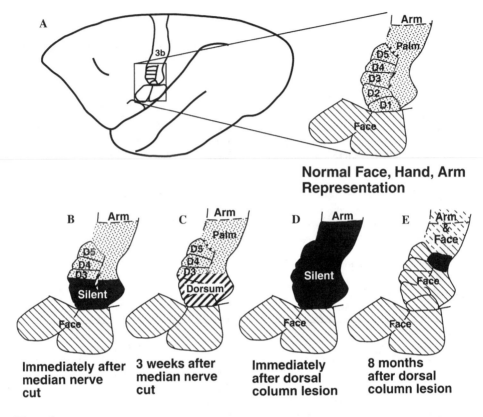

Normal Face, Hand, Arm Representation

Figure 2. Adult plasticity in the somatosensory cortex of owl monkeys. **A,** The location of the primary somatosensory cortex or area 3b on a lateral view of the brain. The body surface is represented from foot to face in an orderly, mediolateral sequence in area 3b. **B,** Part of the hand cortex becomes unresponsive to peripheral stimulation if the median nerve to the hand is cut. The part of the hand representation that becomes silent corresponds to the median nerve–innervated skin of the hand, which is the thumbward half of the palmar skin. **C,** However, after about 3 weeks, this silent cortex begins to respond to stimulation of the skin on the back of the hand. **D,** Even greater plasticity results if a large expanse of cortex is deprived of its normal inputs by cutting dorsal column fibers at the C3–4 level. Immediately after the cut, all of the hand cortex is unresponsive to peripheral stimulation. The face cortex and parts of the arm cortex continue to respond to their normal inputs because these inputs enter the spinal cord and brainstem above the level of the lesion. The deprived cortex remains unresponsive for at least 2 months. **E,** By about 8 months, nearly all of the hand cortex starts responding to the stimulation of the face. Parts of this cortex also respond to stimulation of the skin of the arm. This large-scale reorganization is thought to involve neuronal growth.

stimulation of a digit over just a few hours can increase the territory in cortex that is activated by normal stimuli of that digit. Strong stimulations strengthen the normally weak lateral connections in cortex; thus, they become more effective and recruit a fringe of neurons into their response territory. Similarly, electrical stimulation of a group of neurons in cortex strengthens their lateral connections, so that surrounding neurons respond to the same stimuli as the neurons that were electrically stimulated.

27. How can "silent synapses," or subthreshold inputs, be demonstrated without removing an input?

Neurons in cortex and elsewhere are in a state of tonic inhibition. Thus, only the effects of the most powerful inputs normally are reflected in the receptive fields of neurons. However, the sizes of receptive fields for cortical neurons can be increased simply by blocking local inhibitory influences with drugs. The increases in receptive field sizes result from disinhibition of subthreshold inputs so that they rise above threshold.

28. Do changes in receptive field sizes always reflect disinhibition?

No, enlarged receptive fields also result from the **sensitization** of peripheral afferents. Sensitization is well-known for nociceptors or pain afferents, since painful stimuli often produce inflammation of the skin and the release of factors in the skin that cause an increase in the sensitivity of the nociceptors.

29. The neurotransmitter acetylcholine (ACh) has been called a "permissive factor" in cortical plasticity. Why?

For cortical synapses to be strengthened by LTP (Hebbian mechanisms) during perceptual and motor skill learning, the effectiveness of synaptic contacts needs to be increased enough to activate the NMDA receptors (see Question 19). One way of doing that is to add another signal that helps depolarize cortical neurons when sensory inputs are important enough that they should modify cortical circuits. Projections from nucleus basalis and other parts of the basal forebrain release ACh on cortical neurons during states of attention, arousal, and reward so that cortical neurons are more active and LTP is more likely to occur. If the cholinergic system is suppressed by drugs or damaged, several types of cortical plasticity are greatly reduced or eliminated. Thus, ACh "permits" the plasticity, but its release by itself does not cause plasticity.

30. The larger the area of deprivation, the longer the period required for reactivation of sensory cortex. Why?

The effects of disinhibition are spatially limited, and other mechanisms take time to become effective. The immediate effect of a large sensory loss is that large populations of central neurons are no longer driven, and they are limited to a low level of spontaneous activity. This reduced activity signals a host of cellular changes that tend to restore normal activity levels.

31. What types of changes in neurons follow reduced levels of neural activity?

A number of genes (early genes) are rapidly "turned on" by increases or decreases in levels of neural activity. Such genes produce changes in neurons, including those related to the metabolic functions of cells and to the functions of deprived neurons in local circuits of neurons. For example, gamma-aminobutyric acid (GABA), the major inhibitory neurotransmitter in the brain, is involved in plastic changes that follow persistent changes in activity levels. When activity levels are decreased for a period of days or longer, less GABA is expressed by inhibiting neurons in the deprived regions of cortex, and less inhibition occurs. If higher than normal levels of activity occur and persist for hours to days, more GABA is expressed, and more inhibition occurs. Thus, this mechanism tends to return activity levels toward normal.

Genes also may turn on to make neurotrophic factors that are important in mediating new growth of brain connections and the formation of new synapses.

32. Is the growth of new connections a factor in brain plasticity?

Yes, there is strong evidence for several types of new growth in situations where brain plasticity occurs. The dendrites of neurons have been shown to grow under some conditions, even in adult mammals. Such growth increases the synaptic space and the number of contacts that influence these neurons. Dendrites grow in normal motor cortex of adult rats contralateral to motor cortex with a lesion, probably as a result of increased use of the normal motor area. Dendritic spines also increase in number with use and decrease with disuse. Finally, axons grow under a number of conditions to form new connections.

33. When do axons grow to form new connections?

We do not know all of the conditions and occurrences of axon growth in the central nervous system, as such growth once was thought to be unlikely in the mature brain. However, there have been many demonstrations of axon growth and the formation of new synapses in the hippocampus after lesions. Axon growth has been shown recently in other structures, as well. For example, after injury to peripheral neurons the central processes of the injured neurons may sprout to occupy larger than normal territories in the spinal cord or brainstem. In addition, uninjured axons may grow into the spinal cord territories denervated by nerve injury.

Sprouting and growth of new connections have been described in parts of visual and somatosensory cortex that have reorganized after the loss of part of the corresponding receptor surface. The growth of new connections in the mature brain may be much more common than generally believed.

34. What limits the growth of new connections in the injured, mature brain?

Glial cells in the central nervous system appear to produce substances that inhibit growth. Thus, a chemical block of these growth-inhibiting substances could promote growth. Lesions in the brain also trigger the proliferation of glial cells as part of the recovery process, and the glial scars act as barriers to growth.

35. What promotes the growth of new connections?

The injury to some branches of an axon arbor may trigger growth of remaining parts of the arbor as part of a regeneration process. Growth-promoting molecules are triggered by injury and transported throughout the neuron. Neural tissues and neurons with a substantial decrease in synaptic activity may release chemical signals that diffuse and cause nearby neurons to grow toward the chemical source and into the region of low activity.

36. Can an injured brain add new neurons?

Neurons are added to the mammalian nervous system almost exclusively early in development, and typically before birth. Almost all of your neurons are as old as you are. Yet, new neurons can be generated from stem cells to add neurons in the hippocampus and olfactory bulb throughout life, and the possibility of new neurons in other parts of the brain should be considered. New neurons, however, do not seem to be a major factor in brain plasticity and recovery from damage.

37. What kinds of changes take place in somatosensory cortex after extensive losses of peripheral afferents?

Afferents from cutaneous receptors enter the spinal cord to travel in the dorsal columns to the lower brainstem. When these afferents are damaged high in the spinal cord, all of the afferents from the arm and most of the lower body can be severed. The immediate effect of such damage is to render neurons throughout much of primary somatosensory cortex (S1 or area 3b in monkeys and humans) unresponsive to tactile stimuli. However, the face portion of S1, depending on intact afferents to the brainstem, remain fully responsive. If any afferents, even just a few, from the hand or arm remain intact after the lesion, they take over the hand portion of S1 and reactivate it within weeks. If not, the hand and arm portions of S1 become responsive to the face, but only after 6–8 months (Fig. 2).

Similar cortical changes occur in humans and monkeys with arm amputations. The deprived hand and arm cortex becomes responsive to the inputs from face and the skin of the remaining arm stump.

38. Why does the reactivation of hand cortex by the face take so long?

Part of the reason is that reactivation depends on the growth of afferents from the face into deprived portions of the brainstem nucleus for the hand. The new growth may take some time, and other mechanisms are needed to reinforce and amplify the effects of new growth. The reinnervated brainstem neurons relay face inputs to the thalamus and then to cortex.

39. What are the perceptual consequences of reactivating large parts of hand cortex by inputs from the face?

People with arm amputations, when touched on the stump of the amputated arm or the face on the same side of the body, often feel the touch on both the stump or the face and the hand of the missing arm (the phantom limb). Touch on different parts of the face may lead to the feeling of being touched on different fingers. This suggests that hand and arm cortex has reorganized to represent the face, or stump, or both. Touch on the face activates both face cortex and hand cortex, and the inappropriately activated hand cortex continues to signal touch on the hand.

40. What is a phantom limb?

Individuals with limb amputations, or the loss of other body parts, often have the strong sensation that the missing part is still present. This sensation is thought to be related to spontaneous neural activity in parts of cortex that formerly represented the missing part.

41. Do such extensive reorganizations also take place in the somatosensory thalamus?

Yes. Microelectrode recordings in patients with limb amputations, as part of a treatment for pain, revealed that parts of the somatosensory thalamus formerly devoted to the missing limb had inputs from the stump. The neurons in the deprived part of the thalamus had new receptive fields on the limb stump. Yet, when the neurons were electrically stimulated with the same electrode, the patients felt sensations on the missing limb, not in the stump. The reactivated neurons maintained their old functions. Of course, the thalamic neurons did not produce the sensations themselves, since they relayed to cortex and activated a cortical sequence of processing.

42. Do similar reorganizations occur in visual cortex?

Yes, but perhaps to a more limited extent. If the retina of each eye has a small lesion in "matched" locations (those that are activated by the same location in visual space), then blindness for that space occurs. Recordings from primary visual cortex indicate that the neurons that were formerly activated by the lesioned parts of the eyes come to be activated by parts of the retina around the lesions. Humans with such lesions do have a blind spot or scotoma in their visual field, but they do not see it. Instead, the blind area is filled in with information from the surround of the scotoma. This might be called phantom vision. If the neuronal activity is reversibly blocked by use of drugs such as tetrodotoxin, or by creating a small unstimulated region in the visual field, there is immediate reorganization of the receptive fields of the neurons. However, this reorganization is reversible after the effect of the drug wears off or the normal visual field is restored.

43. And what about the auditory system?

The auditory system is similarly plastic. If part of the cochlea is damaged so that it does not respond to a range of frequencies, parts of the cortex that correspond to that frequency range become nonresponsive. However, over a period of weeks to months the silent cortex starts responding to the adjacent frequencies (Fig. 3).

44. Most of the research on cortical plasticity has been in primary sensory areas. What happens in higher-order sensory areas?

Very little is now known. Since these areas often depend on primary areas for sensory information, any changes in the primary areas are reflected in the higher-order areas. However, the higher-order areas likely add further changes, and they may be even more plastic than the primary areas. As one example, a lesion that removes the hand portion of primary somatosensory cortex in monkeys deprives the hand portion of the second somatosensory area, S2, of activation. After a period of recovery, the hand portion of S2 responds to the foot and other parts of the body. Thus, secondary and higher-order sensory representations are plastic, and they do reorganize.

45. Why should higher-order areas be more plastic?

Areas of the cortex that receive highly processed information are involved in higher cognitive functions, like memory and learning. These areas need to be more plastic to continuously adapt to changes in the environment and to store new information over time. Growth-associated proteins are more numerous in these higher-order areas, such as the frontal cortex, than in primary sensory areas, suggesting that the former may retain more capacity for growth in adulthood.

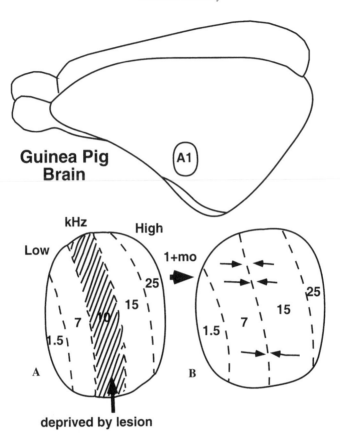

Figure 3.   An example of plasticity in the primary auditory cortex (A1) of adult guinea pigs. **A,** If a part of the cochlea that corresponds to 10 kHz frequency is lesioned, then the part of the cortex that responds to this frequency range becomes silent. **B,** Over a month or more, this cortex starts responding to the adjacent frequencies.

46. Do subcortical nuclei reorganize?

Yes. Massive losses of peripheral receptors, such as in extensive nerve damage, spinal cord injury, or limb amputation, are followed by the reactivations of the deprived portions of the ventro-posterior nucleus of the somatosensory thalamus by remaining inputs from the face and body. Such reactivations appear to depend on the growth of new connections in the dorsal column nuclei of the lower brainstem, which provides the first relay of somatosensory information. Some reactivation of the dorsal column nuclei occurs as a result of this new growth, but the reactivation is incomplete at this level. Other mechanisms amplify the reorganization at thalamic and cortical levels.

Lesions of the retina also are followed by some reactivation of the deprived portions of the lateral geniculate nucleus of the visual thalamus, but the reactivation is limited and incomplete, and there is little new growth. So far, little is known about reorganization in subcortical auditory centers.

47. Does motor cortex reorganize?

There is evidence for motor cortex reorganization after limb amputations or section of motor nerves. Weeks to months after such damage in rats and humans, electrical stimulation of the deprived cortex evokes movements of different body parts. In humans with an arm loss, electrical stimulation of arm and hand motor cortex evokes movements of the arm stump. Experiments in monkeys indicate that higher levels of current often are needed to evoke these movements. Since high levels of current evoke more extensive movements in normal motor cortex, the magnitude of the actual reorganization in motor cortex seems to be limited.

Reorganization of motor cortex also may occur after small lesions of the hand region of motor cortex, especially with extensive use of the impaired hand. Neurons formerly related to other movements begin to participate in the control of hand movements.

48. Does motor cortex organization change with use?

The learning and perfection of any motor skill probably involves changes in the circuits in motor cortex, with more and more neurons becoming involved in the skilled movements. Overlearning may result in extreme changes in motor cortex, and these changes may be involved in the development of some types of focal dystonias, a particular type of involuntary contraction of hand muscles that sometimes follows extensive repetition of a very stereotyped hand movement.

49. Is there plasticity in the vestibular and olfactory systems?

Yes. Most of the evidence in the vestibular system is behavioral. Damage or deafferentation of one labyrinth is followed by disorders in vestibular reflexes, which recover over a period of days. However, the neural mechanisms of recovery are not yet understood.

In the olfactory system, undifferentiated neuroblasts migrate to the olfactory bulb throughout life to provide a substrate for change. There is also a constant turnover of olfactory epithelium. A small olfactory bulb, as a result of long-standing olfactory deprivation, can recover in size even in adult rats if normal olfactory stimulation returns.

50. Does plasticity occur after strokes and damage to nonsensory regions of the brain, such as language centers?

Again, the evidence for plasticity is the considerable behavioral recovery that occurs over time. The brain changes, and the mechanisms of change are more difficult to study in brain regions where normal organization is not well understood.

51. What are the consequences of brain plasticity?

In the normal brain, plasticity has the role of reassigning neurons from one circuit to another to improve performance on some tasks at the probable cost of reduced performance on other, less important tasks. In the damaged brain, such a reassignment of neurons can contribute greatly toward behavioral recovery. In some instances of great plasticity, neurons get reactivated by new sources of sensory input, but they are not integrated into new circuits. Thus, neurons are stimulated by a new source of input, but signal the original source to other neurons. This skewed signaling leads to misperceptions and error. Feedback and experience sometimes can change the perceptual reference of such neurons. While brain plasticity sometimes has negative consequences, it is important in learning sensory and motor skills and in recoveries from brain damage and sensory loss.

52. What is the goal of research on brain plasticity?

Ultimately, the goal of research on brain plasticity is to acquire an understanding of mechanisms that will enable clinicians to promote and foster those types of reorganization that enhance recoveries and facilitate learning, while preventing and restricting those that lead to undesirable outcomes.

BIBLIOGRAPHY

1. Buonomano DV, Merzenich MM: Cortical plasticity: From synapses to maps. Ann Rev Neurosci 21:149–186, 1998.
2. Jain N, Florence SL, Kaas JH: Reorganization of somatosensory cortex after nerve and spinal cord injury. News Physiol Sci 13:143–149, 1998.
3. Kaas JH (ed): Functional Plasticity in Adult Cortex. Semin Neurosci 9:1–67, 1997.
4. Kaas JH: The reorganization of sensory and motor maps after injury in adult mammals. In Gazzaniga MS (ed): The Cognitive Neurosciences, 2nd ed. Cambridge, MA, MIT Press, 1999, pp 109–122.
5. Kolb B, Whishaw IQ: Brain plasticity and behavior. Ann Rev Psych 49:43–64, 1998.
6. Wong-Riley MTT: Primate visual cortex: Dynamic metabolic organization and plasticity revealed by cytochrome oxidase. In Peters A, Rockland KS (eds): Cerebral Cortex. Vol. 10. New York, Plenum Press, 1994, pp 141–200.

26. NEUROBIOLOGY OF PSYCHIATRIC DISORDERS

Harold H. Harsch, M.D.

BACKGROUND

1. Why is it important to understand the historical influences on psychiatry and psychiatric illnesses?

Mental illnesses have been described since the beginning of recorded history. Since they involve changes in behavior and thinking, they often have been equated with frightening, otherworldly domination of the individual. Even today significant stigma surrounds psychiatric illnesses, and misunderstandings continue to exist despite the dramatic progression of our understanding of the neurobiology underlying these illnesses over the last decade.

2. What are the major psychiatric disorders?

Three major groups of psychiatric illnesses are reviewed in this chapter: the psychotic disorders, primarily characterized by schizophrenia; the affective disorders, which are disorders of mood and include major depressive disorder and bipolar disorder; and the anxiety disorders, which include generalized anxiety disorder, panic disorder, and obsessive-compulsive disorder. Many other psychiatric illnesses do not fall into these categories; nevertheless, they are significant because of the suffering they can inflict.

3. What were the perceptions of psychiatric illness before Hippocrates (400 B.C.)?

Although "madness" was well described in early Greek, Chinese, and Hindu literature, the people's understanding was influenced by the spiritual and philosophical beliefs of the particular culture. Across most cultures mental illness was seen as spiritual possession by "noxious spirits" or punishment by a particular "god" for misbehavior. Most interventions before 400 B.C. consisted of either social isolation or religious treatment. In the Hindu culture, for example, treatment consisted of chanting along with fasting and purification rituals performed in temples.

4. What did Hippocrates bring to the understanding of psychiatric illness?

Hippocrates (460–355 B.C.) brought the first radical change to the concept of madness. In addition to classifying mental illness into various categories, he challenged the link to religious phenomena. Hippocrates described hysteria ("wandering of the womb") as an anxiety disorder. He described what he called "melancholia," a term that is still used today to describe major, unipolar depression. He described psychosis, which he called "phrenitis." He also tackled epilepsy, which was considered the "sacred disease." In his writings he outlined a new meaning for this illness: "I do not believe that the 'sacred disease' is any more divine or sacred than any other disease but, on the contrary, has specific characteristics and a definite cause; nevertheless, it is completely different from other diseases, and it has been regarded as a divine visitation by those who, being only human, view it with ignorance and astonishment."

Hippocrates, in essence, accurately described symptoms of major psychiatric illnesses and advocated for them to be understood as diseases of the nervous system rather than religious or spiritual manifestations.

5. What occurred in Europe during the Middle Ages that impacted persons suffering from mental illness?

Christianity spread throughout Europe during the Middle Ages. Unfortunately, a book of the Bible (Deuteronomy) stated that God would punish those who violate his commandments with "madness, and blindness, and astonishment of the heart." The notion that insanity was due to punishment by God was reborn, and it resulted in the persecution of many individuals in medieval Europe. Early in the 14th century, belief in possession by the devil and witchcraft further enflamed the persecution of individuals suffering from a psychiatric illness.

6. What was "Malleus Maleficarium"?

Malleus Maleficarium, "the witch's hammer," was a book written by two Dominican friars that equated symptoms of psychosis with evidence of possession by the devil. This book was published for 29 editions until the middle of the 17th century and was responsible for the deaths of tens of thousands of individuals in medieval Europe.

7. What did Kraeplin and Alzheimer contribute to our knowledge of the major psychiatric illnesses?

Drs. Emil Kraeplin and Alois Alzheimer were colleagues in Germany at the beginning of the 20th century. Alzheimer was interested in what was called "senile dementia," and Kraeplin was interested in several disorders which he called "dementia praecox" (early or premature dementia) and in "cyclical insanity," which later was termed manic depressive illness. With the advent and perfection of a silver staining technique, microscopic examination of neuronal structures in the central nervous system (CNS) was possible. Examining the neuronal tissue of individuals with senile dementia, Alzheimer discovered senile plaques and neurofibrillary tangles, and described the illness that we now know as Alzheimer's disease. Kraeplin attempted similar studies with tissue from individuals suffering from dementia praecox, which we now know as schizophrenia, and found no microscopic pathology. This is one of the reasons that schizophrenia became known as a functional, or nonorganic, illness. Kraeplin also characterized and described manic depressive illness in great detail.

SCHIZOPHRENIA

8. What is schizophrenia?

Schizophrenia, one of the major psychotic illnesses, is manifested by a disturbance of cognitive and sensory processes leading to hallucinatory experiences, delusions, and disturbances of thought. Schizophrenia occurs in 1% of the world's population irrespective of culture, and is found equally in men and women. It is the illness that has been described throughout history as madness. Symptoms of schizophrenia usually become evident in the late teens and early twenties. Current thinking surrounding the etiology of the illness considers both a genetic component and a prenatal or perinatal insult to the developing brain. Damage is thought to occur in the developing dopaminergic system, which leads to clinical symptoms later in life.

9. What are some risk factors for schizophrenia?

Genetic loading is clearly a risk factor for the development of schizophrenia. However, even in monozygotic twins the concordance rate is only about 30–50%, suggesting that some environmental factor is necessary for development of the disorder. Higher incidences of maternal illness during pregnancy and prenatal complications are found in studies of populations with schizophrenia.

10. What is the dopamine theory of schizophrenia?

The dopamine theory of schizophrenia attempts to explain the symptoms of hallucinations and delusions by postulating an excess of dopaminergic neurotransmission in the limbic system. There was no effective treatment for schizophrenia until the advent of chlorpromazine in 1952. Although initially thought to be simply a tranquilizer, the drug's specific antipsychotic properties were soon apparent. It later was discovered that chlorpromazine is a dopamine D2 postsynaptic receptor antagonist. All other pharmacologic agents that possessed antipsychotic activity also were found to be dopamine D2 receptor antagonists. In a 1976 paper by Seeman, et al., the average clinical dose of each antipsychotic agent was plotted against its ability to block the dopamine receptor.

Clinical antipsychotic activity was directly correlated to a drug's ability to block dopamine D2 receptors. The functions of the other dopamine receptor subtypes (D1, D3, and D4) are not well understood.

11. What are the four major dopaminergic tracts in the brain?
- The nigrostriatal system: projects to the basal ganglia; is involved in movement coordination and control of the extrapyramidal motor system.
- The tuberoinfundibular system: a short tract from the hypothalamus to the pituitary gland, where it is involved in the control of prolactin secretion.
- The mesolimbic system: projections to the limbic system; is theorized to be involved in emotional processing and to be responsible for what are considered the "positive" symptoms of schizophrenia.
- The mesofrontal tract: projects to a large portion of the frontal cortex that is thought to be involved in executive functioning; responsible for the deficit or "negative" symptoms seen in schizophrenia (Fig. 1).

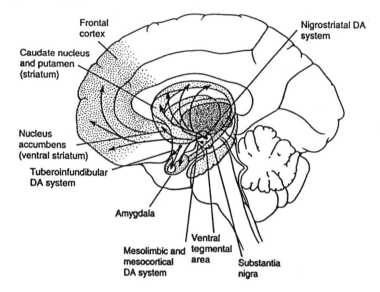

Figure 1. The four major dopaminergic tracts: (1) the nigrostriatal, from the substantia nigra to the basal ganglia; (2) the tuberoinfundibular, from the hypothalamus to the pituitary gland; (3) the mesolimbic, from the ventral tegmental area to the limbic system; (4) the mesocortical, from the ventral tegmental area to the frontal cortex. (Adapted from Kandel ER, Schwartz JH, Jessl TM (eds): Principles of Neural Science, 3rd ed. New York, Elsevier, 1991.)

12. Explain the notion of positive and negative symptoms with regard to schizophrenia.
Current thinking divides symptoms of schizophrenia into two groups. Positive symptoms are thought to be the result of overactivity of the dopaminergic system in the mesolimbic pathway. Positive symptoms include frank hallucinatory experiences featuring auditory, visual, and sometimes tactile and olfactory components; delusions (beliefs that are not based in reality); and psychomotor agitation.

Negative or deficit symptoms in schizophrenia include a flattening of affect, social withdrawal, isolation, a lack of social initiative, and deficiencies in frontal lobe functioning that can be measured by neuropsychological testing. These deficiencies may manifest as impairment in abstraction ability, impairment in reasoning, such as measured by the Wisconsin Card Sort task, and impairment in working memory. Negative symptoms are believed to be partially due to a lack of dopaminergic activity in the mesofrontal dopaminergic tract.

13. Does serotonin neurotransmission affect dopaminergic neurotransmission?

It is known that serotonin (5-hydroxytryptamine) can modulate dopaminergic neurotransmission. Serotonin 5HT3 receptors are found presynpatically on the dopaminergic neurons and regulate dopamine release. There is also evidence that the 5HT2A receptor modulates dopaminergic neurotransmission in several areas of the CNS. This relationship between dopamine and serotonin became apparent when pure serotonin-augmenting agents such as fluoxetine (Prozac) were widely used in clinical populations. Reports began surfacing of extrapyramidal reactions that are due to a suppression of dopamine release in the basal ganglia by increased levels of serotonin.

14. How is schizophrenia treated?

Since the development of chlorpromazine, antipsychotic agents have been the mainstay of treatment in schizophrenia. For many people, these drugs provide good control of the positive symptoms of the illness. Individual and family therapy with a focus on understanding and coping with the illness is also an important treatment factor. Community support programs and sheltered workshops help in maximizing individual functioning. With the 1990 approval of clozapine in the United States, a new generation of "atypical antipsychotics" that may offer greater hope for both positive and negative symptom control in schizophrenia became available.

15. What are atypical antipsychotic agents?

The atypical antipsychotics are a new class of drugs that can be described as combined serotonin and dopamine antagonists. They take advantage of the interplay between serotonin and dopamine to provide improved therapeutic response in schizophrenia with fewer medication-induced side effects. These drugs include clozapine (Clozaril), risperidone (Risperdal), olanzapine (Zyprexa), quetiapine (Seroquel), and ziprasidone (Zeldox). All of these agents offer potent serotonergic 5HT2A blockade and weak dopaminergic D2 blockade—a combination that results in fewer extrapyramidal and parkinsonian effects in schizophrenia.

These agents also provide significant improvement in the negative symptoms of schizophrenia. Blocking the 5HT2A receptor appears to lead to increased dopaminergic neurotransmission in the frontal lobe.

Preliminary evidence demonstrates that individuals with schizophrenia who are maintained on atypical antipsychotics have a lower incidence of suicide, a higher percentage of employment, fewer psychiatric hospitalizations, and a lower incidence of tardive dyskinesia.

16. What is tardive dyskinesia?

Tardive dyskinesia is an involuntary movement disorder caused by the use of antipsychotics that have D2 blockade as their mode of action. It manifests a spectrum of symptoms from mild to severe, which often include choreoathetoid tongue movements and rhythmic jaw movements and can progress to include head, arm, and trunk movements. The exact etiology of this disorder is unclear, but it is directly correlated to years of antipsychotic drug exposure. Preliminary evidence indicates that the atypical antipsychotics produce a much lower incidence of this disorder.

17. What is the evidence that dopamine may be involved in some addictions?

Drugs that cause dopamine release can result in a clinical "high" or euphoria, which may lead to addiction and abuse. Cocaine and amphetamine are two drugs that cause dopamine release, and both have caused significant abuse and addiction problems.

MOOD DISORDERS

18. What is the function of the limbic system?

It is best to think of the limbic structures as a system that modulates certain behaviors and emotions. One mnemonic is that the limbic system controls the four Fs: feeding, fighting, fear, and fornication. Many psychiatric symptoms are thought to be mediated through this system and its projection to other parts of the CNS.

19. What does the card player's "poker face" demonstrate about limbic system control?

The fact that a person can over-ride limbic system emotional signals and continue with a straight face while holding a marvelous poker hand demonstrates that the neocortex can control limbic impulses.

20. What neurotransmitter systems implicated in behavior and emotion project heavily to the limbic system?

The dopamine, serotonin, and norepinephrine neurotransmitter systems project to the limbic structures. These three neurotransmitter systems are implicated in many psychiatric illnesses.

21. How have serotonin and norepinephrine been implicated in neuropsychiatric illness?

While dopamine has been implicated primarily in the psychotic illnesses, such as schizophrenia, other neuropsychiatric illnesses, such as anxiety disorders and mood disorders, seem linked to some dysfunction of either serotonin or norepinephrine neurotransmission.

22. What is the neuroanatomy of the serotonin neurotransmission system?

Serotonin-producing neurons are situated primarily in the midbrain **raphe nuclei**, with axons projecting to a multitude of structures including the frontal cortex, limbic system, basal ganglia, and hypothalamus. It is estimated that one serotonin neuron impacts 500,000 other neurons. In contrast to the dopaminergic system, which is quite focal, the serotonin system is diffuse and is thought to be a major neuromodulator of other neuronal systems (Fig. 2).

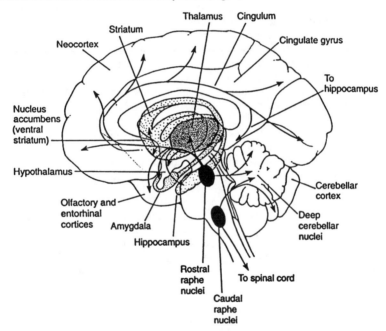

Figure 2. The diffuse projections of the serotonin system. Most anteriorly projecting serotonin neurons have their cell bodies located in the rostral raphe nucleus and have fibers projecting to a large number of limbic and forebrain areas. (Adapted from Kandel ER, Schwartz JH, Jessl TM (eds): Principles of Neural Science, 3rd ed. New York, Elsevier, 1991.)

23. How is serotonin synthesized?

Serotonin is synthesized in the CNS locally by a two-step process involving the amino acid L-tryptophan. Following release into the synaptic cleft, serotonin is inactivated principally by its reuptake into the nerve terminal. Inside the neuron, most of the serotonin is metabolized by monoamine oxidase and other enzymes that produce the primary metabolite 5-hydroxyindoleacetic acid (5HIAA) (Fig. 3).

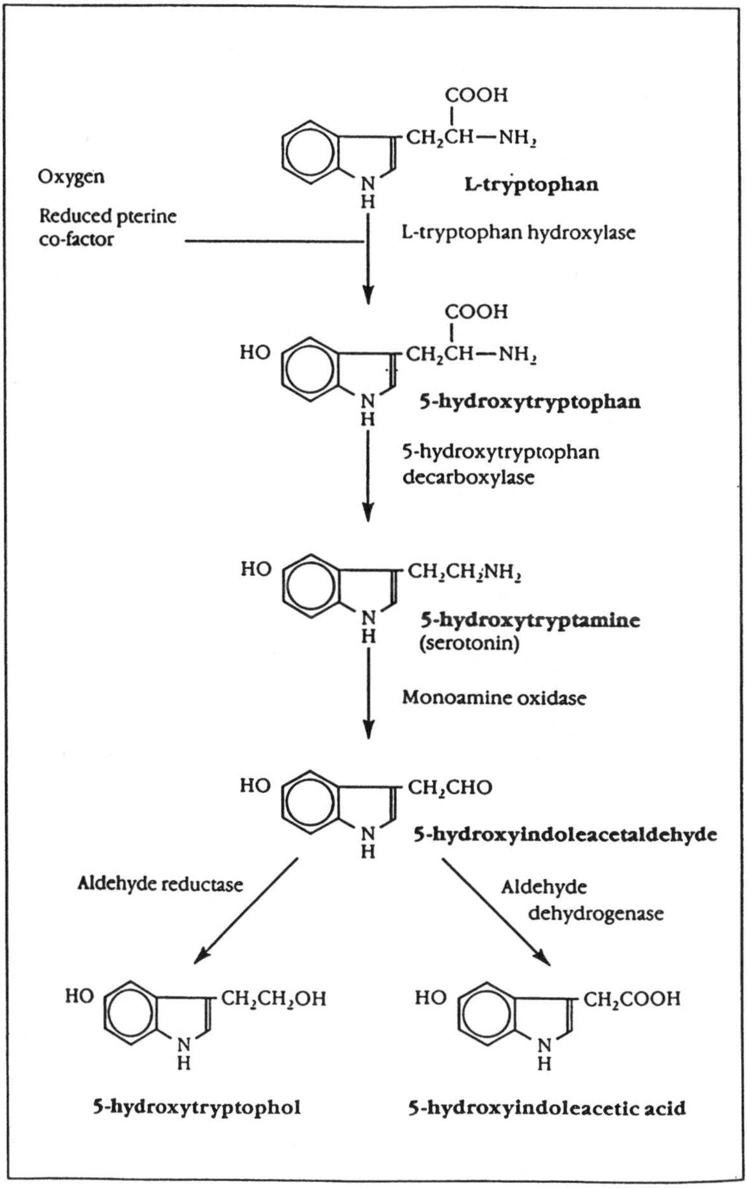

Figure 3. The synthesis and breakdown of serotonin. (Adapted from Feighner JP, Boyer WF (eds): Selective Serotonin Re-uptake Inhibitors. New York, John Wiley, 1991.)

24. How does this diffusely scattered serotonin system allow differential control of various areas of the limbic system and other structures?

The answer to this question lies in the examination of serotonin postsynaptic receptors.

25. What is known about serotonin's pre- and postsynaptic receptors?

There are numerous serotonin receptors that differ in their locations in the brain, secondary messenger systems, and amino acid sequences. The explosion of knowledge concerning serotonin receptors over the last decade has allowed the development of many new pharmaceuticals. Currently, at least 20 unique serotonin receptors have been identified. They are classified from 5HT1 to 5HT7, and some have subtypes designated by a letter.

Laboratories are actively searching for agonists and antagonists for each receptor. Specific agents released for clinical use at this time include buspirone (Buspar), a 5HT1A partial agonist that is used in the treatment of anxiety and also has shown some efficacy in depression, and sumatriptan (Imitrex), a serotonin 5HT1D agonist that is extremely useful in treatment of migraine headaches. 5HT2A blockade is characteristic of all of the atypical antipsychotics and is thought to mediate some symptoms of psychosis. Nonselective 5HT2 blockade by drugs such as nefazadone (Serzone) produces an antidepressant effective in major depression. Blockade of the 5HT3 receptor by agents such as ondansetron (Zofran) reduces dopaminergic neurotransmission, resulting in a clinical antiemetic effect. These agents also are being studied for use in psychosis. The selective serotonin reuptake inhibitors increase serotonin across CNS structures. They have become the most widely used antidepressants and have found utility in a number of psychiatric disorders (Fig. 4).

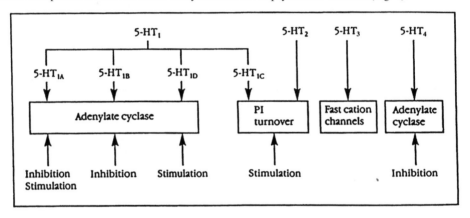

Figure 4. Neuronal effects of some of the known 5HT receptor subtypes. (Adapted from Feighner JP, Boyer WF (eds): Selective Serotonin Re-uptake Inhibitors. New York, John Wiley, 1991.)

26. What is the neuroanatomy of the noradrenergic neurotransmission system?

The majority of norepinephrine in the brain is produced by neurons whose cell bodies are located in the midbrain nucleus, the **locus caeruleus**. The norepinephrine-containing axons project to numerous other areas, including the limbic system structures, the frontal cortex, and the hypothalamus (Fig. 5).

27. Melancholia described by Hippocrates is part of which group of psychiatric illnesses?

What Hippocrates described as melancholia we now know as part of the affective, or mood, disorders. They include major depressive disorder, bipolar illness, minor depression, cyclothymic disorder, seasonal affective disorder, and premenstrual dysphoric disorder.

28. What is major depression?

Major depression, also called unipolar depression, is the most common of the severe mood disorders. It is characterized by the inability to experience pleasure (anhedonia). Major depression also affects sleep, usually in the form of insomnia or oversleeping, and causes a loss of appetite, loss of energy, restlessness or anxiety, feelings of worthlessness, guilt, and thoughts about death and suicide.

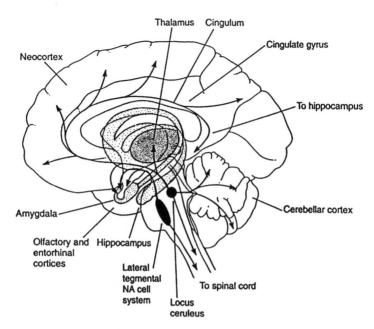

Figure 5. Some main noradrenergic pathways. Most noradrenergic neurons are located in the locus caeruleus, with some in the lateral tegmental area. These neurons project heavily to limbic structures and areas of the neocortex. (Adapted from Kandel ER, Schwartz JH, Jessl TM (eds): Principles of Neural Science, 3rd ed. New York, Elsevier, 1991.)

Cognition also seems to be affected, in that some individuals show significant impairment in attention and concentration. Lifetime prevalence rates are approximately 5%. Major depression is twice as common in women as in men.

29. What is some of the evidence that serotonin and norepinephrine are involved in major depression?

There are many different lines of evidence linking both serotonin and norepinephrine to major depression. The oldest is our experience with drugs effective for major depression. Antidepressant drugs fall into four major classes: (1) tricyclic compounds such as imipramine, (2) serotonin reuptake blockers such as fluoxetine, (3) monoamine oxidase inhibitors such as phenelzine, and (4) other novel agents that are structurally unique or have unique neurochemical properties. Most of these antidepressants act by increasing the synaptic concentration of either serotonin, norepinephrine, or both. One of the most dramatic studies demonstrating the importance of serotonin in mood stability involves depletion in subjects with a well-controlled mood disorder. Serotonin depletion, using an amino acid drink with tryptophan, results in the return of depressive symptoms within hours of depletion. The symptoms resolve when serotonin, via tryptophan, is reintroduced.

Other evidence includes the finding of reduced 5-HIAA levels in the cerebral spinal fluid of patients with severe depression, and lower density of serotonin reuptake sites in platelets and brain of people with major depression.

30. What is manic depressive illness?

Manic depressive illness, also known as bipolar disorder, is a mood disorder that gives rise to periods of mania along with periods of significant depression. The manic episodes often include symptoms of euphoria, irritability, decreased need for sleep, and loss of judgment and may be accompanied by frank psychotic symptoms. Manic-depressive illness occurs in approximately 1% of the population, equally between men and women. It is best treated with lithium salts and a class of drugs called "mood stabilizers." Mood stabilizers are various anticonvulsants, e.g., carbamazepine, gabapentin, lamotrigine, and valproic acid, that were serendipitously found to have mood stabilization properties in manic depressive illness.

ANXIETY DISORDERS

31. What are the anxiety disorders?
There are three major anxiety disorders:
1. panic disorder
2. generalized anxiety disorder (GAD)
3. obsessive compulsive disorder (OCD).

32. What is panic disorder?
Individuals with panic disorder experience brief but intense, spontaneous episodes of terror. These occur without any noticeable stressor and also occur during sleep, at which time the individual wakes up scared and diaphoretic with tachycardia. These episodes produce intense stimulation of the sympathetic nervous system, resulting in trembling, flushing, chest pain, dizziness, and shortness of breath. The frequency and intensity of the attacks vary widely among individuals. One of the consequences of untreated panic disorder is the subsequent development of various phobic avoidance behaviors.

Panic disorder occurs in approximately 2% of the population, and is two to three times more frequent in women. It can be treated with the more potent benzodiazepines, such as alprazolam (Xanax); most antidepressants also are effective. Etiology is speculated to be dysregulation of normal activity of the locus caeruleus.

33. Is there evidence that serotonin is involved in panic disorder?
Fenfluramine is a serotonin-releasing agent that can be used safely as a probe of the serotonin system in human studies. When fenfluramine was given to a group of subjects with panic disorder they quickly developed significant symptoms of anxiety that were not seen in control subjects. In some studies, individuals with panic disorder also show an altered 5-HT uptake in platelets.

34. What is generalized anxiety disorder?
Generalized anxiety disorder is a sustained and excessive motor tension accompanied by psychic anxiety. Individuals often show autonomic hyper-reactivity and symptoms such as an exaggerated startle response. Generalized anxiety disorder may be present in 3–5% of the population. Treatment approaches include the use of benzodiazepines, which increase the chloride ion channel on neurons by binding to the benzodiazepine receptor. Generalized anxiety disorder also responds to treatment with antidepressants, perhaps due to serotonin's modulation of limbic system function.

35. What is obsessive compulsive disorder?
The hallmark of OCD is recurrent obsessions or compulsions to the degree that they cause significant distress or are unduly time consuming. Obsessions typically are marked by intrusive and recurrent thoughts that cause anxiety and distress. Compulsions often take the form of repetitive rituals, such as hand washing, which if stopped result in significant anxiety in the individual. The disorder is thought to occur in approximately 2% of the population. OCD is equally common in men and women. Dual treatment is common: behavioral therapy techniques have been developed to address both the obsessions and compulsions. Recently, serotonergic antidepressants have been shown to be efficacious in the treatment of OCD. Antidepressants that modulate only the norepinephrine system do not seem to be effective in this disorder.

36. What is the evidence that serotonin may be involved with obsessive compulsive disorder?
Drugs that are effective for this disorder are primarily drugs that increase serotonin centrally, such as the selective serotonin reuptake inhibitors. Studies in which serotonin agonists were given to

individuals with OCD found significantly increased symptomatology for hours after administration; these results were not seen in control subjects. One hypothesis is that there is an increased serotonergic responsivity in OCD, which is "down regulated" by the chronic administration of antidepressants that raise serotonin levels.

37. In what other areas of human behavior and psychiatric illness does serotonin seem to play a role?

Serotonin is involved in appetite regulation. Fluoxetine (Prozac) has been approved for use in the treatment of bulimia (an eating disorder). Impulsiveness and aggressiveness associated with some personality disorders and head injuries often are attenuated with agents that increase central serotonin levels. Serotonin also seems to modulate slow wave sleep, and is involved in pain perception. With further study of the various serotonin receptors, many useful pharmaceuticals may be developed.

BIBLIOGRAPHY

1. Baumgarten HG, Grozdanovic Z: The role of serotonin in obsessive-compulsive disorder. Br J Psychiatry 35(suppl):13–20, 1998.
2. Bell CJ, Nutt DJ: Serotonin and panic. Br J Psychiatry 172:465–471, 1998.
3. Charney DS: Monoamine dysfunction and the pathophysiology and treatment of depression. J Clin Psychiatry 59(suppl 14):11–14, 1998.
4. Coccaro EF, Murphy DL (eds): Serotonin in Major Psychiatric Disorders. Washington DC, APA Press, 1990.
5. Feighner JP, Boyer WF (eds): Selective Serotonin Re-uptake Inhibitors. New York, John Wiley, 1991.
6. Fogel BS, Schiffer RB, Rao SM (eds): Neuropsychiatry. Baltimore, Williams & Wilkins, 1996.
7. Kandel ER, Schwartz JH, Jessl TM (eds): Principles of Neural Science, 3rd ed. New York, Elsevier, 1991.
8. Woods BT: Is schizophrenia a progressive neuro-developmental disorder? Am J Psychiatry 155:1661–1670, 1998.

INDEX

Page numbers in **boldface type** indicate complete chapters.